New Frontiers in Regenerative Medicine

New Frontiers in
Regenerative Medicine

Edited by Cedric Pearson

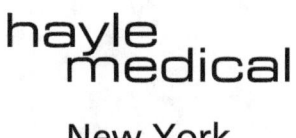

hayle
medical

New York

Hayle Medical,
750 Third Avenue, 9th Floor,
New York, NY 10017, USA

Visit us on the World Wide Web at:
www.haylemedical.com

ISBN: 978-1-63241-893-7

Cataloging-in-Publication Data

New frontiers in regenerative medicine / edited by Cedric Pearson.
   p. cm.
Includes bibliographical references and index.
ISBN 978-1-63241-893-7
1. Regenerative medicine. 2. Stem cells--Therapeutic use.
3. Tissue engineering. I. Pearson, Cedric.
R857.T55 N49 2020
610.28--dc23

Table of Contents

Preface

Regeneration is the process of growth, renewal and restoration that makes cells, genomes, organisms and ecosystems resist events and fluctuations that can cause disturbance or damage. Every species is capable of regeneration, from single-celled organisms like bacteria to complex organisms like humans. Regeneration can be complete such as when new tissue is regenerated similar to the lost tissue, or incomplete when necrotic tissue turns fibrotic. Humans have limited capacity for reparative regeneration, especially in response to injury. An important area of study of regeneration in humans is the hypertrophy of the liver after liver injury. Another vital area of study in reparative regeneration in humans is fingertip regeneration and rib regeneration. The sequence of inflammation and regeneration is however not followed accurately in cancer. There has been rapid progress in the understanding of inflammation and regeneration in recent years. From theories to research to practical applications, case studies related to all contemporary topics of relevance to this domain have been included in this book. It is a complete source of knowledge on the present status of regenerative medicine.

This book is a result of research of several months to collate the most relevant data in the field.

When I was approached with the idea of this book and the proposal to edit it, I was overwhelmed. It gave me an opportunity to reach out to all those who share a common interest with me in this field. I had 3 main parameters for editing this text:

1. Accuracy – The data and information provided in this book should be up-to-date and valuable to the readers.

2. Structure – The data must be presented in a structured format for easy understanding and better grasping of the readers

3. Universal Approach – This book not only targets students but also experts and innovators in the field, thus my aim was to present topics which are of use to all

Thus, it took me a couple of months to finish the editing of this book.

I would like to make a special mention of my publisher who considered me worthy of this opportunity and also supported me throughout the editing process. I would also like to thank the editing team at the back-end who extended their help whenever required.

Editor

Usefulness of nailfold videocapillaroscopy for systemic sclerosis

Satoshi Kubo* and Yoshiya Tanaka

Abstract

Systemic sclerosis is a complex disease that involves "autoimmunity," "inflammation," "fibrosis," and "vasculopathy." Microvascular damage and dysfunction particularly represent the earliest morphological and functional markers of systemic sclerosis. These morphological changes and progressions can be detected by nailfold videocapillaroscopy (NVC).

In 2013, the American College of Rheumatology and European League Against Rheumatism (ACR/EULAR) proposed a new set of criteria for systemic sclerosis for the first time in 30 years. Items are given a weighted score, and a score more than 9 indicates systemic sclerosis. These classification criteria encompass a broader spectrum of systemic sclerosis patients including those with early stage and with excellent sensitivity and specificity. Notably, nailfold capillary abnormalities were one of the new items in the criteria. Moreover, these abnormalities are also markers of systemic sclerosis severity and progression, as reduced capillary density has been associated with a high risk of developing digital skin ulcers and pulmonary arterial hypertension. Since microvascular damage and dysfunction represent early markers of systemic sclerosis, qualitative and semi-quantitative assessment of videocapillaroscopy images is expected in clinical application and treatment outcome assessment.

Despite the potential for targeted therapies in systemic sclerosis, there is no established therapy as yet. This may be due to several reasons. First, no fully validated outcome measures exist. Second, diagnosis of systemic sclerosis is often delayed and early intervention is difficult. Moreover, systemic sclerosis has clinical heterogeneity. Appropriate use of NVC helps to overcome these issues. Moreover, NVC may be useful in evaluating the pathogenesis of systemic sclerosis.

Keywords: Systemic sclerosis, Nailfold videocapillaroscopy, Microvascular changes, Qualitative assessment, Semi-quantitative assessment

Background

In 2013, the American College of Rheumatology and the European League Against Rheumatism (ACR/EULAR) collaborated to propose a new set of criteria for systemic sclerosis for the first time in 30 years [1, 2]. These criteria focused on the early diagnosis of systemic sclerosis. Seven items, namely, skin thickening of the fingers, fingertip lesions, telangiectasia, abnormal nailfold capillaries, pulmonary arterial hypertension and/or interstitial lung disease, Raynaud's phenomenon, and systemic sclerosis-related autoantibodies, are given a weighted score; a score more than 9 indicates systemic sclerosis.

These classification criteria encompass a broader spectrum of systemic sclerosis patients including those with early- and late-stage disease and with excellent sensitivity and specificity. The most significant change in these criteria was the inclusion of nailfold capillary abnormalities as one of the new items. It is now possible to diagnose systemic sclerosis with this scoring system before skin thickening of the fingers is detected.

Role of NVC

Nailfold videocapillaroscopy (NVC) is the best and safest method to detect and analyze morphological microvascular abnormalities. NVC can detect normal capillary morphology in healthy individuals or those experiencing primary Raynaud phenomenon. However,

* Correspondence: kubosato@med.uoeh-u.ac.jp
The First Department of Internal Medicine, School of Medicine, University of Occupational and Environmental Health, 1-1 Iseigaoka, Yahata-nishi-ku, Kitakyushu, Fukuoka 807-8555, Japan

abnormal capillaroscopic findings suggest the possibility of secondary Raynaud phenomenon [3]. Specific NVC changes known as the "systemic sclerosis pattern" are typical of the microvascular involvement in systemic sclerosis [4]. This review will summarize the "systemic sclerosis pattern," which is widely accepted worldwide.

Normal capillary morphology

This section will address the normal morphology of capillaries in healthy individuals [5]. Healthy subjects have numerous thin and linear capillaries (Fig. 1).

Normal capillary morphology has several common characteristics. First, the diameter of normal vessels is less than 20 μm. However, it could be more than 20 μm in some capillaries in healthy individuals. However, the detection of even a single loop with a homogeneous increase to a diameter more than 50 μm should be considered a potential marker of microangiopathy. Second, capillaries are distributed with their major axis running parallel to the skin surface. Finally, there are more than 9 capillaries within 1 mm of the row of the nailfold bed. Abnormalities in these findings (fineness, direction, and number of capillaries) are seen in patients with systemic sclerosis. These sequential capillaroscopic changes are typical of the microvascular involvement in systemic sclerosis. Furthermore, quantitative and semi-qualitative scoring is possible for these findings [6].

Usefulness of NVC for systemic sclerosis diagnosis

The 1980 ACR classification criteria [7, 8] for systemic sclerosis lack sensitivity for the diagnosis of early systemic sclerosis. The new classification criteria encompass a broader spectrum of systemic sclerosis and focus on early diagnosis [1, 2]. Sensitivity and specificity for the new classification criteria were 91 and 92 %, respectively, while they were 75 and 72 %, respectively, for the 1980 ACR classification criteria. The new criteria include "abnormal nailfold capillaries," which are enlarged capillaries and/or capillary loss with or without pericapillary hemorrhages at the nailfold (Fig. 2). Although capillaroscopy can be performed with highly specialized equipment such as in videocapillaroscopy, dermatoscopes (×30 magnifications) suffice for distinguishing between normal and abnormal nailfold capillaries. Therefore, there are no clear definitions of capillary thickness and number for the criteria. However, it is desirable for physicians caring for systemic sclerosis patients to use videocapillaroscopy (×200 magnifications) for an accurate measurement of capillary fineness and number.

Qualitative and semi-quantitative scoring of capillary

Although enlarged capillaries, capillary loss, and pericapillary hemorrhages are included in the new criteria, the severities of these findings are not mentioned. Qualitative and semi-quantitative scoring of systemic sclerosis patterns by NVC has been introduced recently and validated [6, 9].

The following capillaroscopic parameters were scored: presence of enlarged and giant capillaries, hemorrhages, loss of capillaries, disorganization of the microvascular array, and capillary ramifications. The 6 parameters were defined as follows [6]: (a) irregularly enlarged capillaries (Fig. 3a) were defined as an increase in capillary diameter (homogeneous or irregular) >20 μm; (b) giant capillaries (Fig. 3b) as homogeneously enlarged loops with a diameter >50 μm; (c) microhemorrhages (Fig. 3c) as dark masses due to hemosiderin deposits; (d) loss of

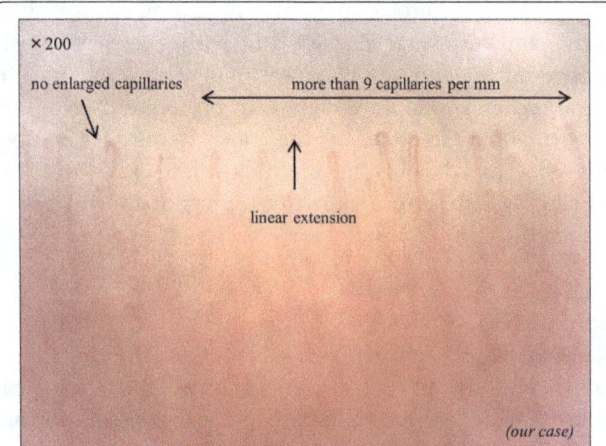

Fig. 1 Representation of the nailfold videocapillaroscopy analysis of healthy donor. The vessels diameter is less than 20μm. Capillaries form a straight line toward distal. The number of capillaries is more than nine with in 1mm of the row of the nailfold bed

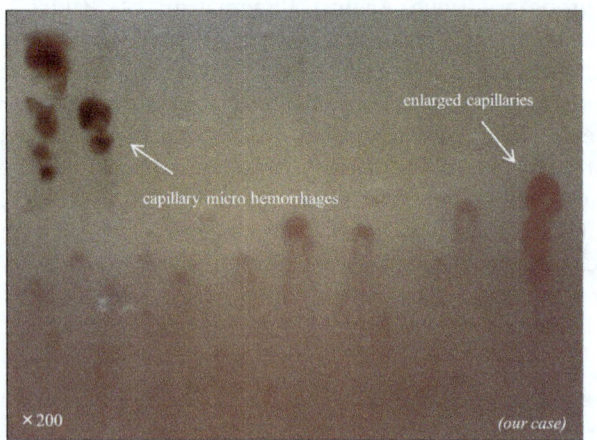

Fig. 2 Representation of the nailfold videocapillaroscopy analysis of patients with systemic sclerosis. Enlarged capillaries and pericapillary hemorrhages at the nailfold are shown

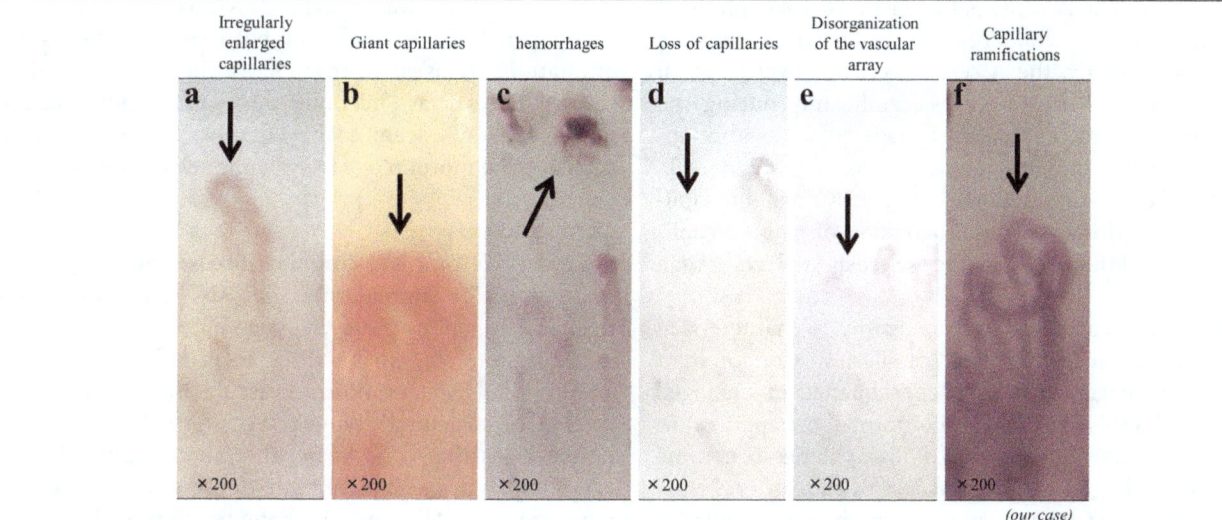

Fig. 3 The six capillaroscopic parameters. **a** Irregularly enlarged capillary. **b** Giant capillary. **c** Micro hemorrhage. **d** Loss of capillaries. **e** Disorganization of the microvascular array. **f** Capillary ramifications

capillaries (Fig. 3d) was indicated by lower than normal capillary numbers (the normal range was adopted from literature; average 9 capillaries per linear mm at the distal row of the nailfold); (e) disorganization of the microvascular array (Fig. 3e) seen as irregular capillary distribution and orientation along with heterogeneity in the loop shape; and (f) capillary ramifications (Fig. 3f) such as branching, bushy, or coiled capillaries that often originated from a single normal sized capillary. Except for irregularly enlarged capillaries, these parameters characterize overt systemic sclerosis. Some habits such as manicures, onychophagia, and guitar playing cause microhemorrhages, which obviously do not depend on any pathological condition. Hence, patients should remove nail polish 2 weeks before the examination.

Qualitative and semi-quantitative assessment can be made by combining these findings. The NVC pattern is classified into three different patterns, namely, early, active, and late, which are clearly distinct from the normal pattern (Table 1). The early pattern is characterized by few giant capillaries, few capillary microhemorrhages, and no evident loss of capillaries. The active pattern comprises many giant capillaries, many capillary microhemorrhages, and moderate loss of capillaries. The late pattern is characterized by irregular enlargement of capillaries, almost no giant capillaries and microhemorrhages, severe loss of capillaries with extensive avascular areas, ramified capillaries, and intense disorganization of the normal capillary array. The natural progression of microvascular damage is from the early pattern to the late pattern [10]. The presence of anti-Scl70 antibodies (also called anti-topoisomerase I) seems to be related to earlier expression of the active and late pattern. On the other hand, anti-centromere antibody positivity seems to be related to delayed expression of the late NVC pattern [11].

A semi-quantitative rating scale (score 0–3) should be adopted to score each of the aforementioned capillary abnormalities (0 = no changes, 1 = less than 33 % capillary alteration, 2 = 33–66 % capillary alteration, 3 = more than 66 % capillary alteration, per linear mm). The mean score value for each parameter should be calculated from the analysis of at least 2 mm in the center of the nailfold of each finger. The scores of irregularly enlarged capillaries, giant capillaries, and microhemorrhages are combined for the "A score." Additionally, the scores for the loss of capillaries, disorganization of the microvascular array, and capillary ramifications are combined for

Table 1 Nailfold videocapillaroscopy analysis of healthy donor

Early pattern	Active pattern	Late pattern
Giant capillaries <33 %	Giant capillaries >33 %	Giant capillaries <33 %
	Capillary microhemorrhage >33 %	Capillary microhemorrhage <33 %
No loss of capillaries	Loss of capillaries < 66 %	Loss of capillaries >66 %
No disorganization of the capillary array	Disorganization of the capillary array <66 %	Disorganization of the capillary array >66 %
No ramified capillaries	Ramified capillaries <33 %	Ramified capillaries >66 %

the "B score." The A score is higher in the early phase of systemic sclerosis, while B score is higher in the late phase. Interestingly, the A score decreases over time. In contrast, the B score increases significantly during the progression of microvascular damage [6]. We also observed this trend in our systemic sclerosis cohort ($n = 89$), and half of the patients showed progressive nailfold capillary changes. Moreover, the progression of nailfold capillary abnormalities in systemic sclerosis reflects organ involvement.

The earliest stage of microangiopathy is characterized by the appearance of giant capillaries. Concomitant microhemorrhages arise as a consequence of damaged microvessel walls. Subsequently, normally shaped capillaries progressively change, with all capillaries becoming irregularly enlarged and evident loss of capillaries. In the advanced stage of microangiopathy, both giant capillaries and microhemorrhages disappear, and neoangiogenesis with ramified capillaries induces microvascular array disorganization.

Several methods such as the Steinbrocker method (qualitative measure of radiographic damage) and the Sharp method (semi-quantitative measure of radiographic damage) have been introduced for scoring plain radiographs in rheumatoid arthritis patients to evaluate the disease course. Likewise, qualitative and semi-quantitative scoring of capillaries will become more important for the evaluation of the systemic sclerosis disease course.

Clinical use of NVC

Multiple candidate therapies such as tocilizumab, rituximab, and autologous stem cell transplantation are being clinically evaluated in systemic sclerosis patients. Especially, tocilizumab is expected to be useful for treating systemic sclerosis. However, none of the targeted therapies has become an established therapy. There are several obstacles for clinical trials in systemic sclerosis. First, there are no fully validated outcome measures. Second, diagnosis of systemic sclerosis is often delayed and early intervention is difficult. Moreover, systemic sclerosis has clinical heterogeneity [12]. To date, early diagnosis of systemic sclerosis can only be made using the new classification criteria. On the other hand, a lack of validated outcome measures was identified in a systemic lupus erythematosus clinical trial. Thus, it is important to have validated outcome measures to obtain good clinical evidence. For example, biological disease-modifying anti-rheumatic drugs revolutionized the treatment of rheumatoid arthritis patients. One of the reasons for this revolution was that highly validated indices such as the simplified disease activity index and 28-joint disease activity scale were widely accepted worldwide for objectively evaluating disease activity, and a lot of

clinical evidence was provided. As we have shown in this paper, NVC is useful for both early diagnosis and evaluation of disease progression. Scoring of capillary abnormalities has become very important because new treatments seem to be effective in modifying the capillary bed morphology in systemic sclerosis patients.

Conclusions

Systemic sclerosis is a complex disease involving "autoimmunity," "inflammation," "fibrosis," and "vasculopathy." Therapeutic goals in systemic sclerosis include minimization of damage from early inflammation and autoimmunity, restoration of vascular homeostasis, promotion of structural connective tissue repair, and resolution of scarring [12]. As in other autoimmune diseases, early diagnosis and intervention are important for achieving these goals. NVC has the potential to provide valuable information for early diagnosis, disease activity, disease progression, qualitative assessment, and pathogenesis of systemic sclerosis. Further clinical application of NVC and its epidemiology are required.

Competing interests

Y. Tanaka has received consulting fees, speaking fees, and/or honoraria from Abbvie, Daiichi-Sankyo, Chugai, Takeda, Mitsubishi-Tanabe, Bristol-Myers, Astellas, Eisai, Janssen, Pfizer, Asahi-kasei, Eli Lilly, GlaxoSmithKline, UCB, Teijin, MSD, and Santen and has received research grants from Mitsubishi-Tanabe, Takeda, Chugai, Astellas, Eisai, Taisho-Toyama, Kyowa-Kirin, Abbvie, and Bristol-Myers.

Authors' contributions

SK contributed to the writing of the manuscript, and YT was involved in the overall review. Both authors read and approved the final manuscript.

Acknowledgements

The author thanks all medical staff at all institutions for providing the data.

References

1. van den Hoogen F, Khanna D, Fransen J, Johnson SR, Baron M, Tyndall A, et al. Classification criteria for systemic sclerosis: an American college of rheumatology/European league against rheumatism collaborative initiative. Arthritis Rheum. 2013;2013(65):2737–47.
2. van den Hoogen F, Khanna D, Fransen J, Johnson SR, Baron M, Tyndall A, et al. Classification criteria for systemic sclerosis: an American college of rheumatology/European league against rheumatism collaborative initiative. Ann Rheum Dis. 2013;2013(72):1747–55.
3. Kahaleh MB. Raynaud phenomenon and the vascular disease in scleroderma. Curr Opin Rheumatol. 2004;16:718–22.
4. Cutolo M, Sulli A, Smith V. Assessing microvascular changes in systemic sclerosis diagnosis and management. Nat Rev Rheumatol. 2010;6:578–87.
5. Kabasakal Y, Elvins DM, Ring EF, McHugh NJ. Quantitative nailfold capillaroscopy findings in a population with connective tissue disease and in normal healthy controls. Ann Rheum Dis. 1996;55:507–12.
6. Sulli A, Secchi ME, Pizzorni C, Cutolo M. Scoring the nailfold microvascular changes during the capillaroscopic analysis in systemic sclerosis patients. Ann Rheum Dis. 2008;67:885–7.
7. Preliminary criteria for the classification of systemic sclerosis (scleroderma). Subcommittee for scleroderma criteria of the American Rheumatism Association Diagnostic and Therapeutic Criteria Committee. Arthritis Rheum. 1980;23:581-90.
8. Preliminary criteria for the classification of systemic sclerosis (scleroderma). Bull Rheum Dis. 1981;31:1-6.

9.   Smith V, Pizzorni C, De Keyser F, Decuman S, Van Praet JT, Deschepper E, et al. Reliability of the qualitative and semiquantitative nailfold videocapillaroscopy assessment in a systemic sclerosis cohort: a two-centre study. Ann Rheum Dis. 2010;69:1092–6.

10. Sulli A, Pizzorni C, Smith V, Zampogna G, Ravera F, Cutolo M. Timing of transition between capillaroscopic patterns in systemic sclerosis. Arthritis Rheum. 2012;64:821–5.

11. Cutolo M, Pizzorni C, Tuccio M, Burroni A, Craviotto C, Basso M, et al. Nailfold videocapillaroscopic patterns and serum autoantibodies in systemic sclerosis. Rheumatology (Oxford). 2004;43:719–26.

12. Denton CP, Ong VH. Targeted therapies for systemic sclerosis. Nat Rev Rheumatol. 2013;9:451–64.

2

Effect of human umbilical cord blood stem cell transplantation on oval cell response in 2-AAF/CCL4 liver injury modell

Hussein Abdellatif[1*], Gamal Shiha[2,3], Dalia M. Saleh[1], Huda Eltahry[1] and Kamal G. Botros[1]

Abstract

Background: Oval cells, specific liver progenitors, are activated in response to injury. The human umbilical cord blood (hUCB) is a possible source of transplantable hepatic progenitors and can be used in cases of severe liver injury. We detected the effect of hUCB stem cell transplantation on natural response of oval cells to injury.

Methods: Twenty-four female albino rats were randomly divided into three groups: (A) control, (B) liver injury with hepatocyte block, and (C) hUCB transplanted group. Hepatocyte block was performed by administration of 2-acetylaminofluorene (2-AAF) for 12 days. CCL4 was administrated at day 5 from experiment start. Animals were sacrificed at 9 days post CCL4 administration, and samples were collected for biochemical and histopathological analysis. Oval cell response to injury was evaluated by the percentage of oval cells in the liver tissue and frequency of cells incorporated into new ducts.

Results: Immunohistochemical analysis of oval cell response to injury was performed. There was significant deviation in the hUCB-transplanted (4.9 ± 1.4) and liver injury groups (2.4 ± 0.9) as compared to control (0.89 ± 0.4) 9 days post injury. Detection of oval cell response was dependant on OV-6 immunoreactivity. For mere localization of cells with human origin, CD34 antihuman immunoreactivity was performed. There was no significant difference in endogenous OV-6 immunoreactivity following stem cell transplantation as compared to the liver injury group.

Conclusions: In vivo transplantation of cord blood stem cells (hUCB) does not interfere with natural oval cell response to liver injury.

Keywords: Liver, Chronic injury, Oval cells, OV-6, CD34, hUCB

Background

Liver stem cell participation in recovery of the severely injured liver have been extensively described. Nevertheless, the exact location of such stem cells is still controversial although bile ducts have been implicated [1]. In experimental carcinogenesis proliferation of the so-called oval cells has been described. These cells are small with oval nuclei that reside in the periphery of the portal tracts in rat models of hepatocarcinogenesis and injury. Oval cells are bi-potent progenitors capable of differentiation into both hepatocytes and cholangiocytes [2]. Their precise nature remains unclear with debate as to whether they are derived from a postulated stem cell or are themselves facultative stem cells. An enormous range of markers has been used for oval cell identification, such as albumin, alpha fetal protein (AFP), epithelial cell adhesion molecule (EpCAM), cytokeratin 7 (CK7), OV-6, and cytokeratin 19 (CK19) [3, 4]. Human umbilical cord blood may be a possible source of transplantable hepatic progenitors. Newsome and his colleagues demonstrated that human umbilical cord blood (hUCB) stem cells could differentiate into hepatocytes after transplantation into immunodeficient

* Correspondence: hussein.abdullatif@hotmail.com
[1]Anatomy and Embryology Department, Faculty of Medicine, University of Mansoura, Mansoura, Egypt

mice [5]. Besides, some antigens traditionally associated with hematopoietic cells (c-kit, flt-3, CD34) can be expressed by oval cells/hepatic progenitor cells (HPCs) as well, leading to the notion that at least some hepatic oval cells are directly derived from a precursor of hematopoietic origin [6]. The underlying mechanism of stem cell plasticity and transdifferentiation into mature hepatocytes is of considerable interest. Exploring the therapeutic potential and role of oval cells in the process of natural repair of the liver is of great value and carries much hope in the future for the treatment of liver disease. Studying cord blood stem cells as a source of transplantable liver progenitors, and whether this may interfere with the natural response of oval cells to injury, to our knowledge is still unclear. Thus the aim of the current work was directed to study the effect of hUCB stem cell transplantation on the natural response of oval cells to liver injury.

Methods
Collection of human umbilical cord blood
Human umbilical cord blood was collected from full-term pregnant women (Department of Obstetrics and Gynecology, Mansoura University) just before placental separation in normal vaginal delivery after taking informative consent. Participants were considered eligible for the study according to the following exclusion (no family history of gene-based disorders or maternal fever during labor) and inclusion (delivery occurring less than 24 h after rupture of membranes) criteria.

Separation of the mononuclear cells
Human umbilical cord blood samples were diluted in Dulbecco's modified Eagle's medium (DMEM) (1:1) supplemented with 10% fetal bovine serum (FBS). Low-density mononuclear cells were collected after centrifugation at $800 \times g$ for 20 min in Ficoll density gradient (Histopaque, 1.077 g ml^{-1}) following the manufacturer's instructions. Mononuclear hematopoietic cells were obtained from the interphase and washed twice with sterilized PBS. Pellets were re-suspended in lysis buffer (150 mM NH$_4$ Cl, 1 mM KHCO$_3$, 0.1 mM Na-EDTA, pH 7.4) and incubated for 5 min at 4 °C to deplete erythrocytes. After washing once with PBS, pellets were again re-suspended. Cell viability, determined by the trypan blue dye exclusion method, was $97.40 \pm 0.43\%$. The total average number of viable cells isolated from one umbilical cord was 8×10^7 [7].

Animal preparation
Twenty-four adult female albino rats (Cux1: HEL1) 12 weeks of age, weighing 200–250 g. Rats were bred and maintained in an air-conditioned animal house (Medical Experimental Research Center, MERC, Mansoura University) (under controlled temperature 25 ± 2 °C) with specific pathogen-free environment and were subjected to a 12:12-h daylight/darkness cycle and allowed free access to rat chow and water. The principles of laboratory animal care were fulfilled in all experimental protocols and were approved by the ethics committee of animal research in MERC.

Animal groups
Rats were randomly divided into the following groups:

- *Control group* ($n = 8$). The rats received corn oil (10 ml kg^{-1} B.W.) orally throughout the whole experiment.
- *Liver injury and hepatocyte block group* ($n = 8$). The rats received acetylaminofluorene (2-AAF) (A7015, Sigma-Aldrich) to inhibit hepatocyte proliferation. The drug was administered in a dose of (10 mg kg^{-1} B.W.) as daily oral gavage for 12 days. 2-AAF was dissolved in a small volume of dimethyl sulfoxide (DMSO; Sigma cat: D8418) and suspended in corn oil to a final concentration of 2 mg ml^{-1}. On day 5 from the start of the experiment, rats received carbon tetrachloride (CCL4) in a dose of 0.6 ml kg^{-1} B.W. dissolved in corn oil (1:1) to induce differentiation of oval cells.
- *Stem cell transplantation group* ($n = 8$). The rats were subjected to 2-AAF/CCL4 liver injury protocol as described before; in addition, they also received human umbilical cord blood stem cells (mononuclear cells, MNCs) as a source of exogenous stem cells to the liver. This group received hUCB MNCs (8×10^6) in 0.3 ml media injection (DMEM) over 3 min through the portal vein on the day following CCL4 administration. Rats in different groups were sacrificed at day 9 post CCL4 injury.

Biochemical analysis
Heparinized blood samples were obtained from all animals at planned time intervals. Aspartate transaminase (AST) and alanine transaminase (ALT) activities and serum albumin and total bilirubin levels in the plasma were determined using commercially available kits (Sigma Chemical Co. kit nos. 58 and 59).

Specimens' collection
The livers were harvested following in situ perfusion through the portal vein using Ca^{++}-free Hank's balanced salt solution (HBSS) (pH 7.4). The initial flow rate was 15–20 ml min^{-1} with the perfusate exiting through the inferior vena cava. The livers were divided into pieces and were used for histopathological studies.

Staining

Small pieces of liver were collected and fixed overnight in 10% neutral-buffered formalin. The fixed liver tissue was then dehydrated in ascending grades of alcohol and then cleaned by xylene then embedded in paraffin. Five-micrometer-thick sections were mounted on clean glass slides. Sections were stained with hematoxylin-eosin (HE) for histopathological changes, antihuman/rat OV-6 antibody (R&D Systems, MAB2020) for the detection of oval cells that may originate from human or rat source, and antihuman CD34 monoclonal antibody (Thermo Scientific, MAI-21937) directed only for the detection of cells that originate from a human source (hUCB-derived cells).

OV-6 and CD34 immunohistochemistry

Tissue sections were rehydrated in decreasing concentrations of ethanol, and endogenous peroxidase activity was blocked with 0.5% hydrogen peroxide in methanol. The tissue was microwaved to boiling for 20 min in 0.1 mol l^{-1} of Tris EDTA pH 9.0 for antigen retrieval. The antibody was diluted in phosphate-buffered saline plus 0.1% nonfat dried milk and applied at 4 °C for 12 h. Primary antibody dilution was 1:10 for OV-6 and 1:80 for CD34. The tissue was incubated with biotinylated anti-mouse secondary antibody in a species-specific manner (R&D Systems, MAB002). The label was peroxidase-conjugated streptavidin. Color development was performed with diaminobenzidine peroxidase substrate (D-4293, Sigma Chemical Co.). Finally, sections were counterstained for 2 min with hematoxylin, dehydrated through graded alcohols, and mounted under glass cover slips.

Image analysis

Analysis of oval cell response was done using an Olympus microscope at a total magnification of 400, captured by digital camera (Olympus LC20) and using the image analyzer software (LC micron). The image analyzer was calibrated at first to convert the measurement units (pixels) produced by the image analyzer program into actual micrometer units. Oval cells were quantified by counting cells positive for OV-6 antigen, relative to total hepatocyte numbers, in 10–15 randomly selected fields of the portal tracts in a blinded way at 400× magnification. The cell count is then expressed as a percentage in relation to the hepatocyte number.

The oval cell response and the frequency of oval cell incorporation into new ducts were scored as (1) oval cells constituting 10% of the field and only 10% of oval cells were incorporated into new ducts, (2) oval cells constituting 20% of the field and only 20% of oval cells were incorporated into new ducts, (3) oval cells constituting 30% of the field and 30% of oval cells were incorporated into new ducts, (4) oval cells constituting 40% of the field and 40% of oval cells were incorporated into new ducts, and (5) oval cells constituting 50% of the field and 50% of oval cells were incorporated into new ducts. Average cell percentages were then pooled for each experimental group, and the overall mean and standard deviation were determined, and then the overall response was scored according to the previously described score.

Statistical analysis

As the oval cell reaction is not uniform around all the portal tracts over their complete size range and the reaction varies between different animals at different time intervals, the coefficient of variation (CV) was calculated and it was statistically significant for all groups. Data are expressed as mean ± SD. Multiple comparisons were done using SPSS 15.0 computer software. Significance of results was considered at P value <0.05.

Results

Biochemical analysis

Nine days post CCL4 injection, ALT and AST levels were estimated in the blood of all experimental groups and were significantly elevated in the liver injury (114 ± 37.5, 265 ± 127.3) and stem cell transplantation groups (132.8 ± 21.1, 162.5 ± 34.8) as compared to the control group (42.6 ± 2.8, 44.3 ± 3.5), respectively. Data are expressed as mean ± SD. Pairwise comparison between sample means reveals significant difference between groups. Data are considered significant at P value <0.05. Serum albumin and bilirubin levels were also estimated in all groups, and no significant difference was found in the liver injury (3.9 ± 0.2, 0.31 ± 0.16) or stem cell transplantation group (3.95 ± 0.13, 0.28 ± 0.11) as compared to the control (3.9 ± 0.3, 0.31 ± 0.18), respectively, as indicated by P value >0.05 (Table 1).

Changes in oval cell response in hematoxylin and eosin stained liver sections

No evidence of oval cells was observed in the control group (Fig. 1a). In the 2-AAF/CCL4 group, oval cells

Table 1 Plasma levels of ALT, AST, albumin, and bilirubin in rats

	Group A control	Group B liver injury group	Group C (2AAF/CCL4 + stem cell transplantation)
At 9 days post CCL4 injury			
ALT	42.6 ± 2.8	114 ± 37.5*	132.8 ± 21.1*
AST	44.3 ± 3.5	265 ± 187.3*	162.5 ± 34.8*
Albumin	3.9 ± 0.3	3.9 ± 0.2	3.95 ± 0.13
Bilirubin	0.31 ± 0.18	0.31 ± 0.16	0.28 ± 0.11

Values are expressed as means ± SD
*Significant deviation from the control group as indicated by $P < 0.05$

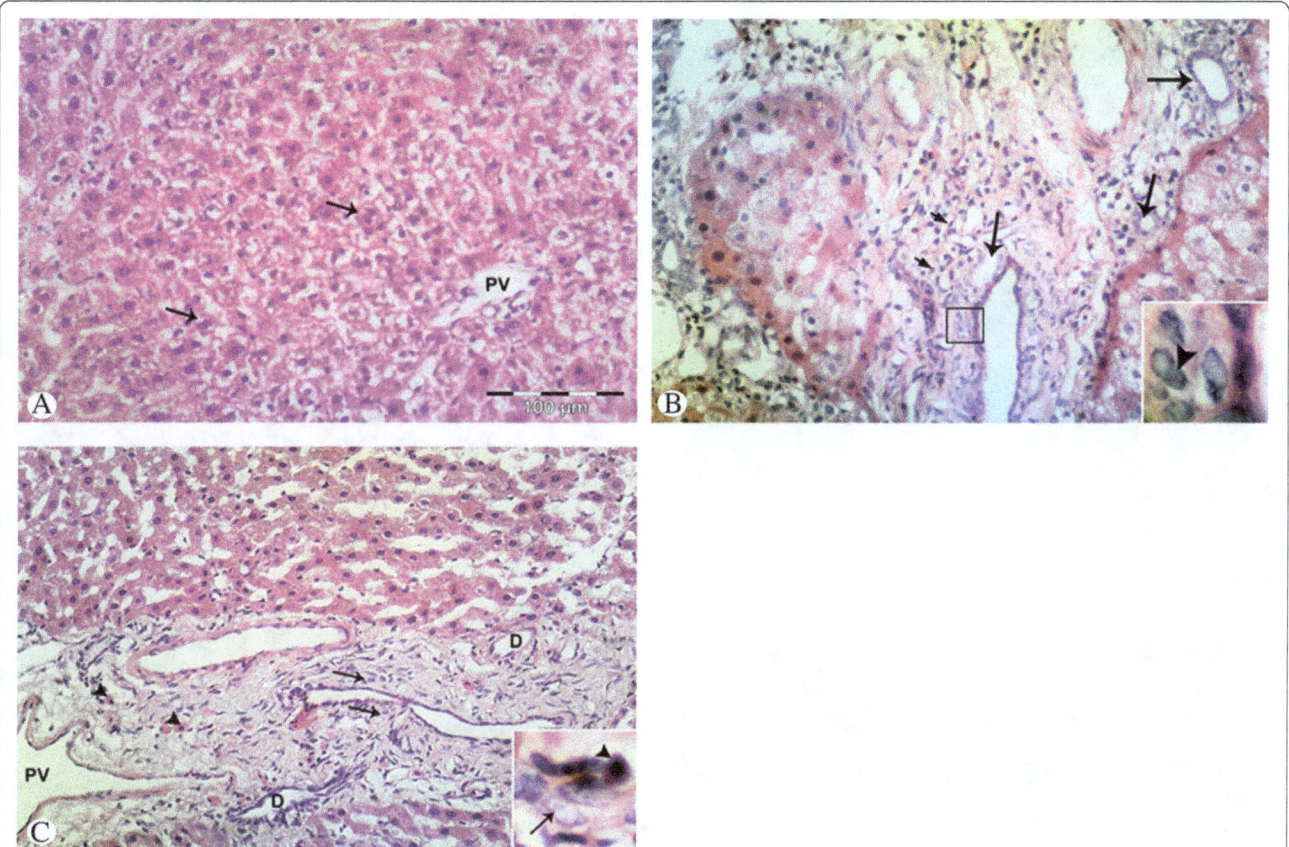

Fig. 1 Photomicrograph of liver tissue in the control (**a**), liver injury (**b**), and stem cell transplantation groups (**c**). **a** Normal liver architecture, some hepatocytes, are binucleated (*arrows*). No signs of oval cell response around the portal vein (*PV*). **b** Oval cell response with ductular reaction (*arrows*) and small hepatocyte-like cells (*short arrows*). **c** Increased oval cell response (*arrows*) with ductular reaction (*D*) around portal vein (*PV*). Small hepatocyte-like cells (*arrowheads*). Inset: high magnification showing oval cells (*arrowhead*) with scanty basophilic cytoplasm (*arrow*) and high nucleo-cytoplasmic ratio (**b**, **c**). H&E, 100×; Inset, 400×

appeared as small oval-shaped cells proliferating in files between hepatocytes in the periportal regions or extending beyond the periportal region. These cells had scanty basophilic cytoplasm, dark staining nucleus with a large nucleo-cytoplasmic ratio (Fig. 1, inset). The cells radiate from the periportal region in the form of individual cells or ductular-like structures (Fig. 1b, arrowheads). Some cells also appeared as individual oval-shaped cells with hepatocyte phenotype (small hepatocyte-like cells) (Fig. 1b, short arrows). In the stem cell transplantation group, there was evident increase in oval cells surrounding the portal tract or emanating from it and invading the liver parenchyma extending far beyond the periportal region (Fig. 1c, arrows). Pairwise comparison between groups reveals a highly significant result in the stem cell transplantation group (4.8 ± 1.5, 4.5 ± 1.4) than in the liver injury (3.5 ± 1.4, 3.3 ± 1.5) and control groups regarding oval cell score and duct formation score, respectively (P value <0.05).

Changes in oval cell response detected by immunoreactivity (IHC methods)

In the control group, mild immunoreactivity to OV-6 antibody was only limited to the intraportal bile duct and terminal duct cells located at the Canals of Hering (Fig. 2d, arrows). No CD34 positive cells were present in the stained liver samples (no cross-reactivity or evidence of human-derived cells). Oval cell response was 0.85 ± 0.4 and 0.78 ± 0.3 regarding the oval cell score and duct formation score, respectively. In the liver injury and hepatocyte block group, marked increase in OV-6 immunoreactivity (2.4 ± 0.9, 2.3 ± 0.8) was observed (Fig. 2e, arrows). No CD34 immunoreactivity was detected. In stem cell transplantation group, significant increase in OV-6 immunoreactivity was observed (4.9 ± 1.4, 4.8 ± 1.2) (Fig. 3) with oval cells forming more reactive ductules (ductular-like oval cells) (Fig. 2f, arrows) or appearing as small hepatocyte-like cells. CD34 (antihuman) immunoreactivity reveals presence of positively stained cells (Fig. 2g, arrows) which demonstrates oval cells derived from

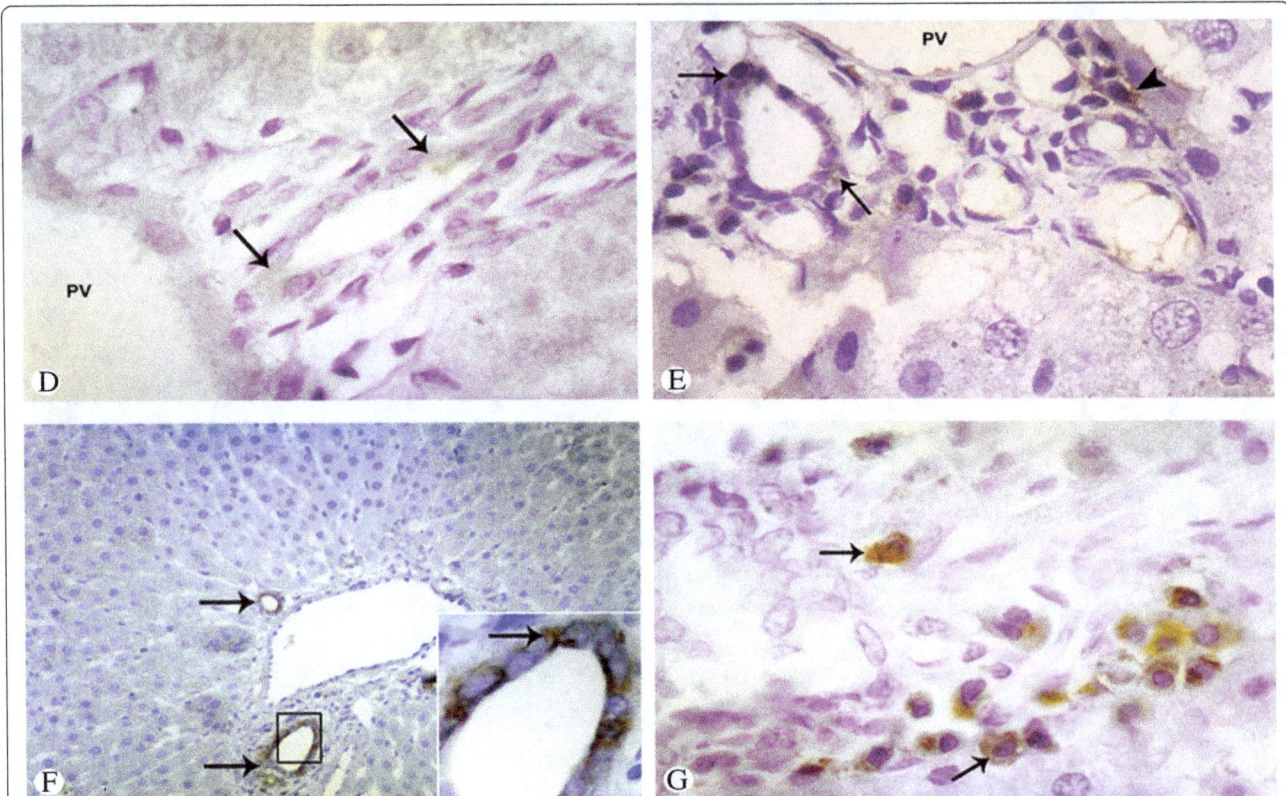

Fig. 2 Photomicrograph of liver tissue in the control (**d**), liver injury (**e**), and stem cell transplantation groups (**f, g**). **d** Mild immunoreactivity to OV-6 antibody limited to intraportal bile duct and terminal duct cells (*arrows*) surrounding the portal vein (*PV*). **e** OV-6 immunoreactivity (cytoplasmic reaction) with oval cells forming more reactive ductules (*arrows*) or appearing as small hepatocyte-like cells (*arrowhead*). The cells are surrounding the portal vein (*PV*) or emanating from it and invading liver parenchyma. **f** Increased OV-6 immunoreactivity with oval cells forming more reactive ductules (*arrows*) around the portal vein. Inset: Positive oval cells in the reactive ductules (*arrow*), 400×. **g** CD34 immunoreactivity of the human oval cells (*arrows*) scattered and invading the liver parenchyma. Immunoperoxidase stain, 400×

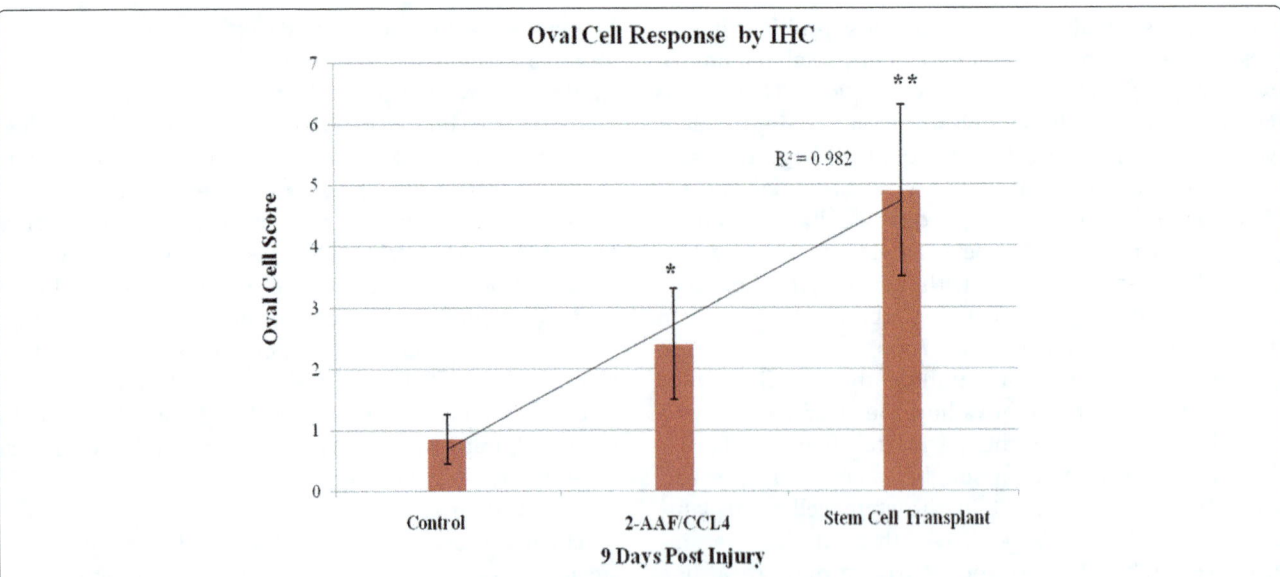

Fig. 3 Oval cell response detected by OV-6 immunoreactivity showing highly significant increase in the stem cell transplantation group (*double asterisk*) as compared to the liver injury (*asterisk*) and control groups (*P* value <0.01). Data are expressed as mean ± SD

human origin (hUCB-derived cells). CD34 oval cell score and frequency of exogenous cells incorporated into new ducts were 3.2 ± 1.2 and 2.2 ± 0.9, respectively. Calculation of the acquired data (oval cells +ve for OV-6, antihuman/ anti-rat Ab - CD34 +ve cells for antihuman Ab = oval cells of only rat origin). No significant difference was found in the acquired data as compared to the response observed in the liver injury and hepatocyte block group. Previously calculated data reveals that hUCB stem cell transplantation has no effect on endogenous response of oval cells to liver injury.

Discussion

The liver can regenerate itself by increasing the rate of hepatocyte mitosis and stem cell differentiation into hepatocytes or cholangiocytes. Stem cells are the principle cell lineage for liver regeneration. However, the exact location of these cells is not yet clear [8].

Oval cells represent the progeny of liver stem cells and function as an amplification compartment for the generation of new hepatocytes [9]. This compartment, consisting of small ovoid cells with scant lightly basophilic cytoplasm, is widely used to describe liver progenitors [10]. Here, we describe whether application of stem cells (hUCB) interferes with the natural response of oval cells to injury (represented by the percentage of oval cells in liver tissue and the frequency of new duct formation) or not.

The general principle underlying oval cell activation is based on a combination of liver injury with inability of hepatocytes to proliferate in response to damage [11]. According to these data, the 2-AAF/CCL4 protocol was used in the current work to induce an oval cell response. CCL4 is a known chemical to induce injury in the hepatic centri-lobular area while 2-AAF has been shown to block proliferation of hepatocytes, thus allowing oval cells to continue to proliferate in large numbers. Oval cells lack the ability to convert the 2-AAF to its toxic metabolite, thus escaping its inhibitory effect. This procedure induces a robust response of oval cells reaching its peak 9 days post CCL4 injury, and this was the time determined to detect for oval cell response in our model [12].

Liver injury is followed by extensive changes in variety of enzyme activities as part of the regenerative process [13] (Table 1). In the current work, the ALT, AST, albumin, and bilirubin levels were estimated in different groups 9 days post injury and compared to the control. ALT and AST were significantly elevated in the liver injury and stem cell transplantation groups (P value <0.05). The most likely explanation for this transaminase elevation is the release of enzymes from damaged liver parenchymal cells. In contrast, the albumin and bilirubin levels were not significantly different from the control level and this was concomitant with the findings stated by Shakoori and his associates who failed to see any

effect on the total protein and bilirubin levels during the first 20 days post injury [14]. The explanation for this may be due to restoration of liver mass and function starting the second week post injury.

In the current work, hUCB was used as a source of hepatic progenitors and this was based on findings noted by Newsome and his colleagues who stated that human umbilical cord blood (hUCB)-derived cells could differentiate into hepatocytes in vivo after their transplantation in immunodeficient mice [5]. This was further modified by Tang and his colleagues who showed that number of positive human AFP and ALB cells in the HUCBSC-treated animals with or without cyclophosphamide did not differ significantly, denoting that immunosuppression had either a mild or no effect on stem cell differentiation in rats [15]. Besides, undifferentiated cells were used in the current work, based on findings of Peters and his colleagues who demonstrated that better results are obtained with undifferentiated stem cells because these cells have very low apoptotic activity responsible for their longer survival. They are lowest in expressing apoptotic proteins, Asp, annexin-V, bax, bad, and bak [16]. These cells derived from the cord blood exhibit higher plasticity than the respective mouse or rat cells [17]. Cell fusion has been implicated as the mechanism by which human cells are seen in the recipient's liver in most cases [18].

Immunohistochemical analysis of oval cell response in all experimental groups has been evaluated (oval cell score and frequency of cells incorporated into new ducts) and revealed highly significant deviation in stem cell transplantation group (4.9 ± 1.4, 4.8 ± 1.2) as compared to the liver injury (2.4 ± 0.9, 2.3 ± 0.8) and control groups (0.85 ± 0.4, 0.78 ± 0.3) (Fig. 3). OV-6 immunoreactivity was only limited to intraportal bile ducts and terminal duct cells with no evident induced oval cell response in the control group. In the liver injury group, response was significantly increased due to 2-AAF-induced mito-inhibitory effect on liver resident hepatocytes and CCL4-induced oval cell activation. Highly significant deviation was found in the stem cell transplantation group, as OV-6 immunoreactivity was directed to cells of both human and rat origin (using antihuman/rat OV-6 antibody). For mere localization of cells with human origin, CD34 antihuman immunoreactivity was performed. Co-staining of OV-6 and CD34 was technically not possible in liver tissue sections as both antigens are membranously expressed to the same extent [19], and this was treated by staining for OV-6 antigen followed by CD34 in the serial parallel liver tissue section, and co-localization of both antigens was done. Analysis of results reveals no significant change in OV-6 immunoreactivity following stem cell transplantation as compared to the liver injury group.

The application of stem cells in liver therapies seems to be a promising feature for treatment of liver diseases.

However, several issues still have to be addressed to fulfill this promise. The fundamental molecular pathways involved in differentiation of hepatocytes and cholangiocytes from stem/progenitor cells need to be explored in more details [20]. Much less is known about the mechanisms of oval cell replication and differentiation [21], and whether the natural response of oval cells to injury is enhanced or decreased by extrahepatic sources of stem cells (like hUCB) is not recently declared. To our knowledge, this is the first time to use an immunohistochemical-based assay to prospectively detect the effect of hUCB stem cells on the natural response of oval cells to liver injury.

Conclusions

Liver regeneration is a well-organized process by hepatocytes and non-parenchymal cells. Oval cells, resident liver progenitors, play a major role in the natural response of the liver to injury. Extrahepatic stem cells (like hUCB) have recently been used as sources of transplantable hepatic progenitors. In the current work, we aimed to detect the effect of stem cell transplantation (hUCB-derived cells) on oval cell response to injury (represented by oval cell score and the frequency of cells incorporated into new ducts). Based on our results, oval cell response to liver injury is not affected by extrahepatic stem cell transplantation. Thus, in vivo differentiation of cord blood stem cells to liver progenitors or hepatocytes (mostly occurring by cell fusion with resident cells) does not interfere with the natural response of oval cells to injury. These molecular pathways for cellular differentiation and signalling need to be further explored.

Abbreviations
2-AAF: Acetylaminofluorene; CCL4: Carbon tetrachloride; DMEM: Dulbecco's modified Eagle's medium; DMSO: Dimethyl sulfoxide; FBS: Fetal bovine serum; HBSS: Hank's balanced salt solution; HPCs: Hepatic progenitor cells; hUCB: Human umbilical cord blood; MNCs: Mononuclear cells

Acknowledgements
We thank the Egyptian Liver Research Institute and Hospital (ELRIAH) for providing suitable laboratories and technical support.

Funding
This research received no specific grant from any funding agency in the public, commercial, or not-for-profit sectors.

Authors' contributions
The authors equally contributed to the preparation of this review. All authors read and approved the final manuscript.

Competing interests
The authors declare that they have no competing interests.

Author details
[1]Anatomy and Embryology Department, Faculty of Medicine, University of Mansoura, Mansoura, Egypt. [2]Internal Medicine Department, Faculty of Medicine, University of Mansoura, Mansoura, Egypt. [3]Egyptian Liver Research Institute and Hospital (ELRIAH), Mansoura, Egypt.

References
1.   Novikoff PM, Yam A, Oikawa I. Blast-like cell compartment in carcinogen-induced proliferating bile ductules. American J Pathol. 1996;148:1473–92.
2.   Fausto N, Lemire JM, Shiojiri N. Oval cells in liver carcinogenesis: cell lineages in hepatic development and the identification of facultative stem cells in normal livers. In: Sirica AE, editor. The role of cell types in hepatocarcinogenesis. Boca Raton: CRC Press; 1992. p. 89–108.
3.   Fausto N, Campbell JS. The role of hepatocytes and oval cells in liver regeneration and repopulation. Mech Dev. 2003;120:117–30.
4.   Lowes KN, Croager EJ, Olynyk JK, Abraham LJ, Yeoh GCT. Oval cell-mediated liver regeneration: role of cytokines and growth factors. J Gastroenterol Hepatol. 2003;18:4–12.
5.   Newsome PN, Johannessen I, Boyle S, Dalakas E, McAulay KA, Samuel K, Rae F, Forrester L, Turner ML, Hayes PC, Harrison DJ, Bickmore WA, Plevris JN. Human cord blood-derived cells can differentiate into hepatocytes in the mouse liver with no evidence of cellular fusion. Gastroenterology. 2003;124:1891–900.
6.   Schmelzer E, Wauthier E, Reid LM. The phenotypes of pluripotent human hepatic progenitors. Stem Cells. 2006;24:1852–8.
7.   Jaatinen T, Laine J. Isolation of mononuclear cells from human cord blood by Ficoll-Paque density gradient. Curr Protoc Stem Cell Biol. 2007;1:2A.1.1–4.
8.   Bae SH. Clinical application of stem cells in liver diseases. Korean J Hepatol. 2008;14:309–17.
9.   Golding M, Sarraf C, Lalani EN, Alison MR. Reactive biliary epithelium: the product of a pluripotential stem cell compartment. Hum Pathol. 1996;27:872–84.
10. Xiao JC, Ruck P, Kaiserling E. Small epithelial cells in extrahepatic biliary atresia: electron microscopic and immunoelectron microscopic findings suggest a close relationship to liver progenitor cells. Histopathology. 1999;35:454–60.
11. Dan YY, Riehle KJ, Lazaro C, Teoh N, Haque J, Campbell JS, Fausto N. Isolation of multipotent progenitor cells from human fetal liver capable of differentiating into liver and mesenchymal lineages. Proceedings of the National Academy of Sciences. 2006;103(26):9912–17.
12. Alison MR, Golding M, Sarraf CE, Edwards RJ, Lalani EN. Liver damage in the rat induces hepatocyte stem cells from biliary epithelial cells. Gastroeneterology. 1996;110:1182–90.
13. Rao KN, Virji MA, Moraca WR, Diven WF, Martin TG, et al. Role of serum markers for liver function and liver regeneration in management of chloroform poisoning. J Analytical toxicol. 1993;17:99–102.
14. Shakoori AR, Kokab R, Mah JG, Anjum F, Ali SS. Effect of mercuric chloride on the activity of some hepatic enzyme of regenerating liver following partial hepatectomy. Apptla. 1995;45:177–84.
15. Tang XP, Zhang M, Yang X, et al. Differentiation of human umbilical cord blood stem cells into hepatocytes in vivo and in vitro. World J Gastroenterol. 2006;12:401.
16. Peters R, Leyvraz S, Perey L. Apoptotic regulation in primitive hematopoietic precursors. Blood. 1998;92:2041–52.
17. Di Campli C, Piscaglia AC, Pierelli L, Rutella S, Bonanno G, Alison MR, Mariotti A, Vecchio FM, Nestola M, Monego G, Michetti F, Mancuso S, Pola P, Leone G, Gasbarrini G, Gasbarrini A. A human umbilical cord stem cell rescue therapy in a murine model of toxic liver injury. Dig Liver Dis. 2004;36:603–13.
18. Fujino H, Hiramatsu H, Tsuchiya A, Niwa A, Noma H, Shiota M, Umeda K, Yoshimoto M, Ito M, Heike T, Nakahata T. Human cord blood CD34+ cells develop into hepatocytes in the livers of NOD/SCID/gamma(c)null mice through cell fusion. FASEB J. 2007;21:3499–510.
19. Pirici D, Mogoanta L, Kumar-Singh S, Pirici I, Margaritescu C, Simionescu C, Stanescu R. Antibody elution method for multiple immunohistochemistry on primary antibodies raised in the same species and of the same subtype. J Histochemistry Cytochemistry. 2009;57(6):567–75.
20. Cantz, Tobias, Michael P. Manns, and Michael Ott. "Stem cells in liver regeneration and therapy." Cell and tissue research. 2008;331(1):271-282.
21. Brooling JT, Campbell JS, Mitchell C, Yeoh GC, Fausto N. Differential regulation of rodent hepatocyte and oval cell proliferation by interferon γ. Hepatology. 2005;41(4):906-15.

3

Complement-targeted therapy: development of C5- and C5a-targeted inhibition

Takahiko Horiuchi[1*] and Hiroshi Tsukamoto[2]

Abstract

The complement system is a major effector of humoral immunity and natural immunity. The complement system has three independent pathways of complement activation: a classical pathway, an alternative pathway, and a lectin pathway. These pathways converge to a common pathway that activates C3. This pathway also leads to the formation of various bioactive molecules such as C5a and the formation of membrane attack complex on the surface of target cells. In the past, the only preparations with anti-complementary action were C1 inhibitors (C1-INH), but an anti-C5 monoclonal antibody (eculizumab) appeared a few years ago, and this antibody has yielded encouraging results. In addition, a C5a receptor (C5aR) antagonist is in the clinical trial phase, and this antagonist should also prove efficacious. Anti-complement agents have garnered attention as a new treatment strategy for refractory inflammatory diseases.

Keywords: Complement, C5, C5a, C5a receptor, Membrane attack complex

Background

The complement system consists of more than 30 proteins. These proteins are activated sequential order in a cascade that produces a variety of molecules that maintain homeostasis in the body by, for example, defending the body from infection. Complement activation results in the formation of membrane attack complex (MAC), and this complex produces holes in the cell membrane, causing the destruction of target cells. Complement fragments such as C3a, C4a, and C5a trigger inflammation as anaphylatoxins and chemotactic factors, and abnormal complement activation leads to various inflammatory diseases [1, 2].

Over the past few years, a monoclonal antibody against complement component C5 (eculizumab) has been approved as a treatment for paroxysmal nocturnal hemoglobinuria and atypical hemolytic uremic syndrome (aHUS), and this antibody has yielded encouraging results [3, 4]. Eculizumab binds to C5 and thus inhibits the cleavage of C5 into C5a and C5b, but its principal action is presumably by inhibiting

the formation of C5b, which precludes the formation of MAC [5]. CCX168 was recently developed to inhibit inflammation caused by C5a. CCX168 is an orally administered C5a receptor antagonist. In a phase II clinical trial of CCX168 to treat anti-neutrophil cytoplasmic antibody (ANCA)-associated renal vasculitis (AARV), administration of CCX168 (+cyclophosphamide) was as efficacious as or more efficacious than the standard treatment (high-dose prednisolone + cyclophosphamide) [6, 7]. CCX168 has garnered attention as a potential replacement for corticosteroids, so CCX168 holds promise.

This paper outlines the mechanisms of complement activation. This paper then describes anti-complement agents that are being put to practical use. Last, this paper describes a C5a receptor antagonist that is in development.

Mechanisms of complement activation

Complements are activated in three independent pathways: a classical pathway, an alternative pathway, and a lectin pathway (Fig. 1). These three pathways ultimately converge to a common pathway where they form a crucial enzyme known as C3 convertase. The classical pathway is triggered when the complement C1 complex

* Correspondence: horiuchi@beppu.kyushu-u.ac.jp
[1]Kyushu University Beppu Hospital, Beppu, Japan
Full list of author information is available at the end of the article

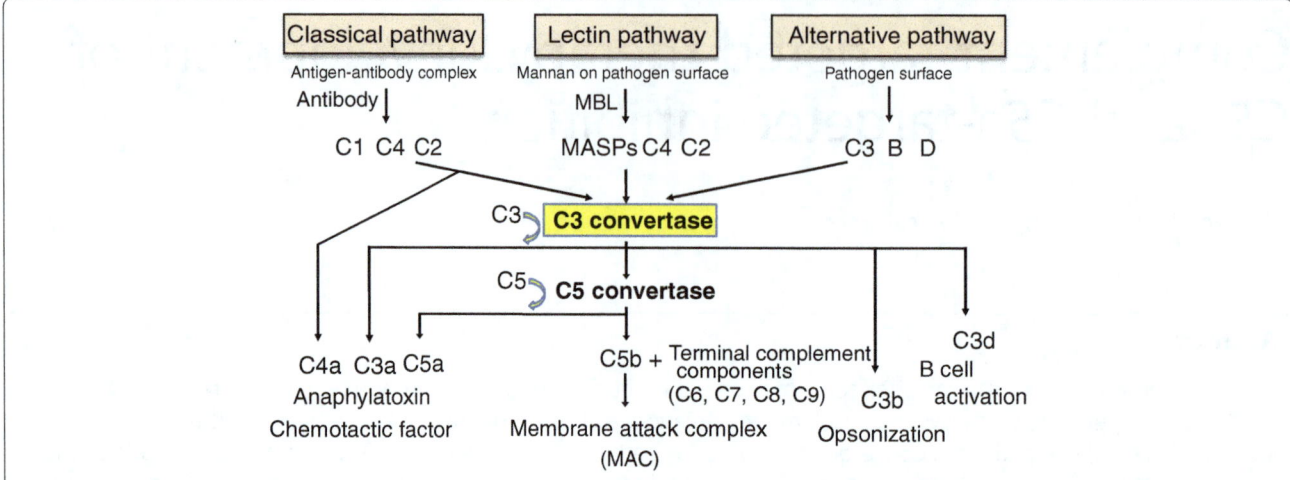

Fig. 1 Complement activation. Three pathways, i.e., classical, lectin, and alternative pathways, are independently activated to form C3 convertase. The activation of this cascade culminates in the generation of various fragments derived from complement proteins and the formation of membrane attack complex (MAC). The former acts as potent mediators of inflammation by binding to their receptors on the cell surface, while the latter is comprised of C5b, C6, C7, C8, and multiple copies of C9 that generate lytic pores in cellular membranes

binds to antibodies that are bound to antigens. Once C1 is activated, C4 and then C2 are activated. In the process, C4b and C2a are produced, and these two fragments combine to form C3 convertase. The lectin pathway is triggered when mannose-binding lectin (MBL) recognizes mannose or other carbohydrate sugar residues on the surface of pathogens. Once MBL-associated serine protease (MASP) is activated, C4 and then C2 are activated. Like in the classical pathway, C4b2a functions as C3 convertase in the lectin pathway. In the alternative pathway, complement factor D is directly activated by the surface of foreign particles. Once factor D is activated, factor B and then complement component C3 are activated. In the process, C3b and Bb are produced, and these two fragments combine to form C3bBb. C3bBb functions as C3 convertase on the surface of foreign substances [1, 2].

C3 is broken down into C3a and C3b by C3 convertase. C3b binds to C3 convertase to form C5 convertase, and C5 is broken down into C5a and C5b. C3a, C4a, and C5a function as potent mediators of inflammation, binding to receptors on the surface of lymphocytes, macrophages, and endothelial cells. Other products of the cleavage of these components have biological functions. C5b binds to the surface of foreign particles. C5b triggers the assembly of complement components C6 to C9 into MAC, which destroys foreign particles [1, 2].

Molecularly targeted therapies with antibodies are yielding dramatic results in the treatment of rheumatoid arthritis (RA) and malignancies. Complement activation by the antibodies themselves is crucial to their action [8, 9].

Complement-targeting drugs that are being put to practical use

Complement activation serves to eliminate pathogens, but abnormal activation is heavily involved in the pathology of various conditions. As of today (February 2016), two drugs targeting specific complement components are being put to practical use. One is a drug that supplements a deficient complement while the other inhibits a complement.

1. C1 inhibitor (C1-INH) (Berinert®)

Hereditary angioedema (HAE) is due to a deficiency in the inhibitor of complement component C1 (C1-INH). A C1-INH has been refined from human plasma to supplement the lacking C1-INH. HAE is an autosomal dominant genetic condition in which an abnormality in the C1-INH gene causes a deficiency of C1-INH that in turn causes transient edema (angioedema) at various sites. The epidemiology of HAE in Japan is unclear, but studies in Europe and the USA estimate that HAE affects 1 in every 50,000 people. If acute edema appears in the eyelids and lips, it can also appear in the bowel and the larynx. Edema of the bowel causes intense abdominal pain, and edema of the larynx can cause asphyxia. Despite its rarity, these symptoms of HAE mean that it must be identified. During an episode of edema, administration of C1-INH can cause the episode to promptly end. Information on diagnosis and treatment of HAE can be found in the guidelines on hereditary angioedema from the Japanese Association for Complement Research [10].

2. Eculizumab, an anti-C5 monoclonal antibody (Soliris®)

Eculizumab is a humanized anti-C5 monoclonal antibody that binds to the α chain of C5. This prevents C5 from being cleaved into C5a and C5b by C5 convertase. As of February 2016, eculizumab is indicated for paroxysmal nocturnal hemoglobinuria (PNH) and atypical hemolytic uremic syndrome (aHUS), but a prospective clinical study is underway to expand its indications to include age-related macular degeneration, myasthenia gravis, optic neuritis, and preventing rejection of a kidney transplant [11].

PNH is a progressive hematologic disorder with a triad of features: complement-mediated intravascular hemolysis, bone marrow failure, and thrombosis. Japan is estimated to have a population of around 430 patients with PNH. The condition is caused by clonal expansion of hematopoietic stem cells with an acquired mutation in the PIG-A gene. In PNH, blood cells lack several types of proteins on their surface because the cells lack an anchor, glycosylphosphatidylinositol (GPI), to hold the proteins to that surface. These missing proteins include CD55 (a decay-accelerating factor, or DAF) and CD59 (a homologous restriction factor, or HRF) that would be present on the surface of various cells, such as red blood cells, to protect them from complement attack [12].

aHUS is defined as a condition with a triad of features: hemolytic anemia, thrombocytopenia, and acute renal insufficiency. The atypical form of aHUS is not associated with Shiga toxin, and the condition is not thrombotic thrombocytopenic purpura (TTP). aHUS has an extremely poor prognosis. aHUS due to genetic complement abnormalities can be treated with eculizumab. When surplus complement is activated in conjunction with abnormalities in various molecules involved in the alternative pathway of complement activation, vascular endothelial cells and platelets are activated and aHUS develops. Administration of eculizumab results in an improved prognosis for patients with aHUS [13]. A study has also suggested that eculizumab would be efficacious in treating HUS associated with Shiga toxin and TTP as well [14].

Eculizumab inhibits two complement functions, the anaphylatoxic action of complement component C5a and interaction with C5b that leads to the formation of MAC. Inhibition of the formation of MAC increases a patient's susceptibility to a meningococcal infection, so caution is required. Thus, vaccination with a meningococcal vaccine prior to administration of eculizumab is recommended. Moreover, vaccination of small children with a pneumococcal vaccine and an influenza type B vaccine is also recommended.

Complement C5a receptor antagonists

Attempts have long been made to develop inhibitors of complement C5 activation besides eculizumab [15]. These inhibitors target factors upstream of C5, including (in order) C5 convertase, complement components C5, C5a, and C5b, and C5a receptor (Fig. 2). Various types of antibodies and compounds such as peptides or nonpeptides have actively been developed, and these substances act as inhibitors of complement components C5 and C5a and antagonists of the C5a receptor. These C5

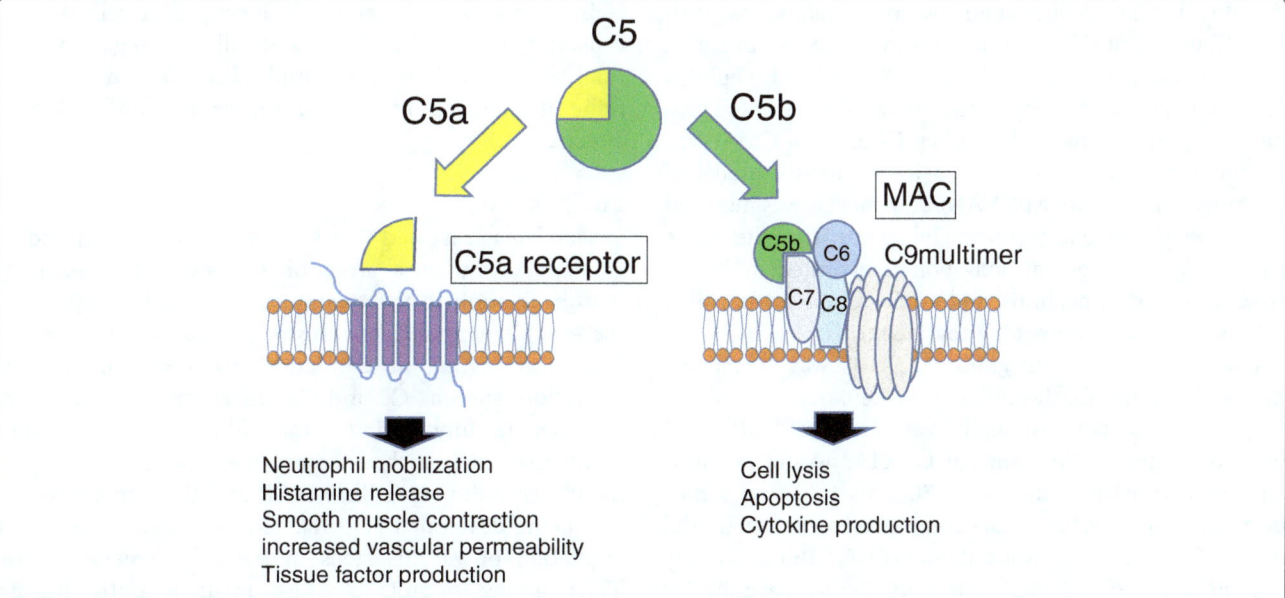

Fig. 2 Activation of C5 by C5 convertase leads to the generation of C5a and C5b. C5a binds to C5a receptor and mediates various biological activities. C5b initiates the formation of MAC, which lyses cells as well as triggers inflammation

and C5a receptor antagonists may be efficacious at treating various inflammatory diseases involving complements.

There is interest in the efficacy of these anti-complement agents on RA. In fact, numerous findings have suggested a relationship between RA and C5 and C5a receptors. C5a levels in synovial fluid are elevated in patients with RA [16], a genome-wide association study (GWAS) indicated that the TRAF1-C5 region is related to RA in humans [17, 18], numerous animal models have indicated that C5 is a gene responsible for causing arthritis [19, 20], and C5 and C5a receptor knockout mice are resistant to arthritis [21, 22]. However, clinical trials indicated that eculizumab (a humanized anti-C5 monoclonal antibody) and PMX53 and MP-435 (C5a receptor antagonists) had little efficacy in treating RA [23, 24].

Research has also suggested that complements are involved in causing ANCA-associated vasculitis (AAV) in humans. Patients with active AAV have significantly elevated C5a levels in plasma and urine in comparison to healthy people and patients with inactive AAV [25]. Bb levels in plasma are correlated with the disease activity of AAV in humans [26]. In a mouse model of nephritis induced with myeloperoxidase anti-neutrophil cytoplasmic antibody (MPO-ANCA), knocking out complement factor B and complement component C5 resulted in the absence of nephritis [27]. In light of these findings, researchers conceived of a model in which neutrophils stimulated by ANCA cause the release of substances that activate the alternative pathway of complement activation [27]. This activation results in the activation of complement factor B. Complement activation proceeds in association with the generation of C5a and MAC, producing nephritis. In fact, administration of an anti-C5 antibody in the mouse model of nephritis induced with MPO-ANCA almost entirely inhibited nephritis [28]. Knocking out the C5a receptor in the mouse model of nephritis induced with MPO-ANCA inhibited nephritis [29]. In addition, knocking in the human C5a receptor produced nephritis in mice [29]. When CCX168 (a C5a receptor antagonist) was administered in the mouse model of nephritis induced with MPO-ANCA, nephritis was inhibited in a dose-dependent manner [29]. Thus, the alternative pathway of complement activation is activated in MPO-ANCA-associated nephritis, and a C5a receptor antagonist may be efficacious in treating that nephritis.

The C5a receptor antagonist CCX168 was efficacious in mice, and the C5aR inhibitor on Leukocytes Exploratory ANCA-associated Renal Vasculitis (CLEAR) trial was conducted to determine if CCX168 would be similarly efficacious in humans [6, 7]. This trial was a randomized, double-blind, placebo-controlled phase II trial in which the C5a receptor antagonist CCX168 was orally administered to patients with ANCA-positive granulomatosis with polyangiitis (GPA), microscopic polyangiitis (MPA), or renal limited vasculitis. Patients were divided into three groups, with one receiving the standard treatment (cyclophosphamide 15 mg/kg IV pulses every 2–3 weeks + high-dose prednisolone 60 mg/day + a placebo; $n = 9$), one receiving CCX168 and prednisolone (cyclophosphamide 15 mg/kg IV pulses every 2–3 weeks + low-dose prednisolone 20 mg/day + 30 mg CCX168 twice daily; $n = 8$), and another receiving CCX168 but not prednisolone (cyclophosphamide 15 mg/kg IV pulses every 2–3 weeks + no prednisolone + 30 mg CCX168 twice daily; $n = 8$). The efficacy of each treatment was compared after 12 weeks. Administration of CCX168 was as efficacious as or more efficacious at inhibiting nephritis as the standard treatment. Moreover, CCX168 was efficacious in treating forms of disease activity besides nephritis. Patients receiving CCX168 were able to tolerate the drug, and they suffered no serious unanticipated adverse events. In addition to the CLEAR trial, the Clinical ANCA Vasculitis Safety and Efficacy Study of Inhibitor of C5aR (CLASSIC) trial is underway. This randomized, double-blind, placebo-controlled phase II trial intends to determine if CCX168 will allow a lower dose or discontinuation of corticosteroids for patients with AAV. Phase II pilot studies of CCX168 to treat aHUS and immunoglobulin A (IgA) nephropathy are also underway.

Eculizumab is an anti-C5 antibody, but C5a receptor antagonists target C5a alone and do not inhibit MAC, so those antagonists may lessen risk of an infection with a pathogen such as *Neisseria meningitidis* seen with eculizumab. However, caution is needed since the C5a receptor is involved in maintaining homeostasis in the body. In specific terms, the C5a receptor is expressed not only by hematopoietic cells but also by various non-immune cells, such as vascular endothelial cells, liver cells, kidney cells, lung cells, spleen cells, and cells of the gastrointestinal tract [30]. Long-term studies are needed to determine if blocking the C5a receptor has unanticipated effects.

Conclusions

Research has revealed that several conditions respond to eculizumab and new attention has focused on eculizumab in relation to the treatment of conditions involving the complement system. This paper has described molecules functioning in the latter stages of complement activation, such as C5 and C5a receptors, but inhibitors of molecules functioning in the earlier stages of complement activation, such as complement factor D, complement factor B, properdin, MASP, and C3 convertase, are also being developed [11, 31]. These inhibitors may allow regulation of various steps in the complement system. Thus far, few attempts have been made to control disease by inhibiting complements, so those attempts hold promise as a new treatment strategy.

Authors' contributions

TH reviewed the literature and interpreted it and drafted the manuscript. HT reviewed the manuscript and made critical comments. Both authors read and approved the final manuscript.

Competing interests

The authors declare that they have no competing interests.

Author details

[1]Kyushu University Beppu Hospital, Beppu, Japan. [2]Kyushu University Graduate School of Medical Sciences, Fukuoka, Japan.

References

1. Ricklin D, Lambris JD. Complement in immune and inflammatory disorders: pathophysiological mechanisms. J Immunol. 2013;190:3831–8.
2. Tsukamoto H, Horiuchi T. Clinical aspects of the complement system. Rinsho Byori. 2006;54:757–62.
3. Hillmen P, Young NS, Schubert J, et al. The complement inhibitor eculizumab in paroxysmal nocturnal hemoglobinuria. N Engl J Med. 2006; 355:1233–43.
4. Gruppo RA, Rother RP. Eculizumab for congenital atypical hemolytic-uremic syndrome. N Engl J Med. 2009;360:544–6.
5. Matis LA, Rollins SA. Complement-specific antibodies: designing novel anti-inflammatories. Nat Med. 1995;1:839–42.
6. Jayne DR, Bruchfeld A, Schaier M, et al. Oral C5a receptor antagonist CCX168 phase II clinical trial in ANCA-associated renal vasculitis. Ann Rheum Dis. 2014;73 Suppl 2:148. abstract.
7. Bekker P, Jayne D, Bruchfeld A, et al. CCX168, an orally administered C5aR inhibitor for treatment of patients with antineutrophil cytoplasmic antibody-associated vasculitis. Arthritis Rheumatol. 2014;66:S820. abstract.
8. Horiuchi T, Mitoma H, Harashima S-I, et al. Transmembrane TNF-alpha: structure, function and interaction with anti-TNF agents. Rheumatology (Oxford). 2010;49:1215–28.
9. Mitoma H, Horiuchi T, Tsukamoto H, et al. Mechanisms for cytotoxic effects of anti-tumor necrosis factor agents on transmembrane tumor necrosis factor alpha-expressing cells. Arthritis Rheum. 2008;58:1248–57.
10. Horiuchi T, Ohi H, Ohsawa I, et al. Guideline for hereditary angioedema (HAE) 2010 by the Japanese Association for Complement Research—secondary publication. Allergol Int. 2012;61:559–62.
11. Reis ES, Mastellos DC, Yancopoulou D, et al. Applying complement therapeutics to rare diseases. Clin Immunol. 2015;161:225–40.
12. Brodsky RA. Complement in hemolytic anemia. Blood. 2015;126:2459–65.
13. Kaplan BS, Ruebner RL, Spinale JM, et al. Current treatment of atypical hemolytic uremic syndrome. Intractable Rare Dis Res. 2014;3:34–45.
14. Noris M, Mescia F, Remuzzi G. STEC-HUS, atypical HUS and TTP are all diseases of complement activation. Nat Rev Nephrol. 2012;8:622–33.
15. Woodruff TM, Nandakumar KS, Tedesco F. Inhibiting the C5-C5a receptor axis. Mol Immunol. 2011;48:1631–42.
16. Jose PJ, Moss IK, Maini RN, et al. Measurement of the chemotactic complement fragment C5a in rheumatoid synovial fluids by radioimmunoassay: role of C5a in the acute inflammatory phase. Ann Rheum Dis. 1990;49:747–52.
17. Plenge RM, Seielstad M, Padyukov L, et al. TRAF1-C5 as a risk locus for rheumatoid arthritis—a genomewide study. N Engl J Med. 2007;357:1199–209.
18. Nishimoto K, Kochi Y, Ikari K, et al. Association study of TRAF1-C5 polymorphism with susceptibility to rheumatoid arthritis and systemic lupus erythematosus in Japanese. Ann Rheum Dis. 2010;69:368–73.
19. Johansson AC, Sundler M, Kjellen P, et al. Genetic control of collagen-induced arthritis in a cross with NOD and C57BL/10 mice is dependent on gene regions encoding complement factor 5 and FcgammaRIIb and is not associated with loci controlling diabetes. Eur J Immunol. 2001;31:1847–56.
20. Lindqvist AK, Johannesson M, Johansson AC, et al. Backcross and partial advanced intercross analysis of nonobese diabetic gene-mediated effects on collagen-induced arthritis reveals an interactive effect by two major loci. J Immunol. 2006;177:3952–9.
21. Wang Y, Kristan J, Hao L, et al. A role for complement in antibody-mediated inflammation: C5-deficient DBA/1 mice are resistant to collagen-induced arthritis. J Immunol. 2000;164:4340–7.
22. Ji H, Gauquier D, Ohmura K, et al. Genetic influences on the end-stage effector phase of arthritis. J Exp Med. 2001;194:321–30.
23. Vergunst CE, Gerlag DM, Dinant H, et al. Blocking the receptor for C5a in patients with rheumatoid arthritis does not reduce synovial inflammation. Rheumatology (Oxford). 2007;46:1773–8.
24. Mojcik CF, Kremer J, Bingham C, et al. Results of a phase 2b study of the humanized anti-C5 antibody eculizumab in patients with rheumatoid arthritis. Ann Rheum Dis. 2004;63 Suppl 1:301. abstract.
25. Yuan J, Gou SJ, Huang J, et al. C5a and its receptors in human anti-neutrophil cytoplasmic antibody (ANCA)-associated vasculitis. Arthritis Res Ther. 2012;14:R140.
26. Gou S-J, Yuan J, Chen M, et al. Circulating complement activation in patients with anti-neutrophil cytoplasmic antibody-associated vasculitis. Kidney Int. 2012;83:129–37.
27. Xiao H, Schreiber A, Heeringa P, et al. Alternative complement pathway in the pathogenesis of disease mediated by anti-neutrophil cytoplasmic autoantibodies. Am J Pathol. 2007;170:52–64.
28. Huugen D, van Esch A, Xiao H, et al. Inhibition of complement factor C5 protects against anti-myeloperoxidase antibody-mediated glomerulonephritis in mice. Kidney Int. 2007;71:646–54.
29. Xiao H, Dairaghi DJ, Powers JP, et al. C5a receptor (CD88) blockade protects against MPO-ANCA GN. J Am Soc Nephrol. 2014;25:225–31.
30. Klos A, Tenner AJ, Johswich K-O, et al. The role of the anaphylatoxins in health and disease. Mol Immunol. 2009;46:2753–66.
31. Ricklin D, Lambris JD. Complement in immune and inflammatory disorders: therapeutic interventions. J Immunol. 2013;190:3839–47.

Liver regeneration and fibrosis after inflammation

Minoru Tanaka[1*] and Atsushi Miyajima[2*]

Abstract

The liver is a unique organ with an extraordinary capacity to regenerate upon various injuries. In acute and transient liver injury by insults such as chemical hepatotoxins, the liver in rodents returns to the original architecture by proliferation and remodeling of the remaining cells within a week. In contrast, chronic liver inflammation due to various etiologies, e.g., virus infection and metabolic and immune disorders, results in liver fibrosis, often leading to cirrhosis and carcinogenesis. In both acute and chronic inflammation, a variety of immune and non-immune cells in the liver is involved in the processes resulting in either regeneration or fibrosis. In addition, chronic hepatitis often accompanies proliferation of atypical biliary cells, also known as liver progenitor cells or oval cells. Although the origin of liver progenitor cells and its contribution to hepatic repair is still under intense debate, recent studies have revealed a regulatory role for immune cells in progenitor proliferation and differentiation. In this review, we summarize recent studies on liver regeneration and fibrosis in the viewpoint of inflammation.

Keywords: Fibrosis, Hepatic stellate cell, Liver sinusoidal endothelial cell, Liver progenitor cell

Background

The liver is a central organ for homeostasis and carries out a wide variety of functions, including metabolism, glycogen storage, drug detoxification, production of various serum proteins, and bile secretion. Most of those liver functions are carried out by hepatocytes, the liver parenchymal cells, which account for approximately 60 % of total liver cells and 80 % of the total liver volume. Hepatocytes are highly polarized epithelial cells and form cords (Fig. 1). Their basolateral surfaces face the sinusoid, a unique form of capillary in the liver, which consists of fenestrated liver sinusoidal endothelial cells (LSECs) and hepatic stellate cells (HSCs). Tight junctions formed between hepatocytes create a canaliculus surrounded by the apical membrane of neighboring hepatocytes. Bile secreted from hepatocytes is exported sequentially through the bile canaliculi, intrahepatic bile ducts, extrahepatic bile ducts, and finally into the duodenum. The bile duct is formed by another type of epithelial cell, biliary epithelial cell (BEC), also known as

cholangiocyte. Hepatocyte and BEC are derived from a common progenitor, "hepatoblast," during development [1]. In the similar context of liver progenitors, the adult liver also harbors a specialized type of cells which proliferates clonally in vitro and gives rise to hepatocyte and BEC depending on culture conditions [2, 3]. It has been believed that such a tissue stem cell-like progenitor contributes to hepatic repair in a case of emergency, e.g., severe or chronic liver injury. However, whether and where stem cells exist in the adult liver is still under debate.

Historically, the regenerative capacity of the liver is well known, and the mechanisms underlying liver regeneration have been investigated for many years. In 1931, Higgins and Anderson developed an experimental model of liver regeneration, i.e., surgical removal of rat median and left lobes that correspond to two thirds of the total liver mass [4]. Since then, the two-thirds partial hepatectomy (PHx) has been used as a standard model for liver regeneration. In this model, the remnant liver lobes enlarge to compensate for the lost mass, which is known as compensatory hyperplasia. After decades of studies on the liver regeneration from two-thirds PHx, it was believed that one or two replications of the remaining hepatocytes should be empirically sufficient to recover

* Correspondence: m-tanaka@ri.ncgm.go.jp; miyajima@iam.u-tokyo.ac.jp
[1]Department of Regenerative Medicine, Research Institute, National Center for Global Health and Medicine, Tokyo, Japan
[2]Institute of Molecular and Cellular Biosciences, The University of Tokyo, Tokyo, Japan

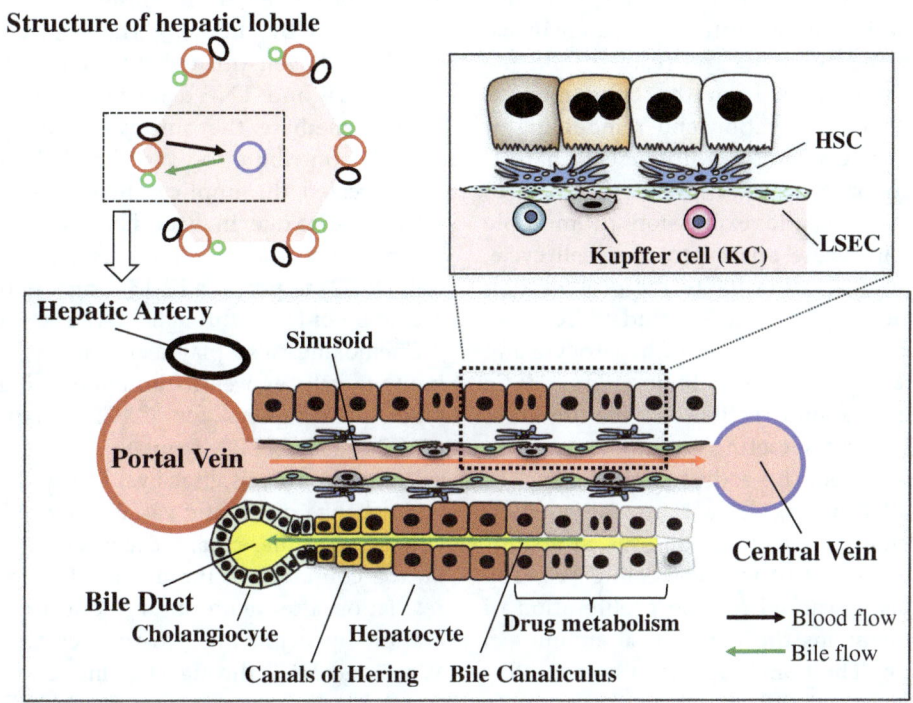

Fig. 1 Schematic overview of the hepatic lobule. Blood flows into the liver from the portal vein and the hepatic artery toward the central vein through the sinusoid surrounded by fenestrated liver sinusoidal endothelial cells (LSECs). Bile produced by hepatocytes is collected into the bile ducts via the bile canaliculi surrounded by the apical membrane of hepatocytes. Kupffer cells (KC), resident macrophages in the liver, are located at the luminal side of the sinusoids, while hepatic stellate cells (HSCs) are positioned in close proximity to LSECs. The canals of Hering is the joint between hepatocytes and the bile ducts

the original mass and function. However, revisiting this old theme by using modern techniques revealed that "hypertrophy" of hepatocytes precedes proliferation and that hypertrophy and proliferation contribute almost equally to the recovery of liver mass [5]. While PHx is an excellent model to study the process of compensatory growth of the liver and provides useful information relevant to liver transplantation, it does not faithfully recapitulate repair processes in human pathological conditions of liver diseases caused by virus infection, metabolic and immune disorders, drug intoxication, and so on. Here, we describe the cellular basis of liver regeneration and fibrosis after inflammation in acute and chronic liver injuries.

Main text
Metabolic zonation, drug-induced acute liver injury, and regeneration
The functional liver unit consists of the hepatic lobule, which has a central vein and hexagonal or polygonal portal triads consisting of the portal vein, hepatic artery, and bile duct. The central vein is connected to portal triads via sinusoids that run through the hepatic plates. Although all hepatocytes are morphologically

similar, their functions are quite diverse and determined by their location along the porto-central axis of the functional liver unit, the hepatic lobule. Periportal hepatocytes are specialized for oxidative liver functions such as gluconeogenesis, ß-oxidation of fatty acids, and cholesterol synthesis, while pericentral hepatocytes are more important for glycolysis, lipogenesis, and cytochrome P450-based drug detoxification. Metabolic zonation is formed by a Wnt/ß-catenin signaling gradient [6, 7]. A recent study revealed that LGR4/5 receptors and their cognate RSPO ligands potentiate Wnt/ß-catenin signaling and control liver zonation [8].

Centrilobular hepatocytes express cytochrome P450s (Cyps) abundantly, which metabolize alcohol and various chemical hepatotoxins such as acetaminophen, carbon tetrachloride (CCl_4), and thioacetamide, to generate highly reactive free radicals that damage hepatocytes. A single administration of drugs such as CCl_4 induces necrosis of hepatocytes and disorganization of sinusoids surrounding the central vein. Proliferation of hepatocytes starts within 24 h, peaks at around 48 h, and terminates by 72 h in mice [9]. Along with proliferation of hepatocytes, sinusoid remodeling occurs in the necrotic area. Prior to these responses, hepatocytes damaged by free radicals produce damage-associated molecular patterns (DAMPs) to induce inflammation, by which the activated non-parenchymal cells contribute to regeneration. The resident and the recruited inflammatory cells from the bone marrow play a crucial role in regeneration and remodeling at the damaged area. The activated Kupffer cell, a resident hepatic macrophage, secretes interleukin-6 (IL-6) that directly induces hepatic expression of multiple genes associated with acute phase proteins, cell-cycle, redox, and anti-apoptosis to facilitate the proliferation of remnant hepatocytes [9–11]. HSCs and LSECs also play crucial roles in the proliferation of hepatocyte and sinusoidal remodeling after liver injury. The HSCs stimulated by inflammation contribute to the initiation of liver regeneration by secreting hepatocyte growth factor (HGF). In addition, the activated HSCs start to produce extracellular matrix (ECM) including collagens to fix the architecture of injured tissue in a similar manner to the process of wound healing [12, 13]. The ECM serves as a scaffold for the proliferation of hepatocytes and maintains the mechanical stability in the damaged region. The LSECs activated by acute inflammation also secrete HGF and Wnt2 to promote liver regeneration [14]. We have reported that Sema3e produced by damaged hepatocytes induces contraction of LSECs, which supports the activation of HSCs and the infiltration of leukocytes into the damaged area [15]. Given that insult of the liver is transient, these cells activated by inflammation will be eventually settled, followed by the resolution of ECM and revascularization. Thus, activation of non-parenchymal cells in the injured area and proliferation of undamaged hepatocytes must be well orchestrated to restore the original mass, functions, and structure of the liver in acute inflammation.

Chronic liver injury and fibrosis

Chronic inflammation is an immune response that persists for months, in which inflammation and tissue remodeling and repair processes occur simultaneously. It can be induced by a number of different insults including hepatitis virus infection, excessive alcohol intake, autoimmune reactions, toxins, and metabolic disorders. However, regardless of etiology, chronic inflammation induces fibrosis that eventually leads to cirrhosis and hepatocellular carcinoma. In chronic hepatitis, activated HSCs become myofibroblasts and play a dominant role in fibrosis by producing a large amount of collagen. In addition, upregulation of a tissue inhibitor of metalloproteinases-1 (TIMP-1) in the fibrotic liver contribute to collagen deposition by inhibiting the resolution of ECM. Persistent production of growth factors for HSCs, fibrogenic cytokines, and chemokines by various types of liver cells are involved in fibrogenesis in chronic inflammation. Among those,

TGF-ß produced by immune cells directly promotes fibrogenesis by inducing the transcription of type I and III collagen through the Smad signaling pathway [16]. IL-1ß and TNF-α do not induce HSC activation instead mediate the survival of activated HSCs and thereby contribute to liver fibrosis [17]. A recent study has revealed the implication of IL-33, an IL-1 family member cytokine in liver fibrosis. IL-33 secreted from damaged hepatocytes stimulates type 2 innate lymphoid cells (ILC2) to produce IL-13, which in turn promotes the activation of HSCs through STAT6 activation [18].

Chemokines also play a role in liver fibrosis via non-immune cells as well as immune cells in the liver. Two types of receptors for CXCL12 (also called SDF1), CXCR4 and CXCR7, regulate a balance between regeneration and fibrosis after liver injury through the phenotypic change of hepatic vascular niche [14]. CXCR4 and CXCR7 are differentially expressed in LSECs depending on the condition of the damaged liver, and CXCR7 upregulation after acute injury contributes to liver regeneration by deploying pro-regenerative factors such as Wnt2 and HGF through the induction of transcription factor Id1. In contrast, constitutive FGFR1 signaling in LSEC under chronic hepatitis induces the predominance of CXCR4 over CXCR7 by augmenting CXCR4 expression, leading to a shift from pro-regenerative vascular niche to pro-fibrotic phenotype accompanied by the proliferation of activated HSCs. On the other hand, CCL2, also called MCP-1 secreted from Kupffer cell and HSC, contributes to the recruitment of CCR2+ Ly6C+ monocytes into the liver. The recruited Ly6C^{hi} macrophages are pro-inflammatory and pro-fibrotic and produce IL-1ß, TNF-α, TGF-ß, and PDGF to induce the survival, activation, and proliferation of myofibroblasts [19–22]. As such, hepatic macrophages contribute to liver fibrogenesis, while they play a crucial role in the resolution of ECM [23]. Ly6C^{lo} restorative macrophages have been reported to exhibit pro-resolution phenotypes with increased expression of fibrinolytic matrix metalloproteinases (MMPs) including MMP9 and MMP12, phagocytosis-related genes, and growth factors [20]. Thus, after acute inflammation, the phenotypic switch of pro-inflammatory macrophages to restorative macrophages together with the disappearance of pro-fibrotic macrophages plays important roles in liver regeneration and ECM resorption. Thus, interactions among immune and non-immune cells in response to persistent inflammatory factors can be a fork toward hepatic regeneration or fibrosis in chronic hepatitis (Fig. 2).

Liver stem/progenitor cells and ductular reaction

Hepatocytes have a long lifespan, and new hepatocytes are derived from pre-existing hepatocytes. Thus, unlike

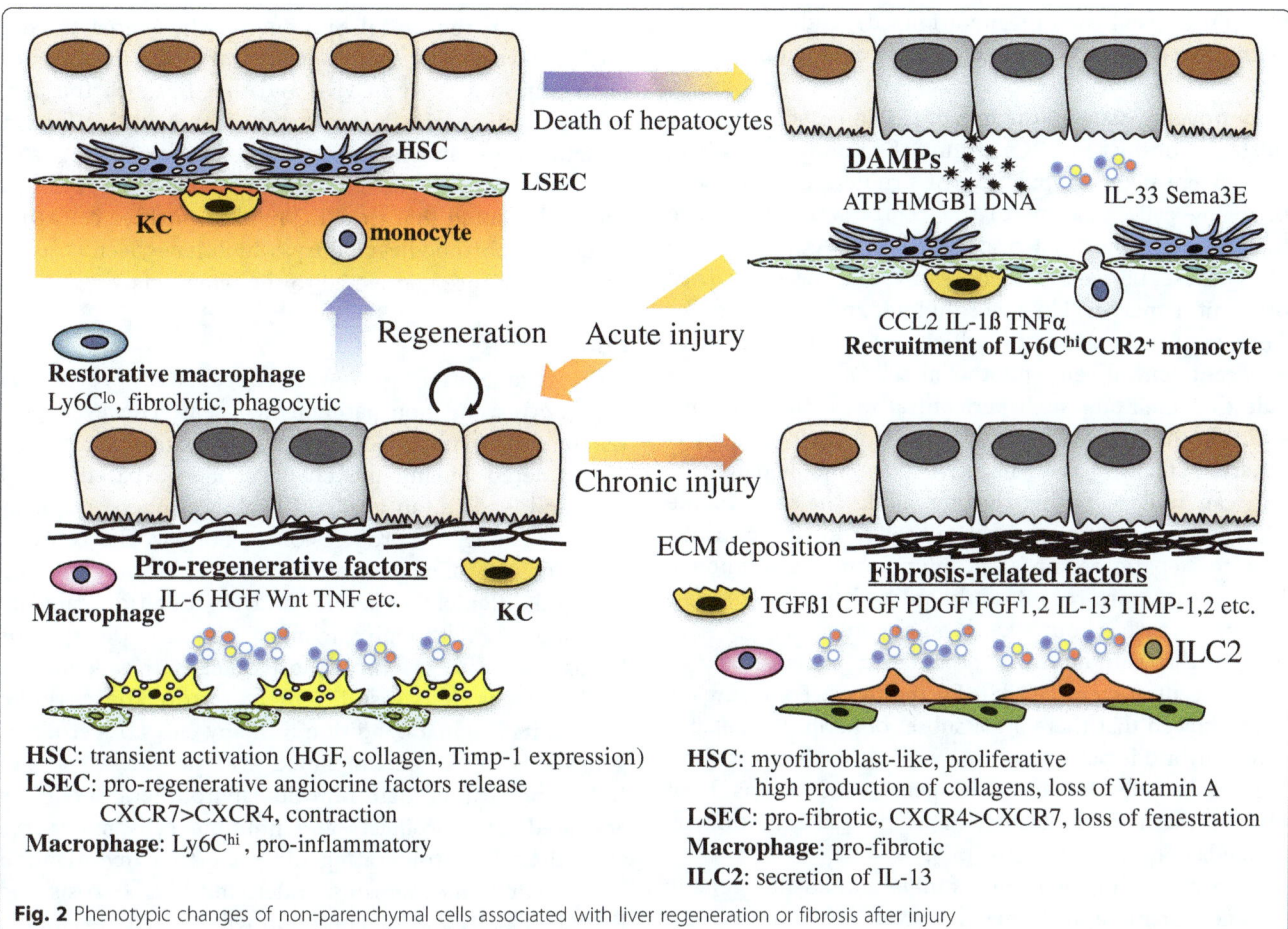

Fig. 2 Phenotypic changes of non-parenchymal cells associated with liver regeneration or fibrosis after injury

intestinal stem cells, the liver homeostasis does not seem to require a resident stem cell population. Also, in acute liver injury, because remnant hepatocytes proliferate to restore the lost cells, stem cells are not necessarily needed. However, in chronic liver injury, it has been believed that liver progenitor cells (LPCs) or oval cells contribute to liver regeneration. Fundamentally, LPCs are defined as bi-potential cells similar to fetal hepatoblast, which can differentiate to both hepatocytes and BECs [1]. Chronic liver injuries often accompany "ductular reaction," which is histologically characterized as ectopic emergence and expansion of bile duct marker-positive cells around the portal vein. It has long been postulated that ductular reaction represents the activation of adult LPCs that may reside in the biliary tree or the canals of Hering, the junctional structure connecting hepatocytes and the bile ducts. The concept of LPCs has been a paradigm in liver regeneration upon chronic injury, and most studies have focused on whether and how LPCs can proliferate and differentiate to hepatocytes to replenish the lost functions of the liver. Considering that LPCs expand in the case of chronic hepatitis, LPCs are supposed to be activated in response to inflammation. In

fact, implications of several inflammatory cytokines, such as tumor necrosis factor (TNF)-alpha, interleukin-6, and interferon-gamma, in LPC proliferation have been reported [24–26]. Among those factors, TNF-related WEAK inducer of apoptosis (TWEAK) and fibroblast growth factor 7 (FGF7) are of particular interest, as they are capable of inducing de novo activation of LPCs without inflammatory insults, suggesting that the cell-of-origin for LPCs is responsive to these extracellular signals [27, 28]. Other growth factors, such as HGF and EGF, have also been implicated in regulating proliferation and/or differentiation of LPCs [29, 30]. Notch signaling is well known to play a pivotal role in the differentiation of fetal hepatoblasts into BECs [31–34]. In line with this notion, Boulter et al. reported that Jagged 1, a Notch ligand expressed by activated myofibroblasts, promoted the specification of LPCs to BECs during biliary regeneration [35]. Notably, macrophages engulfing hepatocyte debris expressed Wnt3a, which enhances canonical Wnt signaling and opposes Notch signaling in LPCs to promote their specification to hepatocytes during liver regeneration. Thus, LPCs are apparently a "facultative" stem/progenitor cell population that emerges around the portal vein for regeneration, depending on the microenvironment generated by chronic inflammation.

A controversy issue on the role of LPC in regeneration

In sharp contrast to LPCs around the portal vein, Wang et al. identified a population of proliferating and self-renewing cells adjacent to the central vein by lineage tracing using the Wnt-responsive gene Axin2 in mice [36]. These pericentral cells expressed the early liver progenitor marker Tbx3, are diploid, and thereby differ from mature hepatocytes, which are mostly polyploid. Adjacent central vein endothelial cells provide Wnt signals that maintain such pericentral cells, thereby constituting the niche. The descendants of pericentral cells differentiate into Tbx3-negative polyploid hepatocytes and can replace all hepatocytes along the liver lobule during homeostatic renewal, although their contribution to hepatic repair after injury remains unknown. However, a more recent study showed that LGR4[+] hepatocytes throughout the lobule contribute to liver homeostasis without zonal dominance, contradictory to the pericentral stem cell [8]. Furthermore, Font-Burgada et al. showed that there are a subset of periportal hepatocytes, "hybrid hepatocytes," that express low levels of Sox9 and some bile duct-enriched genes, and it has been claimed that hybrid hepatocytes are the cells that primarily mediate liver injury repair [37].

In contrast, many recent studies employing genetic lineage-tracing approaches in vivo have shown that LPCs and/or pre-existing BECs do not or rarely contribute to new hepatocytes in mouse models, thereby raising a doubt on the concept that LPCs serve as the backup for hepatocyte regeneration [38–40]. These apparently contradictory results regarding the origin of new hepatocytes in chronic liver injury may be due to the differences in injury models employed. If healthy hepatocytes remain in the injured liver, they proliferate to restore normal functions, but biliary-derived LPCs may give rise to new hepatocytes when most hepatocytes are severely damaged. For instance, hepatocyte-specific genetic deletion of E3 ubiquitin ligase Mdm2 induced hepatocytes to apoptosis, necrosis, and senescence in those cells. Under such severe condition, LPCs are activated to reconstitute functional liver [41].

Lineage-tracing experiments have significantly advanced our understating on LPC and ductular reaction, while the cell-of-origin for LPC is still under intense debate. Using newly established imaging approaches to capture three-dimensional (3D) tissue morphology in situ, we have recently reported that ductular reaction essentially represents the dynamic and adaptive changes of ductal cells maintaining duct-like structure and con-

nection with the portal bile ducts [42]. Clonal tracing further revealed the heterogeneity of BECs in terms of proliferation activity in vivo and that BECs in the periphery proliferate in a stochastic manner [43]. While it remains to be shown whether there is a specific class of BEC that functions as LPC by producing hepatocytes, it should be noted that the BEC marker-positive cells that emerge in chronic liver injury, which have been considered as LPC, are connected to the bile ducts.

Conclusions

Liver regeneration is a well coordinated process by hepatocytes and non-parenchymal cells. However, persistent inflammation in chronic hepatitis alters the well-ordered phenotypic changes of non-parenchymal cells and leads to an aberrant healing process, i.e., liver fibrosis. Along the progression of fibrosis, the replacement of the damaged tissue with ECM impairs the functions, flexible structure, and regeneration capacity of the liver. Although the most effective therapy for fibrosis to date is elimination of causative agents in earlier stages, it is insufficient to restore the cirrhotic liver to its original condition in many cases. Liver fibrogenesis is often accompanied by the emergence of LPCs, suggesting that fibrotic environment including activated myofibroblasts and immune cells may serve as a niche for proliferating LPCs. Further investigation of regulatory mechanisms underlying liver fibrosis and the role of LPCs in regeneration will help in developing therapeutic strategies to counter liver disease.

Abbreviations

BEC, biliary epithelial cell; DAMPs, damage-associated molecular patterns; ECM, extracellular matrix; HSC, hepatic stellate cell; LPC, liver progenitor cell; LSEC, liver sinusoidal endothelial cell; MMP, matrix metalloproteinase; TIMP-1, tissue inhibitor of metalloproteinases-1; TWEAK, TNF-related weak inducer of apoptosis

Acknowledgements

We thank Cindy Kok for her editorial assistance. This work is supported in part by Grants-in-Aid for Scientific Research by Japanese Society for the Promotion of Science and Japan Agency of Medical Research and Development.

Funding

We have received no specific grants.

Authors' contributions

The authors equally contributed to the preparation of this review. All authors read and approved the final manuscript.

Competing interests

The authors declare that they have no competing interests.

References

1. Miyajima A, Tanaka M, Itoh T. Stem/progenitor cells in liver development, homeostasis, regeneration, and reprogramming. Cell Stem Cell. 2014;14:561–74.
2. Suzuki A, Sekiya S, Onishi M, Oshima N, Kiyonari H, Nakauchi H, Taniguchi H. Flow cytometric isolation and clonal identification of self-renewing bipotent hepatic progenitor cells in adult mouse liver. Hepatology. 2008;48:1964–78.
3. Okabe M, Tsukahara Y, Tanaka M, Suzuki K, Saito S, Kamiya Y, Tsujimura T, et al. Potential hepatic stem cells reside in EpCAM+ cells of normal and injured mouse liver. Development. 2009;136:1951–60.
4. Higgins GM, Anderson RM. Experimental pathology of the liver, 1: restoration of the liver of the white rat following partial surgical removal. Arch Pathol. 1931;12:186–202.
5. Miyaoka Y, Ebato K, Kato H, Arakawa S, Shimizu S, Miyajima A. Hypertrophy and unconventional cell division of hepatocytes underlie liver regeneration. Curr Biol. 2012;22:1166–75.
6. Sekine S, Lan BY, Bedolli M, Feng S, Hebrok M. Liver-specific loss of beta-catenin blocks glutamine synthesis pathway activity and cytochrome p450 expression in mice. Hepatology. 2006;43:817–25.
7. Yang J, Mowry LE, Nejak-Bowen KN, Okabe H, Diegel CR, Lang RA, Williams BO, et al. Beta-catenin signaling in murine liver zonation and regeneration: a Wnt-Wnt situation! Hepatology. 2014;60:964–76.
8. Planas-Paz L, Orsini V, Boulter L, Calabrese D, Pikiolek M, Nigsch F, Xie Y, et al. The RSPO-LGR4/5-ZNRF3/RNF43 module controls liver zonation and size. Nat Cell Biol. 2016;18:467–79.
9. Michalopoulos GK, DeFrances MC. Liver regeneration. Science. 1997;276:60–6.
10. Haga S, Terui K, Zhang HQ, Enosawa S, Ogawa W, Inoue H, Okuyama T, et al. Stat3 protects against Fas-induced liver injury by redox-dependent and -independent mechanisms. J Clin Invest. 2003;112:989–98.
11. Taub R. Liver regeneration: from myth to mechanism. Nat Rev Mol Cell Biol. 2004;5:836–47.
12. Raghow R. The role of extracellular matrix in postinflammatory wound healing and fibrosis. Faseb J. 1994;8:823–31.
13. Pellicoro A, Ramachandran P, Iredale JP, Fallowfield JA. Liver fibrosis and repair: immune regulation of wound healing in a solid organ. Nat Rev Immunol. 2014;14:181–94.
14. Ding BS, Cao Z, Lis R, Nolan DJ, Guo P, Simons M, Penfold ME, et al. Divergent angiocrine signals from vascular niche balance liver regeneration and fibrosis. Nature. 2014;505:97–102.
15. Yagai T, Miyajima A, Tanaka M. Semaphorin 3E secreted by damaged hepatocytes regulates the sinusoidal regeneration and liver fibrosis during liver regeneration. Am J Pathol. 2014;184:2250–9.
16. Dooley S, ten Dijke P. TGF-beta in progression of liver disease. Cell Tissue Res. 2012;347:245–56.
17. Pradere JP, Kluwe J, De Minicis S, Jiao JJ, Gwak GY, Dapito DH, Jang MK, et al. Hepatic macrophages but not dendritic cells contribute to liver fibrosis by promoting the survival of activated hepatic stellate cells in mice. Hepatology. 2013;58:1461–73.
18. McHedlidze T, Waldner M, Zopf S, Walker J, Rankin AL, Schuchmann M, Voehringer D, et al. Interleukin-33-dependent innate lymphoid cells mediate hepatic fibrosis. Immunity. 2013;39:357–71.
19. Wynn TA, Barron L. Macrophages: master regulators of inflammation and fibrosis. Semin Liver Dis. 2010;30:245–57.
20. Ramachandran P, Pellicoro A, Vernon MA, Boulter L, Aucott RL, Ali A, Hartland SN, et al. Differential Ly-6C expression identifies the recruited macrophage phenotype, which orchestrates the regression of murine liver fibrosis. Proc Natl Acad Sci U S A. 2012;109:E3186–3195.
21. Karlmark KR, Weiskirchen R, Zimmermann HW, Gassler N, Ginhoux F, Weber C, Merad M, et al. Hepatic recruitment of the inflammatory Gr1+ monocyte subset upon liver injury promotes hepatic fibrosis. Hepatology. 2009;50:261–74.
22. Tacke F, Zimmermann HW. Macrophage heterogeneity in liver injury and fibrosis. J Hepatol. 2014;60:1090–6.
23. Duffield JS, Forbes SJ, Constandinou CM, Clay S, Partolina M, Vuthoori S, Wu S, et al. Selective depletion of macrophages reveals distinct, opposing roles during liver injury and repair. J Clin Invest. 2005;115:56–65.
24. Knight B, Yeoh GC, Husk KL, Ly T, Abraham LJ, Yu C, Rhim JA, et al. Impaired preneoplastic changes and liver tumor formation in tumor necrosis factor receptor type 1 knockout mice. J Exp Med. 2000;192:1809–18.
25. Akhurst B, Matthews V, Husk K, Smyth MJ, Abraham LJ, Yeoh GC. Differential lymphotoxin-beta and interferon gamma signaling during mouse liver regeneration induced by chronic and acute injury. Hepatology. 2005;41:327–35.
26. Yeoh GC, Ernst M, Rose-John S, Akhurst B, Payne C, Long S, Alexander W, et al. Opposing roles of gp130-mediated STAT-3 and ERK-1/ 2 signaling in liver progenitor cell migration and proliferation. Hepatology. 2007;45:486–94.
27. Jakubowski A, Ambrose C, Parr M, Lincecum JM, Wang MZ, Zheng TS, Browning B, et al. TWEAK induces liver progenitor cell proliferation. J Clin Invest. 2005;115:2330–40.
28. Takase HM, Itoh T, Ino S, Wang T, Koji T, Akira S, Takikawa Y, et al. FGF7 is a functional niche signal required for stimulation of adult liver progenitor cells that support liver regeneration. Genes Dev. 2013;27:169–81.
29. Ishikawa T, Factor VM, Marquardt JU, Raggi C, Seo D, Kitade M, Conner EA, et al. Hepatocyte growth factor/c-met signaling is required for stem-cell-mediated liver regeneration in mice. Hepatology. 2012;55:1215–26.
30. Kitade M, Factor VM, Andersen JB, Tomokuni A, Kaji K, Akita H, Holczbauer A, et al. Specific fate decisions in adult hepatic progenitor cells driven by MET and EGFR signaling. Genes Dev. 2013;27:1706–17.
31. Li L, Krantz ID, Deng Y, Genin A, Banta AB, Collins CC, Qi M, et al. Alagille syndrome is caused by mutations in human Jagged1, which encodes a ligand for Notch1. Nat Genet. 1997;16:243–51.
32. McCright B, Lozier J, Gridley T. A mouse model of Alagille syndrome: Notch2 as a genetic modifier of Jag1 haploinsufficiency. Development. 2002;129:1075–82.
33. Kodama Y, Hijikata M, Kageyama R, Shimotohno K, Chiba T. The role of notch signaling in the development of intrahepatic bile ducts. Gastroenterology. 2004;127:1775–86.
34. Tanimizu N, Miyajima A. Notch signaling controls hepatoblast differentiation by altering the expression of liver-enriched transcription factors. J Cell Sci. 2004;117:3165–74.
35. Boulter L, Govaere O, Bird TG, Radulescu S, Ramachandran P, Pellicoro A, Ridgway RA, et al. Macrophage-derived Wnt opposes Notch signaling to specify hepatic progenitor cell fate in chronic liver disease. Nat Med. 2012;18:572–9.
36. Wang B, Zhao L, Fish M, Logan CY, Nusse R. Self-renewing diploid Axin2(+) cells fuel homeostatic renewal of the liver. Nature. 2015;524:180–5.
37. Font-Burgada J, Shalapour S, Ramaswamy S, Hsueh B, Rossell D, Umemura A, Taniguchi K, et al. Hybrid periportal hepatocytes regenerate the injured liver without giving rise to cancer. Cell. 2015;162:766–79.
38. Tarlow BD, Finegold MJ, Grompe M. Clonal tracing of Sox9+ liver progenitors in mouse oval cell injury. Hepatology. 2014;60:278–89.
39. Sekiya S, Suzuki A. Hepatocytes, rather than cholangiocytes, can be the major source of primitive ductules in the chronically injured mouse liver. Am J Pathol. 2014;184:1468–78.
40. Yanger K, Knigin D, Zong Y, Maggs L, Gu G, Akiyama H, Pikarsky E, et al. Adult hepatocytes are generated by self-duplication rather than stem cell differentiation. Cell Stem Cell. 2014;15:340–9.
41. Lu WY, Bird TG, Boulter L, Tsuchiya A, Cole AM, Hay T, Guest RV, et al. Hepatic progenitor cells of biliary origin with liver repopulation capacity. Nat Cell Biol. 2015;17:971–83.
42. Kaneko K, Kamimoto K, Miyajima A, Itoh T. Adaptive remodeling of the biliary architecture underlies liver homeostasis. Hepatology. 2015;61:2056–66.
43. Kamimoto K, Kaneko K, Kok CY, Okada H, Miyajima A, Itoh T. Heterogeneity and stochastic growth regulation of biliary epithelial cells dictate dynamic epithelial tissue remodeling. Elife. 2016;5:e15034.

5

Dissecting cellular senescence and SASP in *Drosophila*

Takao Ito and Tatsushi Igaki[*]

Abstract

Cellular senescence can act as both tumor suppressor and tumor promoter depending on the cellular contexts. On one hand, premature senescence has been considered as an innate host defense mechanism against carcinogenesis in mammals. In response to various stresses including oxidative stress, DNA damage, and oncogenic stress, suffered cells undergo irreversible cell cycle arrest, leading to tumor suppression. On the other hand, recent studies in mammalian systems have revealed that senescent cells can drive oncogenesis by secreting diverse proteins such as inflammatory cytokines, matrix remodeling factors, and growth factors, the phenomenon called senescence-associated secretory phenotype (SASP). However, the mechanisms by which these contradictory effects regulate tumor growth and metastasis in vivo have been elusive. Here, we review the recent discovery of cellular senescence in *Drosophila* and the mechanisms underlying senescence-mediated tumor regulation dissected by *Drosophila* genetics.

Background

Cellular senescence has been considered to be a major defense mechanism against carcinogenesis through the induction of stable cell cycle arrest [1–6]. Aberrant oncogene activation such as Ras activation causes various stresses including oxidative stress and DNA damage, thereby leading to the induction of premature senescence independently of telomere emersion [2, 3, 5–18]. This oncogene-induced senescence (OIS) can block malignant progression of precancerous lesions [5–7, 16]. However, recent studies have indicated that senescent cells can also contribute to tumor progression via the release of secretory components such as inflammatory cytokines, matrix remodeling factors, and growth factors, which is called the senescence-associated secretory phenotype (SASP) [19–22]. Thus, cellular senescence has not only negative effects but also positive effects on tumor development. Therefore, elucidation of how senescent cells drive both tumor suppression and tumor progression through cell–cell communications in vivo is essential if taking into account cellular senescence as a therapeutic target for cancer.

The genetic mosaic technique available in *Drosophila* is a powerful tool to study cell–cell communications in vivo [23, 24]. This technique allows us to analyze in vivo interactions between senescent cells and surrounding cells during tumor progression. In this review, we describe the recent identification of cellular senescence in *Drosophila*, as well as the recent advances in our understanding of the mechanisms by which senescent cells drive tumor progression via SASP in *Drosophila*.

Cellular senescence and SASP in *Drosophila*

Since the first discovery by Hayflick and Moorhead in 1961 [25], cellular senescence has been widely studied in mammalian cells. Cellular senescence is known as a stepwise process from early senescence to full senescence [26–30]. In an early senescence state, senescent cells exhibit senescence-associated β-galactosidase (SA-β-gal) activity [31, 32], elevated expression of cyclin-dependent kinase (CDK) inhibitors such as p16 [12, 33, 34] and p21 [12, 35–37], reversible cell cycle arrest, senescence-associated heterochromatic foci (SAHF) [38–41], and cellular hypertrophy [31]. When matured to a full senescence state, senescent cells exhibit additional phenotypes including irreversible cell cycle arrest and SASP. Despite the extensive studies of cellular senescence in vertebrate models, there has been no evidence that cellular senescence also occurs in invertebrates.

* Correspondence: igaki@lif.kyoto-u.ac.jp
Laboratory of Genetics, Graduate School of Biostudies, Kyoto University, Yoshida-Konoecho-cho, Sakyo-ku, Kyoto 606-8501, Japan

Using *Drosophila* genetics, it has recently been shown that the state of full senescence can be induced by simultaneous activation of the Ras oncogene and mitochondrial dysfunction in *Drosophila* imaginal epithelium [42, 43]. Clones of cells with Ras activation and dysfunction of the mitochondrial electron transport chain (Ras^{V12}/*mito$^{-/-}$* clones), both of which are frequently observed in various types of human cancers [44–48], show elevated SA-β-gal activity, cell cycle arrest accompanied with upregulation of the Cdk inhibitor Dacapo (a *Drosophila* p21/p27 homologue), SAHF, and cellular hypertrophy [42]. In addition, Ras^{V12}/*mito$^{-/-}$* cells present SASP, as these cells excessively secrete the inflammatory cytokine Unpaired (Upd; a *Drosophila* interleukin 6 (IL-6) homologue [49]) and matrix metalloprotease 1 (Mmp1; the *Drosophila* secreted Mmp [50]), thereby causing non-autonomous overgrowth of neighboring cells (Fig. 1) [42, 43]. IL-6 and Mmp are known as SASP factors in mammals [21]. Intriguingly, clones of cells with Ras activation alone (Ras^{V12} clones) show elevated SA-β-gal activity, Dacapo upregulation, SAHF, and cellular hypertrophy but not cell cycle arrest and SASP [42]. Thus, Ras activation alone is insufficient for the induction of full senescence in *Drosophila* imaginal epithelium. Accordingly, mitochondrial dysfunction seems to be crucial for the acceleration of Ras-mediated OIS. These findings indicate that cellular senescence and SASP are evolutionarily conserved in invertebrates and that studies in *Drosophila* could provide novel mechanistic insights into these phenomena.

Regulation of cell cycle arrest in *Drosophila* senescent cells

DNA damage is known to be the major cause of cellular senescence [1, 51]. Studies in mammalian systems have indicated that Ras activation elicits DNA damage mainly through DNA hyper-replication [3, 10] and production of reactive oxygen species (ROS) [13, 51–55]. It has also been well established that the ROS-induced DNA damage triggers cellular senescence. Intriguingly, in *Drosophila* imaginal epithelium, Ras activation and dysfunction of the mitochondrial respiratory chain synergize in inducing ROS production and DNA damage [42, 43]. Ras^{V12}/*mito$^{-/-}$* cells show much larger amount of ROS production and DNA damage than Ras^{V12} cells or *mito$^{-/-}$* cells. A recent study in human cell cultures has indicated that Ras^{V12} cells show elevated mitochondrial respiration via enhanced conversion of pyruvate to acetyl-CoA that is the origin of mitochondrial tricarboxylic acid (TCA) cycle [56]. Therefore, when the mitochondrial electron transport is downregulated in Ras^{V12} cells, large amounts of metabolic intermediates in mitochondrial respiration may be accumulated in mitochondria, which could affect ROS production.

It has been shown in mammals that DNA damage triggers cell cycle arrest and thereby induces cellular senescence [1, 51]. Upon DNA damage, p53 and p16 are upregulated [57–61] and thereby activating the p53/p21/Rb pathway [35, 36, 62, 63] and the p16/Rb pathway [62, 64]. DNA damage stabilizes p53 protein by repressing the ubiquitin ligase Mdm2 [57–59]. p53 directly activates transcription of p21 [35]. Both p21 and p16

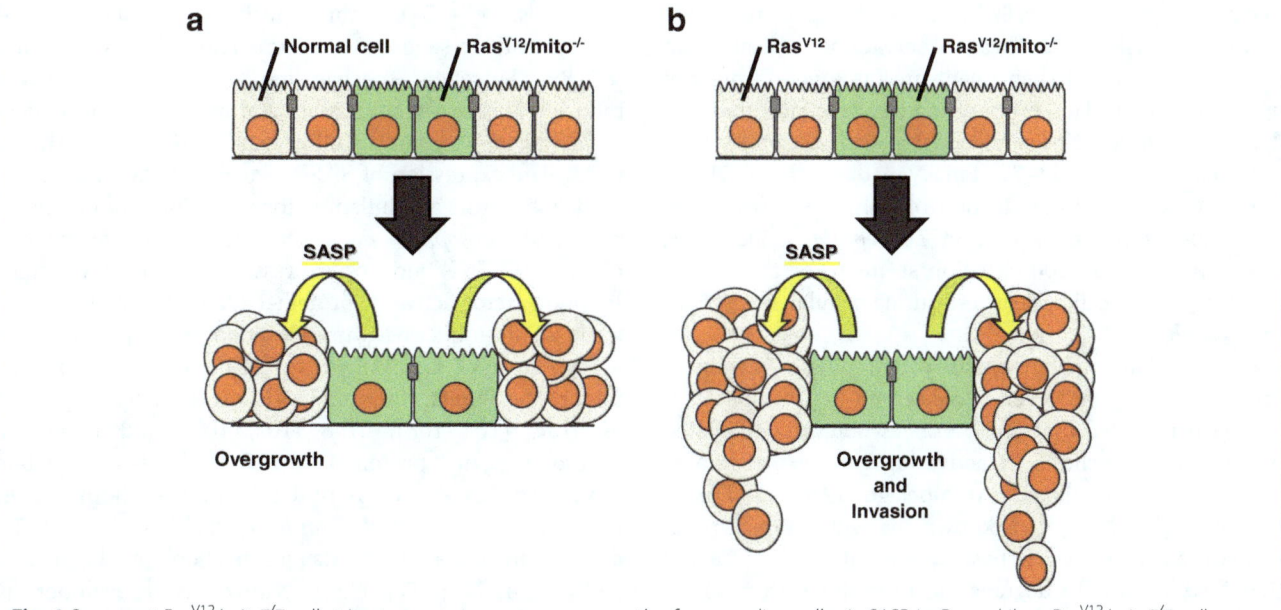

Fig. 1 Senescent Ras^{V12}/*mito$^{-/-}$* cells trigger non-autonomous overgrowth of surrounding cells via SASP in *Drosophila*. **a** Ras^{V12}/*mito$^{-/-}$* cells induce non-autonomous overgrowth of surrounding normal cells. **b** Ras^{V12}/*mito$^{-/-}$* cells induce non-autonomous overgrowth and invasion of surrounding Ras^{V12} cells

positively regulate the function of retinoblastoma 1 (Rb1), a cell cycle keeper, by repressing the activities of CDKs. p21 represses the activity of the Cyclin E-CDK2 complex, while p16 represses the activity of the Cyclin D-CDK4-CDK6 complex, leading to the induction of cell cycle arrest. Intriguingly, the mechanism regulating expression of Cdk inhibitors during cellular senescence in *Drosophila* seems to be distinct from mammals in three ways. First, DNA damage is not involved in stabilization of *Drosophila* p53 (dp53) protein [42, 65]. *Drosophila* Ras^{V12}/*mito*$^{-/-}$ cells, in which huge amount of ROS production and DNA damage occur, present larger elevation of dp53 than Ras^{V12} cells or *mito*$^{-/-}$ cells [42]. Nonetheless, this dp53 elevation is not blocked by suppression of ROS production, suggesting that dp53 protein level is not affected by oxidative DNA damage. Indeed, it has been reported that ionizing radiation (IR)-induced DNA damage does not change dp53 protein level, but it activates dp53 function via Loki (a Chk2 homologue)-dependent phosphorylation [65]. Similarly to mammalian Chk2, Loki acts as a kinase downstream of DNA damage-responsive kinases Tefu (an ATM homologue) and Mei-41 (an ATR homologue) [66, 67]. Thus, an alternative mechanism, not DNA damage, may stabilize dp53 protein, while DNA damage activates dp53 function. Second, dp53 does not regulate expression of *Drosophila* p21/p27, Dacapo [65, 68]. Loss of the dp53 gene in Ras^{V12}/*mito*$^{-/-}$ cells does not block elevation of Dacapo (our unpublished data), which is consistent with previous reports indicating that dp53 does not participate in the regulation of Dacapo expression [65, 68]. Meanwhile, it has been shown that the expression level of Dacapo in Ras^{V12} cells is comparable with that in Ras^{V12}/*mito*$^{-/-}$ cells but is much higher than that in *mito*$^{-/-}$ cells [42]. These observations indicate that Dacapo expression is dependent on Ras function but not dp53 function. In fact, previous studies have indicated that dp53 has a much closer relationship with apoptosis than cell cycle arrest [65, 69–72]. Finally, p16, another CDK inhibitor crucial for the induction of cellular senescence in mammals, is not conserved in *Drosophila*. Collectively, Ras^{V12}-induced Dacapo elevation seems to be the central event triggering cell cycle arrest during cellular senescence in *Drosophila*.

The mechanism by which p53 regulates cyclin E protein stability, however, is conserved in *Drosophila*. It has been reported that dp53 induces ubiquitin-mediated proteolysis of cyclin E by activating gene expression of an E3 ubiquitin ligase Archipelago (Ago; a Fbxw7 homologue) [73–75]. It is known that gene transcription of mammalian Fbxw7 is positively regulated by p53 and that Fbxw7 leads to degradation of cyclin E through its ubiquitin ligase activity [76–78]. Together, these observations suggest that Ras^{V12}-induced Dacapo upregulation and dp53-induced cyclin E degradation may cooperatively drive rigid cell cycle arrest in Ras^{V12}/*mito*$^{-/-}$ cells in *Drosophila*.

Roles of JNK and Hippo signaling in SASP

The c-Jun N-terminal kinase (JNK) pathway is a kinase cascade that mediates stress signaling such as oxidative stress and DNA damage [79–83]. *Drosophila* Ras^{V12}/*mito*$^{-/-}$ senescent cells show much higher *Drosophila* JNK (dJNK; a JNK 1/2/3 homologue) activity than Ras^{V12} cells or *mito*$^{-/-}$ cells, and this dJNK activation is blocked by ROS inhibition [43]. Intriguingly, prominent activation of dJNK in Ras^{V12}/*mito*$^{-/-}$ cells is achieved by cell cycle arrest [42]. Cyclin E overexpression in Ras^{V12}/*mito*$^{-/-}$ cells inhibits dJNK activation without affecting ROS production [42]. In addition, Ras activation, which causes a weak induction of ROS, and loss of cyclin E synergistically trigger excessive activation of dJNK [42, 43]. Ras activation alone slightly increases dJNK activity, while loss of cyclin E alone is insufficient for the induction of dJNK activation. These observations suggest that cell cycle arrest can amplify dJNK activity without changing ROS level. Furthermore, dJNK activation can induce cell cycle arrest [42], which is consistent with a previous report showing that JNK1 stabilizes p21 protein via phosphorylation in a human colon cancer cell line [84]. Taken together, these data suggest the existence of a positive feedback loop between dJNK signaling and cell cycle arrest in Ras^{V12}/*mito*$^{-/-}$ cells, and this loop and oxidative DNA damage may act synergistically to induce excessive activation of dJNK.

Previous reports have suggested a close link between JNK signaling and SASP. SASP is considered to be regulated by NF-κB signaling and epigenetic mechanisms in mammals. NF-κB signaling positively regulates SASP during cellular senescence downstream of Ras signaling [85–89]. Epigenetic mechanisms, such as chromatin remodeling, histone modification, and microRNA, also affect SASP [30, 90–94]. On the other hand, JNK has been shown to regulate expression of SASP factors including matrix remodeling factors and inflammatory cytokines both in mammals and *Drosophila*. As for matrix remodeling factors, mammalian JNK induces expression of Mmps via transcription factor activator protein-1 (AP-1) family [95–100], while dJNK induces Mmp1 elevation via *Drosophila* Fos (dFos), an AP-1 family member [101–103]. As for inflammatory cytokines, mammalian JNK induces elevation of IL-6 [104–106], IL-8 [107, 108], and monocyte chemoattractant protein-1 (MCP-1) [109–111], while dJNK induces elevation of Upd (an IL-6 homologue) [101, 112, 113]. In *Drosophila* Ras^{V12}/*mito*$^{-/-}$ cells, dJNK upregulates Upd via inactivation of the Hippo pathway [42, 43]. The Hippo pathway is an evolutionarily conserved tumor suppressor signaling that regulates cell proliferation and cell death [114, 115]. In mammals, Mst1/2 and Lats1/2, the core components of the Hippo pathway, repress the Hippo effectors Yap1/2 and Taz via phosphorylation [114, 116–120]. Similarly, in *Drosophila*, Hippo (a Mst1/2 homologue) and Warts (a Lats1/2 homologue) inactivate Yorkie (Yki; a Yap1 homologue) via phosphorylation [114, 116, 120–124]. Recent studies have reported that the Hippo pathway negatively regulates expression of SASP factors including IL-6 in mammals [125–128], similarly to *Drosophila* cells [129–132]. Marked upregulation of Upd in *Drosophila* $Ras^{V12}/mito^{-/-}$ cells is blocked by expression of a dominant negative form of dJNK, cyclin E, Warts, or RNAi-mediated knockdown of Yki [42, 43]. Furthermore, it has been shown that dJNK signaling and Ras signaling cooperatively inactivate the Hippo pathway, thereby inducing SASP. Recent studies in *Drosophila* and human cell cultures have shown that JNK signaling and Ras signaling act synergistically to inhibit the Hippo pathway via Ajuba LIM protein (Jub)/Ajuba family proteins, which are known as Warts/LATS inhibitors [133–138]. Thus, Jub/Ajuba family proteins may also act as key regulators of SASP during cellular senescence. These findings indicate the importance of JNK signaling in the induction of SASP.

Senescence or apoptosis?

Apart from cellular senescence, apoptosis also acts as a major defense mechanism against tumorigenesis [139]. Apoptosis is an active cell death program executed by killer proteases called caspases [140–142]. Are there any functional relationships between cellular senescence and apoptosis? Studies in *Drosophila* have indicated that Ras signaling negatively regulates the function of the pro-apoptotic protein head involution defective (Hid) both transcriptionally and post-transcriptionally, thereby suppressing apoptosis [143, 144]. Interestingly, senescent $Ras^{V12}/mito^{-/-}$ cells seem to exhibit apoptosis resistance [42, 43]. On the other hand, in mammals, Ras signaling not only induces cellular senescence but also suppresses apoptosis [145, 146]. Interestingly, it has also been shown in mammals that senescent cells have the resistance to apoptosis [147–150]. Conversely, apoptosis inhibition by the pan-caspase inhibitor accelerates the anticancer agent-induced senescence in human culture cells, suggesting that apoptotic signaling antagonizes cellular senescence [151]. Therefore, two major tumor-suppressive machineries, cellular senescence and apoptosis, seem to counteract each other. Future studies on common signaling involved in both cellular senescence and apoptosis would increase our understanding of how these machineries cooperatively regulate tumorigenesis.

Conclusions

Recent studies in *Drosophila* have revealed that cellular senescence and SASP exist in invertebrates and that Ras activation and mitochondrial dysfunction synergistically

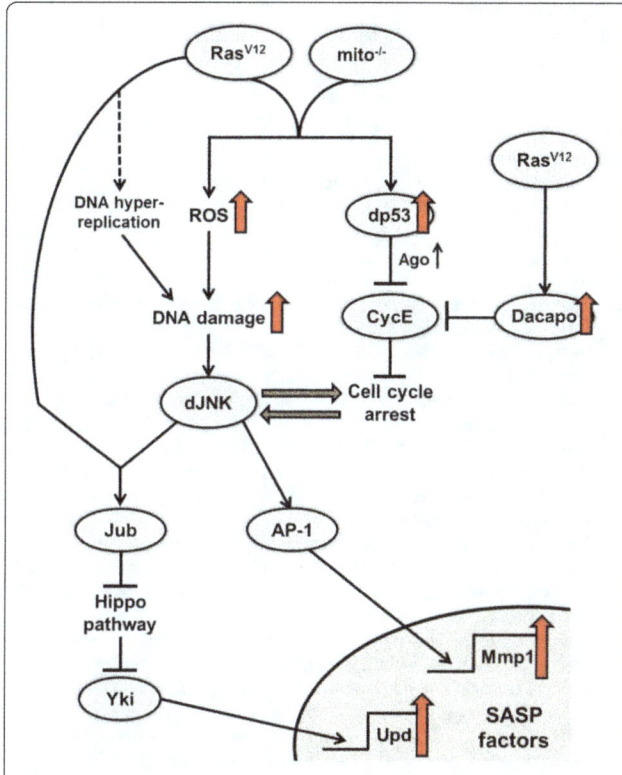

Fig. 2 Scheme of the underlying mechanisms driving cellular senescence and SASP in *Drosophila* $Ras^{V12}/mito^{-/-}$ cells

drive cellular senescence and SASP via complex mechanisms mediated by JNK and Hippo signaling (Fig. 2). These findings have opened a new direction of the research field of cellular senescence. Future studies taking advantages of the powerful genetics of *Drosophila* would provide novel insights into cellular senescence and SASP, as well as new therapeutic strategies against cancers.

Abbreviations
Ago: Archipelago; AP-1: Activator protein-1; CDK: Cyclin-dependent kinase; dFos: *Drosophila* Fos; dJNK: *Drosophila* JNK; dp53: *Drosophila* p53; Hid: Head involution defective; IL-6: Interleukin 6; IR: Ionizing radiation; JNK: c-Jun N-terminal kinase; Mmp: Matrix metalloprotease; OIS: Oncogene-induced senescence; Rb1: Retinoblastoma 1; ROS: Reactive oxygen species; SAHF: Senescence-associated heterochromatic foci; SASP: Senescence-associated secretory phenotype; SA-β-gal: Senescence-associated β-galactosidase; TCA: Tricarboxylic acid; Upd: Unpaired; Yki: Yorkie

Acknowledgements
Not applicable.

Funding
The work in the Igaki laboratory was supported in part by Grant-in-Aid for Scientific Research (A) (16H02505), Grant-in-Aid for Scientific Research on Innovative Areas (26114002), Grant-in-Aid for Challenging Exploratory Research (16K14606), the Takeda Science Foundation, and the Japan Science and Technology Agency.

Authors' contributions

Both authors wrote this paper. Both authors read and approved the final manuscript.

Competing interests

The authors declare that they have no competing interests.

References

1. Campisi J. Cellular senescence as a tumor-suppressor mechanism. Trends Cell Biol. 2001;11(11):S27–31.
2. Bartkova J, Horejsi Z, Koed K, Kramer A, Tort F, Zieger K, Guldberg P, Sehested M, Nesland JM, Lukas C, et al. DNA damage response as a candidate anti-cancer barrier in early human tumorigenesis. Nature. 2005;434(7035):864–70. 861.
3. Bartkova J, Rezaei N, Liontos M, Karakaidos P, Kletsas D, Issaeva N, Vassiliou LV, Kolettas E, Niforou K, Zoumpourlis VC, et al. Oncogene-induced senescence is part of the tumorigenesis barrier imposed by DNA damage checkpoints. Nature. 2006;444(7119):633–7.
4. Bennecke M, Kriegl L, Bajbouj M, Retzlaff K, Robine S, Jung A, Arkan MC, Kirchner T, Greten FR. Ink4a/Arf and oncogene-induced senescence prevent tumor progression during alternative colorectal tumorigenesis. Cancer Cell. 2010;18(2):135–46.
5. Braig M, Lee S, Loddenkemper C, Rudolph C, Peters AH, Schlegelberger B, Stein H, Dorken B, Jenuwein T, Schmitt CA. Oncogene-induced senescence as an initial barrier in lymphoma development. Nature. 2005;436(7051):660–5.
6. Chen Z, Trotman LC, Shaffer D, Lin HK, Dotan ZA, Niki M, Koutcher JA, Scher HI, Ludwig T, Gerald W, et al. Crucial role of p53-dependent cellular senescence in suppression of Pten-deficient tumorigenesis. Nature. 2005;436(7051):725–30. 722.
7. Michaloglou C, Vredeveld LC, Soengas MS, Denoyelle C, Kuilman T, van der Horst CM, Majoor DM, Shay JW, Mooi WJ, Peeper DS. BRAFE600-associated senescence-like cell cycle arrest of human naevi. Nature. 2005;436(7051):720–4.
8. Courtois-Cox S, Jones SL, Cichowski K. Many roads lead to oncogene-induced senescence. Oncogene. 2008;27(20):2801–9. 2804.
9. Mason DX, Jackson TJ, Lin AW. Molecular signature of oncogenic Ras-induced senescence. Oncogene. 2004;23(57):9238–46.
10. Di MR, Fumagalli M, Cicalese A, Piccinin S, Gasparini P, Luise C, Schurra C, Garre' M, Nuciforo PG, Bensimon A, et al. Oncogene-induced senescence is a DNA damage response triggered by DNA hyper-replication. Nature. 2006;444(7119):638–42.
11. Ferbeyre G, de Stanchina E, Lin AW, Querido E, McCurrach ME, Hannon GJ, Lowe SW. Oncogenic ras and p53 cooperate to induce cellular senescence. Mol Cell Biol. 2002;22(10):3497–508.
12. Serrano M, Lin AW, McCurrach ME, Beach D, Lowe SW. Oncogenic ras provokes premature cell senescence associated with accumulation of p53 and p16INK4a. Cell. 1997;88(5):593–602.
13. Lee AC, Fenster BE, Ito H, Takeda K, Bae NS, Hirai T, Yu ZX, Ferrans VJ, Howard BH, Finkel T. Ras proteins induce senescence by altering the intracellular levels of reactive oxygen species. J Biol Chem. 1999;274(12):7936–40.
14. Zhu J, Woods D, McMahon M, Bishop JM. Senescence of human fibroblasts induced by oncogenic Raf. Genes Dev. 1998;12(19):2997–3007.
15. Mallette FA, Gaumont-Leclerc MF, Ferbeyre G. The DNA damage signaling pathway is a critical mediator of oncogene-induced senescence. Genes Dev. 2007;21(1):43–8.
16. Collado M, Gil J, Efeyan A, Guerra C, Schuhmacher AJ, Barradas M, Benguria A, Zaballos A, Flores JM, Barbacid M, et al. Tumour biology: senescence in premalignant tumours. Nature. 2005;436(7051):642.
17. Chen QM, Prowse KR, Tu VC, Purdom S, Linskens MH. Uncoupling the senescent phenotype from telomere shortening in hydrogen peroxide-treated fibroblasts. Exp Cell Res. 2001;265(2):294–303.
18. Ben-Porath I, Weinberg RA. When cells get stressed: an integrative view of cellular senescence. J Clin Invest. 2004;113(1):8–13.
19. Krtolica A, Parrinello S, Lockett S, Desprez PY, Campisi J. Senescent fibroblasts promote epithelial cell growth and tumorigenesis: a link between cancer and aging. Proc Natl Acad Sci U S A. 2001;98(21):12072–7.

20. Coppe JP, Patil CK, Rodier F, Sun Y, Munoz DP, Goldstein J, Nelson PS, Desprez PY, Campisi J. Senescence-associated secretory phenotypes reveal cell-nonautonomous functions of oncogenic RAS and the p53 tumor suppressor. PLoS Biol. 2008;6(12):2853–68.
21. Coppe JP, Desprez PY, Krtolica A, Campisi J. The senescence-associated secretory phenotype: the dark side of tumor suppression. Annu Rev Pathol. 2010;5:99–118.
22. Davalos AR, Coppe JP, Campisi J, Desprez PY. Senescent cells as a source of inflammatory factors for tumor progression. Cancer Metastasis Rev. 2010;29(2):273–83.
23. Xu T, Rubin GM. Analysis of genetic mosaics in developing and adult Drosophila tissues. Development. 1993;117(4):1223–37.
24. Wu JS, Luo L. A protocol for mosaic analysis with a repressible cell marker (MARCM) in Drosophila. Nat Protoc. 2006;1(6):2583–9.
25. HAYFLICK L, MOORHEAD PS. The serial cultivation of human diploid cell strains. Exp Cell Res. 1961;25:585–621.
26. Stein GH, Drullinger LF, Soulard A, Dulic V. Differential roles for cyclin-dependent kinase inhibitors p21 and p16 in the mechanisms of senescence and differentiation in human fibroblasts. Mol Cell Biol. 1999;19(3):2109–17.
27. van Deursen JM. The role of senescent cells in ageing. Nature. 2014;509(7501):439–46.
28. Baker DJ, Jeganathan KB, Cameron JD, Thompson M, Juneja S, Kopecka A, Kumar R, Jenkins RB, de Groen PC, Roche P, et al. BubR1 insufficiency causes early onset of aging-associated phenotypes and infertility in mice. Nat Genet. 2004;36(7):744–9.
29. Meixner A, Karreth F, Kenner L, Penninger JM, Wagner EF. Jun and JunD-dependent functions in cell proliferation and stress response. Cell Death Differ. 2010;17(9):1409–19.
30. Andre T, Meuleman N, Stamatopoulos B, De BC, Pieters K, Bron D, Lagneaux L. Evidences of early senescence in multiple myeloma bone marrow mesenchymal stromal cells. PLoS One. 2013;8(3):e59756.
31. Dimri GP, Lee X, Basile G, Acosta M, Scott G, Roskelley C, Medrano EE, Linskens M, Rubelj I, Pereira-Smith O, et al. A biomarker that identifies senescent human cells in culture and in aging skin in vivo. Proc Natl Acad Sci U S A. 1995;92(20):9363–7.
32. Kurz DJ, Decary S, Hong Y, Erusalimsky JD. Senescence-associated (beta)-galactosidase reflects an increase in lysosomal mass during replicative ageing of human endothelial cells. J Cell Sci. 2000;113(Pt 20):3613–22.
33. Alcorta DA, Xiong Y, Phelps D, Hannon G, Beach D, Barrett JC. Involvement of the cyclin-dependent kinase inhibitor p16 (INK4a) in replicative senescence of normal human fibroblasts. Proc Natl Acad Sci U S A. 1996;93(24):13742–7.
34. Serrano M, Hannon GJ, Beach D. A new regulatory motif in cell-cycle control causing specific inhibition of cyclin D/CDK4. Nature. 1993;366(6456):704–7.
35. el-Deiry WS, Tokino T, Velculescu VE, Levy DB, Parsons R, Trent JM, Lin D, Mercer WE, Kinzler KW, Vogelstein B. WAF1, a potential mediator of p53 tumor suppression. Cell. 1993;75(4):817–825.1.
36. Xiong Y, Hannon GJ, Zhang H, Casso D, Kobayashi R, Beach D. p21 is a universal inhibitor of cyclin kinases. Nature. 1993;366(6456):701–4.
37. Herbig U, Jobling WA, Chen BP, Chen DJ, Sedivy JM. Telomere shortening triggers senescence of human cells through a pathway involving ATM, p53, and p21(CIP1), but not p16(INK4a). Mol Cell. 2004;14(4):501–13.
38. Narita M, Nunez S, Heard E, Narita M, Lin AW, Hearn SA, Spector DL, Hannon GJ, Lowe SW. Rb-mediated heterochromatin formation and silencing of E2F target genes during cellular senescence. Cell. 2003;113(6):703–16.
39. Narita M, Narita M, Krizhanovsky V, Nunez S, Chicas A, Hearn SA, Myers MP, Lowe SW. A novel role for high-mobility group a proteins in cellular senescence and heterochromatin formation. Cell. 2006;126(3):503–14.
40. Narita M. Cellular senescence and chromatin organisation. Br J Cancer. 2007;96(5):686–91.
41. Kosar M, Bartkova J, Hubackova S, Hodny Z, Lukas J, Bartek J. Senescence-associated heterochromatin foci are dispensable for cellular senescence, occur in a cell type- and insult-dependent manner and follow expression of p16(ink4a). Cell Cycle. 2011;10(3):457–68.
42. Nakamura M, Ohsawa S, Igaki T. Mitochondrial defects trigger proliferation of neighbouring cells via a senescence-associated secretory phenotype in Drosophila. Nat Commun. 2014;5:5264.
43. Ohsawa S, Sato Y, Enomoto M, Nakamura M, Betsumiya A, Igaki T.

Mitochondrial defect drives non-autonomous tumour progression through Hippo signalling in Drosophila. Nature. 2012;490(7421):547–51.

44. Brandon M, Baldi P, Wallace DC. Mitochondrial mutations in cancer. Oncogene. 2006;25(34):4647–62.

45. Carew JS, Huang P. Mitochondrial defects in cancer. Mol Cancer. 2002;1:9.

46. Modica-Napolitano JS, Kulawiec M, Singh KK. Mitochondria and human cancer. Curr Mol Med. 2007;7(1):121–31.

47. Pedersen PL. Tumor mitochondria and the bioenergetics of cancer cells. Prog Exp Tumor Res. 1978;22:190–274.

48. Tokarz P, Blasiak J. Role of mitochondria in carcinogenesis. Acta Biochim Pol. 2014;61(4):671–8.

49. Harrison DA, McCoon PE, Binari R, Gilman M, Perrimon N. Drosophila unpaired encodes a secreted protein that activates the JAK signaling pathway. Genes Dev. 1998;12(20):3252–63.

50. Llano E, Pendas AM, Aza-Blanc P, Kornberg TB, Lopez-Otin C. Dm1-MMP, a matrix metalloproteinase from Drosophila with a potential role in extracellular matrix remodeling during neural development. J Biol Chem. 2000;275(46):35978–85.

51. Chen JH, Hales CN, Ozanne SE. DNA damage, cellular senescence and organismal ageing: causal or correlative? Nucleic Acids Res. 2007;35(22):7417–28.

52. Chen Q, Fischer A, Reagan JD, Yan LJ, Ames BN. Oxidative DNA damage and senescence of human diploid fibroblast cells. Proc Natl Acad Sci U S A. 1995;92(10):4337–41.

53. Chen Q, Ames BN. Senescence-like growth arrest induced by hydrogen peroxide in human diploid fibroblast F65 cells. Proc Natl Acad Sci U S A. 1994;91(10):4130–4.

54. Chen JH, Stoeber K, Kingsbury S, Ozanne SE, Williams GH, Hales CN. Loss of proliferative capacity and induction of senescence in oxidatively stressed human fibroblasts. J Biol Chem. 2004;279(47):49439–46.

55. Luo H, Yang A, Schulte BA, Wargovich MJ, Wang GY. Resveratrol induces premature senescence in lung cancer cells via ROS-mediated DNA damage. PLoS One. 2013;8(3), e60065.

56. Kaplon J, Zheng L, Meissl K, Chaneton B, Selivanov VA, Mackay G, van der Burg SH, Verdegaal EM, Cascante M, Shlomi T, et al. A key role for mitochondrial gatekeeper pyruvate dehydrogenase in oncogene-induced senescence. Nature. 2013;498(7452):109–12.

57. Honda R, Tanaka H, Yasuda H. Oncoprotein MDM2 is a ubiquitin ligase E3 for tumor suppressor p53. FEBS Lett. 1997;420(1):25–7.

58. Brooks CL, Gu W. p53 ubiquitination: Mdm2 and beyond. Mol Cell. 2006;21(3):307–15.

59. Maltzman W, Czyzyk L. UV irradiation stimulates levels of p53 cellular tumor antigen in nontransformed mouse cells. Mol Cell Biol. 1984;4(9):1689–94.

60. Wang XQ, Gabrielli BG, Milligan A, Dickinson JL, Antalis TM, Ellem KA. Accumulation of p16CDKN2A in response to ultraviolet irradiation correlates with late S-G(2)-phase cell cycle delay. Cancer Res. 1996;56(11):2510–4.

61. Robles SJ, Adami GR. Agents that cause DNA double strand breaks lead to p16INK4a enrichment and the premature senescence of normal fibroblasts. Oncogene. 1998;16(9):1113–23.

62. Sherr CJ, Roberts JM. CDK inhibitors: positive and negative regulators of G1-phase progression. Genes Dev. 1999;13(12):1501–12.

63. Dulic V, Kaufmann WK, Wilson SJ, Tlsty TD, Lees E, Harper JW, Elledge SJ, Reed SI. p53-dependent inhibition of cyclin-dependent kinase activities in human fibroblasts during radiation-induced G1 arrest. Cell. 1994;76(6):1013–23.

64. Takahashi A, Ohtani N, Yamakoshi K, Iida S, Tahara H, Nakayama K, Nakayama KI, Ide T, Saya H, Hara E. Mitogenic signalling and the p16INK4a-Rb pathway cooperate to enforce irreversible cellular senescence. Nat Cell Biol. 2006;8(11):1291–7.

65. Brodsky MH, Weinert BT, Tsang G, Rong YS, McGinnis NM, Golic KG, Rio DC, Rubin GM. Drosophila melanogaster MNK/Chk2 and p53 regulate multiple DNA repair and apoptotic pathways following DNA damage. Mol Cell Biol. 2004;24(3):1219–31.

66. Abdu U, Brodsky M, Schupbach T. Activation of a meiotic checkpoint during Drosophila oogenesis regulates the translation of Gurken through Chk2/Mnk. Curr Biol. 2002;12(19):1645–51.

67. Song YH. Drosophila melanogaster: a model for the study of DNA damage checkpoint response. Mol Cells. 2005;19(2):167–79.

68. Akdemir F, Christich A, Sogame N, Chapo J, Abrams JM. p53 directs focused genomic responses in Drosophila. Oncogene. 2007;26(36):5184–93.

69. Brodsky MH, Nordstrom W, Tsang G, Kwan E, Rubin GM, Abrams JM. Drosophila p53 binds a damage response element at the reaper locus. Cell. 2000;101(1):103–13.

70. Ollmann M, Young LM, Di Como CJ, Karim F, Belvin M, Robertson S, Whittaker K, Demsky M, Fisher WW, Buchman A, et al. Drosophila p53 is a structural and functional homolog of the tumor suppressor p53. Cell. 2000;101(1):91–101.

71. Fan Y, Lee TV, Xu D, Chen Z, Lamblin AF, Steller H, Bergmann A. Dual roles of Drosophila p53 in cell death and cell differentiation. Cell Death Differ. 2010;17(6):912–21.

72. Marcel V, Dichtel-Danjoy ML, Sagne C, Hafsi H, Ma D, Ortiz-Cuaran S, Olivier M, Hall J, Mollereau B, Hainaut P, et al. Biological functions of p53 isoforms through evolution: lessons from animal and cellular models. Cell Death Differ. 2011;18(12):1815–24.

73. Mandal S, Freije WA, Guptan P, Banerjee U. Metabolic control of G1-S transition: cyclin E degradation by p53-induced activation of the ubiquitin-proteasome system. J Cell Biol. 2010;188(4):473–9.

74. Moberg KH, Bell DW, Wahrer DC, Haber DA, Hariharan IK. Archipelago regulates cyclin E levels in Drosophila and is mutated in human cancer cell lines. Nature. 2001;413(6853):311–6.

75. Mandal S, Guptan P, Owusu-Ansah E, Banerjee U. Mitochondrial regulation of cell cycle progression during development as revealed by the tenured mutation in Drosophila. Dev Cell. 2005;9(6):843–54.

76. Yeh ES, Means AR. PIN1, the cell cycle and cancer. Nat Rev Cancer. 2007;7(5):381–8.

77. Kimura T, Gotoh M, Nakamura Y, Arakawa H. hCDC4b, a regulator of cyclin E, as a direct transcriptional target of p53. Cancer Sci. 2003;94(5):431–6.

78. Mao JH, Perez-Losada J, Wu D, Delrosario R, Tsunematsu R, Nakayama KI, Brown K, Bryson S, Balmain A. Fbxw7/Cdc4 is a p53-dependent, haploinsufficient tumour suppressor gene. Nature. 2004;432(7018):775–9.

79. Roos WP, Kaina B. DNA damage-induced cell death by apoptosis. Trends Mol Med. 2006;12(9):440–50.

80. Essers MA, Weijzen S, de Vries-Smits AM, Saarloos I, de Ruiter ND, Bos JL, Burgering BM. FOXO transcription factor activation by oxidative stress mediated by the small GTPase Ral and JNK. EMBO J. 2004;23(24):4802–12.

81. Karpac J, Jasper H. Insulin and JNK: optimizing metabolic homeostasis and lifespan. Trends Endocrinol Metab. 2009;20(3):100–6.

82. Yoshida K, Yamaguchi T, Natsume T, Kufe D, Miki Y. JNK phosphorylation of 14-3-3 proteins regulates nuclear targeting of c-Abl in the apoptotic response to DNA damage. Nat Cell Biol. 2005;7(3):278–85.

83. Bogoyevitch MA, Kobe B. Uses for JNK: the many and varied substrates of the c-Jun N-terminal kinases. Microbiol Mol Biol Rev. 2006;70(4):1061–95.

84. Kim GY, Mercer SE, Ewton DZ, Yan Z, Jin K, Friedman E. The stress-activated protein kinases p38 alpha and JNK1 stabilize p21(Cip1) by phosphorylation. J Biol Chem. 2002;277(33):29792–802.

85. Acosta JC, O'Loghlen A, Banito A, Guijarro MV, Augert A, Raguz S, Fumagalli M, Da CM, Brown C, Popov N, et al. Chemokine signaling via the CXCR2 receptor reinforces senescence. Cell. 2008;133(6):1006–18.

86. Chien Y, Scuoppo C, Wang X, Fang X, Balgley B, Bolden JE, Premsrirut P, Luo W, Chicas A, Lee CS, et al. Control of the senescence-associated secretory phenotype by NF-kappaB promotes senescence and enhances chemosensitivity. Genes Dev. 2011;25(20):2125–36.

87. Crescenzi E, Pacifico F, Lavorgna A, De PR, D'Aiuto E, Palumbo G, Formisano S, Leonardi A. NF-kappaB-dependent cytokine secretion controls Fas expression on chemotherapy-induced premature senescent tumor cells. Oncogene. 2011;30(24):2707–17.

88. Salminen A, Kauppinen A, Kaarniranta K. Emerging role of NF-kappaB signaling in the induction of senescence-associated secretory phenotype (SASP). Cell Signal. 2012;24(4):835–45.

89. Karin M, Greten FR. NF-kappaB: linking inflammation and immunity to cancer development and progression. Nat Rev Immunol. 2005;5(10):749–59.

90. Kozlowski M, Ladurner AG. ATM, MacroH2A.1, and SASP: the checks and balances of cellular senescence. Mol Cell. 2015;59(5):713–5.

91. Zhang H, Pan KH, Cohen SN. Senescence-specific gene expression fingerprints reveal cell-type-dependent physical clustering of up-regulated chromosomal loci. Proc Natl Acad Sci U S A. 2003;100(6):3251–6.

92. Shah PP, Donahue G, Otte GL, Capell BC, Nelson DM, Cao K, Aggarwala V, Cruickshanks HA, Rai TS, McBryan T, et al. Lamin B1 depletion in senescent cells triggers large-scale changes in gene expression and the chromatin landscape. Genes Dev. 2013;27(16):1787–99.

93. Iliopoulos D, Hirsch HA, Struhl K. An epigenetic switch involving NF-kappaB, Lin28, Let-7 MicroRNA, and IL6 links inflammation to cell transformation. Cell. 2009;139(4):693–706.

94. Olivieri F, Rippo MR, Monsurro V, Salvioli S, Capri M, Procopio AD, Franceschi C. MicroRNAs linking inflamm-aging, cellular senescence and cancer. Ageing Res Rev. 2013;12(4):1056–68.

95. Byun HJ, Hong IK, Kim E, Jin YJ, Jeoung DI, Hahn JH, Kim YM, Park SH, Lee H. A splice variant of CD99 increases motility and MMP-9 expression of human breast cancer cells through the AKT-, ERK-, and JNK-dependent AP-1 activation signaling pathways. J Biol Chem. 2006;281(46):34833–47. 34831.

96. Chakraborti S, Mandal M, Das S, Mandal A, Chakraborti T. Regulation of matrix metalloproteinases: an overview. Mol Cell Biochem. 2003;253(1-2):269–85.

97. Cheung LW, Leung PC, Wong AS. Gonadotropin-releasing hormone promotes ovarian cancer cell invasiveness through c-Jun NH2-terminal kinase-mediated activation of matrix metalloproteinase (MMP)-2 and MMP-9. Cancer Res. 2006;66(22):10902–10.

98. Lin SJ, Lee IT, Chen YH, Lin FY, Sheu LM, Ku HH, Shiao MS, Chen JW, Chen YL. Salvianolic acid B attenuates MMP-2 and MMP-9 expression in vivo in apolipoprotein-E-deficient mouse aorta and in vitro in LPS-treated human aortic smooth muscle cells. J Cell Biochem. 2007;100(2):372. 371-384.

99. Mengshol JA, Vincenti MP, Brinckerhoff CE. IL-1 induces collagenase-3 (MMP-13) promoter activity in stably transfected chondrocytic cells: requirement for Runx-2 and activation by p38 MAPK and JNK pathways. Nucleic Acids Res. 2001;29(21):4361–72. 4362.

100. Westermarck J, Kahari VM. Regulation of matrix metalloproteinase expression in tumor invasion. FASEB J. 1999;13(8):781. 797-792.

101. Bunker BD, Nellimoottil TT, Boileau RM, Classen AK, Bilder D. The transcriptional response to tumorigenic polarity loss in Drosophila. Elife. 2015;4:1.

102. Page-McCaw A. Remodeling the model organism: matrix metalloproteinase functions in invertebrates. Semin Cell Dev Biol. 2008;19(1):14. 13-23.

103. Uhlirova M, Bohmann D. JNK- and Fos-regulated Mmp1 expression cooperates with Ras to induce invasive tumors in Drosophila. EMBO J. 2006;25(22):5294–304. 5292.

104. An J, Sun Y, Sun R, Rettig MB. Kaposi's sarcoma-associated herpes virus encoded vFLIP induces cellular IL-6 expression: the role of the NF-kappaB and JNK/AP1 pathways. Oncogene. 2003;22(22):3371–85.

105. Jang S, Kelley KW, Johnson RW. Luteolin reduces IL-6 production in microglia by inhibiting JNK phosphorylation and activation of AP-1. Proc Natl Acad Sci U S A. 2008;105(21):7534. 7536-7539.

106. Das M, Garlick DS, Greiner DL, Davis RJ. The role of JNK in the development of hepatocellular carcinoma. Genes Dev. 2011;25(6):634–45.

107. Li LF, Ouyang B, Choukroun G, Matyal R, Mascarenhas M, Jafari B, Bonventre JV, Force T, Quinn DA. Stretch-induced IL-8 depends on c-Jun NH2-terminal and nuclear factor-kappaB-inducing kinases. Am J Physiol Lung Cell Mol Physiol. 2003;285(2):L464–75. 463.

108. Schmeck B, Moog K, van Laak V, Zahlten J, N'Guessan PD, Opitz B, Rosseau S, Suttorp N, Hippenstiel S. Streptococcus pneumoniae induced c-Jun-N-terminal kinase- and AP-1 -dependent IL-8 release by lung epithelial BEAS-2B cells. Respir Res. 2006;7:98.

109. Yamana J, Santos L, Morand E. Enhanced induction of LPS-induced fibroblast MCP-1 by interferon-gamma: involvement of JNK and MAPK phosphatase-1. Cell Immunol. 2009;255(1-2):26. 26-32.

110. Wu J, Mei C, Vlassara H, Striker GE, Zheng F. Oxidative stress-induced JNK activation contributes to proinflammatory phenotype of aging diabetic mesangial cells. Am J Physiol Renal Physiol. 2009;297(6):F1622–31.

111. Nomura J, Busso N, Ives A, Tsujimoto S, Tamura M, So A, Yamanaka Y. Febuxostat, an inhibitor of xanthine oxidase, suppresses lipopolysaccharide-induced MCP-1 production via MAPK phosphatase-1-mediated inactivation of JNK. PLoS One. 2013;8(9):e75527.

112. Jiang H, Patel PH, Kohlmaier A, Grenley MO, McEwen DG, Edgar BA. Cytokine/Jak/Stat signaling mediates regeneration and homeostasis in the Drosophila midgut. Cell. 2009;137(7):1343–55.

113. Santabarbara-Ruiz P, Lopez-Santillan M, Martinez-Rodriguez I, Binagui-Casas A, Perez L, Milan M, Corominas M, Serras F. ROS-induced JNK and p38 signaling is required for unpaired cytokine activation during drosophila regeneration. PLoS Genet. 2015;11(10):e1005595–1005591.

114. Badouel C, McNeill H. SnapShot: the hippo signaling pathway. Cell. 2011;145(3):484–484.e1. 481.

115. Pan D. The hippo signaling pathway in development and cancer. Dev Cell. 2010;19(4):491–505.

116. Zhao B, Wei X, Li W, Udan RS, Yang Q, Kim J, Xie J, Ikenoue T, Yu J, Li L, et al. Inactivation of YAP oncoprotein by the Hippo pathway is involved in cell contact inhibition and tissue growth control. Genes Dev. 2007;21(21):2747–61.

117. Lei QY, Zhang H, Zhao B, Zha ZY, Bai F, Pei XH, Zhao S, Xiong Y, Guan KL. TAZ promotes cell proliferation and epithelial-mesenchymal transition and is inhibited by the hippo pathway. Mol Cell Biol. 2008;28(7):2426–36. 2426.

118. Zhao B, Li L, Tumaneng K, Wang CY, Guan KL. A coordinated phosphorylation by Lats and CK1 regulates YAP stability through SCF (beta-TRCP). Genes Dev. 2010;24(1):72–85. 73.

119. Liu CY, Zha ZY, Zhou X, Zhang H, Huang W, Zhao D, Li T, Chan SW, Lim CJ, Hong W, et al. The hippo tumor pathway promotes TAZ degradation by phosphorylating a phosphodegron and recruiting the SCF{beta}-TrCP E3 ligase. J Biol Chem. 2010;285(48):37159–69. 37158.

120. Dong J, Feldmann G, Huang J, Wu S, Zhang N, Comerford SA, Gayyed MF, Anders RA, Maitra A, Pan D. Elucidation of a universal size-control mechanism in Drosophila and mammals. Cell. 2007;130(6):1120–33. 1121.

121. Staley BK, Irvine KD. Hippo signaling in Drosophila: recent advances and insights. Dev Dyn. 2012;241(1):3–15. 11.

122. Grusche FA, Richardson HE, Harvey KF. Upstream regulation of the hippo size control pathway. Curr Biol. 2010;20(13):R574–82.

123. Ren F, Zhang L, Jiang J. Hippo signaling regulates Yorkie nuclear localization and activity through 14-3-3 dependent and independent mechanisms. Dev Biol. 2010;337(2):303–12. 314.

124. Oh H, Irvine KD. In vivo regulation of Yorkie phosphorylation and localization. Development. 2008;135(6):1081–8.

125. Lu L, Li Y, Kim SM, Bossuyt W, Liu P, Qiu Q, Wang Y, Halder G, Finegold MJ, Lee JS, et al. Hippo signaling is a potent in vivo growth and tumor suppressor pathway in the mammalian liver. Proc Natl Acad Sci U S A. 2010;107(4):1437–42. 1431.

126. Zhang W, Nandakumar N, Shi Y, Manzano M, Smith A, Graham G, Gupta S, Vietsch EE, Laughlin SZ, Wadhwa M, et al. Downstream of mutant KRAS, the transcription regulator YAP is essential for neoplastic progression to pancreatic ductal adenocarcinoma. Sci Signal. 2014;7(324):ra42–18.

127. Kim T, Yang SJ, Hwang D, Song J, Kim M, Kyum KS, Kang K, Ahn J, Lee D, Kim MY, et al. A basal-like breast cancer-specific role for SRF-IL6 in YAP-induced cancer stemness. Nat Commun. 2015;6:10186–1.

128. Zhang J, Ji JY, Yu M, Overholtzer M, Smolen GA, Wang R, Brugge JS, Dyson NJ, Haber DA. YAP-dependent induction of amphiregulin identifies a non-cell-autonomous component of the Hippo pathway. Nat Cell Biol. 2009;11(12):1444–50. 1442.

129. Ren F, Wang B, Yue T, Yun EY, Ip YT, Jiang J. Hippo signaling regulates Drosophila intestine stem cell proliferation through multiple pathways. Proc Natl Acad Sci U S A. 2010;107(49):21064–9.

130. Shaw RL, Kohlmaier A, Polesello C, Veelken C, Edgar BA, Tapon N. The Hippo pathway regulates intestinal stem cell proliferation during Drosophila adult midgut regeneration. Development. 2010;137(24):4147–58. 4141.

131. Karpowicz P, Perez J, Perrimon N. The Hippo tumor suppressor pathway regulates intestinal stem cell regeneration. Development. 2010;137(24):4135–45. 4138.

132. Staley BK, Irvine KD. Warts and Yorkie mediate intestinal regeneration by influencing stem cell proliferation. Curr Biol. 2010;20(17):1580–7. 1582.

133. Sun G, Irvine KD. Ajuba family proteins link JNK to Hippo signaling. Sci Signal. 2013;6(292):ra81.

134. Reddy BV, Irvine KD. Regulation of Hippo signaling by EGFR-MAPK signaling through Ajuba family proteins. Dev Cell. 2013;24(5):459–71.

135. Sun S, Reddy BV, Irvine KD. Localization of Hippo signalling complexes and Warts activation in vivo. Nat Commun. 2015;6:8402.

136. Sun G, Irvine KD. Regulation of Hippo signaling by Jun kinase signaling during compensatory cell proliferation and regeneration, and in neoplastic tumors. Dev Biol. 2011;350(1):139–51.

137. Codelia VA, Sun G, Irvine KD. Regulation of YAP by mechanical strain through Jnk and Hippo signaling. Curr Biol. 2014;24(17):2012–7.

138. Enomoto M, Kizawa D, Ohsawa S, Igaki T. JNK signaling is converted from anti- to pro-tumor pathway by Ras-mediated switch of Warts activity. Dev Biol. 2015;403(2):162–71.

139. Lowe SW, Cepero E, Evan G. Intrinsic tumour suppression. Nature. 2004;432(7015):307–15.

140. Kerr JF, Wyllie AH, Currie AR. Apoptosis: a basic biological phenomenon with wide-ranging implications in tissue kinetics. Br J Cancer. 1972;26(4):239–57.

141. Haake AR, Polakowska RR. Cell death by apoptosis in epidermal biology. J Invest Dermatol. 1993;101(2):107–12.

142. Nicholson DW, Thornberry NA. Caspases: killer proteases. Trends Biochem Sci. 1997;22(8):299–306.

143. Bergmann A, Agapite J, McCall K, Steller H. The Drosophila gene hid is a direct molecular target of Ras-dependent survival signaling. Cell. 1998;95(3):331–41.

144. Kurada P, White K. Ras promotes cell survival in Drosophila by downregulating hid expression. Cell. 1998;95(3):319–29.

145. Cox AD, Der CJ. The dark side of Ras: regulation of apoptosis. Oncogene. 2003;22(56):8999–9006.

146. Karnoub AE, Weinberg RA. Ras oncogenes: split personalities. Nat Rev Mol Cell Biol. 2008;9(7):517–31.

147. Hampel B, Wagner M, Teis D, Zwerschke W, Huber LA, Jansen-Durr P. Apoptosis resistance of senescent human fibroblasts is correlated with the absence of nuclear IGFBP-3. Aging Cell. 2005;4(6):325–30.

148. Ryu SJ, Oh YS, Park SC. Failure of stress-induced downregulation of Bcl-2 contributes to apoptosis resistance in senescent human diploid fibroblasts. Cell Death Differ. 2007;14(5):1020–8.

149. Pasillas MP, Shields S, Reilly R, Strnadel J, Behl C, Park R, Yates III JR, Klemke R, Gonias SL, Coppinger JA. Proteomic analysis reveals a role for Bcl2-associated athanogene 3 and major vault protein in resistance to apoptosis in senescent cells by regulating ERK1/2 activation. Mol Cell Proteomics. 2015;14(1):1–14.

150. Childs BG, Baker DJ, Kirkland JL, Campisi J, van Deursen JM. Senescence and apoptosis: dueling or complementary cell fates? EMBO Rep. 2014;15(11):1139–53.

151. Rebbaa A, Zheng X, Chou PM, Mirkin BL. Caspase inhibition switches doxorubicin-induced apoptosis to senescence. Oncogene. 2003;22(18):2805–11.

6

Roles of hepatic stellate cells in liver inflammation

Tomoko Fujita* and Shuh Narumiya

Abstract

Connected with the intestinal tract through the portal circulation, liver sinusoids function as the first line of defense against extrahepatic stimuli such as bacterial products and other toxic substances. Hepatic stellate cells (HSCs) are pericytes residing in the perisinusoidal space, between sinusoidal endothelial cells and hepatocytes, store vitamin A, and regulate sinusoidal circulation. Following chronic hepatitis, HSCs actively produce extracellular matrices and cause liver fibrosis. In spite of their close position to the liver sinusoids, however, whether HSCs contribute to liver inflammation has remained elusive. Evidence now accumulates to suggest that HSCs actively take part in the regulation of various forms of liver inflammation. Upon inflammatory stimuli from the sinusoids, HSCs produce various inflammatory molecules and interact with other liver cells, thereby recruiting and then activating infiltrating leukocytes and ultimately causing hepatocyte death. On the other hand, HSCs also exert hepatoprotective effects through inhibition of cytokine and chemokine production or induction of immunosuppressive cell population. HSCs therefore integrate cytokine-mediated inflammatory responses in the sinusoids and relay them to the liver parenchyma, either amplifying liver inflammation or suppressing parenchymal damage through immunoregulatory signaling depending on the context.

Keywords: Hepatic stellate cells, Liver sinusoids, Inflammatory cytokines, Hepatitis

Background

The liver is not only an organ of metabolism and detoxification but also the site where active immune responses take place. It is supplied by both systemic and portal circulation; 20 % of the blood comes from the hepatic artery and 80 % from the portal vein [1]. Various toxic substances, such as bacterial components and food antigens, are absorbed from the gut and first carried into the liver via the portal vein. Indeed, the concentrations of bacterial endotoxin in the systemic circulation were significantly lower than those of the portal vein [2], showing the potent filtering capacity of the liver.

Liver sinusoids, connected directly to the portal circulation, serve as the first barrier against these noxious stimuli. They contain various cell types, including sinusoidal endothelial cells, Kupffer cells (liver macrophages), and hepatic stellate cells (HSCs). Kupffer cells and sinusoidal endothelial cells, facing the sinusoidal lumen and

in direct contact with the portal circulation, serve as the first line of defense against immune and inflammatory challenges [1, 3], producing inflammatory chemokines and cytokines and thereby attracting inflammatory cells from the systemic circulation and lymphoid organs.

HSCs reside in the space of Disse, the abluminal side of the sinusoids between liver sinusoidal endothelium and hepatocytes. They represent 5–8 % of all liver cells and 13 % of sinusoidal cells [4]. Physiological roles of HSCs include storage of vitamin A, synthesis of extracellular matrices (ECM) and matrix-degrading metalloproteinases, and regulation of sinusoidal blood flow. HSCs are regarded as pericyte equivalents in the liver. Like pericytes in other organs, HSCs are responsible for the regulation of blood flow and the production of ECM in inflammatory states. Upon liver injury, HSCs are activated, lose lipid-rich granules and transdifferentiate into α-smooth muscle actin (α-SMA)-positive myofibroblasts, which produce increased amount of ECM, and proinflammatory as well as profibrogenic cytokines, and cause liver fibrosis.

---

* Correspondence: ftom@ak.med.kyoto-u.ac.jp
Center for Innovation in Immunoregulatory Technology and Therapeutics, Faculty of Medicine, Kyoto University, Yoshida Konoecho, Sakyo-ku, Kyoto 606-8501, Japan

While the involvement of HSCs in liver fibrosis is well-recognized and attracts much attention [5], their role in liver inflammation has been little documented. Considering their anatomical position, HSCs appear to respond to inflammatory signaling from the sinusoids. HSCs from both human [6] and rodents [6, 7] produce cytokines and chemokines upon aberrant stimuli such as lipopolysaccharide (LPS) and other toxic substances, suggesting that HSCs can potentially regulate hepatic immune and inflammatory responses through their own gene expression. However, whether HSCs take part in the development of liver inflammation, and if so, whether they take on pro- or anti-inflammatory roles, is still controversial. We will review the recent findings on the roles of HSCs in acute and chronic liver inflammation.

HSCs in immune-induced hepatitis

Concanavalin A (ConA) and LPS first activate immune cells in the sinusoids upon entry into the circulation and induce liver injury through massive production of inflammatory cytokines and chemokines by intra- and extrahepatic immune cells, followed by intraparenchymal infiltration of inflammatory cells [8]. Here, we discuss the roles of HSCs in these immune-mediated liver inflammation models.

ConA-induced hepatitis

ConA is a lectin, a member of the family of carbohydrate-binding proteins. Intravenously injected ConA constitutively activates intrahepatic and systemic immune cells [9, 10]. Upon entry into the sinusoids, ConA binds to glycoproteins on the surface of Kupffer cells and sinusoidal endothelial cells. Sinusoidal endothelial cell barrier is disrupted by ConA [11, 12], which allows access of cytokines and sinusoidal cells to HSCs and hepatocytes. Inflammatory cytokines thus produced along with cells thus recruited in the liver cause massive liver injury. Among the numerous cytokines and chemokines produced in the liver, tumor necrosis factor (TNF)-α and interferon-γ (IFN-γ) are of high importance. Genetic deletion of TNF receptors [13] or IFN-γ [14] or neutralizing anti-TNF (TNF-α, lymphotoxin-α, and lymphotoxin-β) [15] or anti-IFN-γ antibody [16] attenuates ConA hepatitis in mice. In contrast to the above described roles of Kupffer cells and sinusoidal endothelial cells, contribution of HSCs to ConA hepatitis has not been investigated.

Our recent work [6] shows that HSCs receive inflammatory signals generated in the sinusoids and relay them to the liver parenchyma. In this work to clarify the role of prostaglandin D_2 (PGD$_2$) in liver pathophysiology, we found that mice deficient in PGD receptor DP1 showed exacerbated hepatitis after ConA injection, whereas administration of a DP1-specific agonist BW245C significantly suppressed liver inflammation induced by

ConA. Bone marrow chimera studies suggested that DP1 expressed in non-hematopoietic cells is the target of BW245C. Consistently, DP1 is expressed exclusively in HSCs in the liver, while PGD synthase is induced in Kupffer cells after ConA injection, suggesting that PGD$_2$ produced by Kupffer cells acts locally on HSCs to exert the protective effects. BW245C significantly suppressed intrahepatic and serum concentrations of TNF-α and IFN-γ, and DNA microarray analysis of the liver cDNA showed DP1 stimulation in HSC-inhibited expression of numerous TNF-α- and/or IFN-γ-inducible proinflammatory genes, which include *Nos2* (inducible nitric oxide synthase (iNOS)), *Tf* (tissue factor), *Edn1* (endothelin-1), *Vcam1* (vascular cell adhesion molecule-1 (VCAM-1)), and *Sele* (E-selectin). Decreased expression of these genes may have ameliorated hepatocyte damage, sinusoidal leukocyte accumulation, and hemostasis in ConA- and BW245C-treated mice.

In addition, our study also indicates that HSCs control CD4$^+$ T cell trafficking to liver parenchyma. While CD4$^+$ T cells were scattered in the parenchyma of the liver of ConA-treated mice, the cells failed to enter the liver parenchyma and formed clusters in periportal connective tissues in BW245C-administered, ConA-treated mice. Similar to skin pericytes which navigate neutrophils to the site of inflammation through intercellular adhesion molecule-1 (ICAM-1) [17], HSCs may serve as the hub for the intraparenchymal migration of CD4$^+$ T cells. Since VCAM-1 is essential in CD4$^+$ T cell adhesion on hepatic sinusoidal walls [18, 19], DP1-mediated suppression of lymphocyte migration from the periportal space to the liver parenchyma could in part be due to the decreased VCAM-1 expression by BW245C.

These findings suggest the role of HSCs in ConA-induced hepatitis as follows. Upon ConA injection, massive production of inflammatory cytokines such as TNF-α and IFN-γ occurs in the sinusoids first by Kupffer cells and T cells and secondarily by HSCs in a paracrine manner. This amplification of cytokine production leads to a series of deleterious events (see Fig. 1), all of which contribute to massive liver injury. At the same time, PGD$_2$ is produced by Kupffer cells, acts on DP1 of HSCs, and suppresses inflammatory responses to limit the amplification loop of liver inflammation. PGD$_2$-DP1 system in the liver may thus serve as the brake on constitutive hepatic inflammation that would otherwise take place due to continuous external inflammatory stimuli carried into the liver via enterohepatic circulation.

LPS/GalN-induced hepatitis

Intraperitoneal injection of LPS binds to TLR4 expressed in immune cells in the circulation and the sinusoids and activates them, which causes massive hemorrhagic liver injury through enhanced production of inflammatory

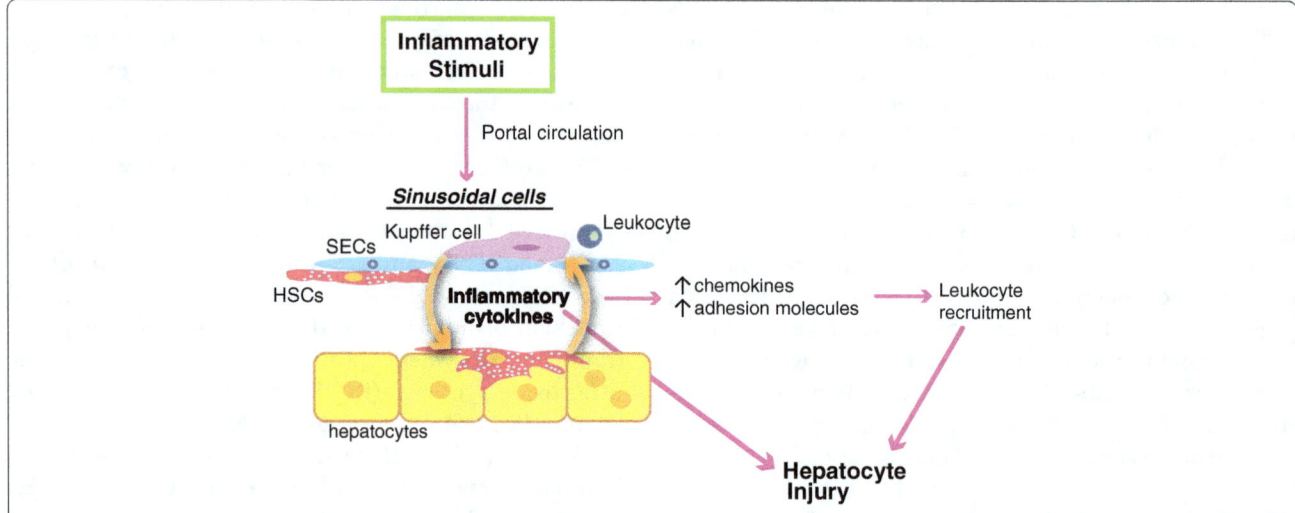

Fig. 1 Schematic diagram of the proinflammatory effects of HSCs in liver inflammation. Inflammatory signals, such as bacterial products or toxic substances entering the liver through the portal circulation, first encounter immune cells and endothelial cells in the sinusoids. Immune cells (Kupffer cells and leukocytes) produce large amount of inflammatory cytokines and chemokines, which in turn damage endothelial cells and act on HSCs. Sinusoidal inflammation amplifies in a paracrine manner, causing hepatocyte injury through cytokines themselves or through infiltration of leukocytes into the liver parenchyma

cytokines and chemokines [20]. LPS is often injected simultaneously with a hepatotoxic agent D-galactosamine (GalN) to inhibit the protein synthesis and to promote cell death in hepatocytes, and this model of hepatitis is termed LPS and D-galactosamine (LPS/GalN) liver injury [20]. We found the suppression of LPS/GalN liver injury by DP1 stimulation and concomitant decrease in systemic and intrahepatic TNF-α levels [6]. Others observed attenuated liver injury after LPS administration in HSC-depleted mice, with decreased cytokine and chemokine expression [21]. These data, along with those of ConA-induced hepatitis, suggest that HSCs are involved in the pathogenesis of liver injury initiated by sinusoidal inflammation.

HSCs in I/R liver injury

Ischemia and reperfusion (I/R) injury is a major complication of liver transplantation. It is induced by temporary liver ischemia of dissected liver graft and restoration of hepatic blood flow after transplantation. In liver transplantation, it is one of the major problems that affect the clinical outcomes [22]. During the ischemic period, hepatocytes are primarily affected by ischemia through mitochondrial damage and imbalances in pH and electrolytes. Endothelial cell damage, disturbance of microcirculation through up-regulation of a vaso-constrictive peptide endothelin-1 and its receptor endothelin-A receptor, and Kupffer cell activation also ensue. These lead to liver inflammation and injury through massive increase in reactive oxygen species and inflammatory mediators [22]. Reperfusion injury mainly involves reactive oxygen species generation by

endothelial cells and neutrophils triggered by the reentry of oxygen into the liver tissue. During I/R liver injury, HSCs contribute to microcirculatory disturbances by acquiring a contractile phenotype through activation by inflammatory mediators [22].

Although HSCs have direct access to immune cells in the sinusoids due to endothelial cell damage, their role in the regulation of sinusoidal inflammation has not been studied in detail. However, several recent reports point to the proinflammatory properties of HSCs in I/R liver injury. A model for depleting HSCs was developed to elucidate the role of HSCs in I/R liver injury [21]. Transgenic mice expressing the herpes simplex virus thymidine kinase gene driven by the mouse GFAP promotor were treated with carbon tetrachloride to induce HSC proliferation and render them susceptible to cell killing induced by subsequent ganciclovir treatment. This method resulted in depletion of 64–72 % of HSCs. Liver injury caused by I/R, along with TNF-α, CXCL1, and endothelin-A receptor expression, was attenuated in HSC-depleted mice compared with controls. Histological studies further revealed decreased neutrophil infiltration and parenchymal cell death. These findings suggest that HSCs are, at least in part, involved in hepatic production of CXCL1 and contribute to neutrophil recruitment and microcirculatory failure caused by endothelin-A receptor stimulation.

Another group activated or depleted HSCs through pharmacological activation of endocannabinoid receptors CB1 or CB2, respectively [23], and examined their roles in I/R liver injury. CB1 stimulation activates HSCs and enhances liver fibrosis whereas that of CB2 causes

HSC apoptosis [24], as evaluated by immunostaining for α-SMA. They first found that, after reperfusion, more than 25 % of CD4+ T cells adhering to the sinusoidal walls colocalized with HSCs in vehicle-treated mice. Activation of HSCs with a CB1 agonist increased non-perfused liver areas with no significant changes in CD4+ T cell recruitment, whereas their depletion with a CB2 agonist resulted in the attenuation of CD4+ T cell infiltration and reduced sinusoidal perfusion failure and liver enzyme activities. These data show that CD4+ T cells interact with HSCs before entering the hepatic parenchyma and suggest the possibility that HSCs may serve as sentinels in T cell migration into the parenchyma [23]. Hepatoprotective property of HSCs is also observed [25]. Adoptive transfer of HSCs induced the expansion of regulatory T cells (Treg cells) in the liver and provided partial protection against I/R liver injury, and depletion of Treg cells abolished the protective effect of HSCs, suggesting the cross talk between HSCs and Treg cells in hepatoprotection [25]. Further studies are required to define the precise roles of HSCs in I/R liver injury and delineate the spatiotemporal regulation of their actions.

HSCs in NASH

Nonalcoholic steatohepatitis (NASH) is distinguished from nonalcoholic fatty liver in that NASH is characterized by the presence of intrahepatic inflammation accompanied by hepatocyte damage with or without fibrosis [26]. Upon liver injury, various liver resident cells such as Kupffer cells and HSCs are activated and, at the same time, inflammatory cells are recruited into the liver. This results in the amplification of intrahepatic inflammation and hepatocyte damage progresses further, leading to tissue fibrosis in some cases. Increased intestinal permeability is recently highlighted as a primary cause of liver injury in NASH [27]. Gut microbiota easily flow into the liver through the portal circulation, thus activating Toll-like receptors (TLRs) in liver cells, TLR4 in particular [28]. There have been numerous reports on the important roles of TLR4, which binds LPS. Serum LPS levels are elevated in patients with NASH and in animal models of NASH [29, 30], suggesting the activation of TLR4. TLR4 activation in HSCs induces the production of chemokines and the expression of adhesion molecules ICAM-1 and VCAM-1 [31, 32]. Furthermore, TLR4 signaling in HSCs promotes the interaction between HSCs and Kupffer cells by promoting the chemotaxis of Kupffer cells and up-regulating the expression of adhesion molecules in HSCs [32]. Down-regulation of transforming growth factor (TGF)-β pseudoreceptor BAMBI also occurs in HSCs by TLR4 ligation and activates TGF-β signaling, resulting in increased ECM production by HSCs and resulting fibrosis [32]. These findings provide evidence that HSCs are actively involved in the intrahepatic inflammation in NASH.

HSCs in viral hepatitis

Hepatitis B and C virus (HBV and HCV, respectively) are main causes of chronic hepatitis and cirrhosis. In some patients, hepatocellular carcinoma (HCC) ensues, which in many cases is difficult to treat [33]. Hepatitis viruses replicate primarily in hepatocytes, causing mitochondrial injury and reactive oxygen species (ROS) formation [34]. Then, viral peptides presented with HLA elicit acquired immune responses by T cells [35]. Resident macrophages (Kupffer cells) and other immune cells recruited into the liver produce ROS and inflammatory as well as fibrogenic mediators. This results in the activation of HSCs accompanied by increased collagen synthesis [34].

Accumulating evidence suggests that HSCs play a role in HCV-induced chronic hepatitis [36]. The cross talk between HCV-infected hepatocytes and HSCs is demonstrated in an in vitro study [37]. Coculture of HSCs and HCV-infected hepatocytes induced CCL3 production by HCV-infected hepatocytes, which was mediated by HSC-derived IL-1α. IL-1α induces acute-phase response in the liver [38], and its expression is augmented in the liver of HCV-infected patients [39]. HCV proteins themselves can also elicit inflammatory and fibrogenic responses by HSCs [40]. HCV core protein induces cell proliferation and nonstructural proteins augment ICAM-1 expression and chemokine production through the NF-κB and c-Jun N-terminal kinase pathways in activated HSCs [40]. Finally, in the liver of chronic hepatitis C patients, CCR7 on HSCs induced cell migration and activation of several inflammatory pathways in response to CCL21 secreted by activated dendritic cells, resulting in induction of proinflammatory genes in HSCs [41].

HSCs in HCC

HCC develops from several underlying diseases, such as viral hepatitis, alcoholic liver diseases, and NASH. The vast majority of HCC cases are preceded by liver fibrosis, with 90 % of hepatoma arising from cirrhotic livers [42]. Activated HSCs residing in the fibrous tissue, along with immune cells, contribute to the formation of tumor microenvironment favorable for tumor growth [43]. Tumor microenvironment is a mixture of tumor cells, stromal cells, and inflammatory molecules and ECM produced from the stromal cells, mainly HSCs in the case of HCC. Activated HSCs in the tumor stroma continuously produce ECM. Dysregulation of tissue inhibitor of metalloproteinases 1 (TIMP-1), which favors matrix deposition, and matrix metalloproteinases (MMPs), which degrade ECM, leads to increased collagen I deposition in the stroma and contributes to HCC progression [42, 44, 45]. HSCs in active state also produce soluble factors favoring tumor growth, such as hepatocyte growth factor and TGF-β [42], and proangiogenic factors such as vascular endothelial growth factor-A (VEGF-A) and MMP9 [46]. Malignant hepatocytes, in turn, produce inflammatory cytokines and chemokines that promote the survival of activated HSCs. HCC-HSC cross talk is vital in forming a tumor microenvironment that contributes to HCC survival and progression. In another concept, HSCs favor the survival and expansion of immunosuppressive cell populations. HSCs cause imbalance of T cell population by accelerating activated T cell apoptosis and expanding Treg cells [47–49]. Consistent with the above findings, HSCs cotransplanted with HCC cells support the implantation and growth of implanted tumor cells [47, 50].

HCC emerges from non-cirrhotic liver as well, notably in nonalcoholic fatty liver diseases including NASH [51]. Here, carcinogenesis has been linked to the secretion of inflammatory cytokines from adipose tissue, lipid accumulation in hepatocytes, and resulting hyperinsulinemia [51]. Unlike HCC resulting from chronic viral hepatitis, hepatoma cells in non-cirrhotic HCC are well-differentiated and tumors grow in a large nodular pattern [52]. It has been argued that HSCs may play only a minor role in this type of HCC, since larger liver nodules may be associated with diminished formation of fibrotic septa and therefore attenuation of HSC activation [51]. However, a recent study by Yoshimoto et al. associates prolonged activation of HSC and HCC development in obese mice without preceding cirrhosis [53]. They found that obesity alters gut microbiota and their metabolic product entered the liver through enterohepatic circulation, thus promoting hepatocarcinogenesis through sustained secretion of inflammatory mediators by HSCs. It should be noted that, in this model, chronic inflammation mainly contributes to hepatocarcinogenesis. This study shows the crucial role of HSCs as a bridge connecting intestinal flora and liver parenchyma in chronic liver inflammation.

Conclusions

HSCs have traditionally been studied in the context of liver fibrosis. However, as reviewed here, recent studies show that they actively participate in liver inflammation by sensing external signals, producing inflammatory cytokines, and navigating T lymphocytes into the parenchyma (Fig. 1). In some context, HSCs can elicit anti-inflammatory actions as seen in DP1 stimulation in ConA-induced hepatitis and expansion of immunosuppressive cells in I/R liver injury and HCC. Further studies are required to elucidate the unexplored roles of HSCs in the development of hepatitis and clarify the factors that regulate different phenotypes of HSCs. As pericyte equivalents, further understanding of the physiology and inflammatory responses of HSCs will provide deeper insights into the actions of pericytes also in other organs and provide novel therapeutic targets in the treatment of inflammatory diseases of many organs including liver.

Abbreviations

ConA: concanavalin A; ECM: extracellular matrix; HBV: hepatitis B virus; HCC: hepatocellular carcinoma; HCV: hepatitis C virus; HSCs: hepatic stellate cells; I/R: ischemia and reperfusion; ICAM-1: intercellular adhesion molecule-1; IFN-γ: interferon-γ; iNOS: inducible nitric oxide synthase; LPS: lipopolysaccharide; LPS/GalN: LPS and D-galactosamine; MMP: metalloproteinase; NASH: nonalcoholic steatohepatitis; PGD$_2$: prostaglandin D$_2$; ROS: reactive oxygen species; TGF-β: transforming growth factor-β; TIMP-1: tissue inhibitor of metalloproteinases-1; TLR: Toll-like receptor; TNF: tumor necrosis factor; Treg cells: regulatory T cells; VCAM-1: vascular cell adhesion molecule-1; VEGF-A: vascular endothelial growth factor-A; α-SMA: α-smooth muscle actin.

Competing interests

The authors are employed by the Coordination Fund from the Japan Science and Technology Agency and Astellas Pharma. The authors have no additional conflict of interests.

Authors' contributions

TF planned and conducted the research [6] and wrote the manuscript. SN supervised the research [6] and wrote the manuscript. This review was written by TF and SN. Both authors read and approved the final manuscript.

Acknowledgements

The authors thank Dr. Keiko Iwaisako (Target Therapy Oncology, Faculty of Medicine, Kyoto University), Dr. Masataka Asagiri, and Dr. Catharina Sagita Moniaga (Center for Innovation in Immunoregulatory Technology and Therapeutics, Faculty of Medicine, Kyoto University) for their helpful discussion.

Funding

Studies by Fujita et al. [6] were funded by the Coordination Fund from the Japan Science and Technology Agency and Astellas Pharma.

References

1. Jenne CN, Kubes P. Immune surveillance by the liver. Nat Immunol. 2013;14:996–1006.
2. Lumsden AB, Henderson JM, Kutner MH. Endotoxin levels measured by a chromogenic assay in portal, hepatic and peripheral venous blood in patients with cirrhosis. Hepatology. 1988;8:232–6.
3. Vollmar B, Menger MD. The hepatic microcirculation: mechanistic contributions and therapeutic targets in liver injury and repair. Physiol Rev. 2009;89:1269–339.
4. Reynaert H, Thompson MG, Thomas T, Geerts A. Hepatic stellate cells: role in microcirculation and pathophysiology of portal hypertension. Gut. 2002;50:571–81.
5. Bataller R, Brenner DA. Liver fibrosis. J Clin Invest. 2005;115:209–18.
6. Fujita T, Soontrapa K, Ito Y, Iwaisako K, Moniaga CS, Asagiri M, et al. Hepatic stellate cells relay inflammation signaling from sinusoids to parenchyma in mouse models of immune-mediated hepatitis. Hepatology. 2016;63:1325–39.
7. Harvey SA, Dangi A, Tandon A, Gandhi CR. The transcriptomic response of rat hepatic stellate cells to endotoxin: implications for hepatic inflammation and immune regulation. PLoS ONE. 2013;8:e82159.
8. Schumann J, Tiegs G. Pathophysiological mechanisms of TNF during intoxication with natural or man-made toxins. Toxicology. 1999;138:103–26.
9. Heymann F, Hamesch K, Weiskirchen R, Tacke F. The concanavalin A model of acute hepatitis in mice. Lab Anim. 2015;49:12–20.
10. Tiegs G, Hentschel J, Wendel A. A T cell-dependent experimental liver injury in mice inducible by concanavalin A. J Clin Invest. 1992;90:196–203.
11. Yang MC, Chang CP, Lei HY. Endothelial cells are damaged by autophagic induction before hepatocytes in Con A-induced acute hepatitis. Int Immunol. 2010;22:661–70.
12. Knolle PA, Gerken G, Loser E, Dienes HP, Gantner F, Tiegs G, et al. Role of sinusoidal endothelial cells of the liver in concanavalin A-induced hepatic injury in mice. Hepatology. 1996;24:824–9.
13. Maeda S, Chang L, Li ZW, Luo JL, Leffert H, Karin M. IKKbeta is required for prevention of apoptosis mediated by cell-bound but not by circulating TNFalpha. Immunity. 2003;19:725–37.

14. Tagawa Y, Sekikawa K, Iwakura Y. Suppression of concanavalin A-induced hepatitis in IFN-gamma(-/-) mice, but not in TNF-alpha(-/-) mice: role for IFN-gamma in activating apoptosis of hepatocytes. J Immunol. 1997;159:1418–28.

15. Mizuhara H, O'Neill E, Seki N, Ogawa T, Kusunoki C, Otsuka K, et al. T cell activation-associated hepatic injury: mediation by tumor necrosis factors and protection by interleukin 6. J Exp Med. 1994;179:1529–37.

16. Mizuhara H, Uno M, Seki N, Yamashita M, Yamaoka M, Ogawa T, et al. Critical involvement of interferon gamma in the pathogenesis of T-cell activation-associated hepatitis and regulatory mechanisms of interleukin-6 for the manifestations of hepatitis. Hepatology. 1996;23:1608–15.

17. Stark K, Eckart A, Haidari S, Tirniceriu A, Lorenz M, von Bruhl ML, et al. Capillary and arteriolar pericytes attract innate leukocytes exiting through venules and 'instruct' them with pattern-recognition and motility programs. Nat Immunol. 2013;14:41–51.

18. Morikawa H, Hachiya K, Mizuhara H, Fujiwara H, Nishiguchi S, Shiomi S, et al. Sublobular veins as the main site of lymphocyte adhesion/transmigration and adhesion molecule expression in the porto-sinusoidal-hepatic venous system during concanavalin A-induced hepatitis in mice. Hepatology. 2000;31:83–94.

19. Wolf D, Hallmann R, Sass G, Sixt M, Kusters S, Fregien B, et al. TNF-alpha-induced expression of adhesion molecules in the liver is under the control of TNFR1—relevance for concanavalin A-induced hepatitis. J Immunol. 2001;166:1300–7.

20. Hamesch K, Borkham-Kamphorst E, Strnad P, Weiskirchen R. Lipopolysaccharide-induced inflammatory liver injury in mice. Lab Anim. 2015;49:37–46.

21. Stewart RK, Dangi A, Huang C, Murase N, Kimura S, Stolz DB, et al. A novel mouse model of depletion of stellate cells clarifies their role in ischemia/reperfusion- and endotoxin-induced acute liver injury. J Hepatol. 2014;60:298–305.

22. Peralta C, Jimenez-Castro MB, Gracia-Sancho J. Hepatic ischemia and reperfusion injury: effects on the liver sinusoidal milieu. J Hepatol. 2013;59:1094–106.

23. Reifart J, Rentsch M, Mende K, Coletti R, Sobocan M, Thasler WE, et al. Modulating CD4+ T cell migration in the postischemic liver: hepatic stellate cells as new therapeutic target? Transplantation. 2015;99:41–7.

24. Siegmund SV, Schwabe RF. Endocannabinoids and liver disease. II. Endocannabinoids in the pathogenesis and treatment of liver fibrosis. Am J Physiol Gastrointest Liver Physiol. 2008;294:G357–62.

25. Feng M, Wang Q, Wang H, Wang M, Guan W, Lu L. Adoptive transfer of hepatic stellate cells ameliorates liver ischemia reperfusion injury through enriching regulatory T cells. Int Immunopharmacol. 2014;19:267–74.

26. Sharma M, Mitnala S, Vishnubhotla RK, Mukherjee R, Reddy DN, Rao PN. The riddle of nonalcoholic fatty liver disease: progression from nonalcoholic fatty liver to nonalcoholic steatohepatitis. J Clin Exp Hepatol. 2015;5:147–58.

27. Seki E, Schnabl B. Role of innate immunity and the microbiota in liver fibrosis: crosstalk between the liver and gut. J Physiol. 2012;590:447–58.

28. Ganz M, Szabo G. Immune and inflammatory pathways in NASH. Hepatol Int. 2013;7 Suppl 2:771–81.

29. Miele L, Valenza V, La Torre G, Montalto M, Cammarota G, Ricci R, et al. Increased intestinal permeability and tight junction alterations in nonalcoholic fatty liver disease. Hepatology. 2009;49:1877–87.

30. Cani PD, Amar J, Iglesias MA, Poggi M, Knauf C, Bastelica D, et al. Metabolic endotoxemia initiates obesity and insulin resistance. Diabetes. 2007;56:1761–72.

31. Paik YH, Schwabe RF, Bataller R, Russo MP, Jobin C, Brenner DA. Toll-like receptor 4 mediates inflammatory signaling by bacterial lipopolysaccharide in human hepatic stellate cells. Hepatology. 2003;37:1043–55.

32. Seki E, De Minicis S, Osterreicher CH, Kluwe J, Osawa Y, Brenner DA, et al. TLR4 enhances TGF-beta signaling and hepatic fibrosis. Nat Med. 2007;13:1324–32.

33. Bartosch B, Thimme R, Blum HE, Zoulim F. Hepatitis C virus-induced hepatocarcinogenesis. J Hepatol. 2009;51:810–20.

34. Bataller R, Lemon SM. Fueling fibrosis in chronic hepatitis C. Proc Natl Acad Sci U S A. 2012;109:14293–4.

35. Walker CM. Adaptive immunity to the hepatitis C virus. Adv Virus Res. 2010;78:43–86.

36. Seki E, Schwabe RF. Hepatic inflammation and fibrosis: functional links and key pathways. Hepatology. 2015;61:1066–79.

37. Nishitsuji H, Funami K, Shimizu Y, Ujino S, Sugiyama K, Seya T, et al. Hepatitis C virus infection induces inflammatory cytokines and chemokines mediated by the cross talk between hepatocytes and stellate cells. J Virol. 2013;87:8169–78.

38. Moshage H. Cytokines and the hepatic acute phase response. J Pathol. 1997;181:257–66.

39. Kasprzak A, Zabel M, Biczysko W, Wysocki J, Adamek A, Spachacz R, et al. Expression of cytokines (TNF-alpha, IL-1alpha, and IL-2) in chronic hepatitis C: comparative hybridocytochemical and immunocytochemical study in children and adult patients. J Histochem Cytochem. 2004;52:29–38.

40. Bataller R, Paik YH, Lindquist JN, Lemasters JJ, Brenner DA. Hepatitis C virus core and nonstructural proteins induce fibrogenic effects in hepatic stellate cells. Gastroenterology. 2004;126:529–40.

41. Bonacchi A, Petrai I, Defranco RM, Lazzeri E, Annunziato F, Efsen E, et al. The chemokine CCL21 modulates lymphocyte recruitment and fibrosis in chronic hepatitis C. Gastroenterology. 2003;125:1060–76.

42. Thompson AI, Conroy KP, Henderson NC. Hepatic stellate cells: central modulators of hepatic carcinogenesis. BMC Gastroenterol. 2015;15:63.

43. Hernandez-Gea V, Toffanin S, Friedman SL, Llovet JM. Role of the microenvironment in the pathogenesis and treatment of hepatocellular carcinoma. Gastroenterology. 2013;144:512–27.

44. Zhou X, Jamil A, Nash A, Chan J, Trim N, Iredale JP, et al. Impaired proteolysis of collagen I inhibits proliferation of hepatic stellate cells: implications for regulation of liver fibrosis. J Biol Chem. 2006;281:39757–65.

45. Theret N, Musso O, Turlin B, Lotrian D, Bioulac-Sage P, Campion JP, et al. Increased extracellular matrix remodeling is associated with tumor progression in human hepatocellular carcinomas. Hepatology. 2001;34:82–8.

46. Coulouarn C, Corlu A, Glaise D, Guenon I, Thorgeirsson SS, Clement B. Hepatocyte-stellate cell cross-talk in the liver engenders a permissive inflammatory microenvironment that drives progression in hepatocellular carcinoma. Cancer Res. 2012;72:2533–42.

47. Zhao W, Su W, Kuang P, Zhang L, Liu J, Yin Z, et al. The role of hepatic stellate cells in the regulation of T-cell function and the promotion of hepatocellular carcinoma. Int J Oncol. 2012;41:457–64.

48. Zhao W, Zhang L, Xu Y, Zhang Z, Ren G, Tang K, et al. Hepatic stellate cells promote tumor progression by enhancement of immunosuppressive cells in an orthotopic liver tumor mouse model. Lab Invest. 2014;94:182–91.

49. Xu Y, Zhao W, Xu J, Li J, Hong Z, Yin Z, et al. Activated hepatic stellate cells promote liver cancer by induction of myeloid-derived suppressor cells through cyclooxygenase-2. Oncotarget. 2016.

50. Amann T, Bataille F, Spruss T, Muhlbauer M, Gabele E, Scholmerich J, et al. Activated hepatic stellate cells promote tumorigenicity of hepatocellular carcinoma. Cancer Sci. 2009;100:646–53.

51. Baffy G, Brunt EM, Caldwell SH. Hepatocellular carcinoma in non-alcoholic fatty liver disease: an emerging menace. J Hepatol. 2012;56:1384–91.

52. Hytiroglou P, Park YN, Krinsky G, Theise ND. Hepatic precancerous lesions and small hepatocellular carcinoma. Gastroenterol Clin North Am. 2007;36:867–87. vii.

53. Yoshimoto S, Loo TM, Atarashi K, Kanda H, Sato S, Oyadomari S, et al. Obesity-induced gut microbial metabolite promotes liver cancer through senescence secretome. Nature. 2013;499:97–101.

7

The roles of RGMa-neogenin signaling in inflammation and angiogenesis

Yuki Fujita[*] and Toshihide Yamashita[*]

Abstract

Repulsive guidance molecule (RGM) is a glycosylphosphatidylinositol (GPI)-anchored glycoprotein that has diverse functions in the developing and pathological central nervous system (CNS). The binding of RGM to its receptor neogenin regulates axon guidance, neuronal differentiation, and survival during the development of the CNS. In the pathological state, RGM expression is induced after spinal cord injury, and the inhibition of RGM promotes axon growth and functional recovery. Furthermore, RGM expression is also observed in immune cells, and RGM regulates inflammation and neurodegeneration in autoimmune encephalomyelitis. RGMa induces T cell activation in experimental autoimmune encephalomyelitis (EAE), which is the animal model of multiple sclerosis (MS). RGM is expressed in pathogenic Th17 cells and induces neurodegeneration by binding to neogenin. Angiogenesis is an additional key factor involved in the pathophysiology of EAE. Via neogenin, treatment with RGMa can suppress endothelial tube formation; this finding indicates that RGMa inhibits neovascularization. These observations suggest the feasibility of utilizing the RGMa-neogenin signaling pathway as a therapeutic target to overcome inflammation and neurodegeneration. This review focuses on the molecular mechanisms of inflammation and angiogenesis via RGM-neogenin signaling.

Keywords: RGMa, Neogenin, Immune response, Angiogenesis, Multiple sclerosis

Background

Repulsive guidance molecule (RGM) is a glycosylphosphatidylinositol (GPI)-anchored glycoprotein with an N-terminal signal peptide, an Arg-Gly-Asp site, a partial von Willebrand type D domain, and a hydrophobic domain of unknown function [1]. RGM was originally identified as an axon repellent in the chick retinotectal system [2, 3]. Neogenin, the receptor for RGM and netrins, is widely expressed in both embryonic and adult tissues and mediates various functions [4, 5]. There are three homologs of RGM in vertebrates: RGMa, RGMb (DRAGON), and RGMc (hemojuvelin). The homologies of chick RGM to mouse RGMa, RGMb, and RGMc are 78, 43, and 40%, respectively.

The binding of RGMa to neogenin regulates axon guidance, neuronal differentiation, and survival during the development of the central nervous system (CNS) [6–8]. Although RGMa expression levels are relatively low in the adult CNS, RGMa expression is induced following ischemic stroke in humans and spinal cord injury in rats [9, 10]. In an animal model of spinal cord injury, treatment with an RGMa-neutralizing antibody at the lesion site significantly enhances axon regeneration and motor function recovery [11]. Because the stimulation of neurons with RGMa induces RhoA and ROCK (Rho-associated coiled-coil-containing protein kinase), resulting in axon growth inhibition, the effect of this antibody may be dependent on the inhibition of this signaling pathway.

In addition to its aforementioned roles, RGMa is involved in neuroinflammatory diseases. The notion that the pathogenesis of multiple sclerosis (MS) is associated with acquired autoimmunity to the CNS has been widely accepted. In MS, immune cells infiltrate the CNS and attack myelin sheaths, leading to demyelination, axonal damage, and neurological disabilities [12, 13]. CD4+ T cells are critical effector cells in CNS inflammation [14]. Interestingly, the inhibition of RGMa via a neutralizing antibody reduces cytokine production, demyelination, and neurodegeneration and relieves neurological deficits

* Correspondence: yuki-fujita@molneu.med.osaka-u.ac.jp;
yamashita@molneu.med.osaka-u.ac.jp
Department of Molecular Neuroscience, Graduate School of Medicine, Osaka University, 2-2 Yamadaoka, Suita, Osaka, Japan

in experimental autoimmune encephalomyelitis (EAE) [15, 16]. In addition to its role in neuroimmune interactions, RGMa inhibits angiogenesis, which is often accompanied by inflammation, as mentioned below.

Thus, these findings indicate that the RGM-neogenin signaling pathway is strongly associated with disease severity in neuroinflammatory diseases. In this review, we introduce the pivotal role of RGMa in inflammation and angiogenesis and discuss the potential therapeutic implications of targeting this signaling.

The RGMa-neogenin pathway mediates auto-immune encephalomyelitis

Although the RGM-neogenin interaction mediates diverse functions in the developing and adult CNS, we also found that RGMa was expressed in bone marrow-derived dendritic cells and that neogenin was expressed in CD4+ T cells. Based on these observations, we assessed the role of RGMa in immune systems and found that the inhibition of RGMa suppressed the T cell response and attenuated the severity of EAE [15]. RGMa treatment of CD4+ T cells induces the activation of the small GTPase Rap1 and increases the adhesion of CD4+ T cells to intracellular adhesion molecule-1 (ICAM-1). Treatment with an RGMa-neutralizing antibody attenuates the clinical severity of myelin oligodendrocyte glycoprotein (MOG)-induced EAE and diminishes relapses in proteolipid protein (PLP)-induced EAE. In humans, an RGMa-specific antibody reduces T cell proliferation and pro-inflammatory cytokine production in peripheral blood mononuclear cells (PBMCs) from individuals with MS. Thus, the RGMa-neogenin signaling pathway is involved in T cell-mediated autoimmune processes in MS (Fig. 1).

Interferon-gamma (IFN-γ)-producing Th1 cells were initially regarded as a predominant effector CD4+ T cell subset that induces the pathogenesis of MS [17]. More recently, interleukin-23 (IL-23) has been shown to be required for the induction of EAE [18] and the pathogenic activity of T helper type 17 (Th17) cells. The key role of IL-17-producing Th17 cells in the pathogenesis of EAE has been established [19]. Indeed, a deficiency of IL-17, IL-17 receptor, or IL-23 receptor diminishes clinical signs in EAE [20–22]. Interestingly, among T cell subsets, including Th0, Th1, Th17, and Treg cells, Th17 cells highly express RGMa. The specific function of RGMa in Th17 cells was determined to be involved in neurodegeneration in EAE [16]. In particular, in Th17 cells, RGMa binds to neogenin and induces Akt dephosphorylation and axonal degeneration (Fig. 2). An RGMa-specific neutralizing antibody diminished neuronal damage and alleviated clinical symptoms of Th17-induced EAE. Taken together, these observations suggest that RGMa could be a therapeutic target for MS. Polymorphisms of RGMa have been correlated with expression changes in IFN-γ and tumor necrosis factor (TNF) in MS patients [23]. This finding raises the intriguing possibility of an association between genetic susceptibility in MS pathogenesis and RGMa.

Angiogenesis via the RGMa-neogenin pathway

In MS, in addition to various prominent features, such as inflammation, demyelination, and axonal damage, neovascularization is found in inflammatory lesions. In EAE, an angiogenic response is observed following alterations in blood-brain barrier (BBB) permeability and the release of vascular endothelial growth factor (VEGF) [24, 25]. Both detrimental and beneficial effects have been reported in angiogenesis. Since the angiogenic response is related to excess energy consumption and the expansion of inflammation, this response's pathological contributions to the disease progression of MS and EAE are widely accepted [26]. However, trophic factors from new vessels exert positive effects on the nervous systems. VEGF derived from new blood vessels exhibits pro-inflammatory effects

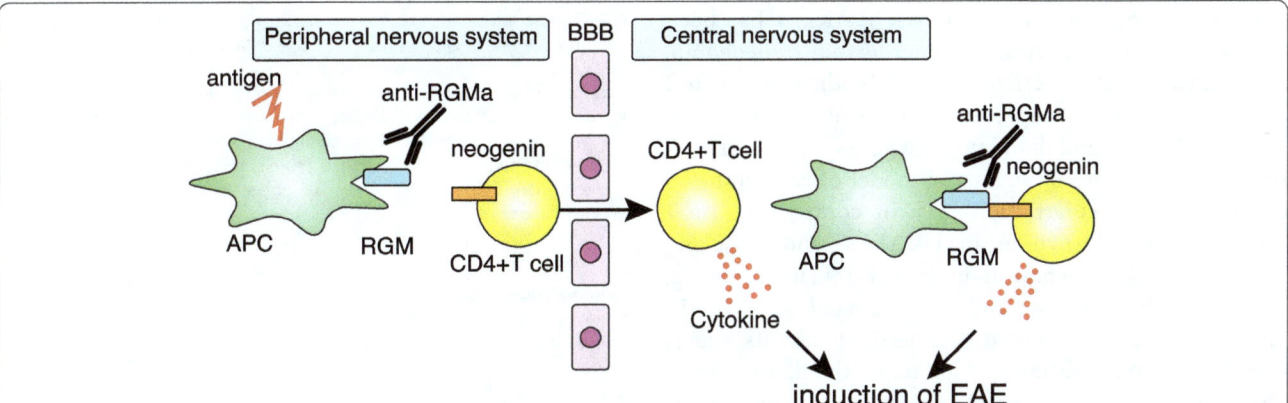

Fig. 1 RGMa-neogenin signaling mediates autoimmune encephalomyelitis. RGMa in antigen-presenting cells (APCs) binds to neogenin, leading to the activation of CD4+ T cells in both the peripheral and the central nervous systems. Blocking RGMa with a neutralizing antibody diminishes immune responses and ameliorates the severity of EAE

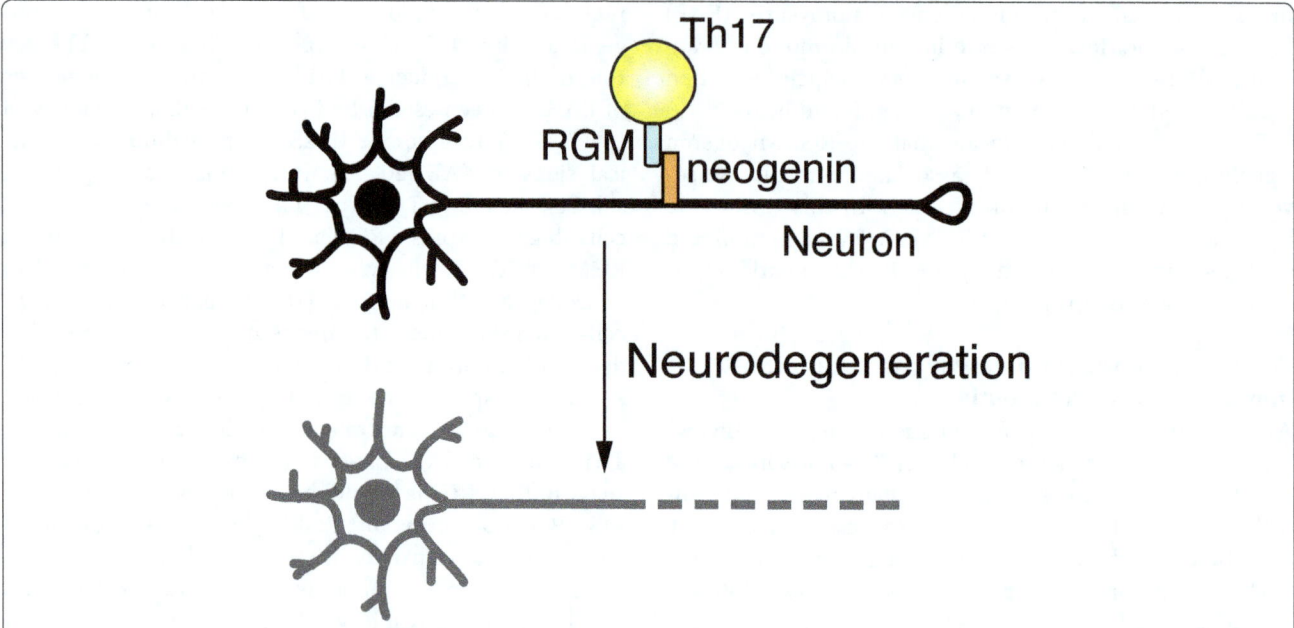

Fig. 2 RGMa in Th17 cells induces neurodegeneration. RGMa is preferentially expressed in Th17 cells. The association of RGMa with neogenin in neurons induces neurodegeneration through the dephosphorylation of Akt

during the early phase of EAE but is involved in repair processes during the late phase of EAE. VEGF mediates the proliferation, migration, and differentiation of neural progenitors and the survival and migration of oligodendrocyte precursor cells [27, 28]. Prostaglandin I_2 (PGI$_2$) produced from new blood vessels is associated with motor recovery in EAE [29]. Thus, specific molecules derived from new vascular cells can be therapeutic targets for MS.

We have shown that RGMa inhibits angiogenesis via neogenin [30]. In the presence of VEGF, RGMa suppresses endothelial tube formation by human umbilical artery endothelial cells (HUAECs), and this effect could be partially reversed by knocking down neogenin. RGMa treatment of HUAECs decreased VEGF-induced phosphorylation of focal adhesion kinase (FAK). It has been demonstrated that netrins, the other ligands of neogenin, also regulate neovascularization. The binding of netrin-4 to neogenin causes neogenin to associate with its co-receptor Unc5b and inhibits angiogenesis both in cultured HUAECs and in an animal model of laser-induced choroidal neovascularization [31]. In contrast, netrin-1 promotes tube formation in HUAECs, and knocking down netrin-1 in zebrafish inhibits vascular sprouting, suggesting that netrin-1 induces angiogenesis [32–34]. However, it is also reported that netrin-1 inhibits angiogenesis via the activation of Unc5b and the disruption of Unc5b induces excess vessel branching and the extension of endothelial filopodia [35, 36]. Netrin-4 binds only to neogenin, whereas netrin-1 is predicted to interact with neogenin, Unc5b, and Unc5c. Differences in

binding affinity to neogenin might be responsible for these proteins' different effects on angiogenesis.

Conclusions

Here, we reviewed the role of RGMa in inflammation and angiogenesis, particularly in MS. Since RGMa mediates both immune responses and neurodegeneration in EAE, the inhibition of RGMa could be a promising therapeutic intervention for MS. Further research will establish the feasibility of an anti-RGMa antibody for treating MS.

Abbreviations
BBB: Blood-brain barrier; CNS: Central nervous systems; EAE: Experimental autoimmune encephalomyelitis; FAK: Focal adhesion kinase; GPI: Glycosylphosphatidylinositol; HUAECs: Human umbilical artery endothelial cells; ICAM-1: Intracellular adhesion molecule-1; IFN-γ: Interferon-gamma; IL: Interleukin; MOG: Myelin oligodendrocyte glycoprotein; MS: Multiple sclerosis; PBMCs: Peripheral blood mononuclear cells; PGI₂: Prostaglandin I₂; PLP: Proteolipid protein; RGM: Repulsive guidance molecule; Th1: T helper type 1; TNF: Tumor necrosis factor; VEGF: Vascular endothelial growth factor

Acknowledgements
We are grateful to all the Yamashita's lab members for the critical discussions.

Funding
This work was supported by funding to TY from the Practical Research Project for Rare/Intractable Diseases from the Japan Agency for Medical Research and Development (AMED).

Authors' contributions
YF and TY wrote the manuscript. Both authors read and approved the final manuscript.

Competing interests
The authors declare that they have no competing interests.

References
1. Yamashita T, Mueller BK, Hata K. Neogenin and repulsive guidance molecule signaling in the central nervous system. Curr Opin Neurobiol. 2007;17:29–34.
2. Monnier PP, Sierra A, Macchi P, Deitinghoff L, Andersen JS, Mann M, Flad M, Hornberger MR, Stahl B, Bonhoeffer F, et al. RGM is a repulsive guidance molecule for retinal axons. Nature. 2002;419:392–5.
3. Stahl B, Muller B, von Boxberg Y, Cox EC, Bonhoeffer F. Biochemical characterization of a putative axonal guidance molecule of the chick visual system. Neuron. 1990;5:735–43.
4. De Vries M, Cooper HM. Emerging roles for neogenin and its ligands in CNS development. J Neurochem. 2008;106:1483–92.
5. Mueller BK, Yamashita T, Schaffar G, Mueller R. The role of repulsive guidance molecules in the embryonic and adult vertebrate central nervous system. Philos Trans R Soc Lond B Biol Sci. 2006;361:1513–29.
6. Matsunaga E, Tauszig-Delamasure S, Monnier PP, Mueller BK, Strittmatter SM, Mehlen P, Chedotal A. RGM and its receptor neogenin regulate neuronal survival. Nat Cell Biol. 2004;6:749–55.
7. Rajagopalan S, Deitinghoff L, Davis D, Conrad S, Skutella T, Chedotal A, Mueller BK, Strittmatter SM. Neogenin mediates the action of repulsive guidance molecule. Nat Cell Biol. 2004;6:756–62.
8. Wilson NH, Key B. Neogenin interacts with RGMa and netrin-1 to guide axons within the embryonic vertebrate forebrain. Dev Biol. 2006;296:485–98.
9. Schwab JM, Conrad S, Monnier PP, Julien S, Mueller BK, Schluesener HJ. Spinal cord injury-induced lesional expression of the repulsive guidance molecule (RGM). Eur J Neurosci. 2005;21:1569–76.
10. Schwab JM, Monnier PP, Schluesener HJ, Conrad S, Beschorner R, Chen L, Meyermann R, Mueller BK. Central nervous system injury-induced repulsive guidance molecule expression in the adult human brain. Arch Neurol. 2005;62:1561–8.
11. Hata K, Fujitani M, Yasuda Y, Doya H, Saito T, Yamagishi S, Mueller BK, Yamashita T. RGMa inhibition promotes axonal growth and recovery after spinal cord injury. J Cell Biol. 2006;173:47–58.
12. Hauser SL, Oksenberg JR. The neurobiology of multiple sclerosis: genes, inflammation, and neurodegeneration. Neuron. 2006;52:61–76.
13. Trapp BD, Nave KA. Multiple sclerosis: an immune or neurodegenerative disorder? Annu Rev Neurosci. 2008;31:247–69.
14. Goverman J. Autoimmune T cell responses in the central nervous system. Nat Rev Immunol. 2009;9:393–407.
15. Muramatsu R, Kubo T, Mori M, Nakamura Y, Fujita Y, Akutsu T, Okuno T, Taniguchi J, Kumanogoh A, Yoshida M, et al. RGMa modulates T cell responses and is involved in autoimmune encephalomyelitis. Nat Med. 2011;17:488–94.
16. Tanabe S, Yamashita T. Repulsive guidance molecule-a is involved in Th17-cell-induced neurodegeneration in autoimmune encephalomyelitis. Cell Rep. 2014;9:1459–70.
17. Sospedra M, Martin R. Immunology of multiple sclerosis. Annu Rev Immunol. 2005;23:683–747.
18. Becher B, Durell BG, Noelle RJ. Experimental autoimmune encephalitis and inflammation in the absence of interleukin-12. J Clin Invest. 2002;110:493–7.
19. Bettelli E, Carrier Y, Gao W, Korn T, Strom TB, Oukka M, Weiner HL, Kuchroo VK. Reciprocal developmental pathways for the generation of pathogenic effector TH17 and regulatory T cells. Nature. 2006;441:235–8.
20. Hu Y, Ota N, Peng I, Refino CJ, Danilenko DM, Caplazi P, Ouyang W. IL-17RC is required for IL-17A- and IL-17F-dependent signaling and the pathogenesis of experimental autoimmune encephalomyelitis. J Immunol. 2010;184:4307–16.
21. Komiyama Y, Nakae S, Matsuki T, Nambu A, Ishigame H, Kakuta S, Sudo K, Iwakura Y. IL-17 plays an important role in the development of experimental autoimmune encephalomyelitis. J Immunol. 2006;177:566–73.
22. McGeachy MJ, Chen Y, Tato CM, Laurence A, Joyce-Shaikh B, Blumenschein WM, McClanahan TK, O'Shea JJ, Cua DJ. The interleukin 23 receptor is essential for the terminal differentiation of interleukin 17-producing effector T helper cells in vivo. Nat Immunol. 2009;10:314–24.
23. Nohra R, Beyeen AD, Guo JP, Khademi M, Sundqvist E, Hedreul MT, Sellebjerg F, Smestad C, Oturai AB, Harbo HF, et al. RGMA and IL21R show association with experimental inflammation and multiple sclerosis. Genes Immun. 2010;11:279–93.
24. Girolamo F, Coppola C, Ribatti D, Trojano M. Angiogenesis in multiple sclerosis and experimental autoimmune encephalomyelitis. Acta Neuropathol Commun. 2014;2:84.
25. Kirk S, Frank JA, Karlik S. Angiogenesis in multiple sclerosis: is it good, bad or an epiphenomenon? J Neurol Sci. 2004;217:125–30.
26. Putnam TJ. The pathogenesis of multiple sclerosis: a possible vascular factor. N Engl J Med. 1933;209:786–90.
27. Jin K, Zhu Y, Sun Y, Mao XO, Xie L, Greenberg DA. Vascular endothelial growth factor (VEGF) stimulates neurogenesis in vitro and in vivo. Proc Natl Acad Sci U S A. 2002;99:11946–50.
28. Hayakawa K, Pham LD, Som AT, Lee BJ, Guo S, Lo EH, Arai K. Vascular endothelial growth factor regulates the migration of oligodendrocyte precursor cells. J Neurosci. 2011;31:10666–70.
29. Muramatsu R, Takahashi C, Miyake S, Fujimura H, Mochizuki H, Yamashita T. Angiogenesis induced by CNS inflammation promotes neuronal remodeling through vessel-derived prostacyclin. Nat Med. 2012;18:1658–64.
30. Harada K, Fujita Y, Yamashita T. Repulsive guidance molecule A suppresses angiogenesis. Biochem Biophys Res Commun. 2016;469:993–9.
31. Lejmi E, Leconte L, Pedron-Mazoyer S, Ropert S, Raoul W, Lavalette S, Bouras I, Feron JG, Maitre-Boube M, Assayag F, et al. Netrin-4 inhibits angiogenesis via binding to neogenin and recruitment of Unc5B. Proc Natl Acad Sci U S A. 2008;105:12491–6.
32. Park KW, Crouse D, Lee M, Karnik SK, Sorensen LK, Murphy KJ, Kuo CJ, Li DY. The axonal attractant netrin-1 is an angiogenic factor. Proc Natl Acad Sci U S A. 2004;101:16210–5.
33. Wilson BD, Ii M, Park KW, Suli A, Sorensen LK, Larrieu-Lahargue F, Urness LD, Suh W, Asai J, Kock GA, et al. Netrins promote developmental and therapeutic angiogenesis. Science. 2006;313:640–4.
34. Nguyen A, Cai H. Netrin-1 induces angiogenesis via a DCC-dependent ERK1/2-eNOS feed-forward mechanism. Proc Natl Acad Sci U S A. 2006;103:6530–5.
35. Lu X, Le Noble F, Yuan L, Jiang Q, De Lafarge B, Sugiyama D, Breant C, Claes F, De Smet F, Thomas JL, et al. The netrin receptor UNC5B mediates guidance events controlling morphogenesis of the vascular system. Nature. 2004;432:179–86.
36. Larrivee B, Freitas C, Trombe M, Lv X, Delafarge B, Yuan L, Bouvree K, Breant C, Del Toro R, Brechot N, et al. Activation of the UNC5B receptor by netrin-1 inhibits sprouting angiogenesis. Genes Dev. 2007;21:2433–47.

8

The pathophysiological role of acute inflammation after spinal cord injury

Seiji Okada[1,2]

Abstract

Traumatic spinal cord injury (SCI) causes irreparable severe motor and sensory dysfunction. Mechanical trauma rapidly leads to blood-spinal cord barrier disruption, neural cell death, axonal damage, and demyelination, followed by a cascade of secondary injury that expands the additional inflammatory reaction at the lesion site. Although the role of inflammation in this phase is complex, a number of studies have suggested that inflammatory responses spread the damage to the surrounding tissue, induce apoptotic cell death, and impair spontaneous regeneration and functional recovery. However, recent advances in experimental technology, such as the depletion antibodies for a specific fraction of inflammatory cells and the genetically engineered mice deficient only in specific cells, suggest the beneficial aspects of inflammatory cells, such as a neuroprotective effect, the removal of cellular debris, and the attenuation of the inflammatory reaction in general. In this review, I summarize our recent findings about the biological role of inflammatory cells, especially infiltrating neutrophils and activated microglia after SCI. A better understanding of the pathophysiological role of inflammation in the acute phase of SCI will aid in the development of therapeutic strategy to enhance the functional recovery after SCI.

Keywords: Spinal cord injury, Neutrophil, Microglia

Abbreviations: BLT1, Leukotriene B4 receptor 1; CCR2, C-C chemokine receptor type 2; CNS, Central nervous system; CX3CR1, Chemokine (C-X3-C motif) receptor 1; CXCL1, Chemokine (C-X-C motif) ligand 1; FACS, Fluorescence activated cell sorting; HO-1, Heme oxygenase 1; IL-6, Interleukin-6; iNOS, Inducible nitric oxide synthase; LTB4, Leukotriene B4; MDSC, Myeloid-derived suppressor cells; NADPF, Nicotinamide adenine dinucleotide phosphate; NF-kB, Nuclear factor-kappa B; ROS, Reactive oxygen species; SCI, Spinal cord injury; TGFβ, Transforming growth factor β; TNFα, Tumor necrosis factor α; VEGF, Vascular endothelial growth factor

Background

Traumatic spinal cord injury (SCI) is a major public health problem and a devastating event for individuals that causes permanent severe motor/sensory dysfunction and significantly degrades the quality of life. SCI is known to result in neurological deficits through both the primary and secondary damage. The "primary" injury encompasses the immediate mechanical damage to the spinal cord tissue that occurs at the moment of impact, which is irreversible and not preventable. The "secondary" injury, by contrast, is incurred as a result of the pathological processes initiated at the time of the primary injury and continues for several days or months after injury and is amenable to therapy.

Main text

Inflammatory reaction and the secondary injury

In the secondary injury process of SCI, the infiltration of leukocytes and activation of glial cells can aggravate tissue damage by releasing proteases, reactive oxygen intermediates, lysosomal enzymes, and proinflammatory cytokines/chemokines [1, 2]. Although the role of inflammation in this phase is complex, with certain beneficial aspects as well, such as the removal of cellular debris, a number of studies have suggested that inflammatory responses spread the damage to surrounding tissue, induce apoptotic cell death, and impair spontaneous regeneration and functional recovery [3]. To protect the injured spinal cord from these secondary pathological processes, several

Correspondence: seokada@ortho.med.kyushu-u.ac.jp
[1]Department of Advanced Initiatives, Graduate School of Medical Sciences, Kyushu University, 3-1-1 Maidashi, Higashi-ku, Fukuoka 812-8582, Japan
[2]Orthopaedics, Graduate School of Medical Sciences, Kyushu University, Fukuoka, Japan

approaches to manipulate the inflammatory responses have been assessed and found effective. These approaches include the blockage or neutralization of specific cytokine signaling using a monoclonal antibody, the delivery of anti-inflammatory drugs, and the use of genetically modified animals. Indeed, we previously examined whether or not the administration of IL-6 receptor antibody immediately after SCI attenuated the secondary injury and caused a therapeutic effect, since IL-6 is a principal proinflammatory cytokine in SCI [4].

IL-6 signaling plays roles in regulating various steps in inflammatory reactions, such as the activation and infiltration of neutrophils, monocytes, macrophages, and lymphocytes. Indeed, previous studies from other research groups have reported that the delivery of the IL-6/sIL-6R fusion protein to spinal cord injury sites induced a sixfold increase in neutrophils and a twofold increase in macrophages and microglial cells and expanded the damaged area [5]. We therefore speculated that blockage of IL-6 signaling would suppress the inflammatory response and ameliorate the secondary injury after SCI. We found that the number of infiltrated macrophages as well as scar tissue formation was significantly reduced, resulting in improved functional recovery [4]. The same strategy conducted later by other groups also demonstrated that the temporary inhibition of IL-6 signaling reduced the infiltration of hematogenous macrophages and the activation of the phagocytic activity of microglial cells [6, 7]. In addition to the anti-inflammatory effect, this approach also had a number of additional effects, including the attenuation of glial scar formation and preservation of neuroprotective phosphatidylcholine [8]. Moreover, a clinical merit of this strategy is that humanized antibody to human IL-6R (ACTEMRA®, tocilizumab) has already been in widespread use for rheumatoid arthritis and its efficacy as well as safety profile was confirmed.

However, in contrast to these reports, IL-6 itself was reported to enhance spinal cord repair by modifying the migration of reactive astrocytes or enhancing axonal regrowth [9, 10]. Although these results seem inconsistent, this contributes to the consequence of the context-dependent pleiotropic actions of IL-6 in SCI. During the acute phase of SCI, IL-6 family cytokines act primarily as potent proinflammatory mediators and cause secondary injury but also enhance the repair process after the subacute phase of SCI. These findings for IL-6 signaling suggest that the inflammatory response in SCI is very complicated and has context-dependent pleiotropic actions.

Flow cytometric evaluation of infiltrating leukocytes in SCI

In the research field of SCI, the conventional evaluation of inflammatory cell infiltration has been mainly limited to histological analyses. However, accurate quantification with histology is relatively difficult, as the lesion site is too fragile to treat in the acute phase of injury when the most prominent cell infiltration is observed. We therefore have induced flow cytometry, which enables the accurate detection and direct isolation of these cells for the evaluation of inflammatory cells after SCI [11]. With this method, we were able to quantitatively examine the detailed profile of infiltrated leukocytes into the lesion area (Fig. 1). The infiltrated neutrophil population had increased dramatically 12 h after SCI and remained at a high level for up to 1 day before gradually decreasing thereafter. Although the peak monocyte/macrophage infiltration is commonly understood to occur at a later phase than neutrophil infiltration, including in human SCI [12–14], we found that that monocyte/macrophage infiltration also peaked at 12 h after SCI. In addition, the temporal change in the number of infiltrated monocytes/macrophages was completely different from that of the microglial cells, which dramatically increased at 7 days after SCI. We attribute this discrepancy between the present and previous reports to the shortcomings of the immunohistological analyses, which have difficulty in discriminating infiltrated monocytes/macrophages from resident microglial cells. This methodology enables us to quantify not only the accurate number of the cells at multiple time points after SCI but also the secretory activity of the inflammatory mediators by sorting the inflammatory cell fractions [11].

Modulation of infiltrating neutrophils after SCI

Among the infiltrating leukocytes in the acute phase of SCI, neutrophils are considered to be one of the most potent triggers of post-traumatic spinal cord damage, which occurs through the release of proteases, reactive oxygen intermediates, nitric oxide, and lysosomal enzymes. Despite the fact that neutrophils are essential for innate immunity and important as anti-infectious factors in host defense, several studies focusing on the suppression of neutrophil infiltration have reported reduced severity of secondary injury and better functional recovery after SCI [15, 16].

The process of neutrophil infiltration to the lesion site is enhanced and amplified by variety of factors, such as proinflammatory cytokines, eiconosides, and adhesion molecules. Of these factors, leukotriene B4 (LTB4) is a highly potent lipid chemoattractant for neutrophils. LTB4 is produced rapidly by arachidonic acid cascade from membrane phospholipids without any requirement of transcription or translation and is mediated by its high-affinity specific receptor LTB4 receptor 1 (BLT1) [17]. In addition to this effect, LTB4 activates neutrophils that promote lysosomal enzyme release and superoxide production. This LTB4 biosynthesis system exerts its effect on the injured tissue faster than other inflammatory cytokines and chemokines, implying that LTB4

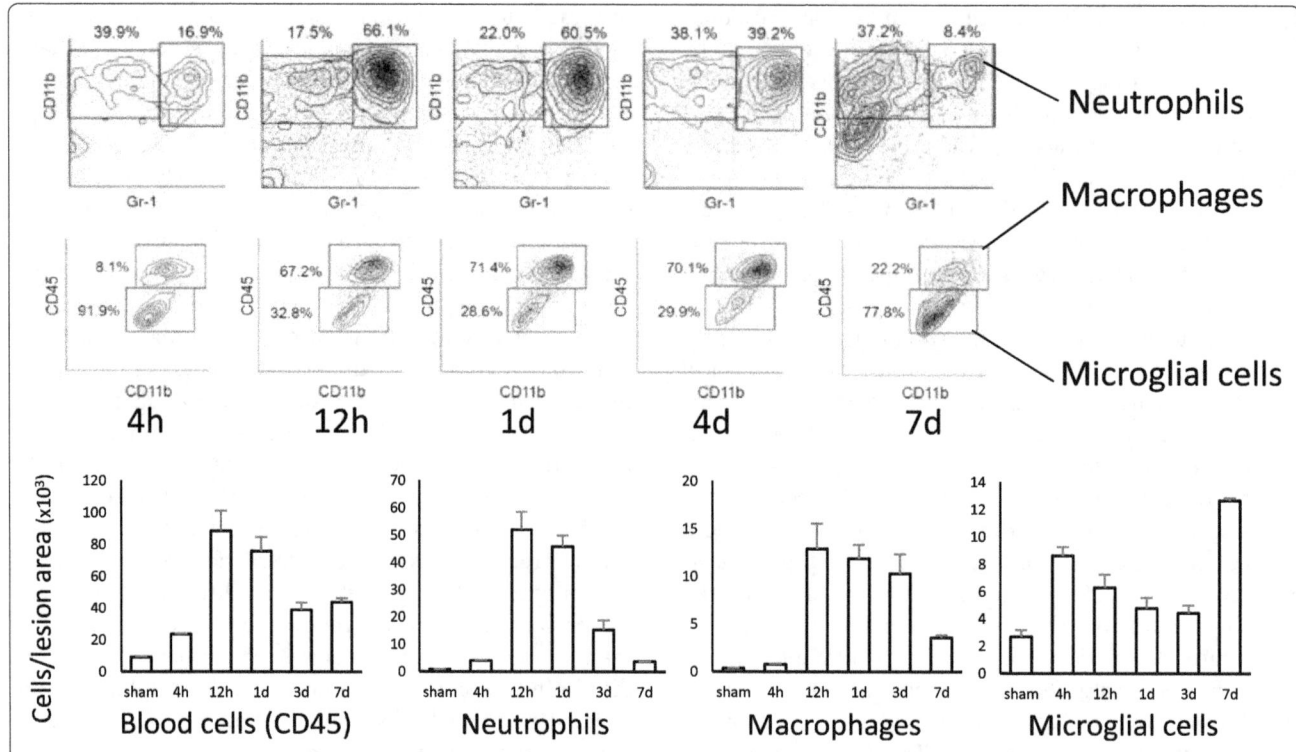

Fig. 1 Time course of infiltrating inflammatory cells in injured spinal cord. A quantitative time course evaluation of the infiltrated neutrophils (CD45$^+$CD11b$^+$Gr-1$^+$ fraction), macrophages (CD11b$^+$Gr-1$^-$CD45^{high}), and microglial cells (CD11b$^+$Gr-1$^-$CD45^{int}) in the SCI mice (Th9 contusion injury, 70 kdyn). Dot plots and graph data ($n=6$ in each time point) were quoted from [13]

might have a superior influence on the inflammatory cascade [18].

Previous studies have demonstrated that LTB4 is not only an important mediator in the regulation of microbial infection but also deeply related to several inflammatory diseases, autoimmune diseases, and atherosclerosis [19–22]. However, as for traumatic injury, the physiological role of LTB4 is not yet well understood. In addition, few analyses have examined the relationship between LTB4 and pathophysiology after SCI, although LTB4 may be a major contributive factor for inflammatory cell infiltration.

We therefore analyzed the pathophysiological involvement of LTB4 in a mouse SCI model using BLT1-deficient mice. Our results showed that BLT1-knockout mice exhibited a 23 % decrease in neutrophils and 10 % decrease in macrophages after SCI compared to the wild-type mice [11]. These reduced numbers of infiltrated leukocytes resulted in the suppression of neural apoptosis, less demyelination, and reduced proinflammatory cytokine expression as well as better functional recovery in BLT1-knockout mice than in wild-type mice [11]. These results showed that the LTB4-BLT1 pathway was indeed involved in the pathogenesis of traumatic secondary damage through the amplification of neutrophils and macrophages infiltration, suggesting that neutralizing

LTB4 has potential as a therapeutic strategy during the acute phase of SCI.

Pathophysiological role of microglia in SCI

Microglial cells constitute about 10 % of the adult central nervous system (CNS) cell population and represent the innate immune system of the spinal cord. Under pathological conditions such as neurodegenerative disease, stroke, tumor invasion, and traumatic injury, these cells become activated, surround damaged and dead cells, and clear cellular debris from the area, much like the phagocytic macrophages of the immune system [23]. In healthy mammalian brain tissue, microglia display characteristically elongated cell bodies with spine-like processes that often branch perpendicularly. Although microglia were initially believed to be essentially quiescent cells, recent studies have revealed that they are continually surveying their microenvironment and represent the first line of defense against invading pathogens or other types of CNS tissue injury [24, 25]. Indeed, we found that the spinal microglial secretory activity was quickly stimulated at 3 h post SCI in response to pathological changes, while the infiltration of other leukocytes peaked at 12 h post SCI [11, 26]. In addition, we demonstrated that microglial activity was significantly attenuated in young mice compared to adult mice, with reduced leukocyte infiltration and neural damage as well as better functional recovery in the younger mice than in the older ones [26]. The expressions of potent chemo-attractant for neutrophil infiltration, IL-6, and CXCL1 were also significantly reduced in the microglia isolated from the young mice. Considering that these chemoat-tractants are dominantly secreted by activated microglia and that microglial activation occurred prior to the infiltration of leukocytes, microglial activity appears to be critical for the trigger of propagation and enhancement of the inflammatory response. Leukocytes that infiltrate the lesion site also produce cytokines/chemokines by interaction with the other immune cells or microglial cells, leading to the amplification of the chemotactic gradient and to further infiltration of leukocytes to the lesion site [27]. We therefore believe that the reduced immediate activation of microglial cells in young mice results in the decreased infiltration of neutrophils, leading to reduced amplification/exaggeration of the inflammatory response in SCI.

Although the precise mechanisms of microglial activation remains unclear, several basic research studies have reported that hyperglycemia is involved in the activation of resident monocytic cells, including microglia. For example, the number of pancreatic resident monocytes is increased in hyperglycemic rodents, leading to the up-regulation of islet-derived inflammatory factors, such as IL-6 and IL-8 [28]. In addition, peritoneal monocytes are activated under hyperglycemic conditions, subsequently inducing a greater production of TNFα than that associated with a normo-glycemic state [29]. Furthermore, hyperglycemia correlates with worsening of tactile allodynia accompanied by the hyperactivation of dorsal horn microglia [30].

Because microglial activation is associated with secondary injury after SCI, we hypothesized that hypergly-cemia may also influence the pathophysiology of SCI by altering microglial responses. We thus investigated the effects of hyperglycemia on the pathophysiological processes and motor functional outcomes in two experimental mouse models of hyperglycemia in the acute phase of injury [31]. An in vivo cell type-specific gene expression analysis with flow cytometry revealed enhanced the proinflammatory reactivity in the microglial cells of the hyperglycemic mice. We found that hyperglycemia induced the overactivation of NF-kB in microglial cells as well as excessive inflammation, resulting in a poor functional recovery after SCI [31]. We also conducted a multivariable linear regression analysis of the clinical data obtained from 528 human SCI subjects, which provided entirely new evidence showing that acute phase hyperglycemia is a critical factor in the poor functional outcomes of SCI. Finally, we showed that achieving glycemic control can ameliorate the pathological and functional outcomes of hyperglycemic mice, thus supporting the existence of a direct relationship between acute hyperglycemia and the exacerbation of SCI outcomes [31] (Fig. 2).

With regard to the mechanisms involved in the hyperglycemia-related overactivation of NF-kB in microglia, NADPH oxidase is considered to possibly play a role. NADPH oxidase is present in several types of phagocytes, including microglia, causing inflammatory activation of these cells [32]. In addition, several studies have reported that hyperglycemia enhances the NADPH oxidase activity in innate immune cells [33, 34]. Furthermore, NADPH oxidase is known to produce reactive

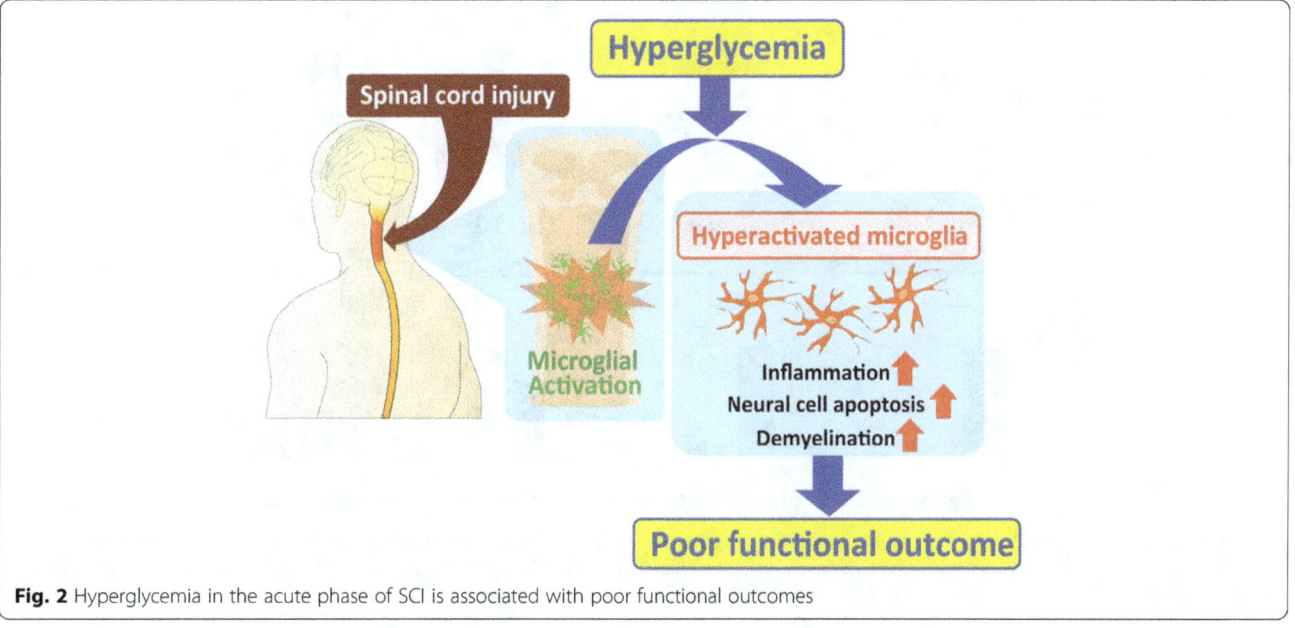

Fig. 2 Hyperglycemia in the acute phase of SCI is associated with poor functional outcomes

oxygen species (ROS) [35], which may promote the translocation of NF-kB [36]. Therefore, hyperglycemia may promote the translocation of NF-kB in microglial cells via the NADPH oxidase/ROS/NF-kB pathway. The fact that the increased expression of NADPH oxidase and ROS has been confirmed in spinal microglial cells after injury also supports the role of this pathway [37]. These findings shed light on the importance of achieving tight glycemic control in acute human SCI to obtain better neurological outcomes, also providing a better understanding of the inflammatory machinery after SCI.

Resolution of acute inflammation after SCI

Although the acute inflammation after SCI spontaneously diminishes within a short period of time, the mechanism underlying this inflammatory resolution is largely unknown. Recently, we demonstrated that the infiltrating $Ly6C^+Ly6G^-$ immature monocyte fraction exhibited the same characteristics as myeloid-derived

suppressor cells (MDSCs) and played a critical role in the resolution of acute inflammation and in the subsequent tissue repair after SCI [38].

Immediately after SCI, a large number of $CD11b^+Gr-1^+$ inflammatory cells infiltrated the lesion area and led to the secondary damage of neural tissue. Although Gr-1 surface antigen is a common epitope on Ly6C and Ly6G, which express monocytic and granulocytic subsets, respectively, the detailed role of each subset at the lesion areas remains elusive. We therefore evaluated the temporal change in the infiltration of $Ly6C^+Ly6G^-$, $Ly6C^-Ly6G^-$, and $Ly6C^-Ly6G^+$ cell subsets in the $CD45^+CD11b^+$ fraction by flow cytometry from 4 h until 7 days after SCI [38]. The flow cytometry analysis revealed that the infiltrating $Ly6C^-Ly6G^+$ and $Ly6C^+Ly6G^-$ fractions had similar patterns of change, peaking at 12 h after injury, whereas the $Ly6C^-Ly6G^-$ fraction increased gradually with time. To investigate the physiological roles of these myeloid-derived inflammatory cell subsets after SCI, we used FACS to

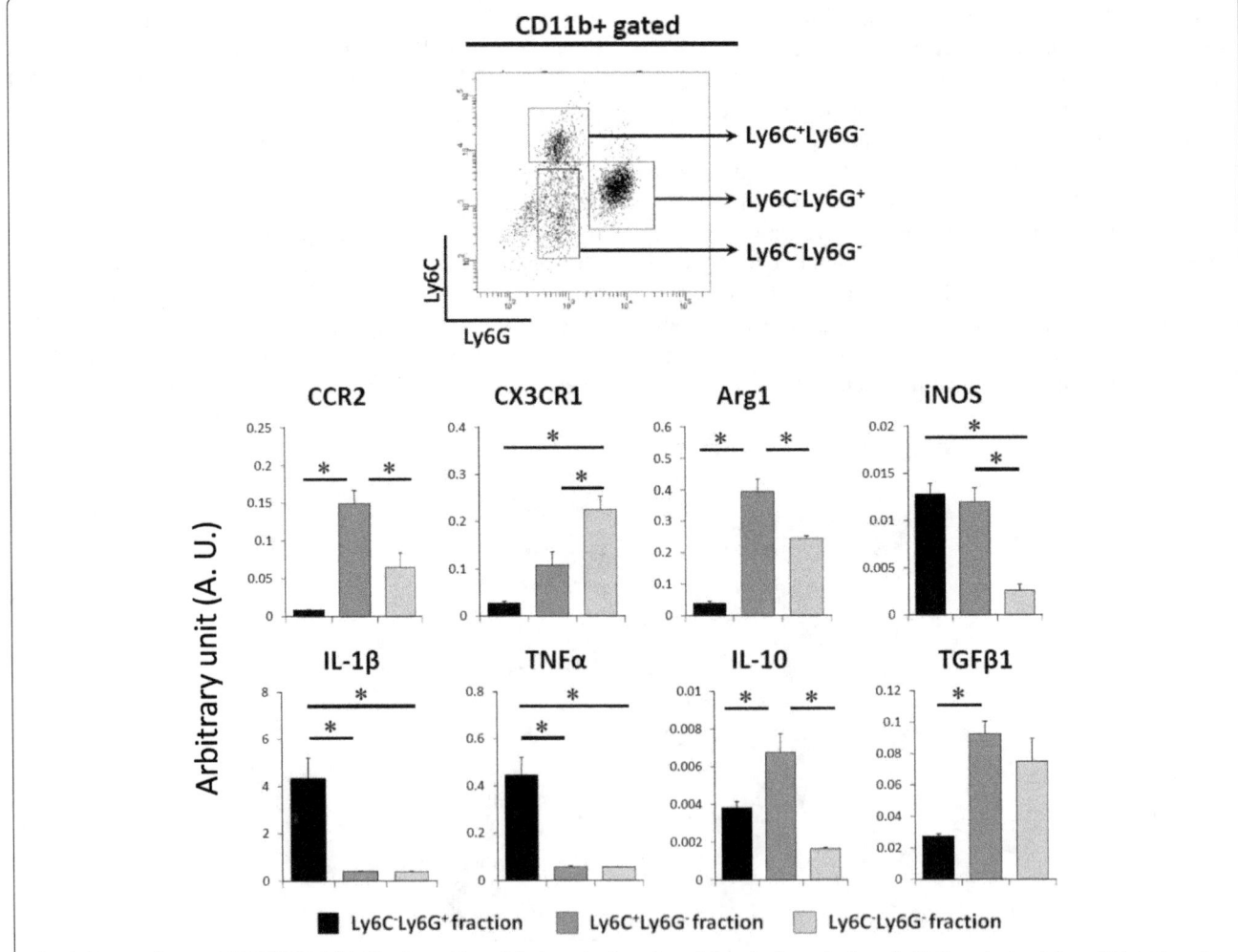

Fig. 3 Three subsets of $CD45^+CD11b^+$ infiltrating cells and their each phenotype. Injured mice spinal cords (Th9 contusion injury, 70 kdyn) were harvested at 4 days after injury and subjected to a flow cytometric analysis. $Ly6C^+Ly6G^-$, $Ly6C^-Ly6G^+$, and $Ly6C^-Ly6G^-$ fractions were analyzed by quantitative RT-PCR. *$p < 0.05$ using a Kruskal–Wallis H test, with Bonferroni's post hoc correction. Data were quoted from [38]

isolate each subset based on their expression of Ly6C and Ly6G cell surface antigens. We confirmed that the flow cytometry-sorted Ly6C-Ly6G$^+$ fraction expressed significantly higher levels of CXCR1 and CXCR2, the Ly6C$^+$Ly6G$^-$ fraction expressed a higher level of CCR2, and the Ly6C$^-$Ly6G$^-$ fraction expressed higher levels of CX3CR1 than the other fractions, which indicated that each subset was regulated by different chemokines. The infiltrating Ly6C$^-$Ly6G$^+$ fraction showed proinflammatory properties with elevated expression of IL-1β and TNFα. In contrast, we confirmed that the Ly6C$^+$Ly6G$^-$ fraction had elevated expression of both iNOS and arginase 1 (Fig. 3). This expression pattern is a typical feature of MDSCs, which exert immunosuppressive effects by modulating macrophage activation toward an immunosuppressive phenotype. In addition, the Ly6C$^+$Ly6G$^-$ fraction had elevated expression of anti-inflammatory mediators such as IL-10, TGFβ, and VEGF, which is also consistent with the typical features of MDSCs. We also demonstrated that complete depletion of this population resulted in prolonged inflammation and significantly exacerbated tissue edema, vessel permeability, and hemorrhaging, causing impaired neurological outcomes. Furthermore, the transplantation of MDSCs at lesion areas significantly attenuated acute inflammation and promoted tissue repair, which improved neurological outcomes after SCI [38].

Among the anti-inflammatory factors from Ly6C$^+$ MDSCs, IL-10 functions as a potent inducer of HO-1 in macrophages [39]. HO-1 is a heme-degrading enzyme that protects tissues from free heme toxicity. In addition, it also has a direct effect of attenuating inflammation [40]. We confirmed that transplantation of MDSCs significantly up-regulated HO-1 expression, suggesting that MDSCs created an environment favorable for tissue repair. In addition, the expression of both arginase 1 and iNOS was enhanced in the lesion areas after MDSC transplantation for 1 week after SCI [38]. This up-regulation of both arginase 1 and iNOS was a determining factor for defining the characteristics of MDSCs. These findings clarified the role of MDSCs after traumatic SCI and suggested the potential utility of an MDSC-based therapeutic strategy for the acute phase of SCI.

Conclusions

Although inflammatory reactions lead to further damage and dysfunction after SCI, we confirmed that complete neutrophil depletion using the Gr-1 antibody severely impaired the functional recovery in a mouse SCI model. Thus, whether or not neuroinflammation after SCI has a neurotoxic or neuroprotective effect remains highly controversial. Although only minor attention has been paid to the role of inflammation in tissue protection after SCI thus far, it could be an essential factor for a well-balanced inflammatory reaction under pathological conditions.

Nevertheless, more basic research should be conducted to clarify the detailed pathophysiological role of inflammation after SCI, which suggest a new approach for SCI treatment by modifying the inflammatory response in SCI.

Funding
This work was supported by Grants-in-Aid for Scientific Research to SO (16H05450) from the Japan Society for the Promotion of Science (JSPS).

Author's contributions
SO wrote the review and approved to submit the final manuscript.

Competing interests
The author declares that he has no competing interests.

References

1. Beattie MS. Inflammation and apoptosis: linked therapeutic targets in spinal cord injury. Trends Mol Med. 2004;10:580-3.
2. Ren Y, Young W. Managing inflammation after spinal cord injury through manipulation of macrophage function. Neural Plast. 2013;2013:945034.
3. Okada S, Nakamura M, Fenault-Mihara F, et al. The role of cytokine signaling in pathophysiology for spinal cord injury. Inflamm Regen. 2008;28:440-6.
4. Okada S, Nakamura M, Mikami Y, et al. Blockade of interleukin-6 receptor suppresses reactive astrogliosis and ameliorates functional recovery in experimental spinal cord injury. J Neurosci Res. 2004;76:265-76.
5. Lacroix S, Chang L, Rose-John S, et al. Delivery of hyper-interleukin-6 to the injured spinal cord increases neutrophil and macrophage infiltration and inhibits axonal growth. J Comp Neurol. 2002;454:213-28.
6. Mukaino M, Nakamura M, Yamada O, et al. Anti-IL-6-receptor antibody promotes repair of spinal cord injury by inducing microglia-dominant inflammation. Exp Neurol. 2010;224:403-14.
7. Guerrero AR, Uchida K, Nakajima H, et al. Blockade of interleukin-6 signaling inhibits the classic pathway and promotes an alternative pathway of macrophage activation after spinal cord injury in mice. J Neuroinflammation. 2012;9:40.
8. Arima H, Hanada M, Hayasaka T, et al. Blockade of IL-6 signaling by MR16-1 inhibits reduction of docosahexaenoic acid-containing phosphatidylcholine levels in a mouse model of spinal cord injury. Neuroscience. 2014;269:1-10.
9. Cafferty WB, Gardiner NJ, Das P, et al. Conditioning injury-induced spinal axon regeneration fails in interleukin-6 knock-out mice. J Neurosci. 2004;24:4432-43.
10. Penkowa M, Giralt M, Lago N, et al. Astrocyte-targeted expression of IL-6 protects the CNS against a focal brain injury. Exp Neurol. 2003;181:130-48.
11. Saiwai H, Ohkawa Y, Yamada H, et al. The LTB4-BLT1 axis mediates neutrophil infiltration and secondary injury in experimental spinal cord injury. Am J Pathol. 2010;176:2352-66.
12. Fleming JC, Norenberg MD, Ramsay DA, et al. The cellular inflammatory response in human spinal cords after injury. Brain. 2006;129:3249-69.
13. Popovich PG, Guan Z, Wei P, et al. Depletion of hematogenous macrophages promotes partial hindlimb recovery and neuroanatomical repair after experimental spinal cord injury. Exp Neurol. 1999;158:351-65.
14. Longbrake EE, Lai W, Ankeny D, et al. Characterization and modeling of monocyte-derived macrophages after spinal cord injury. J Neurochem. 2007;102:1083-94.
15. Taoka Y, Okajima K, Uchiba M, et al. Activated protein C reduces the severity of compression induced spinal cord injury in rats by inhibiting activation of leukocytes. J Neurosci. 1998;18:1393-8.
16. Genovese T, Mazzon E, Crisafulli C, et al. TNF-alpha blockage in a mouse model of SCI: evidence for improved outcome. Shock. 2008;29:32-41.
17. Yokomizo T, Izumi T, Chang K, et al. A G-protein-coupled receptor for leukotriene B4 that mediates chemotaxis. Nature. 1997;387:620-4.
18. Okuno T, Yokomizo T, Hori T, et al. Leukotriene B4 receptor and the function of its helix 8. J Biol Chem. 2005;280:32049-52.

19. Matsukawa A, Hogaboam CM, Lukacs NW, et al. Endogenous monocyte chemoattractant protein-1 protects mice in a model of acute septic peritonitis: cross-talk between MCP-1 and leukotriene B4. J Immunol. 1999;163:6148–54.

20. Dahlen SE, Kumlin M, Bjorck T, et al. Lipoxins and other lipoxygenase products with relevance to inflammatory reactions in the lung. Ann NY Acad Sci. 1991;629:262–73.

21. Heller EA, Liu E, Tager AM, et al. Inhibition of atherogenesis in BLT1-deficient mice reveals a role for LTB4 and BLT1 in smooth muscle cell recruitment. Circulation. 2005;112:578–86.

22. Back M, Bu D, Branstrom R, et al. Leukotriene B4 signaling through NF-kB-dependent BLT1 receptors on vascular smooth muscle cells in atherosclerosis and intimal hyperplasia. Proc Natl Acad Sci U S A. 2005;102:17501–6.

23. Bernhardi V, Tichauer JE, Eugenin J. Aging-dependent changes of microglial cells and their relevance for neurodegenerative disorders. J Neurochem. 2010;112:1099–114.

24. Davalos D, Grutzendler J, Yang G, et al. ATP mediates rapid microglial response to local brain injury in vivo. Nat Neurosci. 2005;8:752–8.

25. Nimmerjahn A, Kirchhoff F, Helmchen F. Resting microglial cells are highly dynamic surveillants of brain parenchyma in vivo. Science. 2005;308:1314–8.

26. Kumamaru H, Saiwai H, Ohkawa Y, et al. Age-related differences in cellular and molecular profiles of inflammatory responses after spinal cord injury. J Cell Physiol. 2012;227:1335–46.

27. Letellier E, Kumar S, Sancho-Martinez I, et al. CD95-ligand on peripheral myeloid cells activates Syk kinase to trigger their recruitment to the inflammatory site. Immunity. 2010;32:240–52.

28. Ehses JA, Perren A, Eppler E, et al. Increased number of islet-associated macrophages in type 2 diabetes. Diabetes. 2007;56:2356–70.

29. Sherry CL, O'Connor JC, Kramer JM, et al. Augmented lipopolysaccharide-induced TNF-alpha production by peritoneal macrophages in type 2 diabetic mice is dependent on elevated glucose and requires p38 MAPK. J Immunol. 2007;178:663–70.

30. Tsuda M, Ueno H, Kataoka A, et al. Activation of dorsal horn microglia contributes to diabetes-induced tactile allodynia via extracellular signal-regulated protein kinase signaling. Glia. 2008;56:378–86.

31. Kobayakawa K, Kumamaru H, Saiwai H, et al. Acute hyperglycemia impairs functional improvement after spinal cord injury in mice and humans. Sci Transl Med. 2014;6:256ra137.

32. Brown GC. Mechanisms of inflammatory neurodegeneration: iNOS and NADPH oxidase. Biochem Soc Trans. 2007;35:1119–21.

33. Hayek T, Kaplan M, Kerry R, et al. Macrophage NADPH oxidase activation, impaired cholesterol fluxes, and increased cholesterol biosynthesis in diabetic mice: a stimulatory role for D-glucose. Atherosclerosis. 2007;195:277–86.

34. Ayilavarapu S, Kantarci A, Fredman G, et al. Diabetes-induced oxidative stress is mediated by Ca2+-independent phospholipase A2 in neutrophils. J Immunol. 2010;184:1507–15.

35. Jackson SH, Gallin JI, Holland SM. The p47phox mouse knock-out model of chronic granulomatous disease. J Exp Med. 1995;182:751–8.

36. Schreck R, Rieber P, Baeuerle PA. Reactive oxygen intermediates as apparently widely used messengers in the activation of the NF-kappa B transcription factor and HIV-1. Embo J. 1991;10:2247–58.

37. Kim D, You B, Jo EK, et al. NADPH oxidase 2-derived reactive oxygen species in spinal cord microglia contribute to peripheral nerve injury-induced neuropathic pain. Proc Natl Acad Sci U S A. 2010;107:14851–6.

38. Saiwai H, Kumamaru H, Ohkawa Y, et al. Ly6C$^+$ Ly6G$^-$ myeloid-derived suppressor cells play a critical role in the resolution of acute inflammation and the subsequent tissue repair process after spinal cord injury. J Neurochem. 2013;125:74–88.

39. Lee TS, Chau LY. Heme oxygenase-1 mediates the anti-inflammatory effect of interleukin-10 in mice. Nat Med. 2002;8:240–6.

40. Otterbein LE, Soares MP, Yamashita K, et al. Heme oxygenase-1: unleashing the protective properties of heme. Trends Immunol. 2003;24:449–55.

9

Pharmacological targeting of bone marrow mesenchymal stromal/stem cells for the treatment of hematological disorders

Noriko Sugino[1,2], Tatsuo Ichinohe[3], Akifumi Takaori-Kondo[2], Taira Maekawa[1] and Yasuo Miura[1*]

Abstract

The therapeutic effects of mesenchymal stromal/stem cells (MSCs) are mainly based on three characteristics: immunomodulation, tissue regeneration, and hematopoietic support. Cell therapy using culture-expanded MSCs is effective in some intractable bone and hemato-immune disorders; however, its efficacy is limited. In this article, we review the previous efforts to improve the clinical outcomes of cell therapy using MSCs for such disorders. We describe pharmacological targeting of endogenous bone marrow-derived MSCs as a crucial quality-based intervention to establish more effective MSC-based therapies.

Keywords: Mesenchymal stromal/stem cell, Hematopoiesis, Regeneration, Immunomodulation, Pharmacological modification, Cell therapy

Background

There are two types of multipotent cells in bone marrow (BM): hematopoietic stem/progenitor cells (HSCs) and mesenchymal stromal/stem cells (MSCs). HSCs produce all types of hematopoietic cells and are established as a central player in BM. MSCs support hematopoiesis in the BM microenvironment and have been considered to be a second-class player in BM, despite their ability to differentiate into a variety of mesenchymal cells [1–4]. Nevertheless, emerging evidence has revealed the active contribution of BM-derived MSCs (BM-MSCs) to the pathogenesis of hematological diseases. More importantly, culture-expanded MSCs are practically available in clinics as off-the-shelf stem cell products for the treatment of some intractable refractory diseases. This review describes the basic characteristics of human MSCs and their clinical applications in the past and present and looks ahead toward the new horizon of MSC-based therapy.

Main text

Characteristics of human MSCs

The International Society of Cellular Therapy (ISCT) has proposed the following minimal criteria of human MSCs to define their characteristics [5]: (1) the ability to adhere to plastic plates; (2) the ability to differentiate into osteoblasts, adipocytes, and chondroblasts in vitro; and (3) the positive surface expression of CD105, CD73, and CD90 in the absence of surface human leukocyte antigen (HLA)-DR molecules and hematopoietic lineage markers of pan-leukocytes (CD45), endothelial/primitive cells (CD34), myeloid lineage cells (CD14 or CD11b), and B cell lineage cells (CD79α or CD19). MSCs are isolated from various tissues/organs via diverse methods in multiple institutions [6, 7]. Therefore, it is critical to determine the common characteristics of MSCs in order to discuss clinical and basic studies using these cells. The minimal criteria for MSCs proposed by the ISCT are appropriate for product identity but have no relevance to functions including hematopoietic support, immunomodulation, and tissue regeneration (Fig. 1).

There are two principal methods to isolate MSCs: classical isolation and prospective isolation. The classical isolation method selects cells that adhere to plastic dishes and form colonies. This method is simple and convenient; however, the isolated cells are heterogeneous.

* Correspondence: ym58f5@kuhp.kyoto-u.ac.jp
[1]Department of Transfusion Medicine and Cell Therapy, Kyoto University Hospital, 54 Kawaharacho, Shogoin, Sakyo-ku, Kyoto 606-8507, Japan
Full list of author information is available at the end of the article

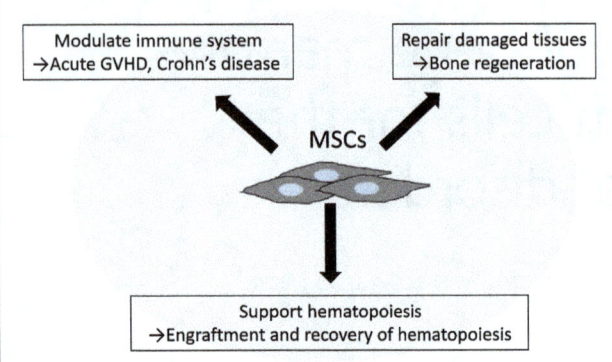

Fig. 1 The main characteristics of MSCs. MSCs are multipotent stromal cells that have the ability to modulate the immune system, support hematopoiesis, and repair damaged tissues. These characteristics are applied to treat acute GVHD and Crohn's disease, to regenerate bone, and to induce engraftment and recovery of hematopoiesis by infusing ex vivo expanded MSCs

The prospective isolation method is based on cell sorting using surface markers that are expressed on MSCs [8, 9]. This method has the advantage of isolating a homogenous and high-quality cell population. According to the database provided by the National Institutes of Health (USA) at http://www.clinicaltrials.gov/, the conventional isolation method has been generally used in clinical trials using MSCs.

Clinical applications of human MSCs
Acute graft-versus-host disease (GVHD)
A substantial proportion of patients who undergo allogeneic hematopoietic stem/progenitor cell transplantation (HSCT) develop intractable acute graft-versus-host disease (GVHD). The European Group for Blood and Marrow Transplantation conducted a multi-institutional phase II study and showed that infusion of MSCs from multiple donor sources conferred an overall response rate of 71% (39 of 55 cases), with a complete response rate of 55% and a partial response rate of 16%, in cases with steroid-resistant acute GVHD [10]. The 2-year overall survival rate in cases with a complete response was 52%, which was better than that in historical controls (about 10%). These results suggested that intravenous infusion of MSCs is an effective therapy for patients with steroid-resistant acute GVHD.

In clinical trials using commercial off-the-shelf MSC products, their infusion was tolerable overall and they showed an efficacy to improve acute GVHD, especially in pediatric patients and gastrointestinal GVHD patients [11–15]. However, the preliminary results of a phase III study that was conducted outside of Japan showed that infusion of MSCs had an initial effect, but conferred no significant advantage in the longer term for acute GVHD

patients [16]. A recent meta-analysis of 13 studies (336 patients) revealed that 241 (72%) patients achieved an overall response, with a 6-month overall survival rate of 63% in responders versus 16% in non-responders [17]. The overall response rate of individual organs was 49% for the gastrointestinal tract, 49% for the skin, and 28% for the liver. Although MSCs are certainly effective for the treatment of acute GVHD, the results of long-term follow-up are needed.

Skeletal disorders
Osteogenesis imperfecta (OI) is an inherited skeletal dysplasia characterized by osteopenia and frequent bone fractures. The molecular mechanism underlying this disease is a defect of type I collagen (COL1a1 and COL1a2) in progenies of MSCs, namely, osteoblasts. Allogeneic BM transplantation effectively improved the histological and clinical manifestations of OI in children [18, 19]. However, the engraftment of donor cells was not ensured via this strategy. In 2005, Le Blanc et al. performed in utero transplantation (IUT) of MSCs into a female fetus with severe OI [20]. A bone biopsy after delivery showed the engraftment of donor cells, suggesting that IUT is a promising strategy to solve the problem of engraftment and settlement of donor-derived MSCs.

Hypophosphatasia (HPP) is an inherited metabolic disorder characterized by low alkaline phosphatase activity and impaired bone formation. BM transplantation transiently improved the clinical features of HPP, but a boost of donor BM cells was required [21]. Tadokoro et al. reported successful BM and MSC transplantation into an 8-month-old patient with perinatal HPP [22]. Subsequently, the same group reported that transplantation of ex vivo expanded allogeneic MSCs following BM transplantation improved bone mineralization, muscle mass, respiratory function, and mental development in patients with HPP [23]. Combined BM and MSC transplantation may be effective to prevent the rejection of allogeneic donor-derived MSCs.

Cell therapy using MSCs has been applied for bone regeneration in adults. One important application is the repair of bone fractures or defects due to malignant bone tumors or external injuries. Quatro et al. reported three cases of successful autologous BM stromal cell transplantation to treat large bone defects in the tibia, ulna, and humerus [24]. They expanded osteoprogenitor cells isolated from BM cells and implanted them into the lesion sites with macroporous hydroxyapatite scaffolds. All three patients achieved improvement of bone function and radiographic examination findings. Following this report, many studies of local MSC transplantation for bone repair were conducted. However, the osteogenic differentiation potential of implanted MSCs in defected lesions was not certified in these reports.

Hematopoietic engraftment and recovery after HSCT

Attempts have been made to use MSCs to support hematopoiesis upon HSCT. For this purpose, two major interventions were applied: co-transplantation of HSCs and MSCs and transplantation of HSCs that were expanded ex vivo in the presence of MSCs.

In an early phase I/II trial of co-transplantation of autologous peripheral blood stem/progenitor cells (PBSCs) and culture-expanded autologous MSCs in advanced breast cancer patients that received high-dose chemotherapy, engraftment was effectively accelerated [25]. Following this report, clinical trials of co-transplantation of allogeneic BM or PBSCs and MSCs for patients with hematological malignant diseases were conducted (Table 1) [26–28]. Lazarus et al. co-administered HSCs and culture-expanded MSCs from the same donor (HLA-identical siblings) after myeloablative conditioning; however, acceleration of engraftment was not observed [26]. Le Blanc et al. conducted a pilot study of co-transplantation of MSCs and HSCs for patients with graft failure [27]. All patients achieved engraftment, indicating that such co-transplantation improves engraftment of cells from the second donor in salvage HSCT. MacMillan et al. reported that co-transplantation of MSCs supported rapid engraftment of unrelated cord blood cells in children with high-risk leukemia [28]. In summary, although co-transplantation of MSCs is not effective in a standard risk transplantation setting, it could be effective in cases of engraftment failure or delayed hematopoietic recovery, such as HSCT from HLA-haploidentical donors, cord blood transplantation, and retransplantation.

MSCs support the expansion of cord blood cells in vitro [29]. de Lima et al. studied whether cord blood cells culture-expanded in the presence of MSCs effectively induce hematopoietic recovery upon double cord blood cell transplantation [30]. Cord blood cells from one unit with a smaller cell number were expanded in co-culture with MSCs. These manipulated cells were co-transplanted with non-manipulated cord blood cells from another unit with a larger cell number. The time-to-engraftment of neutrophils and platelets was shorter in these patients than in the historical controls, indicating that ex vivo expansion of cord blood cells with MSCs is an effective strategy to improve engraftment.

Pharmacological targeting of endogenous BM-MSCs

In most clinical trials using allogeneic human MSCs, these cells were isolated from tissues/organs of volunteer donors, culture-expanded ex vivo, and intravenously infused into recipients. This intervention is a "quantity"-based approach to achieve therapeutic effects of MSCs. However, ex vivo expansion of MSCs might change their characteristics and reduce their quality. More importantly, a substantial proportion of intravenously infused donor MSCs become trapped within the lungs and are not distributed to the damaged tissues/organs of recipients [31]. There is obviously a limitation in the current strategy employed for cell therapy using MSCs because their effects are not dependent on the sustained settlement of infused cells or on proximate interactions with the target cells [32].

In a series of preclinical studies using model mice, we suggested that pharmacological treatment modifies the functions of endogenous BM-MSCs to achieve their therapeutic effects (Table 2) [33–37]. Acetylsalicylic acid (ASA), also known as aspirin, is a medication used to treat pain, fever, and inflammation. These therapeutic effects are mediated through inhibition or modification of cyclooxygenases [38, 39]. We showed that treatment with ASA ameliorates bone loss in osteoporotic mice due to the increased bone-forming capability of ASA-treated BM-MSCs [33]. Telomerase activity is enhanced in ASA-treated BM-MSCs [33]. This observation is consistent with a previous report that ASA contributes to the improvement of bone mineral density, although the contribution of MSCs is unknown [40]. These preclinical

Table 1 Clinical studies of co-infusion of MSCs with HSCs for hematopoietic recovery after hematopoietic stem/progenitor cell transplantation

Number of patients	Median age of patients, years (range)	HSC donor	MSC donor	MSC dose (×10^6/kg)	Median time for Neut recovery (range)	Median time for Plt recovery (range)	Reference
46	44.5 (19–61)	HLA-matched sibling	HSC donor	1.0, 2.5, or 5.0	Neut >500/µl at day 14 (11–26)	Plt >20,000/µl at day 20 (15–36)	[26]
7	12 (1–44)	HLA-matched sibling in three cases Unrelated donor in three cases Cord blood in one case	HLA-matched sibling or HLA-haploidentical donor	1.0	Neut >500/µl at day 12 (10–28)	Plt >30,000/µl at day 12 (8–36)	[27]
8	7.5 (0.25–16)	Cord blood	HLA-haploidentical parent	0.9–5.0	Neut >500/µl at day 19 (9–28)	Plt >50,000/µl at day 53 (36–98)	[28]

HLA human leukocyte antigen, *HSC* hematopoietic stem/progenitor cell, *MSC* mesenchymal stromal/stem cell, *Neut* neutrophil, *Plt* platelet

Table 2 The effects of pharmacological treatment of MSCs

Drug	Target cells	Clinical effect	MSC-mediated hematopoiesis	MSC-mediated bone regeneration	Mechanism(s) in MSCs	References
ASA	Broad cells	Anti-inflammation	N/T	↑	Telomerase activity↑	[33]
EPO	Erythroid progenitors	Erythropoiesis	↑	↑	EPOR/Stat5 pathway↑	[34]
PTH	Osteoblasts/Osteoclasts	Osteoporosis	↑	→	CDH11 expression↑	[35]
VK2	Osteoblasts	Osteoporosis	↑	↑	CXCL12 expression↓	[37]
OICS	N/A	Osteoporosis	↑	→	CXCL12 and VCAM1 expression↓	[36]

Up arrows indicate up-regulation or activation. Down arrows indicate down-regulation or inactivation

ASA acetylsalicylic acid (aspirin), *EPO* erythropoietin, *EPOR* erythropoietin receptor, *MSC* mesenchymal stromal/stem cell, *N/T* not tested, *OICS* osteo-inductive cocktail (dexamethasone, phosphate, and vitamin C), *PTH* parathyroid hormone, *VCAM1* vascular cell adhesion protein 1, *VK2* vitamin K2

and clinical studies indicate the efficacy of ASA treatment for bone repair in patients with skeletal disorders through activation of endogenous BM-MSCs.

Parathyroid hormone (PTH) is clinically used to treat osteoporosis because it has anabolic effects on bone formation though activating osteoblasts [41]. We demonstrated that short-term administration of PTH prolongs the survival of lethally irradiated mice that undergo BM transplantation, which is accompanied by enhanced hematopoietic marrow formation in BM [35]. PTH acts on human BM-MSCs to enhance their hematopoietic cell expansion capability through upregulation of the adhesion molecule cadherin-11 in BM-MSCs [35]. In another study, we showed that an erythropoicsis-stimulating agent, erythropoietin, acts on human BM-MSCs to enhance not only bone formation but also hematopoietic marrow formation in vivo, by using ectopically xeno-grafted mice [34]. The erythropoietin receptor/Stat5 pathway is enhanced in BM-MSCs as well as in erythroblast progenitor cells [34, 42]. Vitamin K2 (VK2) is clinically approved for the treatment of patients with osteoporosis. It is known that VK2 improves

hematopoiesis in some patients with hematological diseases although the underlining mechanisms are not fully understood [43, 44]. In our study, the expression of CXCL12 in VK2-treated BM-MSCs was low, which suggested that CXCL12-CXCR4-mediated interaction between BM-MSCs and HSCs is released, thereby HSCs expand and differentiate into mature hematopoietic cells [37].

We have proposed that pharmacological targeting of endogenous MSCs is a quality-based intervention to achieve therapeutic effects in patients (Fig. 2). This strategy may enhance the therapeutic capability of MSCs to act closely on target cells through secretion of soluble factors and adherence in microenvironments, without requiring the redistribution of externally infused MSCs to damaged tissues/organs. However, attention needs to be paid to unexpected off-target effects of drugs in patients. To avoid this, we have sought drugs that act on MSCs and elicit therapeutic effects among compounds developed for medical purposes. We believe that this drug repositioning strategy shortens the drug development period, reduces medical costs, and provides

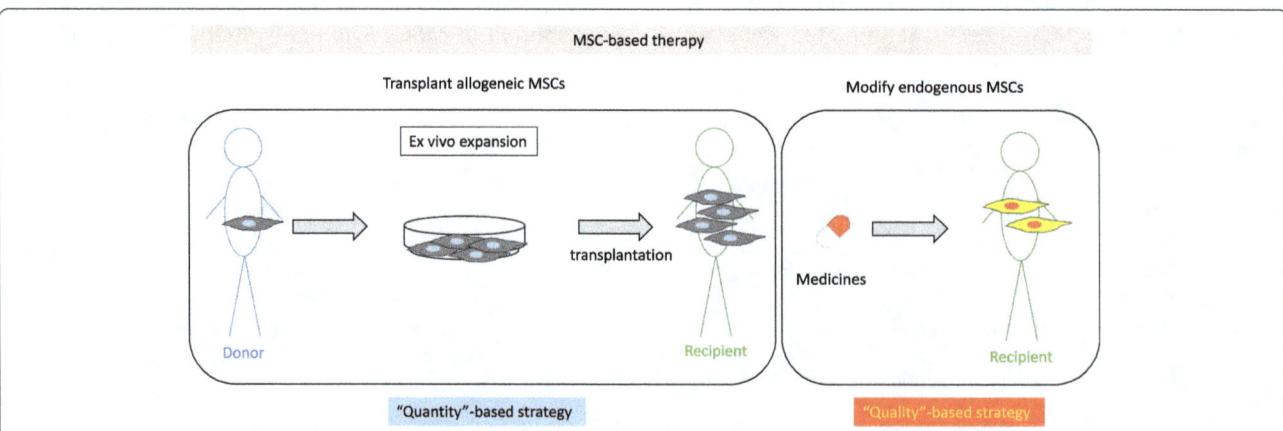

Fig. 2 MSC-based therapy with pharmacological modification of endogenous MSCs. In a conventional approach, MSCs are isolated from donors, culture-expanded ex vivo, and then infused into recipients, mainly intravenously. This intervention is a "quantity"-based strategy to achieve the therapeutic effects of MSCs (*left panel*). We have proposed a strategy in which pharmacological treatment activates or modifies the functions of endogenous MSCs. This intervention is a "quality"-based strategy to achieve the therapeutic effects of MSCs (*right panel*)

patients with safe medications. In addition, there is a possibility that the characteristics of MSCs in patients might be affected [45]. Therefore, pharmacological stimulation of such affected MSCs may have unexpected effects on the pathogenesis of diseases. Thus, further investigations are needed to establish a quality-based, pharmacological, MSC-targeted strategy.

Perspectives of MSC-based therapy

We recently reported that short-term treatment with ascorbic acid, inorganic phosphate, and dexamethasone (osteogenesis-inducing cocktails) accelerates hematopoietic recovery in mice that undergo BM transplantation, with altered chemotaxis- and adhesion-related gene expression profiles in BM-MSCs [36]. As well as treatment with a single pharmacological agent, combination treatment is also effective to achieve a therapeutic effect.

Recent studies reveal that MSCs are associated not only with normal hematopoiesis but also with the pathogenesis and progression of hematological malignant diseases. Our laboratory previously reported that defective MSCs are responsible for the impaired physiological early B cell lymphopoiesis in C/EBPβ-knockout mice [46]. Furthermore, MSC-mediated resistance to anti-cancer drugs in B cell precursor acute lymphoblastic leukemia cells can be ameliorated by pharmacological treatment of MSCs [47]. Raaijmakers et al. showed that deletion of *Dicer1* in mouse osteoprogenitors causes myelodysplasia [48]. Balderman et al. suggested a novel therapeutic strategy to target the BM microenvironment for the treatment of myelodysplastic syndromes using model mice [49]. Collectively, the BM microenvironment is closely related to the pathogenesis and progression of hematological malignant diseases; therefore, targeting MSCs in this microenvironment is a crucial therapeutic strategy.

Conclusions

MSCs have a variety of biological characteristics. Cell therapy using MSCs is effective in a substantial proportion of intractable diseases; however, it is still in the process of development. Further investigations are needed to establish more effective MSC-based therapies.

Abbreviations

ASA: Acetylsalicylic acid; BM: Bone marrow; BM-MSC: Bone marrow-derived mesenchymal stromal/stem cell; GVHD: Graft-versus-host disease; HLA: Human leukocyte antigen; HPP: Hypophosphatasia; HSC: Hematopoietic stem/progenitor cell; HSCT: Hematopoietic stem/progenitor cell transplantation; ISCT: International Society of Cellular Therapy; IUT: In utero transplantation; MSC: Mesenchymal stromal/stem cell; OI: Osteogenesis imperfecta; PBSC: Peripheral blood stem/progenitor cells; PTH: Parathyroid hormone

Acknowledgements
We thank Dr. Masaki Iwasa, Dr. Aya Fujishiro, Dr. Sumie Fujii, Ms. Yoko Nakagawa, Dr. Satoshi Yoshioka, and Dr. Hisayuki Yao for their excellent work. The authors are grateful to Prof. Songtao Shi (University of Pennsylvania) for his mentorship on MSC studies.

Funding
This study was supported in part by a Grant-in-Aid from the Ministry of Education, Culture, Sports, Science, and Technology in Japan (#26293277 and #15K09453, YM and TI; #16H00656, NS). This work was also supported in part by the Program of the network-type Joint Usage/Research Disaster Medical Science of Hiroshima University, Nagasaki University, and Fukushima Medical University (YM).

Authors' contributions
NS and YM wrote the manuscript. TI, ATK, and TM provided the intellectual input to the manuscript. All authors read and approved the final manuscript.

Competing interests
The authors declare that they have no competing interests.

Author details
[1]Department of Transfusion Medicine and Cell Therapy, Kyoto University Hospital, 54 Kawaharacho, Shogoin, Sakyo-ku, Kyoto 606-8507, Japan. [2]Department of Hematology/Oncology, Graduate School of Medicine, Kyoto University, Kyoto 606-8507, Japan. [3]Department of Hematology and Oncology, Research Institute for Radiation Biology and Medicine, Hiroshima University, Hiroshima 734-8553, Japan.

References
1. Pittenger MF, Mackay AM, Beck SC, Jaiswal RK, Douglas R, Mosca JD, Moorman MA, Simonetti DW, Craig S, Marshak DR. Multilineage potential of adult human mesenchymal stem cells. Science. 1999;284:143–7.
2. Gerson SL. Mesenchymal stem cells: no longer second class marrow citizens. Nat Med. 1999;5:262–4.
3. Miura Y, Gao Z, Miura M, Seo BM, Sonoyama W, Chen W, Gronthos S, Zhang L, Shi S. Mesenchymal stem cell-organized bone marrow elements: an alternative hematopoietic progenitor resource. Stem Cells. 2006;24:2428–36.
4. Miura Y. Human bone marrow mesenchymal stromal/stem cells: current clinical applications and potential for hematology. Int J Hematol. 2016; 103:122–8.
5. Dominici M, Le Blanc K, Mueller I, Slaper-Cortenbach I, Marini F, Krause D, Deans R, Keating A, Prockop D, Horwitz E. Minimal criteria for defining multipotent mesenchymal stromal cells. The International Society for Cellular Therapy position statement. Cytotherapy. 2006;8:315–7.
6. Yoshioka S, Miura Y, Iwasa M, Fujishiro A, Yao H, Miura M, Fukuoka M, Nakagawa Y, Yokota A, Hirai H, Ichinohe T, Takaori-Kondo A, Maekawa T. Isolation of mesenchymal stromal/stem cells from small-volume umbilical cord blood units that do not qualify for the banking system. Int J Hematol. 2015;102:218–29.
7. Miura M, Gronthos S, Zhao M, Lu B, Fisher LW, Robey PG, Shi S. SHED: stem cells from human exfoliated deciduous teeth. Proc Natl Acad Sci U S A. 2003;100:5807–12.
8. Morikawa S, Mabuchi Y, Niibe K, Suzuki S, Nagoshi N, Sunabori T, Shimmura S, Nagai Y, Nakagawa T, Okano H, Matsuzaki Y. Development of mesenchymal stem cells partially originate from the neural crest. Biochem Biophys Res Commun. 2009;379:1114–9.
9. Mabuchi Y, Matsuzaki Y. Prospective isolation of resident adult human mesenchymal stem cell population from multiple organs. Int J Hematol. 2016;103:138–44.
10. Le Blanc K, Frassoni F, Ball L, Locatelli F, Roelofs H, Lewis I, Lanino E, Sundberg B, Bernardo ME, Remberger M, Dini G, Egeler RM, Bacigalupo A, Fibbe W, Ringden O. Mesenchymal stem cells for treatment of steroid-resistant, severe, acute graft-versus-host disease: a phase II study. Lancet (London, England). 2008;371:1579–86.

11. Kebriaei P, Isola L, Bahceci E, Holland K, Rowley S, McGuirk J, Devetten M, Jansen J, Herzig R, Schuster M, Monroy R, Uberti J. Adult human mesenchymal stem cells added to corticosteroid therapy for the treatment of acute graft-versus-host disease. Biol Blood Marrow Transplant. 2009;15:804–11.

12. Prasad VK, Lucas KG, Kleiner GI, Talano JA, Jacobsohn D, Broadwater G, Monroy R, Kurtzberg J. Efficacy and safety of ex vivo cultured adult human mesenchymal stem cells (Prochymal) in pediatric patients with severe refractory acute graft-versus-host disease in a compassionate use study. Biol Blood Marrow Transplant. 2011;17:534–41.

13. Kurtzberg J, Prockop S, Teira P, Bittencourt H, Lewis V, Chan KW, Horn B, Yu L, Talano JA, Nemecek E, Mills CR, Chaudhury S. Allogeneic human mesenchymal stem cell therapy (remestemcel-L, Prochymal) as a rescue agent for severe refractory acute graft-versus-host disease in pediatric patients. Biol Blood Marrow Transplant. 2014;20:229–35.

14. Muroi K, Miyamura K, Ohashi K, Murata M, Eto T, Kobayashi N, Taniguchi S, Imamura M, Ando K, Kato S, Mori T, Teshima T, Mori M, Ozawa K. Unrelated allogeneic bone marrow-derived mesenchymal stem cells for steroid-refractory acute graft-versus-host disease: a phase I/II study. Int J Hematol. 2013;98:206–13.

15. Muroi K, Miyamura K, Okada M, Yamashita T, Murata M, Ishikawa T, Uike N, Hidaka M, Kobayashi R, Imamura M, Tanaka J, Ohashi K, Taniguchi S, Ikeda T, Eto T, Mori M, Yamaoka M, Ozawa K. Bone marrow-derived mesenchymal stem cells (JR-031) for steroid-refractory grade III or IV acute graft-versus-host disease: a phase II/III study. Int J Hematol. 2016;103:243–50.

16. Remberger M, Ringden O. Treatment of severe acute graft-versus-host disease with mesenchymal stromal cells: a comparison with non-MSC treated patients. Int J Hematol. 2012;96:822–4.

17. Hashmi S, Ahmed M, Murad MH, Litzow MR, Adams RH, Ball LM, Prasad VK, Kebriaei P, Ringden O. Survival after mesenchymal stromal cell therapy in steroid-refractory acute graft-versus-host disease: systematic review and meta-analysis. The Lancet Haematology. 2016;3:e45–52.

18. Horwitz EM, Prockop DJ, Fitzpatrick LA, Koo WW, Gordon PL, Neel M, Sussman M, Orchard P, Marx JC, Pyeritz RE, Brenner MK. Transplantability and therapeutic effects of bone marrow-derived mesenchymal cells in children with osteogenesis imperfecta. Nat Med. 1999;5:309–13.

19. Horwitz EM, Prockop DJ, Gordon PL, Koo WW, Fitzpatrick LA, Neel MD, McCarville ME, Orchard PJ, Pyeritz RE, Brenner MK. Clinical responses to bone marrow transplantation in children with severe osteogenesis imperfecta. Blood. 2001;97:1227–31.

20. Le Blanc K, Gotherstrm C, Ringden O, Hassan M, McMahon R, Horwitz E, Anneren G, Axelsson O, Nunn J, Ewald U, Norden-Lindeberg S, Jansson M, Dalton A, Astrom E, Westgren M. Fetal mesenchymal stem-cell engraftment in bone after in utero transplantation in a patient with severe osteogenesis imperfecta. Transplantation. 2005;79:1607–14.

21. Whyte MP, Kurtzberg J, McAlister WH, Mumm S, Podgornik MN, Coburn SP, Ryan LM, Miller CR, Gottesman GS, Smith AK, Douville J, Waters-Pick B, Armstrong RD, Martin PL. Marrow cell transplantation for infantile hypophosphatasia. J Bone Miner Res. 2003;18:624–36.

22. Tadokoro M, Kanai R, Taketani T, Uchio Y, Yamaguchi S, Ohgushi H. New bone formation by allogeneic mesenchymal stem cell transplantation in a patient with perinatal hypophosphatasia. J Pediatr. 2009;154:924–30.

23. Taketani T, Oyama C, Mihara A, Tanabe Y, Abe M, Hirade T, Yamamoto S, Bo R, Kanai R, Tadenuma T, Michibata Y, Yamamoto S, Hattori M, Katsube Y, Ohnishi H, Sasao M, Oda Y, Hattori K, Yuba S, Ohgushi H, Yamaguchi S. Ex vivo expanded allogeneic mesenchymal stem cells with bone marrow transplantation improved osteogenesis in infants with severe hypophosphatasia. Cell Transplant. 2015;24:1931–43.

24. Quarto R, Mastrogiacomo M, Cancedda R, Kutepov SM, Mukhachev V, Lavroukov A, Kon E, Marcacci M. Repair of large bone defects with the use of autologous bone marrow stromal cells. N Engl J Med. 2001;344:385–6.

25. Koc ON, Gerson SL, Cooper BW, Dyhouse SM, Haynesworth SE, Caplan AI, Lazarus HM. Rapid hematopoietic recovery after coinfusion of autologous-blood stem cells and culture-expanded marrow mesenchymal stem cells in advanced breast cancer patients receiving high-dose chemotherapy. Journal of clinical oncology: official journal of the American Society of Clinical Oncology. 2000;18:307–16.

26. Lazarus HM, Koc ON, Devine SM, Curtin P, Maziarz RT, Holland HK, Shpall EJ, McCarthy P, Atkinson K, Cooper BW, Gerson SL, Laughlin MJ, Loberiza Jr FR, Moseley AB, Bacigalupo A. Cotransplantation of HLA-identical sibling culture-expanded mesenchymal stem cells and hematopoietic stem cells in hematologic malignancy patients. Biol Blood Marrow Transplant. 2005;11:389–98.

27. Le Blanc K, Samuelsson H, Gustafsson B, Remberger M, Sundberg B, Arvidson J, Ljungman P, Lonnies H, Nava S, Ringden O. Transplantation of mesenchymal stem cells to enhance engraftment of hematopoietic stem cells. Leukemia. 2007;21:1733–8.

28. Macmillan ML, Blazar BR, DeFor TE, Wagner JE. Transplantation of ex-vivo culture-expanded parental haploidentical mesenchymal stem cells to promote engraftment in pediatric recipients of unrelated donor umbilical cord blood: results of a phase I-II clinical trial. Bone Marrow Transplant. 2009;43:447–54.

29. Robinson SN, Ng J, Niu T, Yang H, McMannis JD, Karandish S, Kaur I, Fu P, Del Angel M, Messinger R, Flagge F, de Lima M, Decker W, Xing D, Champlin R, Shpall EJ. Superior ex vivo cord blood expansion following co-culture with bone marrow-derived mesenchymal stem cells. Bone Marrow Transplant. 2006;37:359–66.

30. de Lima M, McNiece I, Robinson SN, Munsell M, Eapen M, Horowitz M, Alousi A, Saliba R, McMannis JD, Kaur I, Kebriaei P, Parmar S, Popat U, Hosing C, Champlin R, Bollard C, Molldrem JJ, Jones RB, Nieto Y, Andersson BS, Shah N, Oran B, Cooper LJ, Worth L, Qazilbash MH, Korbling M, Rondon G, Ciurea S, Bosque D, Maewal I, Simmons PJ, Shpall EJ. Cord-blood engraftment with ex vivo mesenchymal-cell coculture. N Engl J Med. 2012;367:2305–15.

31. Schrepfer S, Deuse T, Reichenspurner H, Fischbein MP, Robbins RC, Pelletier MP. Stem cell transplantation: the lung barrier. Transplant Proc. 2007;39:573–6.

32. Miura Y, Yoshioka S, Yao H, Takaori-Kondo A, Maekawa T, Ichinohe T. Chimerism of bone marrow mesenchymal stem/stromal cells in allogeneic hematopoietic cell transplantation. Chimerism. 2013;4:78–83.

33. Yamaza T, Miura Y, Bi Y, Liu Y, Akiyama K, Sonoyama W, Patel V, Gutkind S, Young M, Gronthos S, Le A, Wang CY, Chen W, Shi S. Pharmacologic stem cell based intervention as a new approach to osteoporosis treatment in rodents. PLoS One. 2008;3, e2615.

34. Yamaza T, Miura Y, Akiyama K, Bi Y, Sonoyama W, Gronthos S, Chen W, Le A, Shi S. Mesenchymal stem cell-mediated ectopic hematopoiesis alleviates aging-related phenotype in immunocompromised mice. Blood. 2009;113: 2595–604.

35. Yao H, Miura Y, Yoshioka S, Miura M, Hayashi Y, Tamura A, Iwasa M, Sato A, Hishita T, Higashi Y, Kaneko H, Ashihara E, Ichinohe T, Hirai H, Maekawa T. Parathyroid hormone enhances hematopoietic expansion via upregulation of cadherin-11 in bone marrow mesenchymal stromal cells. Stem Cells. 2014;32:2245–55.

36. Sugino N, Miura Y, Yao H, Iwasa M, Fujishiro A, Fujii S, Hirai H, Takaori-Kondo A, Ichinohe T, Maekawa T. Early osteoinductive human bone marrow mesenchymal stromal/stem cells support an enhanced hematopoietic cell expansion with altered chemotaxis- and adhesion-related gene expression profiles. Biochem Biophys Res Commun. 2016;469:823–9.

37. Fujishiro A, Miura Y, Iwasa M, Fujii S, Tamura A, Sato A, Yokota A, Sugino N, Hirai H, Ando A, Ichinohe T, Maekawa T. Vitamin K2 supports hematopoiesis through acting on bone marrow mesenchymal stromal/stem cells [Abstract]. Blood. 2015;126:1192.

38. Cashman J, McAnulty G. Nonsteroidal anti-inflammatory drugs in perisurgical pain management. Mechanisms of action and rationale for optimum use. Drugs. 1995;49:51–70.

39. Buttar NS, Wang KK. The "aspirin" of the new millennium: cyclooxygenase-2 inhibitors. Mayo Clin Proc. 2000;75:1027–38.

40. Carbone LD, Tylavsky FA, Cauley JA, Harris TB, Lang TF, Bauer DC, Barrow KD, Kritchevsky SB. Association between bone mineral density and the use of nonsteroidal anti-inflammatory drugs and aspirin: impact of cyclooxygenase selectivity. J Bone Miner Res. 2003;18:1795–802.

41. Neer RM, Arnaud CD, Zanchetta JR, Prince R, Gaich GA, Reginster JY, Hodsman AB, Eriksen EF, Ish-Shalom S, Genant HK, Wang O, Mitlak BH. Effect of parathyroid hormone (1-34) on fractures and bone mineral density in postmenopausal women with osteoporosis. N Engl J Med. 2001;344:1434–41.

42. Kuhrt D, Wojchowski DM. Emerging EPO and EPO receptor regulators and signal transducers. Blood. 2015;125:3536–41.

43. Takami A, Nakao S, Ontachi Y, Yamauchi H, Matsuda T. Successful therapy of myelodysplastic syndrome with menatetrenone, a vitamin K2 analog. Int J Hematol. 1999;69:24–6.

44. Nishimaki J, Miyazawa K, Yaguchi M, Katagiri T, Kawanishi Y, Toyama K, Ohyashiki K, Hashimoto S, Nakaya K, Takiguchi T. Vitamin K2 induces apoptosis of a novel cell line established from a patient with myelodysplastic syndrome in blastic transformation. Leukemia. 1999;13:1399–405.

45. Ferrer RA, Wobus M, List C, Wehner R, Schonefeldt C, Brocard B, Mohr B, Rauner M, Schmitz M, Stiehler M, Ehninger G, Hofbauer LC, Bornhauser M,

Platzbecker U. Mesenchymal stromal cells from patients with myelodyplastic syndrome display distinct functional alterations that are modulated by lenalidomide. Haematologica. 2013;98:1677–85.

46. Yoshioka S, Miura Y, Yao H, Satake S, Hayashi Y, Tamura A, Hishita T, Icinohe T, Hirai H, Takaor-Kondo A, Maekawa T. CCAAT/enhancer-binding protein beta expressed by bone marrow mesenchymal stromal cells regulates early B-cell lymphopoiesis. Stem Cells. 2014;32:730–40.

47. Iwasa M, Miura Y, Fujishiro A, Fujii S, Sugino N, Yoshioka S, Tamura A, Sato A, Yokota A, Kito K, Ando A, Hirai H, Takaori-Kondo A, Ichinohe T, Maekawa T. Bortezomib attenuates adhesion of B cell precursor acute lymphoblastic lleukemia cells to bone marrow mesenchymal stromal/stem cells via regulating SPARC expression [Abstract]. Blood. 2015;126:786.

48. Raaijmakers MH, Mukherjee S, Guo S, Zhang S, Kobayashi T, Schoonmaker JA, Ebert BL, Al-Shahrour F, Hasserjian RP, Scadden EO, Aung Z, Matza M, Merkenschlager M, Lin C, Rommens JM, Scadden DT. Bone progenitor dysfunction induces myelodysplasia and secondary leukaemia. Nature. 2010;464:852–7.

49. Balderman SR, Li AJ, Hoffman CM, Frisch BJ, Goodman AN, LaMere MW, Georger MA, Evans AG, Liesveld JL, Becker MW, Calvi LM. Targeting of the bone marrow microenvironment improves outcome in a murine model of myelodysplastic syndrome. Blood. 2016;127:616–25.

10

BAFF- and APRIL-targeted therapy in systemic autoimmune diseases

Shingo Nakayamada and Yoshiya Tanaka*

Abstract

B cells play a pivotal role in autoimmunity not only by producing pathogenic autoantibodies but also by modulating immune responses via the production of cytokines and chemokines. The B cell-activating factor/a proliferation-inducing ligand (BAFF/APRIL) system promotes B cell survival and differentiation and thus plays a prominent role in the pathogenesis of autoimmune diseases. Currently, BAFF and APRIL inhibitors are in clinical trials for systemic lupus erythematosus with significant efficacy. However, several studies have demonstrated the efficacy of the BAFF/APRIL blockade which showed considerable variability in the response to B cell-targeted therapy. This may indicate substantial heterogeneity in the pathogenesis of autoimmune diseases. Therefore, objective markers that can predict the effect of BAFF/APRIL-blocking agents could be valuable to the precision medicine linked clinically and to cost-effective therapy.

Keywords: BAFF, APRIL, B cells, Tfh cells, Autoimmune diseases

Background

Systemic autoimmune diseases are pathologically characterized by immune complexes consisting of antigens, the activation of dendritic cells and autoreactive T cells, and the overproduction of autoantibodies secreted from activated B cells, which cause severe inflammation in various organs [1]. Although the survival of patients with autoimmune diseases has improved over the past 50 years with conventional treatments such as immunosuppressants and corticosteroids, these drugs are limited by inefficacy and intolerance in some patients. Since several autoimmune diseases such as systemic lupus erythematosus (SLE) and ANCA-associated vasculitis (AAV) remain an important cause of mortality and morbidity, innovative therapeutic approaches need to be developed.

B cells play a pivotal role in the pathogenesis of autoimmune diseases not only by producing pathogenic autoantibodies but also by modulating immune responses via production of cytokines and chemokines [2]. The potential efficacy of B cell depletion therapy has been reported in several autoimmune diseases. Rituximab, a chimeric anti-CD20 antibody, eliminates CD20-expressing pre-B and mature B cells through antibody- and complement-dependent cytotoxic activities [3]. In Japan, rituximab is approved for clinical use in childhood refractory nephrotic syndrome and AAV such as granulomatosis with polyangiitis (GPA) and microscopic polyangiitis (MPA). Despite expectations, large randomized controlled clinical trials of rituximab for non-renal and renal SLE (EXPLORER and LUNAR, respectively) did not achieve the primary goal [4, 5]. In addition, adverse reactions such as hepatitis B virus reactivation, opportunistic infections, malignancies, and inefficacy in AAV patients who were treated with rituximab have been reported in a Japanese cohort (RiCRAV) [6].

Currently, the TNF family ligands, B cell-activating factor (BAFF), a proliferation-inducing ligand (APRIL), and those receptors (BAFF receptor (BAFF-R), transmembrane activator and calcium modulator and cytophilin ligand interactor (TACI), B cell maturation antigen (BCMA), and proteoglycans) are found to play a prominent role in the pathogenesis of and are known as the potential therapeutic target for autoimmune diseases. In this review, we highlight the recent advance in the BAFF/APRIL-targeted therapy in systemic autoimmune diseases.

* Correspondence: tanaka@med.uoeh-u.ac.jp
The First Department of Internal Medicine, School of Medicine, University of Occupational and Environmental Health, 1-1 Iseigaoka, Yahata-nishi, Kitakyushu 807-8555, Japan

Pathological significance of the interaction between B cells and Tfh cells

Disturbances of T cell and B cell functions are involved in the development of autoimmune diseases [2, 7–11]. Activated B cells function as potent antigen-presenting cells and activate autoreactive T cells. The expression of co-stimulatory molecules, such as CD40 and CD80, is enhanced on B cells in autoimmune diseases such as SLE and is involved in the interactive activation with surrounding immunocompetent cells including autoreactive T cells [8, 9]. In addition, RNA- or DNA-containing autoantigens co-ligate B cell receptors (BCRs) and Toll-like receptor (TLR)-7/9, leading to robust activation, proliferation, and differentiation of autoreactive B cells [12]. In SLE, autoantibodies produced by autoreactive B cells form immune complexes that deposit in tissues, leading to persistent inflammation and organ damage. Furthermore, it is well known that the number of memory B cells and plasmablasts correlate with disease activity in SLE [13–15]. We reported previously that the proportions of $CD19^+IgD^-CD27^+$ class-switched memory B cells and $CD19^+IgD^-CD27^-$ effector memory B cells tended to be higher in the peripheral blood of refractory SLE patients than in that of the control [16–18]. In contrast, B regulatory (Breg) cells, which produce interleukin (IL)-10 and transforming growth factor-β (TGF-β) and suppress effector T cells, are defective in patients with SLE [19].

The differentiation of $CD4^+$ T helper cells into functionally distinct helper T subsets is critical for the pathogenesis of autoimmune diseases [20, 21], especially since the active involvement of T helper (Th) 17 and T follicular helper (Tfh) cells and the dysfunction of T regulatory (Treg) cells have been reported [20, 22–27]. Among these subsets, the Tfh cells have emerged as a critical regulator of autoimmunity [22]. The Tfh cells provide B cell help by promoting the class switching of B cells and are defined by the expression of the master regulator Bcl6 and effector cytokine IL-21, along with key surface molecules, such as PD-1, CXCR5, CD40L, and ICOS [22, 28]. The CXCR5 expression allows Tfh cells to migrate from the T cell zone to the B cell follicle where they localize in the germinal center (GC) and mediate B cell help via cell-cell contact using the co-stimulatory molecules CD40L and ICOS [22]. Thus, B-Tfh cell interaction is necessary for autoantibody production. In mice, the excessive activity of Tfh cells induces hyperactive GC formation and autoantibody production, leading to a SLE-like phenotype [29, 30]. While we and others have reported the mechanism of Tfh differentiation, the exact role of this subset in patients remains elusive. High proportions of circulating Tfh cells, which are characterized as $CD4^+CXCR5^+ICOS^{high}PD-1^{high}$, have been described in SLE patients, and their level in the peripheral blood correlates with titers of autoantibodies and with disease severity [31, 32].

Taken together, these findings highlight the notion that activated T cells, in addition to activated B cells, may also be potentially involved in the pathogenesis of autoimmunity and that the interaction between activated B and Tfh cells may play an important role in autoantibody-driven autoimmune diseases.

Pathological role of BAFF and APRIL in autoimmune diseases

BAFF, also called B lymphocyte stimulator (BLyS), is a B cell activation factor which is mainly expressed by monocytes, macrophages, and activated T cells. BAFF can be expressed on the cell surface as a membrane-bound form or released as a soluble form after cleavage by furin. BAFF binds to three receptors, the BAFF-R, BCMA, or TACI, and regulates B cell survival, differentiation, maturation, immunoglobulin class switching, and antibody production (Fig. 1) [33, 34]. BAFF-R is mainly expressed in immature B cells, whereas TACI and BCMA are expressed in matured memory B cells and plasma cells, respectively. In addition, APRIL, which is a homologous factor to BAFF, binds to TACI, BCMA, and proteoglycans (Fig. 1). APRIL forms heterotrimers with BAFF and enhances BAFF-mediated B cell activation [35]. TACI binds with higher affinity to APRIL but lower affinity to BAFF, compared with other BAFF receptors. Although both BAFF and APRIL promote B cell survival and differentiation, there are complicated regulatory mechanisms according to the varieties of the receptors (BAFF-R, BCMA, or TACI) and the differentiation stage of B cells, as described above. In addition to its effect on B cells, recent works have demonstrated that BAFF can promote T cell activation, proliferation, and differentiation [36]. Interestingly, Coquery et al. reported that BCMA negatively regulates Tfh cell expansion, while BAFF-R-mediated signaling promotes Tfh cell accumulation into GC in lupus-prone mice [37]. Thus, the balance between BCMA and BAFF-R signaling may control the development of Tfh cells, indicating that BAFF/APRIL regulate autoimmunity not only via survival and differentiation of B cell but also via expansion of Tfh cells.

Animal studies have shown that BAFF-deficient mice lack B cell maturation and the knockout of BAFF in lupus-prone mice showed a reduction of mortality and disease severity [38]. The transgenic mice for BAFF show an expanded B cell maturation and develop severe SLE, which is supported by evidence on increased concentrations of anti-double-stranded DNA (dsDNA) antibodies and immune complex deposition in the mesangium [34, 39–41]. In humans, the serum level of BAFF and APRIL is both elevated in patients with SLE and positively correlates with disease activity and serological markers such as anti-

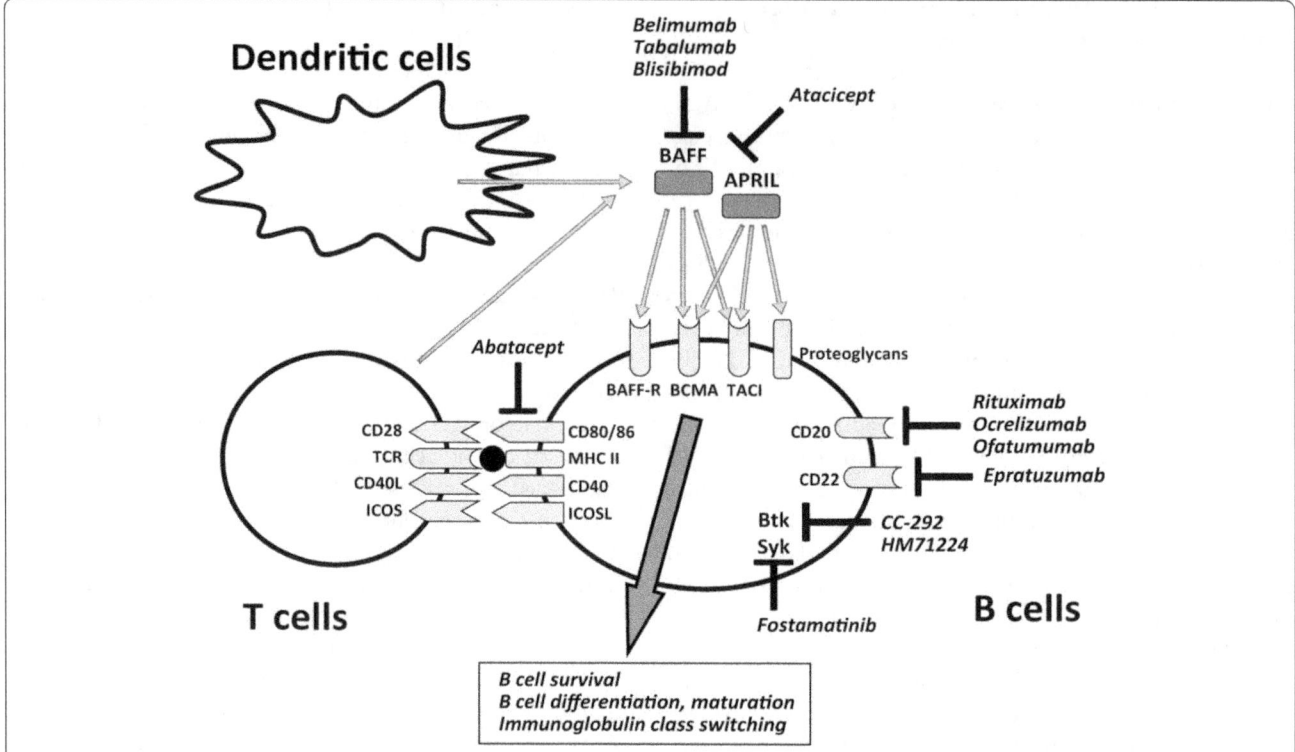

Fig. 1 Emerging B cell-targeted therapy including BAFF/APRIL inhibition in autoimmune diseases. Current strategies for autoimmune diseases include appropriate targets for therapeutic modulation such as B cell surface antigens (CD20 and CD22), co-stimulatory molecules (CTLA-4, CD40/CD40L, ICOS/ICOSL, and BAFF/APRIL/BAFF-R/BCMA/TACI), and various intracellular signal transduction pathways (Syk and Btk)

dsDNA antibody levels [42, 43]. There is a correlation between BAFF levels and circulating autoantibody levels in Sjogren's syndrome (SS) [44]. In addition, BAFF has been found to be elevated in the serum of AAV patients [45, 46]. These results suggest a potential therapeutic strategy for patients with systemic autoimmune diseases by BAFF and/or APRIL blockade.

Targeting BAFF and APRIL in systemic autoimmune diseases

1. BAFF blockers

Current strategies for autoimmune diseases include appropriate targets for therapeutic modulation such as B cell surface antigens (CD20 and CD22), co-stimulatory molecules (CTLA-4, CD40/CD40L, ICOS/ICOSL, and BAFF/APRIL/BAFF-R/BCMA/TACI), and various intracellular signal transduction pathways (Syk and Btk) (Fig. 1) [47, 48]. Selective inhibitors of BAFF and APRIL, which should ameliorate the pathogenesis by inhibiting autoreactive B cell activation and autoantibody production, are in clinical trials for autoimmune diseases (Fig. 1).

Belimumab is a fully human monoclonal antibody that antagonizes BAFF, thus inhibiting B cell survival and

differentiation [49]. Belimumab directly reduces activation of naïve and transitional B cells and indirectly inhibits development of IgD⁻CD27⁺ class-switched memory B cells, plasmablasts, and plasma cells. The multicenter, randomized placebo-controlled double-blind phase III trials, BLISS-52 and BLISS-76, were performed to investigate the efficacy of belimumab at 1 or 10 mg/kg compared to placebo in the treatment of active SLE [50–52]. The primary end point was amelioration in SRI (SLE responder index), a composite measurement of SELENA-SLEDAI (Safety of Estrogens in Lupus Erythematosus National Assessment-Systemic Lupus Erythematosus Disease Activity Index), BILAG (British Isles Lupus Assessment Group) score, and physician global assessment. The BLISS-52 trial demonstrated that SRI rates at 52-week posttreatment were 44 %, 51 % ($p = 0.01$), and 58 % ($p < 0.01$) in the placebo, belimumab 1 mg/kg, and belimumab 10 mg/kg groups, respectively, suggesting a significant improvement of disease activity with an increased dose of this drug [51]. Belimumab has greater therapeutic benefit in patients with higher disease activity (SLEDAI ≥10), anti-dsDNA positivity, or low complement [53]. No significant difference between the frequency of serious adverse reactions between the belimumab group and the placebo group was observed. Collectively, these results highlighted the efficacy and tolerability of belimumab as a novel biologic agent for the treatment of SLE, and the FDA approved this drug in 2011. However, the patients with active lupus nephritis were excluded in these trials. Therefore, it would be useful to investigate in future trials to elucidate the efficacy of belimumab in the patients with major organ involvements. Currently, the phase III trials to examine the efficacy and safety of belimumab in active lupus nephritis (NCT01639339) and in SLE patients located in Northeast Asia (NCT01345253) are ongoing.

Furthermore, belimumab is currently undergoing clinical trials in SS and AAV. In the phase II trial in 30 patients with primary SS (BELISS), 60 % of the patients were responders and systemic activity scores measured by the EULAR SS disease activity index (ESSDAI) were significantly improved [54, 55]. Since this is an open-label trial, further randomized controlled trials are warranted. The phase III multicenter, randomized, double-blind study to evaluate the efficacy and safety of belimumab in combination with azathioprine for the maintenance of remission in GPA and MPA (BREVAS) is ongoing (NCT01663623) [56, 57].

Other anti-BAFF agents, tabalumab and blisibimod, are also being assessed in phase III randomized placebo-controlled trials to evaluate their efficacy in SLE. Tabalumab is a monoclonal antibody that neutralizes BAFF in both membrane-bound form and soluble form, whereas belimumab is thought to target the soluble form only. In rheumatoid arthritis (RA), tabalumab showed clinical efficacy in phase II trials in patients with an inadequate response to methotrexate (MTX) [58, 59]. However, the phase III trial demonstrated that tabalumab did not provide the degree of clinical efficacy in moderate-severe RA, taking the MTX observed with other approved biological agents [60]. Based on these findings, the pharmaceutical company discontinued the phase III trial for RA. In addition, the phase III clinical trials for tabalumab in moderate to severe SLE (ILLUMINATE-2) met its primary end point only at higher doses but failed to meet secondary end points [61]. The pharmaceutical company also discontinued the development of this drug for SLE.

Blisibimod is a human "peptibody," which binds to both cell membrane-expressed and soluble BAFF and antagonizes BAFF, and has recently been evaluated in a phase II clinical trial (PEARL-SC) [62]. In this study, the significant reductions in proteinuria and anti-dsDNA and significant increases in C3 were observed with the blisibimod group. Currently, a phase III study to examine the efficacy and safety of blisibimod in patients with active SLE (NCT01395745) is under way.

Briobacept, a protein containing both IgG and the ligand of BAFF-R, which antagonizes BAFF did not show sufficient efficacy in a phase II trial (ATLAS) (NCT01499355) and was terminated.

2. TACI-Ig: atacicept

Atacicept, a recombinant fusion protein containing both the Fc portion of the human IgG1 and the extracellular domain of TACI [63, 64], binds to APRIL and BAFF and inhibits activation of TACI-mediated signaling. The phase I trial in moderately active SLE showed that atacicept resulted in a 60 % reduction in mature B cells and a 45 % attenuation of immunoglobulin compared to placebo [65]. There were no significant differences in the levels of adverse reactions between atacicept and placebo. However, the phase II clinical trial in patients with active lupus nephritis who are taking steroids and MMF was terminated due to severe infection [66]. Isenberg et al. reported recently the results of a randomized phase II/III trial of atacicept that sought to determine the efficacy and safety of atacicept in the prevention of flares in SLE [67]. The results with a high dose of atacicept were encouraging, but there are severe concerns about the infections. Currently, the phase III clinical trials for atacicept in patients who have no major organ involvements (ADDRESS II) (NCT01972568, NCT02070978) are under way. In Japan, a phase IIb trial in patients with SLE is in progress.

Conclusions

BAFF and APRIL play a prominent role in the pathogenesis of autoimmune diseases. Indeed, a certain number of patients receive benefit from BAFF/APRIL-blocking therapies. On the other hand, several clinical trials have demonstrated the efficacy of the BAFF/APRIL blockade which showed considerable variability in the response to B cell-targeted therapy. Furthermore, increasing evidence points to substantial heterogeneity in the pathogenesis of autoimmune diseases; thus, B cell-targeted therapy may be ineffective in some patients but effective in others. Therefore, objective markers that can predict the effect of BAFF/APRIL-blocking agents should be valuable to the precision medicine linked clinically and to cost-effective therapy.

Abbreviations

AAV: ANCA-associated vasculitis; APRIL: a proliferation-inducing ligand; BAFF: B cell-activating factor; BCMA: B cell maturation antigen; BCR: B cell receptor; BILAG: British Isles Lupus Assessment Group; BLyS: B lymphocyte stimulator; Breg: B regulatory; ESSDAI: EULAR SS disease activity index; GC: germinal center; GPA: granulomatosis with polyangitis; IL: interleukin; MPA: microscopic polyangitis; MTX: methotrexate; RA: rheumatoid arthritis; SELENA: Safety of Estrogens in Lupus Erythematosus National Assessment; SLE: systemic lupus erythematosus; SLEDAI: Systemic Lupus Erythematosus Disease Activity Index; SRI: SLE responder index; SS: Sjogren's syndrome; TACI: transmembrane activator and calcium modulator and cytophilin ligand interactor; Tfh: T follicular helper; TGF: transforming growth factor; TLR: Toll-like receptor; Treg: T regulatory.

Competing interests

Y. Tanaka has received consulting fees, lecture fees, and/or honoraria from Mitsubishi-Tanabe, Eisai, Chugai, Abbott Japan, Astellas, Daiichi-Sankyo, Abbvie, Janssen, Pfizer, Takeda, Astra-Zeneca, Eli Lilly Japan, GlaxoSmithKline, Quintiles, MSD, and Asahi-Kasei and has received research grants from Bristol-Myers, Mitsubishi-Tanabe, Abbvie, MSD, Chugai, Astellas, and Daiichi-Sankyo. S. Nakayamada declares no conflict of interest.

Authors' contributions

SN and YT contributed to the overall review and writing of the manuscript. All authors enrolled and clinically managed the study patients, and Both authors read and approved the final manuscript.

Funding

This work was supported in part by Research on Rare and Intractable Diseases and Research Grant-In-Aid for Scientific Research by the Ministry of Health, Labor and Welfare of Japan; the Ministry of Education, Culture, Sports, Science and Technology of Japan; and the University of Occupational and Environmental Health, Japan, and UOEH Grant for Advanced Research.

References

1. Arbuckle MR, McClain MT, Rubertone MV, et al. Development of autoantibodies before the clinical onset of systemic lupus erythematosus. N Engl J Med. 2003; 349:1526–33.
2. Liu Z, Davidson A. Taming lupus-a new understanding of pathogenesis is leading to clinical advances. Nat Med. 2012;18:871–82.
3. Tanaka Y, Yamamoto K, Takeuchi T, et al. A multicenter phase I/II trial of rituximab for refractory systemic lupus erythematosus. Mod Rheumatol. 2007;17:191–7.
4. Merrill JT, Neuwelt CM, Wallace DJ, et al. Efficacy and safety of rituximab in moderately-to-severely active systemic lupus erythematosus: the randomized, double-blind, phase II/III systemic lupus erythematosus evaluation of rituximab trial. Arthritis Rheum. 2010;62:222–33.
5. Rovin BH, Furie R, Latinis K, et al. Efficacy and safety of rituximab in patients with active proliferative lupus nephritis: the Lupus Nephritis Assessment with Rituximab study. Arthritis Rheum. 2012;64:1215–26.
6. Nagafuchi H, Atsumi T, Hatta K, et al. Long-term safety and efficacy of rituximab in 7 Japanese patients with ANCA-associated vasculitis. Mod Rheumatol. 2015;25:603–8.
7. Nakayamada S, Saito K, Nakano K, Tanaka Y. Activation signal transduction by beta1 integrin in T cells from patients with systemic lupus erythematosus. Arthritis Rheum. 2007;56:1559–68.
8. Desai-Mehta A, Lu L, Ramsey-Goldman R, Datta SK. Hyperexpression of CD40 ligand by B and T cells in human lupus and its role in pathogenic autoantibody production. J Clin Invest. 1996;97:2063–73.
9. Grammer AC, Slota R, Fischer R, et al. Abnormal germinal center reactions in systemic lupus erythematosus demonstrated by blockade of CD154-CD40 interactions. J Clin Invest. 2003;112:1506–20.
10. Crispin JC, Kyttaris V, Juang YT, Tsokos GC. Systemic lupus erythematosus: new molecular targets. Ann Rheum Dis. 2007;66 Suppl 3:iii65–9.
11. Tsokos GC. Systemic lupus erythematosus. N Engl J Med. 2011;365:2110–21.
12. Avalos AM, Busconi L, Marshak-Rothstein A. Regulation of autoreactive B cell responses to endogenous TLR ligands. Autoimmunity. 2010;43:76–83.
13. Jacobi AM, Reiter K, Mackay M, et al. Activated memory B cell subsets correlate with disease activity in systemic lupus erythematosus: delineation by expression of CD27, IgD, and CD95. Arthritis Rheum. 2008;58:1762–73.
14. Jacobi AM, Odendahl M, Reiter K, et al. Correlation between circulating CD27high plasma cells and disease activity in patients with systemic lupus erythematosus. Arthritis Rheum. 2003;48:1332–42.
15. Anolik JH, Barnard J, Owen T, et al. Delayed memory B cell recovery in peripheral blood and lymphoid tissue in systemic lupus erythematosus after B cell depletion therapy. Arthritis Rheum. 2007;56:3044–56.
16. Iwata S, Saito K, Tokunaga M, Tanaka Y. Persistent memory B cell down-regulation after 6-year remission induced by rituximab therapy in patients with systemic lupus erythematosus. Lupus. 2013;22:538–40.
17. Iwata S, Saito K, Tokunaga M, et al. Phenotypic changes of lymphocytes in patients with systemic lupus erythematosus who are in longterm remission after B cell depletion therapy with rituximab. J Rheumatol. 2011;38:633–41.
18. Tokunaga M, Fujii K, Saito K, et al. Down-regulation of CD40 and CD80 on B cells in patients with life-threatening systemic lupus erythematosus after successful treatment with rituximab. Rheumatology (Oxford). 2005;44:176–82.
19. Blair PA, Norena LY, Flores-Borja F, et al. CD19(+)CD24(hi)CD38(hi) B cells exhibit regulatory capacity in healthy individuals but are functionally impaired in systemic lupus erythematosus patients. Immunity. 2010;32:129–40.
20. Nakayamada S, Takahashi H, Kanno Y, O'Shea JJ. Helper T cell diversity and plasticity. Curr Opin Immunol. 2012;24:297–302.

21. O'Shea JJ, Paul WE. Mechanisms underlying lineage commitment and plasticity of helper CD4+ T cells. Science. 2010;327:1098–102.
22. Crotty S. Follicular helper CD4 T cells (TFH). Annu Rev Immunol. 2011;29:621–63.
23. Nakayamada S, Kanno Y, Takahashi H, et al. Early Th1 cell differentiation is marked by a Tfh cell-like transition. Immunity. 2011;35:919–31.
24. Shin MS, Lee N, Kang I. Effector T-cell subsets in systemic lupus erythematosus: update focusing on Th17 cells. Curr Opin Rheumatol. 2011;23:444–8.
25. Tangye SG, Ma CS, Brink R, Deenick EK. The good, the bad and the ugly—TFH cells in human health and disease. Nat Rev Immunol. 2013;13:412–26.
26. Bonelli M, Smolen JS, Scheinecker C. Treg and lupus. Ann Rheum Dis. 2010;69 Suppl 1:i65–6.
27. Miyara M, Gorochov G, Ehrenstein M, Musset L, Sakaguchi S, Amoura Z. Human FoxP3+ regulatory T cells in systemic autoimmune diseases. Autoimmun Rev. 2011;10:744–55.
28. Schwartzberg PL, Mueller KL, Qi H, Cannons JL. SLAM receptors and SAP influence lymphocyte interactions, development and function. Nat Rev Immunol. 2009;9:39–46.
29. Vinuesa CG, Cook MC, Angelucci C, et al. A RING-type ubiquitin ligase family member required to repress follicular helper T cells and autoimmunity. Nature. 2005;435:452–8.
30. Linterman MA, Rigby RJ, Wong RK, et al. Follicular helper T cells are required for systemic autoimmunity. J Exp Med. 2009;206:561–76.
31. Simpson N, Gatenby PA, Wilson A, et al. Expansion of circulating T cells resembling follicular helper T cells is a fixed phenotype that identifies a subset of severe systemic lupus erythematosus. Arthritis Rheum. 2010;62:234–44.
32. Le Coz C, Joublin A, Pasquali JL, Korganow AS, Dumortier H, Monneaux F. Circulating TFH subset distribution is strongly affected in lupus patients with an active disease. PLoS One. 2013;8, e75319.
33. Bossen C, Schneider P. BAFF, APRIL and their receptors: structure, function and signaling. Semin Immunol. 2006;18:263–75.
34. Chan VS, Tsang HH, Tam RC, Lu L, Lau CS. B-cell-targeted therapies in systemic lupus erythematosus. Cell Mol Immunol. 2013;10:133–42.
35. Mackay F, Ambrose C. The TNF family members BAFF and APRIL: the growing complexity. Cytokine Growth Factor Rev. 2003;14:311–24.
36. Chen M, Lin X, Liu Y, et al. The function of BAFF on T helper cells in autoimmunity. Cytokine Growth Factor Rev. 2014;25:301–5.
37. Coquery CM, Loo WM, Wade NS, et al. BAFF regulates follicular helper t cells and affects their accumulation and interferon-gamma production in autoimmunity. Arthritis Rheumatol. 2015;67:773–84.
38. Jacob CO, Pricop L, Putterman C, et al. Paucity of clinical disease despite serological autoimmunity and kidney pathology in lupus-prone New Zealand mixed 2328 mice deficient in BAFF. J Immunol. 2006;177:2671–80.
39. Groom JR, Fletcher CA, Walters SN, et al. BAFF and MyD88 signals promote a lupuslike disease independent of T cells. J Exp Med. 2007;204:1959–71.
40. Mackay F, Schneider P, Rennert P, Browning JBAFFAND. APRIL: a tutorial on B cell survival. Annu Rev Immunol. 2003;21:231–64.
41. Shulga-Morskaya S, Dobles M, Walsh ME, et al. B cell-activating factor belonging to the TNF family acts through separate receptors to support B cell survival and T cell-independent antibody formation. J Immunol. 2004;173:2331–41.
42. Chu VT, Enghard P, Schurer S, et al. Systemic activation of the immune system induces aberrant BAFF and APRIL expression in B cells in patients with systemic lupus erythematosus. Arthritis Rheum. 2009;60:2083–93.
43. Zollars E, Bienkowska J, Czerkowicz J, et al. BAFF (B cell activating factor) transcript level in peripheral blood of patients with SLE is associated with same-day disease activity as well as global activity over the next year. Lupus Sci Med. 2015;2, e000063.
44. Mariette X, Roux S, Zhang J, et al. The level of BLyS (BAFF) correlates with the titre of autoantibodies in human Sjogren's syndrome. Ann Rheum Dis. 2003;62:168–71.
45. Nagai M, Hirayama K, Ebihara I, Shimohata H, Kobayashi M, Koyama A. Serum levels of BAFF and APRIL in myeloperoxidase anti-neutrophil cytoplasmic autoantibody-associated renal vasculitis: association with disease activity. Nephron Clin Pract. 2011;118:c339–45.
46. Bader L, Koldingsnes W, Nossent J. B-lymphocyte activating factor levels are increased in patients with Wegener's granulomatosis and inversely correlated with ANCA titer. Clin Rheumatol. 2010;29:1031–5.
47. Kamal A, Khamashta M. The efficacy of novel B cell biologics as the future of SLE treatment: a review. Autoimmun Rev. 2014;13:1094–101.
48. Nakayamada S, Iwata S, Tanaka Y. Relevance of lymphocyte subsets to B cell-targeted therapy in systemic lupus erythematosus. Int J Rheum Dis. 2015;18:208–18.

49. Sanz I, Lee FE. B cells as therapeutic targets in SLE. Nat Rev Rheumatol. 2010;6:326–37.

50. Furie R, Petri M, Zamani O, et al. A phase III, randomized, placebo-controlled study of belimumab, a monoclonal antibody that inhibits B lymphocyte stimulator, in patients with systemic lupus erythematosus. Arthritis Rheum. 2011;63:3918–30.

51. Navarra SV, Guzman RM, Gallacher AE, et al. Efficacy and safety of belimumab in patients with active systemic lupus erythematosus: a randomised, placebo-controlled, phase 3 trial. Lancet. 2011;377:721–31.

52. Manzi S, Sanchez-Guerrero J, Merrill JT, et al. Effects of belimumab, a B lymphocyte stimulator-specific inhibitor, on disease activity across multiple organ domains in patients with systemic lupus erythematosus: combined results from two phase III trials. Ann Rheum Dis. 2012;71:1833–8.

53. van Vollenhoven RF, Petri MA, Cervera R, et al. Belimumab in the treatment of systemic lupus erythematosus: high disease activity predictors of response. Ann Rheum Dis. 2012;71:1343–9.

54. Mariette X, Seror R, Quartuccio L, et al. Efficacy and safety of belimumab in primary Sjogren's syndrome: results of the BELISS open-label phase II study. Ann Rheum Dis. 2015;74:526–31.

55. Seror R, Nocturne G, Lazure T, et al. Low numbers of blood and salivary natural killer cells are associated with a better response to belimumab in primary Sjogren's syndrome: results of the BELISS study. Arthritis Res Ther. 2015;17:241.

56. Lenert A, Lenert P. Current and emerging treatment options for ANCA-associated vasculitis: potential role of belimumab and other BAFF/APRIL targeting agents. Drug Des Devel Ther. 2015;9:333–47.

57. Lutalo PM, D'Cruz DP. Biological drugs in ANCA-associated vasculitis. Int Immunopharmacol. 2015;27:209–12.

58. Genovese MC, Lee E, Satterwhite J, et al. A phase 2 dose-ranging study of subcutaneous tabalumab for the treatment of patients with active rheumatoid arthritis and an inadequate response to methotrexate. Ann Rheum Dis. 2013;72:1453–60.

59. Genovese MC, Bojin S, Biagini IM, et al. Tabalumab in rheumatoid arthritis patients with an inadequate response to methotrexate and naive to biologic therapy: a phase II, randomized, placebo-controlled trial. Arthritis Rheum. 2013;65:880–9.

60. Smolen JS, Weinblatt ME, van der Heijde D, et al. Efficacy and safety of tabalumab, an anti-B-cell-activating factor monoclonal antibody, in patients with rheumatoid arthritis who had an inadequate response to methotrexate therapy: results from a phase III multicentre, randomised, double-blind study. Ann Rheum Dis. 2015;74:1567–70.

61. Merrill JT, van Vollenhoven RF, Buyon JP, et al. Efficacy and safety of subcutaneous tabalumab, a monoclonal antibody to B-cell activating factor, in patients with systemic lupus erythematosus: results from ILLUMINATE-2, a 52-week, phase III, multicentre, randomised, double-blind, placebo-controlled study. Ann Rheum Dis. 2016;75:332–40.

62. Furie RA, Leon G, Thomas M, et al. A phase 2, randomised, placebo-controlled clinical trial of blisibimod, an inhibitor of B cell activating factor, in patients with moderate-to-severe systemic lupus erythematosus, the PEARL-SC study. Ann Rheum Dis. 2015;74:1667–75.

63. Gregersen JW, Jayne DR. B-cell depletion in the treatment of lupus nephritis. Nat Rev Nephrol. 2012;8:505–14.

64. La Cava A. Targeting B cells with biologics in systemic lupus erythematosus. Expert Opin Biol Ther. 2010;10:1555–61.

65. Dall'Era M, Chakravarty E, Wallace D, et al. Reduced B lymphocyte and immunoglobulin levels after atacicept treatment in patients with systemic lupus erythematosus: results of a multicenter, phase Ib, double-blind, placebo-controlled, dose-escalating trial. Arthritis Rheum. 2007;56:4142–50.

66. Ginzler EM, Wax S, Rajeswaran A, et al. Atacicept in combination with MMF and corticosteroids in lupus nephritis: results of a prematurely terminated trial. Arthritis Res Ther. 2012;14:R33.

67. Isenberg D, Gordon C, Licu D, Copt S, Rossi CP, Wofsy D. Efficacy and safety of atacicept for prevention of flares in patients with moderate-to-severe systemic lupus erythematosus (SLE): 52-week data (APRIL-SLE randomised trial). Ann Rheum Dis. 2015;74:2006–15.

11

Joint-preserving regenerative therapy for patients with early-stage osteonecrosis of the femoral head

Yutaka Kuroda[1*], Shuichi Matsuda[1] and Haruhiko Akiyama[2]

Abstract

Osteonecrosis of the femoral head is an intractable disease often occurring in patients aged 30–40 years that can cause femoral head collapse, pain, and gait disturbance. Background factors, including corticosteroid use, alcohol intake, and idiopathic causes, have been indicated. It is estimated that 70–80 % of osteonecrosis patients experience femoral head collapse, for which total hip arthroplasty is considered the most effective treatment, even in young patients. Thus, there is a crucial need for developing a minimally invasive regenerative therapy as a preventive surgery for femoral head collapse: this has been an important area of research in the past decades. Core decompression, the most popular minimally invasive surgery for osteonecrosis of the femoral head, has been used for a long time; however, it has been insufficient to prevent femoral head collapse. For further improvement in therapeutic efficacy, cell transplantation and the use of artificial bone and growth factors have been proposed in addition to core decompression. Since 2000, newer therapies such as autologous bone marrow cell transplantation and the embedding of metal implant rods have been developed in Europe and the USA; however, these approaches have yet to become a global standard. This practical review summarizes applied state-of-the-art regenerative therapy-based core decompression. We introduce the clinical application of recombinant human fibroblast growth factor (rhFGF)-2-impregnated gelatin hydrogel for patients with precollapse osteonecrosis of the femoral head. Radiography and computed tomography have confirmed bone regeneration inside the femoral heads around the region of rhFGF-2 gelatin hydrogel administration. With further development, the minimally invasive method, which can be expected to promote bone regeneration in necrotic areas, could become a useful early-stage treatment for osteonecrosis of the femoral head. Patients can resume their daily routine soon after surgery, and the procedure is inexpensive. As such, it is a promising regenerative therapy that can be actively employed in osteonecrosis of the femoral head before femoral head collapse.

Keywords: Osteonecrosis, Femoral head, Regenerative therapy, Growth factor, Fibroblast growth factor, Clinical trial

Background

Osteonecrosis of the femoral head (ONFH) is a destructive disease of the hip joint caused by a critical decrease in the vascular supply to the femoral head. Several causative factors have been indicated, including corticosteroid use, alcohol intake, hypercoagulation, bone marrow fat embolisms, elevation of intraosseous pressure in the femoral head, and vascular endothelial dysfunction [1–4]. However, the pathogenesis of ONFH is poorly understood. ONFH often occurs in young adults who are in their 30s, and it occurs bilaterally in approximately half of the cases. Steroid-induced ONFH is commonly encountered by orthopedic surgeons and in other medical departments (such as collagen disease, rheumatology, hematology, nephrology, transplant surgery, respiratory, dermatology, and ophthalmology departments) where steroid pulse therapies are performed. Thus, magnetic resonance imaging (MRI) can be performed for early diagnosis, especially for patients receiving steroid pulse therapy.

Core decompression, which is frequently used in Europe and the USA [2, 3, 5], is a minimally invasive surgery; however, if the necrotic area is large, the effect of core decompression may be limited, and femoral head

* Correspondence: ykuromd@kuhp.kyoto-u.ac.jp
[1]Department of Orthopaedic Surgery, Graduate School of Medicine, Kyoto University, Shogoin, Kawahara-cho 54, Sakyo-ku, Kyoto 606-8507, Japan
Full list of author information is available at the end of the article

collapse often occurs regardless. This procedure is almost never performed in Japan, except for biopsy purposes. Other conventional joint-preserving therapies, such as trochanteric rotational osteotomy (the most common hip joint surgery in Japan) and vascularized bone grafts, are difficult, highly invasive, and entail several months of recovery before the patient can resume a daily routine. Considering the age at which ONFH commonly occurs, opting for such operations while the patient is still asymptomatic is difficult. Both the patients and surgeons have difficulty in deciding on a method and the timing of these operations.

Femoral head collapse occurs in 70–80 % of ONFH cases, depending on the size and location [6, 7]. After femoral head collapse, the ONFH site develops secondary osteoarthritis (OA), destroying both the femoral head and the acetabulum [2, 3, 8]. Total hip arthroplasty (THA) is considered an effective treatment for secondary osteoarthritis, even in young patients [3, 7]. As THA is invasive and requires a revision surgery, it is crucial to develop a minimally invasive regenerative therapy that can preserve the femoral head, thus preventing collapse. This has been a research focus for many years [2, 3, 9–11].

Cell therapy [12–16], proteins, and other bone substitutes [9, 17, 18] have been proposed, and various types of cell therapies using autologous marrow cells or stem cells are already being attempted, though they have not yet become standardized. Non-cellular therapeutic strategies using growth factors have also been proposed; however, verification in animal experiments has made little progress, primarily because of the absence of an animal model for femoral head-specific necrosis [9, 19, 20] and secondarily because of the lack of a technique to locally deliver the growth factor [21].

To help address this problem, we reported a new rabbit model in which early ONFH progresses to femoral head collapse and OA, similar to that in humans. While animal models of corticosteroid treatment alone do not develop the characteristics of advanced ONFH seen in humans [22], we applied a rabbit model of ONFH induced by a combination of methylprednisolone administration and vascular occlusion of the capital femoral epiphysis by electrocoagulation. The rabbits started to develop ONFH around 4 weeks after the ONFH procedure and established ONFH within 8 weeks [23]. In this model, we showed that a single local injection of recombinant human fibroblast growth factor (rhFGF)-2-impregnated gelatin hydrogel, which has superior slow-release characteristics, suppresses the progression of femoral head necrosis. To translate this research to humans, the clinical application of controlled release rhFGF-2 for precollapse ONFH patients was performed at the Department of Orthopaedic Surgery in Kyoto University Hospital starting in March 2013 [24]. In this review article, we present the local application of rhFGF-2 in human ONFH and its clinical benefit compared to other treatments.

Treatment strategy for ONFH

Conventional surgical treatment, mainly core decompression, is used widely in Europe and the USA [2, 3, 5]; in contrast, in Japan, a variety of surgical osteotomy procedures have been performed. However, clinical results vary: the collapse rate of the femoral head was more than 70 % in core decompression with precollapse ONFH in one study [13], while others have reported a collapse rate of 50 % with rotational osteotomy [25]. A variety of surgical methods have also been reported, including free or vascularized methods with fibular and iliac bone grafts, allogeneic bone grafts, and bone cartilage transplantation (mosaicplasty); bone cement injection to the femoral head has also been reported, although it is not common. Currently, there is no consensus regarding the standard treatment (Fig. 1).

The use of MRI improves early diagnosis, especially in patients receiving steroid pulse therapy. Accordingly, the treatment target has emphasized aggressive early prevention of femoral head collapse. Core decompression alone is challenging [13, 26, 27]; therefore, cell transplantation and artificial bone or metal implants in the core site have also been attempted. In addition, a deliverable, growth factor-containing, bone-promoting substitute has also been proposed [2, 3, 9, 17, 18].

Osteotomy

Over 40 years, various types of osteotomies have been performed for the treatment of ONFH. The concept of surgery consists of moving the necrotic region from the weight-bearing surface of the femoral head. These involve three-axis directions, varus-valgus, flexion-extension, and anterior-posterior rotation. These procedures are technically demanding and are popular in Asia, though less in other regions [3, 28].

Bone grafting

Various surgical techniques have been reported for the use of bone grafts for the treatment of ONFH. In the 1930s, Phemister first reported a surgical procedure of a non-vascularized bone graft from the tibia for the treatment of ONFH [28]. Since then, newer techniques such as the lightbulb and trapdoor non-vascularized bone graft have been used with good results [29]. Another technique for bone grafting is vascularized option. Vascularized fibular graft was introduced in 1979 and consists of a fibular graft together with its vascular supply and harvested directly into the necrotic lesion of the femoral head [28]. Vascularized fibular graft is one of the technically difficult orthopedic surgeries which require technique of microvascular surgery. More recently, the

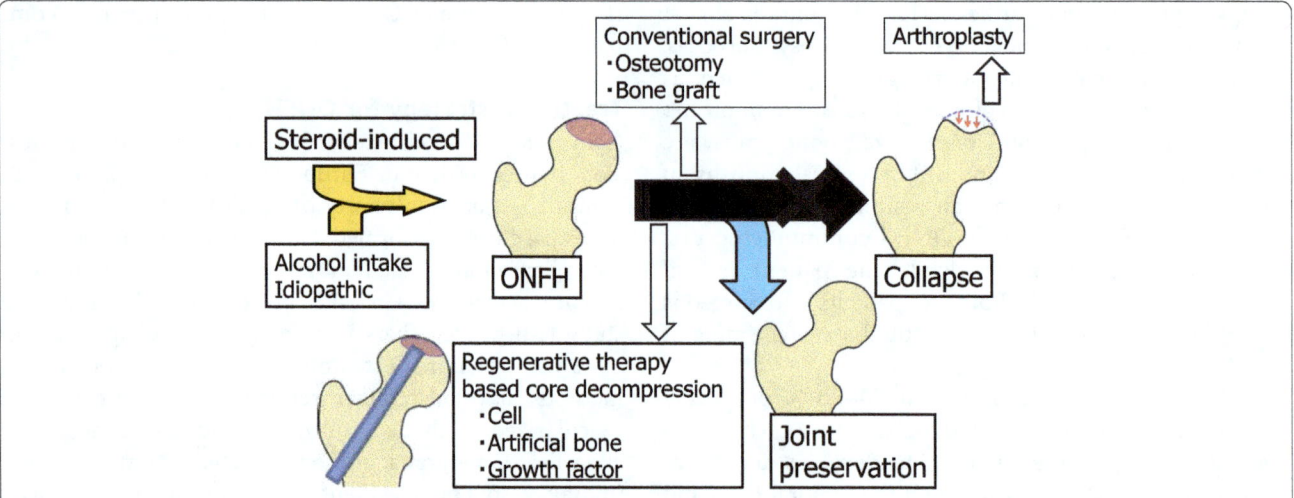

Fig. 1 Treatment strategy for osteonecrosis of the femoral head. Scheme of treatment strategy for osteonecrosis of the femoral head (*ONFH*) is shown. In daily clinical cases, even if a patient is diagnosed with ONFH, most cases experience femoral head collapse without surgical treatments and finally have to undergo total hip arthroplasty. The ultimate goal for ONFH therapy is to prevent femoral head collapse. Surgical alternatives for preservation include osteotomy and vascularized bone grafting, but the procedures are difficult, technically demanding, and require long-term hospitalization. Therefore, there has been a great desire for a minimally invasive regenerative therapy that can prevent femoral head collapse. Several regenerative treatment options, including cell or stem cell transplantation, artificial bone substitutes, and administration of growth and differentiation factors, have been recently reported

addition of biological reagents has demonstrated positive results [30].

Pure conservative therapy

A recent prospective, double-blind study showed that with conservative therapy using an oral bisphosphonate agent to prevent femoral head collapse, there was no difference in collapse progress between the placebo and treatment groups [31]. In Japan, novel clinical trials as a pure conservative therapy are performed and are registered to the public Japanese clinical trials registry, the University Hospital Medical Information Network (UMIN) Clinical Trials Registry. In recent years, bisphosphonates and parathyroid hormone have also started to be used to prevent collapse (UMIN000017582). In addition, for systemic lupus erythematosus patients undergoing steroid pulse therapy, a three-drug combination of the enzyme 3-hydroxy-3-methylglutaryl coenzyme A reductase inhibitor (pitavastatin), adenosine diphosphate receptor blocking antiplatelet (clopidogrel), and antioxidant (tocopherol) is co-administered (UMIN000008230). Other types of conservative treatment using an external device, such as hyperbaric oxygen therapy and extracorporeal shock wave lithotrity (UMIN000020197), have also been developed [32].

Core decompression

Core decompression is a minimally invasive surgery for ONFH dating back to the 1960s [28]. It was originally used to create a single large bone hole >10-mm diameter and had a high femoral head collapse rate. Over time,

the method improved and now involves multiple bone holes of a smaller diameter (3 mm); this method has been popular since the 2000s. With the improved method, collapse rates are now 30 % for precollapse ONFH [33]. To further improve therapeutic efficacy to prevent femoral head collapse, cell transplantation, artificial bone, and growth factors have been used (Fig. 2).

Regenerative therapy-based core decompression
Metal implants

A preventive treatment involving the placement of cylindrical artifacts in the core decompression site has been developed in Europe and the USA. Such artifacts include implant rods made of Zimmer Trabecular Metal (porous tantalum, manufactured by Zimmer, Warsaw, IN, USA), which are available in both small and large diameters. Tsao et al. used a large-diameter rod in 113 joints from 97 patients with precollapse ONFH; over 4 years, 19 joints (19.6 %) underwent THA [34]. Similarly, Veillette et al. reported that of 48 joints from 42 patients, 16 (33.3 %) experienced a collapsed femoral head over 4 years [35]. In addition, Floerkemeier et al. reported that in 23 joints with ONFH, 13 (56.5 %) required THA after an average of 1.45 years. In contrast to other studies, the outcome after core decompression combined with tantalum rod insertion was not superior compared to core decompression alone [36].

Artificial bones

Yu et al. reported that injectable calcium phosphate-based artificial bone ($CaSO_4$/$CaPO_4$ composite) was used alone

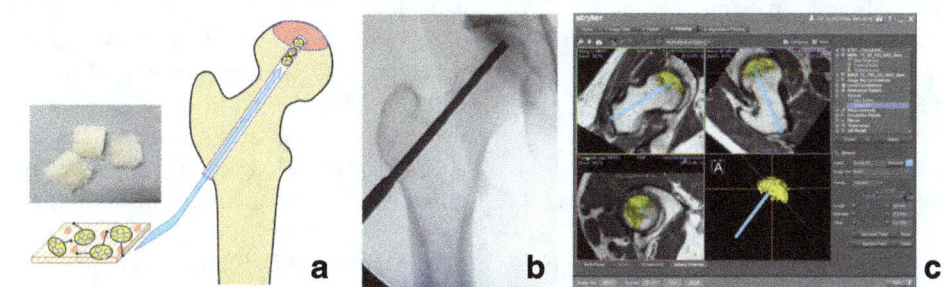

Fig. 2 Regenerative therapy using controlled release of recombinant human fibroblast growth factor. Schematic views and photographs of the surgical procedure using recombinant human fibroblast growth factor (rhFGF)-2-impregnated gelatin hydrogel for patients with precollapse stage of osteonecrosis of the femoral head (ONFH) are shown. **a** A schema of the surgical procedure administering the rhFGF-2 gelatin hydrogel. The rhFGF-2-impregnated gelatin hydrogel is embedded percutaneously over the lateral aspect of the femur near the level of the lesser trochanter. A *small photograph* on the *left side* shows the actual gelatin hydrogel, which is a superior slow-release carrier for growth factors. **b** A representative intraoperative fluoroscopic image at drilling. **c** A screenshot of the preoperative planning using navigation software is shown. The *yellow area* shows the area of ONFH. The surgeon planned the suitable route of drilling (*blue screw*)

Table 1 Joint-preserving regenerative therapy-based core decompression

First author year/design	Technique	Number of hips (precollapse)	Background factors for ONFH (%)	Mean age (years)	Mean follow-up (years)	Hip survivorship (%)
Tsao [34] 2005/P	CD TR	94	S 41, A 24, I 30, others 5	43	4.0	80.4
Veillette [35] 2006/R	CD TR	50	S 45, A 3, I 26, T 10, others 16	35	4.0	66.7
Floerkemeier [36] 2011/P	CD TR	23	NR	40	1.4	43.5
Yu [37] 2015/P	CD CaSO$_4$/CaPO$_4$	6	S 5, A 68, I 21, T 5	48	1.4	50.0
Hernigou [16] 2009/P	CD BMMNC	534	S 19, SCD 31, I 28	39	13.0	82.4
Gangji [13] 2011/RCT	CD	11	S 82, A 9, I 9	45.7	5.0	27.3
Gangji [13] 2011/RCT	CD BMMNC	13	S 85, A 8, I 8	42.2	5.0	76.9
Civinini [41] 2012/P	CD, BMC, CaSO$_4$/CaPO$_4$	30	S 49, A 35, I 16	43.9	1.7	83.3
Yamasaki [42] 2010/R	CD HA	9	S 22, A 44, I 33	49	2.4	0
Yamasaki [42] 2010/R	CD, BMMNC, HA	27	S 73, A 20, I 7	41	2.4	56.7
Lieberman [17] 2004/P	CD, FBG rhBMP 50 mg	16	S 76, A 18, S&A 6	47	4.4	87.5
Papanagiotou [43] 2014/P	CD, FBG rhBMP 3.5 g	5	S 40, A 20, I 40	32	4.0	80.0
Kuroda [23] 2015/P	CD rhFGF-2 800 μg	10	S 80, A 20	39.8	1.0	90.0

P prospective study, *R* retrospective study, *RCT* randomized clinical trial, *CD* core decompression, *TR* tantalum rod, *BMMNC* bone marrow mononuclear cell, *BMC* bone marrow cell, *HA* hydroxyapatite, *FBG* fibular bone graft, *rhBMP* recombinant human bone morphogenetic protein, *ONFH* osteonecrosis of the femoral head, *S* steroid use, *A* alcohol intake, *I* idiopathic, *T* trauma, *NR* not reported, *SCD* sickle cell disease

for ONFH. In 19 joints from 18 patients, 3/6 joints (50 %) with precollapse ONFH and 8/13 joints (61.5 %) with early collapsed ONFH were reported to have undergone THA after an average of 8.5 months post-surgery [37].

Cell transplantation

In ONFH, progression of the necrotic area and occurrence of additional necrotic areas are extremely rare [38]. Therefore, regeneration of the necrotic bone to normal bone tissue could make it possible to cure ONFH. To regenerate the necrotic bone, there is a need to promote remodeling and angiogenesis as well as absorption of the necrotic bone. However, clinical results for free bone grafts do not indicate significant improvement over core decompression. Thus, a new treatment strategy has been attempted in which cell transplantation, such as autologous bone marrow mononuclear cells, was employed to regenerate the necrotic bone directly. As reported by Hernigou and Beaujean, bone marrow was taken from the iliac crest, and the mononuclear cell-containing fraction was separated using a cell centrifugal separation device [12]. The cells were injected into the necrotic bone area from the core decompression site that promotes the remodeling of

cancellous bone regeneration and necrosis. After 8–18 years, only 94 of the 534 patients (17.6 %) with precollapse ONFH were reported to have femoral head collapse [16]. In addition, Gangji et al. conducted a prospective double-blind study on 24 hips, in which core decompression and autologous bone marrow mononuclear cell transplantation combination were compared over 5 years. Progress and structural destruction of the subchondral bone were noted in 8 of the 11 joints (72.7 %) in the core decompression group and in 3 of the 13 joints (23.1 %) in the combination group [13]. Furthermore, in a systematic review, Papakostidis et al. reported that in the precollapse stage, core decompression with autologous bone marrow cell implantation into the femoral head is clinically effective and can improve survivorship of the femoral heads and reduce the need for THA [39]. Another systemic review by Lau et al. reported that cell therapy is considered a reliable regenerative approach to engraft more cells in the necrotic area and that further development of a method promoting differentiation is needed [40].

In combination with cell therapy, the use of artificial bone in the core decompression site has also been

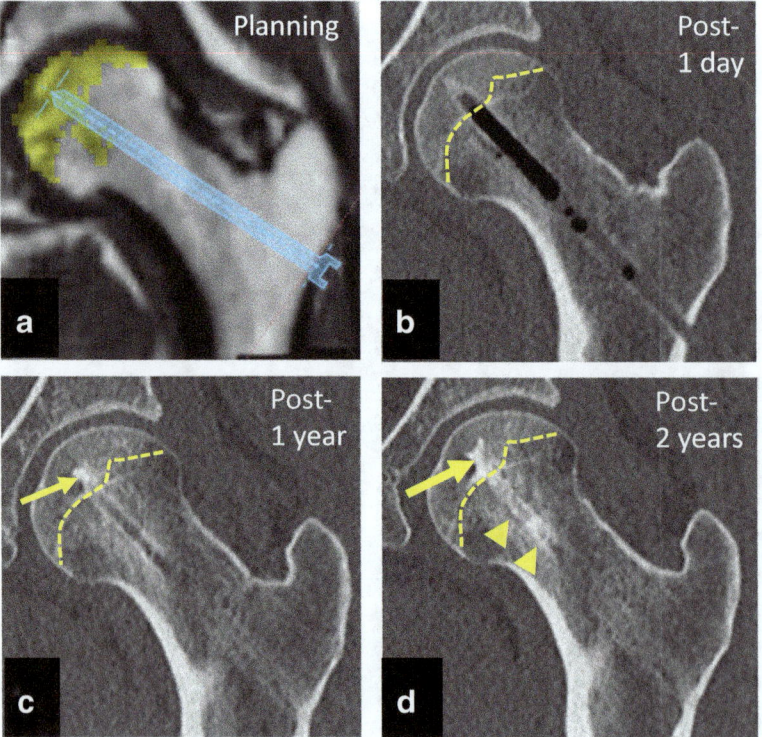

Fig. 3 Planning and representative computed tomography images. **a** A screenshot of the preoperative planning. **b** Coronal computed tomography image shows a bone defect at the drilling route and implanted region 1 day postoperatively. The *yellow dashed line* shows the border of the osteonecrotic area of the femoral head. **c** In contrast, apparent bone regeneration of the osteonecrotic area is observed at 1 year postoperatively (*yellow arrow*). The normal contour of the femoral head is maintained. **d** Apparent bone regeneration of the osteonecrotic area is observed in the implanted region (*yellow arrow*) and drilling route (*yellow arrowheads*) at 2 years postoperatively. Normal contour, thick trabecular bone, and bone regeneration of the drilling route can be observed

developed. For instance, Civinini et al. reported that, with a combination of bone marrow cell transplantation and artificial bone, 5/30 joints (16.6 %) with precollapse ONFH and 3/7 joints (42.8 %) with early collapsed ONFH further collapsed or progressed further an average of 20.6 months post-surgery [41]. Yamasaki et al. reported that 30 joints from 22 patients received transplanted bone marrow mononuclear cells with interconnected porous calcium hydroxyapatite into the femoral head; over an average of 29 months, 13 (43.3 %) experienced femoral head collapse [42].

Autologous bone marrow cell transplantation may be reliable in early-stage ONFH patients [12, 13, 16, 39, 40]. Ex vivo amplification of bone marrow cells has been proposed to increase the number of injected stem cells [13–15, 30].

Growth factors

Bone regeneration in joint areas using cell growth factors, another treatment approach, has become an important topic of research. Problems with protein therapy include an extremely short half-life and side effects with systemic or high-dose administration. The use of rhFGF-2-impregnated gelatin hydrogel has the advantage of sustained release over rhFGF-2 solution because its biologic half-life period is short [21]. A slow-release system built around a bioabsorbable gelatin hydrogel enables local

administration with excellent controlled release, greatly contributing to establishing practical use for protein therapy. Such factors useful for bone regeneration include transforming growth factor-β, bone morphogenetic protein (BMP), FGF-2, vascular endothelial growth factor, and insulin-like growth factor [2, 3, 9]. For ONFH, the use of BMP in combination with bone grafts has been reported. For example, Lieberman et al. co-administered rhBMP (50 mg) with an allogeneic fibular graft after core decompression. Of 16 cases with precollapse ONFH, two (12.5 %) collapsed after an average of 53 months [17]. Moreover, Papanagiotou et al. co-administered rhBMP 3.5 mg with an autologous fibular graft; of five cases with precollapse ONFH, one (20 %) experienced femoral head collapse over an average of 4 years [43].

In the field of bone and joint medicine, the angiogenic and osteogenic actions of rhFGF-2 have been the subject of numerous reports [21, 23, 24, 44, 45]. In particular, the use of gelatin hydrogel as a superior slow-release carrier has produced increased bone mass in areas of bone deficit [21]. Furthermore, rhFGF-2 administration produced rapid osteogenesis and increased bone mass in humans with lower leg fracture [44] and osteotomy surface [45]. A strategy using growth factors has also been proposed to treat ONFH. We reported the first clinical application of rhFGF-2-impregnated gelatin hydrogel for patients with precollapse stage of ONFH (Fig. 2) [24].

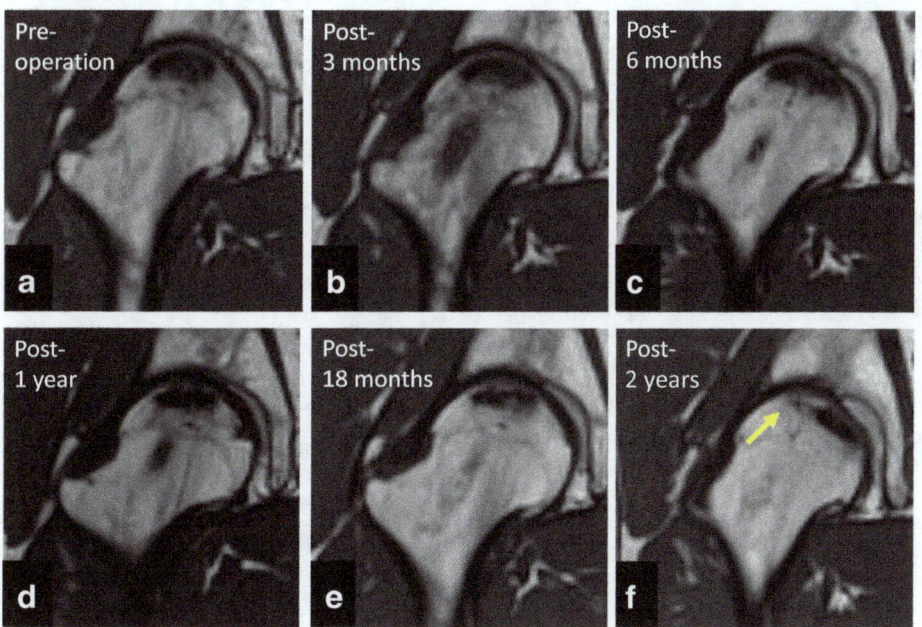

Fig. 4 Representative magnetic resonance images. **a** Preoperative coronal T1-weighted magnetic resonance imaging (MRI) showing osteonecrosis of the femoral head (ONFH) that occupied the weight-bearing portion and extended laterally to the acetabular edge. **b–d** MRI scan of the ONFH area and the femoral neck region 6 months and 1 year postoperatively, showing continued low signal intensity, indicating the influence of the traumatic procedure. **e** MRI scan 18 months postoperatively, showing the first change of signal intensity at the drilling route. The drilling site at the femoral neck is changing to the normal signal intensity of the bone. **f** Most recent MRI scan 2 years postoperatively, showing almost normal signal intensity at the ONFH area. The area and size of ONFH decreased at the weight-bearing surface (*yellow arrow*)

Ten patients with femoral heads up to precollapse stage 2 underwent a single local administration of 800-μg rhFGF-2-impregnated gelatin hydrogel and followed up for 1 year. Primary outcomes included adverse events and complications. Secondary outcomes included changes in Harris Hip Scores, visual analog scale pain scores, and UCLA activity rating scores, radiological changes as determined via radiographs, computed tomography scans, and MRI of the hip joint. One-year short-term results of this pilot study indicated the approach was safe and feasible. During 1-year follow-up of 10 patients, there was only one case of femoral head collapse; however, this occurred in a hip with extensive necrosis. Stage progression and collapse did not occur in the other nine cases. The results of previous joint-preserving regenerative therapy-based core decompression are presented in Table 1.

The minimally invasive therapy (1-cm skin incision) attempted to prevent femoral head collapse through direct administration of rhFGF-2, which has both angiogenic and osteogenic actions. Computed tomography (Fig. 3) and recent MRI (Fig. 4) confirmed bone regeneration and reduction of the necrotic area. Additionally, hospitalization costs were dramatically reduced to 10 % of that for THA. From an economic standpoint, avoiding the need for artificial joints could greatly reduce medical expenses. However, it is still unclear whether rhFGF-2 administration or conservative treatment has a better efficacy. Further studies with longer follow-up are needed to analyze and evaluate the survival rates of femoral heads treated with rhFGF-2 administration or conservative treatment.

Conclusions

The most recent regenerative therapy for ONFH has aimed to induce bone regeneration to prevent femoral head collapse. To develop the practical clinical application for regenerative ONFH therapies, suitable sources, including cell sources, artificial materials, specific proteins, or combinations thereof, must be identified. With the use of various regenerative therapies, including cell therapy, implants, and recombinant growth factors, the treatment for ONFH will reach a turning point in the near future.

Abbreviations
BMP: bone morphogenetic protein; MRI: magnetic resonance imaging; OA: osteoarthritis; ONFH: osteonecrosis of the femoral head; rhFGF: recombinant human fibroblast growth factor; THA: total hip arthroplasty.

Competing interests
The authors declare that they have no competing interests.

Authors' contributions
YK, SM, and HA conceived and designed the experiments. YK and HA performed the experiments. KY, SM, and HA contributed to the writing of the manuscript. All authors read and approved the final manuscript.

Acknowledgements
We thank T. Ito-Ihara and R. Aasda for the clinical trial design and management.

Funding
This work was supported in part by grants from The Uehara Memorial Foundation (to HA).

Author details
[1]Department of Orthopaedic Surgery, Graduate School of Medicine, Kyoto University, Shogoin, Kawahara-cho 54, Sakyo-ku, Kyoto 606-8507, Japan. [2]Department of Orthopaedic Surgery, Gifu University, Gifu, Japan.

References
1. Fukushima W, Fujioka M, Kubo T, Tamakoshi A, Nagai M, Hirota Y. Nationwide epidemiologic survey of idiopathic osteonecrosis of the femoral head. Clin Orthop Relat Res. 2010;468(10):2715–24.
2. Moya-Angeler J, Gianakos AL, Villa JC, Ni A, Lane JM. Current concepts on osteonecrosis of the femoral head. World J Orthop. 2015;6(8):590–601. 18.
3. Mont MA, Cherian JJ, Sierra RJ, Jones LC, Lieberman JR. Nontraumatic osteonecrosis of the femoral head: where do we stand today? A ten-year update. J Bone Joint Surg Am. 2015;97(19):1604–27.
4. Seamon J, Keller T, Saleh J, Cui Q. The pathogenesis of nontraumatic osteonecrosis. Arthritis. 2012;2012:601763.
5. Johnson AJ, Mont MA, Tsao AK, Jones LC. Treatment of femoral head osteonecrosis in the United States: 16-year analysis of the Nationwide Inpatient Sample. Clin Orthop Relat Res. 2014;472(2):617–23.
6. Mont MA, Carbone JJ, Fairbank AC. Core decompression versus nonoperative management for osteonecrosis of the hip. Clin Orthop Relat Res. 1996;324:169–78.
7. Hernigou P, Ooignard A, Nogier A, Manicom O. Fate of very small asymptomatic stage-I osteonecrotic lesions of the hip. J Bone Joint Surg Am. 2004;86:2589–93.
8. Jawad MU, Haleem AA, Scully SP. In brief: Ficat classification: avascular necrosis of the femoral head. Clin Orthop Relat Res. 2012;470(9):2636–9.
9. Mont MA, Jones LC, Einhorn TA, Hungerford DS, Reddi AH. Osteonecrosis of the femoral head—potential treatment with growth and differentiation factors. Clin Orthop Relat Res. 1998;355:S314–35.
10. Mont MA, Jones LC, Hungerford DS. Nontraumatic osteonecrosis of the femoral head: ten years later. J Bone Joint Surg Am. 2006;88:1117–32.
11. Bakhshi H, Rasouli MR, Parvizi J. Can local Erythropoietin administration enhance bone regeneration in osteonecrosis of femoral head? Med Hypotheses. 2012;79:154–6.
12. Hernigou P, Beaujean F. Treatment of osteonecrosis with autologous bone marrow grafting. Clin Orthop Relat Res. 2002;405:14–23.
13. Gangji V, De Maertelaer V, Hauzeur JP. Autologous bone marrow cell implantation in the treatment of non-traumatic osteonecrosis of the femoral head: five year follow-up of a prospective controlled study. Bone. 2011;49:1005–9.
14. Rastogi S, Sankineani SR, Nag HL, Mohanty S, Shivanand G, Marimuthu K, et al. Intralesional autologous mesenchymal stem cells in management of osteonecrosis of femur: a preliminary study. Musculoskelet Surg. 2013;97:223–8.
15. Houdek MT, Wyles CC, Martin JR, Sierra RJ. Stem cell treatment for avascular necrosis of the femoral head: current perspectives. Stem Cells Cloning. 2014;7:65–70.
16. Hernigou P, Poignard A, Zilber S, Rouard H. Cell therapy of hip osteonecrosis with autologous bone marrow grafting. Indian J Orthop. 2009;43:40–5.
17. Lieberman JR, Conduah A, Urist MR. Treatment of osteonecrosis of the femoral head with core decompression and human bone morphogenetic protein. Clin Orthop Relat Res. 2004;429:139–45.

18. Sun W, Li Z, Gao F, Shi Z, Zhang Q, Guo W. Recombinant human bone morphogenetic protein-2 in debridement and impacted bone graft for the treatment of femoral head osteonecrosis. PLoS One. 2014;9:e100424.

19. Manggold J, Sergi C, Becker K, Lukoschek M, Simank HG. A new animal model of femoral head necrosis induced by intraosseous injection of ethanol. Lab Anim. 2002;36:173–80.

20. Boss JH, Misselevich I. Osteonecrosis of the femoral head of laboratory animals: the lessons learned from a comparative study of osteonecrosis in man and experimental animals. Vet Pathol. 2003;40:345–54.

21. Tabata Y, Yamada K, Miyamoto S, Nagata I, Kikuchi H, Aoyama I, et al. Bone regeneration by basic fibroblast growth factor complexed with biodegradable hydrogel. Biomaterials. 1998;19:807–15.

22. Jones LC, Tucci MA, Haile A, Wang D. Animal models of corticosteroid-associated bone diseases. In: Koo K-H, Mont MA, Jones LC, editors. Osteonecrosis. Heidelberg, New York, Dordrecht, London: Springer; 2014. p. 493–505.

23. Kuroda Y, Akiyama H, Kawanabe K, Tabata Y, Nakamura T. Treatment of experimental osteonecrosis of the hip in adult rabbits with a single local injection of recombinant human FGF-2 microspheres. J Bone Miner Metab. 2010;28:608–16.

24. Kuroda Y, Asada R, So K, Yonezawa A, Nankaku M, Mukai K, et al. A pilot study of regenerative therapy using controlled release of rhFGF-2 for patients with precollapse osteonecrosis of the femoral head. Int Orthop. 2015; doi: 10.1007/s00264-015-3083-1

25. Rijnen WH, Gardeniers JW, Westrek BL, Buma P, Schreurs BW. Sugioka's osteotomy for femoral-head necrosis in young Caucasians. Int Orthop. 2005;29:140–4.

26. Koo KH, Kim R, Ko GH, Song HR, Jeong ST, Cho SH. Preventing collapse in early osteonecrosis of the femoral head. A randomised clinical trial of core decompression. J Bone Joint Surg (Br). 1995;77(6):870–4.

27. Soohoo NF, Vyas S, Manunga J, Sharifi H, Kominski G, Lieberman JR. Cost-effectiveness analysis of core decompression. J Arthroplasty. 2006;21:670–81.

28. Steinberg ME, Steinberg DR. Historical perspective. In: Koo K-H, Mont MA, Jones LC, editors. Osteonecrosis. Heidelberg, New York, Dordrecht, London: Springer; 2014. p. 3–15.

29. Jauregui JJ, Banerjee S, Kapadia BH, Cherian JJ, Issa K, Mont MA. Principles of bone grafting for osteonecrosis of the hip. In: Koo K-H, Mont MA, Jones LC, editors. Osteonecrosis. Heidelberg, New York, Dordrecht, London: Springer; 2014. p. 307–13.

30. Aoyama T, Goto K, Kakinoki R, Ikeguchi R, Ueda M, Kasai Y, et al. An exploratory clinical trial for idiopathic osteonecrosis of femoral head by cultured autologous multipotent mesenchymal stromal cells augmented with vascularized bone grafts. Tissue Eng Part B Rev. 2014;20(4):233–42.

31. Chen CH, Chang JK, Lai KA, Hou SM, Chang CH, Wang GJ. Alendronate in the prevention of collapse of the femoral head in nontraumatic osteonecrosis: a two-year multicenter, prospective, randomized, double-blind, placebo-controlled study. Arthritis Rheum. 2012;64:1572–8.

32. Wang C, Peng J, Lu S. Summary of the various treatments for osteonecrosis of the femoral head by mechanism: a review. Exp Ther Med. 2014;8(3):700–6.

33. Marker DR, Seylee TM, McGrath MS, Delanois RE, Ulrich SD, Mont MA. Treatment of early stage osteonecrosis of the femoral head. J Bone Joint Surg Am. 2008;90:175–87.

34. Tsao AK, Roberson JR, Christie MJ, Dore DD, Heck DA, Robertson DD, et al. Biomechanical and clinical evaluations of a porous tantalum implant for the treatment of early-stage osteonecrosis. J Bone Joint Surg Am. 2005;87(S2):22–7.

35. Veillette CJ, Mehdian H, Schemitsch EH, McKee MD. Survivorship analysis and radiographic outcome following tantalum rod insertion for osteonecrosis of the femoral head. J Bone Joint Surg Am. 2006;88(S3):48–55.

36. Floerkemeier T, Thorey F, Daentzer D, Lerch M, Klages P, Windhagen H, et al. Clinical and radiological outcome of the treatment of osteonecrosis of the femoral head using the osteonecrosis intervention implant. Int Orthop. 2011;35(4):489–95.

37. Yu PA, Peng KT, Huang TW, Hsu RW, Hsu WH, Lee MS. Injectable synthetic bone graft substitute combined with core decompression in the treatment of advanced osteonecrosis of the femoral head: a 5-year follow-up. Biomed J. 2015;38(3):257–61.

38. Nam KW, Kim YL, Yoo JJ, Koo KH, Yoon KS, Kim HJ. Fate of untreated asymptomatic osteonecrosis of the femoral head. J Bone Joint Surg Am. 2008;90(3):477–84.

39. Papakostidis C, Tosounidis TH, Jones E, Giannoudis PV. The role of "cell therapy" in osteonecrosis of the femoral head. Acta Orthop. 2015;29:1–7.

40. Lau RL, Perruccio AV, Evans HM, Mahomed SR, Mahomed NN, Gandhi R. Stem cell therapy for the treatment of early stage avascular necrosis of the femoral head: a systematic review. BMC Musculoskelet Disord. 2014;15:156.

41. Civinini R, De Biase P, Carulli C, Matassi F, Nistri L, Capanna R, et al. The use of an injectable calcium sulphate/calcium phosphate bioceramic in the treatment of osteonecrosis of the femoral head. Int Orthop. 2012;36(8):1583–8.

42. Yamasaki T, Yasunaga Y, Ishikawa M, Hamaki T, Ochi M. Bone-marrow-derived mononuclear cells with a porous hydroxyapatite scaffold for the treatment of osteonecrosis of the femoral head: a preliminary study. J Bone Joint Surg (Br). 2010;92(3):337–41.

43. Papanagiotou M, Malizos KN, Vlychou M, Dailiana ZH. Autologous (non-vascularised) fibular grafting with recombinant bone morphogenetic protein-7 for the treatment of femoral head osteonecrosis: preliminary report. Bone Joint J. 2014;96-B(1):31–5.

44. Kawaguchi H, Oka H, Jingushi S, Izumi T, Fukunaga M, Sato K, et al. A local application of recombinant human fibroblast growth factor 2 for tibial shaft fractures: a randomized, placebo-controlled trial. J Bone Miner Res. 2010;25:2735–43.

45. Kawaguchi H, Jingushi S, Izumi T, Fukunaga M, Matsushita T, Nakamura T, et al. Local application of recombinant human fibroblast growth factor-2 on bone repair: a dose-escalation prospective trial on patients with osteotomy. J Orthop Res. 2007;25:480–7.

12

Isolation of dental pulp stem cells with high osteogenic potential

Takazumi Yasui[1,2,3], Yo Mabuchi[2,4], Satoru Morikawa[1], Katsuhiro Onizawa[3], Chihiro Akazawa[4], Taneaki Nakagawa[1], Hideyuki Okano[2] and Yumi Matsuzaki[2,5*]

Abstract

Dental pulp stem cells/progenitor cells (DPSCs) can be easily obtained and can have excellent proliferative and mineralization potentials. Therefore, many studies have investigated the isolation and bone formation of DPSCs. In most previous reports, human DPSCs were traditionally isolated by exploiting their ability to adhere to plastic tissue culture dishes. DPSCs isolated by plastic adherence are frequently contaminated by other cells, which limits the ability to investigate their basic biology and regenerative properties. Additionally, the proliferative and osteogenic potentials vary depending on the isolated cells. It is very difficult to obtain cells of a sufficient quality to elicit the required effect upon transplantation. Considering clinical applications, stem cells used for regenerative medicine need to be purified in order to increase the efficiency of bone regeneration, and a stable supply of these cells must be generated. Here, we review the purification of DPSCs and studies of cranio-maxillofacial bone regeneration using these cells. Additionally, we introduce the prospective isolation of DPSCs using specific cell surface markers: low-affinity nerve growth factor and thymocyte antigen 1.

Keywords: Bone regeneration, Dental pulp stem/progenitor cell, Flow cytometry, Isolation, Osteogenic potential, Low-affinity nerve growth factor receptor, THY-1, Transplantation, Cranio-maxillofacial

Background

Dental pulp, which contains connective tissue, mesenchymal cells, neural fibers, blood vessels, and lymphatics, is located at the center of the pulp chamber enclosed in mineralized dentin. The main functions of dental pulp are to produce dentin and to maintain the biological and physiological vitality of dentin [1]. Dental pulp stem cells/progenitor cells (DPSCs) in adult dental pulp tissue are induced to differentiate into odontoblasts to form reparative dentin in order to protect dental pulp [2, 3]. DPSCs and stem cells from human exfoliated deciduous teeth (SHEDs) have a high proliferative potential, an extensive self-renewal ability, and a multilineage differentiation capacity, with osteogenic, chondrogenic, adipogenic, neurogenic, and myogenic potentials [3–5]. In particular, DPSCs and SHEDs have a high mineralization potential and are considered to be useful in bone regenerative

therapy [6–8]. Many studies regarding DPSCs have been reported because dental pulp tissue is easily obtained. In most previous reports, DPSCs were traditionally isolated by exploiting their ability to adhere to plastic tissue culture dishes [3]. However, adherent culture conditions on plastic dishes inevitably change the expression of surface markers and the biological properties of stem cells. Consequently, stem cell properties may diminish during adherent culture on plastic tissue culture dishes [9, 10]. Furthermore, DPSCs isolated based on their adherence to plastic are frequently contaminated by cells with different phenotypes. Additionally, the proliferative and osteogenic potentials vary depending on the isolated cells. It is very difficult to obtain cells of a sufficient quality to elicit the required effect upon transplantation. Considering clinical applications, stem cells used for regenerative medicine need to be purified in order to increase the efficiency of bone regeneration, and a stable supply of these cells must be generated. Here, we review the purification of DPSCs and the studies of cranio-maxillofacial bone regeneration using these cells. Additionally, we introduce the prospective isolation of DPSCs with high osteogenic potential.

* Correspondence: matsuzak@med.shimane-u.ac.jp
[2]Department of Physiology, Keio University School of Medicine, 35 Shinanomachi, Shinjuku-ku, Tokyo 160-8582, Japan
[5]Department of Cancer Biology, Faculty of Medicine, Shimane University, 89-1 Enya-cho, Izumo, Shimane 693-8501, Japan
Full list of author information is available at the end of the article

Bone regenerative therapy in the cranio-maxillofacial region

Bone regenerative therapies are required to treat many diseases affecting the cranio-maxillofacial region such as craniofacial abnormalities, bone defects following mandible tumor surgery, trauma, jaw bone necrosis, and bone augmentation for dental implants. Bone regeneration plays significant roles in the recovery of function and improvement of aesthetic disorders in the cranio-maxillofacial area. Autogenous bones harvested from the patient's own body, such as the iliac bone, scapula, and fibula, have been used for major reconstruction of the maxillofacial area [11]. This bone grafting requires large-scale surgery, e.g., reconstruction using vascular pedicle bone grafts and particulate cancellous bone marrow with a titanium mesh [11, 12]. Autogenous bone from the chin and ramus of the mandible, allogenic bone, and xenogenic bone have been used for minor bone augmentation [13, 14].

Regenerative medicine studies have used various approaches such as osteoinductive chemical factors, osteoinductive growth factors, osteoinductive materials, extracellular matrix, and cell-based tissue engineering. Many studies of adult stem cell-based tissue engineering have sought to effectively regenerate bone in the maxillofacial area. One recent line of progress in stem cell research is bone regeneration using stem cells from bone marrow (BMMSCs). BMMSCs not only have high osteogenic and chondrogenic potentials, but also have an excellent regenerative potential to treat bone defects in vivo [15]. Therefore, these cells are considered to be very useful for bone regenerative therapies in the maxillofacial area. Several groups showed that tissue-engineered bone constructed with BMMSCs elicits beneficial effects in a mandibular defect model, a maxillary sinus floor elevation model, and a jaw malformation model [16–18]. In humans, injectable tissue-engineered bone formation using BMMSCs and platelet-rich plasma was applied to 14 cases for ridge augmentation and dental implant placement [19]. Furthermore, another group applied BMMSCs seeded onto β-tricalciumphosphate to upper jaw bone defects for dental implant placement after trauma [20].

Dental stem cells are an attractive option for regenerative therapy because they can be easily expanded to generate the number required for generation of graft materials. Furthermore, dental stem cells can be easily obtained in comparison with BMMSCs because exfoliated deciduous teeth and impacted third molar teeth are often extracted for clinical or orthodontic reasons. All dental stem cells (including DPSCs, SHEDs, periodontal ligament stem cells, dental follicle stem cells, and stem cells isolated from the apical papilla) are considered to be obtained via minimally invasive methods when isolated from these extracted teeth. They can give rise to proliferative cells and osteogenic cells under appropriate conditions [3, 4, 21–23].

Characterization of stem cells from dental pulp

DPSCs are traditionally isolated from dental pulp by exploiting their ability to adhere to plastic tissue culture dishes after enzyme digestion [3] (Fig. 1a). This technique gives rise to heterogeneous cell populations that are frequently contaminated by other cells, including osteoblasts, osteoprogenitor cells, fat cells, reticular cells, macrophages, endothelial cells, and hematopoietic cells. There is a pressing need to enrich regenerative DPSCs. The study of DPSCs has been profoundly influenced by earlier studies of BMMSCs because DPSCs are positive for cell surface markers similar to those of BMMSCs, including CD44, CD73, CD105, STRO-1, and CD146, but are negative for CD45, CD34, CD14, C11b, CD79, CD19, and HLA-DR [5]. SHEDs also highly express MSC markers, including CD105, CD146, STRO-1, and CD29, but are negative for CD31 and CD34 [5]. Various methods have been tested to isolate and purify clonal subsets of stem cells from dental pulp, including immunoselection of cell surface markers by fluorescence-activated cell sorting (FACS) and magnetic-activated cell sorting (MACS) (Table 1).

DPSCs were first isolated from dental pulp tissue using cell surface markers, mainly STRO-1. Several studies reported that STRO-1$^+$ cells have a high colony-forming ability and a multilineage differentiation capability [4, 24–26] and express CD146, and a pericyte marker (3G5) in perivascular and perineural sheath regions [24]. STRO-1$^+$ and CD146$^+$ cells in pulp of deciduous teeth are also located in perivascular regions [4]. c-Kit$^+$CD34$^+$CD45$^-$ cells isolated from dental pulp by flow cytometry have a potent proliferative potential and readily differentiate into osteogenic precursors capable of generating three-dimensional woven bone tissue chips in vitro [27]. Although STRO-1$^+$c-Kit$^+$CD34$^+$ human DPSCs (hDPSCs), which reside in a perivascular niche, have a lower proliferative capacity than STRO-1$^+$c-Kit$^+$CD34$^-$ hDPSCs; they strongly express Nestin and the surface antigen low-affinity nerve growth factor (LNGFR, also called CD271) [28]. STRO-1$^+$c-Kit$^+$CD34$^+$ hDPSCs show a stronger tendency toward neurogenic commitment than STRO-1$^+$c-Kit$^+$CD34$^-$ hDPSCs, even though no significant differences between the two subpopulations arise after differentiation toward mesoderm lineages (osteogenic, adipogenic, and myogenic). c-Kit$^+$FLK-1$^+$CD34$^+$STRO-1$^+$ stem cells isolated from a plastic-adherent population by FACS have a potent growth potential (92% colony formation from 3–4 seeded cells) and are multipotent [9]. Other groups have demonstrated that colony-derived populations of DPSCs

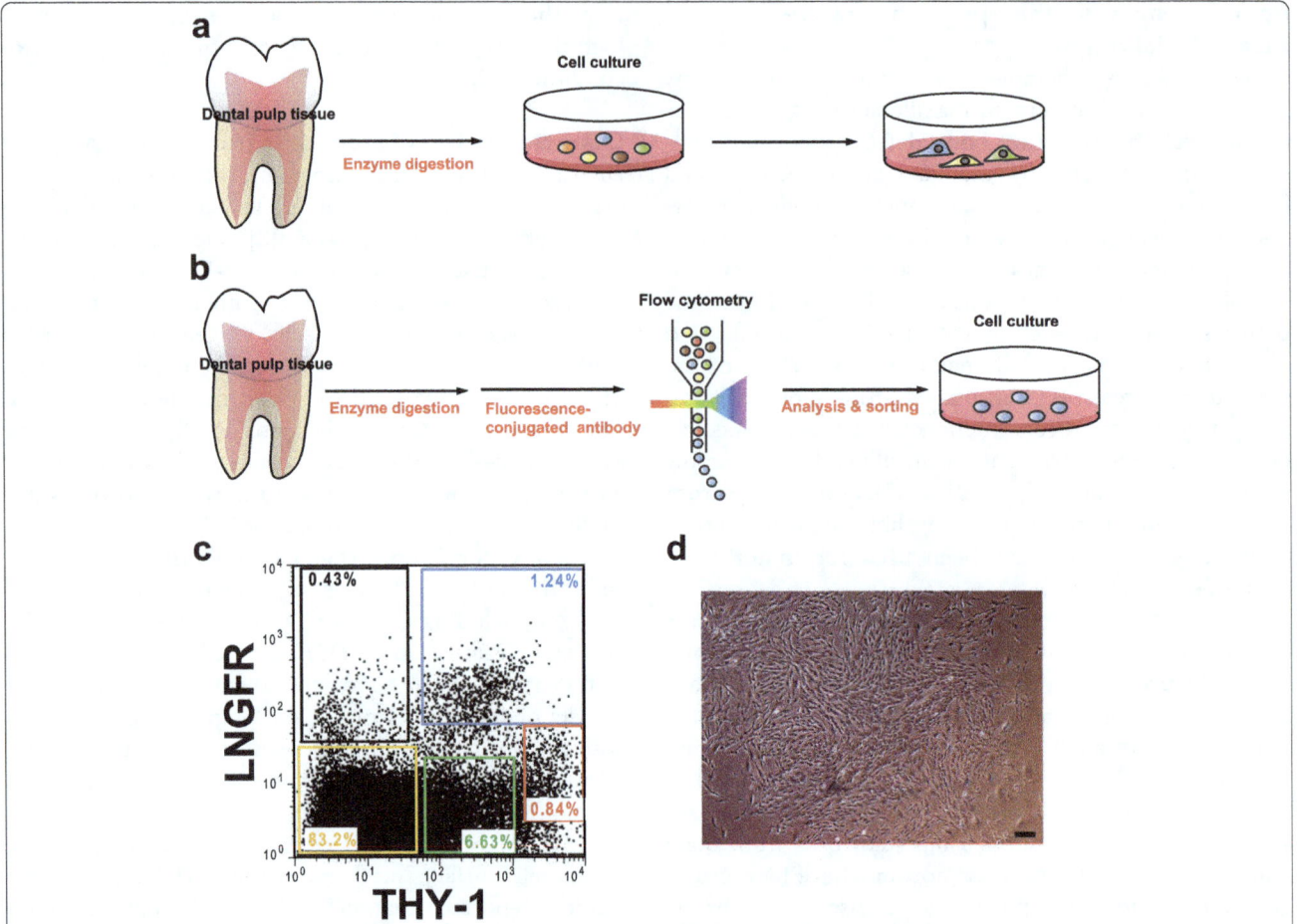

Fig. 1 a Traditional isolation of dental pulp stem/progenitor cells (DPSCs) by adherent culture on dishes. **b** Prospective isolation of DPSCs by flow cytometric identification of cell surface markers. **c** Representative fluorescence-activated cell sorting profiles of dental pulp cells. **d** A representative phase-contrast micrograph of plastic-adherent colony-forming LNGFR^{Low+}THY-1^{High+} cells with fibroblast morphologies. *Scale bars* = 100 μm

express typical mesenchymal markers, including CD29, CD44, CD90, CD166, and CD105 [29].

Subsequently, a side population (SP) was isolated from dental pulp based on efflux of the fluorescent dye Hoechst 33342 detected by FACS [30, 31]. This method, which has been used on SP cell populations from hematopoietic bone marrow, highly enriches cells with stem cell activity [32]. SP cells from dental pulp exhibit a self-renewal capacity with a long proliferative lifespan and differentiate into odontoblast-like cells, neurons, chondrocytes, and adipocytes [30, 31]. Furthermore, CD31$^-$CD146$^-$ SP cells and CD105$^+$ cells from dental pulp have high proliferative and migration activities and a multilineage differentiation potential in vitro, including adipogenic, dentinogenic, angiogenic, and neurogenic potentials [33, 34]. In a whole dental pulp removal model, transplantation of canine CD31$^-$CD146$^-$ SP and CD105$^+$ DPSCs expressing angiogenic and neurotrophic factors promotes regeneration of pulp in permanent teeth [33, 35]. Immature dental pulp stem cells express various embryonic stem cell markers [36]. A recent study

of SHEDs demonstrated that stage-specific embryonic antigen-4$^+$ cells derived from human deciduous dental pulp tissue have a multilineage differentiation potential in vitro [37].

Dental pulp originates from migrating neural crest cells; therefore, stem cells have been isolated from dental pulp using LNGFR, an embryonic neural crest marker [38, 39]. LNGFR has been used to prospectively isolate neural crest stem cells (NCSCs) from mammalian fetal peripheral nerves [40]. NCSCs can self-renew and differentiate into neurons, Schwann cells, and smooth muscle-like myofibroblasts in vitro. The characteristics of NCSCs are similar to those of MSCs. Cranial neural crest-derived cells contribute to ectomesenchymal cells in the developing dental papilla during tooth development [41, 42]. Cranial neural crest-derived LNGFR$^+$ ectomesenchymal stem cells have odonto-differentiation potential [43]. Multipotent NCSCs have been identified not only in the early embryonic stage, but also in adulthood. Neural crest-related stem cells were isolated from mature dental pulp in several studies [39, 44, 45]. The enriched cell population expresses

Table 1 Purification of dental pulp stem/progenitor cells (DPSCs) and stem cells from human exfoliated deciduous teeth (SHEDs)

Authors	Year	Cell source	Enzyme digestion	Selection	Differentiation	Result
Shi et al. [24]	2003	Human DPSCs	3 mg/ml collagenase type I, 4 mg/ml dispase	STRO-1$^+$ (MACS)	Odontogenic/osteogenic cells	Production of osteodentin-like structures and fibrous connective tissues
Laino et al. [27]	2006	Human DPSCs/SHEDs	3 mg/ml collagenase type I, 4 mg/ml dispase	c-Kit$^+$CD34$^+$STRO-1$^+$CD45$^-$ (FACS)	Osteogenic cells	High positivity for CD44, RUNX2, and osteocalcin
Iohara et al. [31]	2006	Human, bovine, canine, and porcine DPSCs	–	Hoechst 33342 (FACS)	Odontogenic, chondrogenic, adipogenic, and neurogenic cells	SP cells are enriched for stem cell properties and useful for cell therapy with BMP2 to regenerate dentin
Yang et al. [25]	2007	Rat DPSCs	–	STRO-1$^+$ (FACS)	Odontogenic, neurogenic, adipogenic, myogenic, and chondrogenic cells	STRO-1 selection obtains a more homogeneous cell population with a multilineage differentiation capacity
Honda et al. [30]	2007	Human DPSCs	–	Hoechst 33342 (FACS)	Odontogenic cells	SP cells expressing ABCG2 in human adult dental pulp that differentiate into odontoblast-like cells
Waddington et al. [39]	2009	Rat DPSCs	4 mg/ml collagenase, 4 mg/ml dispase	LNGFR (MACS)	Osteogenic, adipogenic, and chondrogenic cells	LNGFR$^+$ DPSCs express CD105 and Notch 2
Ricco et al. [87]	2010	Human DPSCs	3 mg/ml collagenase type I, 4 mg/ml dispase	CD34$^+$c-Kit$^+$STRO-1$^+$ (MACS)	Osteogenic cells	CD34$^+$c-Kit$^+$STRO-1$^+$ DPSCs produce mineralized matrix in 2D and 3D cultures
Iohara et al. [33]	2011	Dog DPSCs	–	CD105 (FACS)	Odontogenic/osteogenic, adipogenic, angiogenic, and neurogenic cells	Transplantation of CD105$^+$ DPSCs with SDF-1 completely regenerates dental pulp in a pulpectomy model
Mikami et al. [38]	2011	Human SHEDs	2 mg/ml collagenase type I	CD271$^+$CD90$^+$CD44 (FACS)	Osteogenic, adipogenic, chondrogenic, and myogenic cells	LNGFR positivity inhibits the differentiation of DPSCs into osteogenic, adipogenic, chondrogenic, and myogenic lineages
Hosoya et al. [58]	2012	Rat DPSCs	2 mg/ml collagenase, 0.25% trypsin	THY-1^{High+} (FACS)	Osteogenic cells	Hard tissue formation upon subcutaneous transplantation of THY-1$^+$ cells
Kawanabe et al. [37]	2015	Human SHEDs	5 mg/ml collagenase type II, 2.5 mg/ml dispase I	SSEA-4$^+$ (FACS)	Osteogenic, adipogenic, and chondrogenic cells	SSEA-4$^+$ SHEDs have a multilineage potential.
Yasui et al. [50]	2016	Human DPSCs	2 mg/ml collagenase, 4 mg/ml dispase	LNGFR^{Low+}THY-1^{High+} (FACS)	Osteogenic, adipogenic, and chondrogenic cells	LNGFR^{Low+}THY-1^{High+} DPSCs promote osteogenic differentiation.

BMP2 bone morphogenetic protein 2, FACS fluorescence-activated cell sorting, LNGFR low-affinity nerve growth factor, MACS magnetic-activated cell sorting, SDF-1 stromal cell-derived factor-1, SP side population, SSEA-4 stage-specific embryonic antigen-4, THY-1 thymocyte antigen 1

Nestin, LNGFR, and SOX10 and can be induced to differentiate into osteoblasts, melanocytes, and Schwann cells [45]. Thymocyte antigen 1 (THY-1, also called CD90)$^+$ glial cells generate multipotent MSCs that produce dental pulp cells and odontoblasts [46]. LNGFR$^+$THY-1$^+$ neural crest-like cells derived from human pluripotent stem cells can differentiate into both mesenchymal and neural crest lineages [47]. Therefore, LNGFR and THY-1 could be useful to isolate clonogenic DPSCs from neural crest-derived dental pulp tissue.

Prospective isolation of DPSCs using surface makers

Although many methods to enrich DPSCs have been devised, most assume that plastic-adherent cells are stem cells. Adherent culture on plastic dishes inevitably changes the expression of surface markers and gradually diminishes the differentiation, proliferation, and migration potencies of stem cells [9, 10]. These methods may not be able to reproduce the experimental results or reveal the biological properties of DPSCs. It is important to establish a method that can be used to prospectively isolate purified DPSC populations without cell culture. Therefore, specific cell surface markers need to be identified in order to isolate highly regenerative DPSCs. LNGFR and THY-1 have been identified as selective markers for the purification and phenotypic characterization of MSCs from various sources such as bone marrow, decidua, adipose tissue, and synovium [48, 49]. Especially in human bone marrow, LNGFR$^+$THY-1$^+$ cells are extremely enriched with clonogenic cells (2×10^5-fold enrichment vs. whole bone marrow cells) [48]. Our study demonstrated that these markers can also be used to prospectively isolate hDPSC populations, thereby avoiding the need for prolonged cell culture [50] (Fig. 1b). Flow cytometric analyses revealed five cell populations, namely, LNGFR$^+$THY-1$^+$, LNGFR^{Low+}THY-1^{High+}, LNGFR$^-$THY-1^{Low+}, LNGFR$^+$THY-1$^-$, and LNGFR$^-$THY-1$^-$ (Fig. 1c). Although LNGFR$^+$THY-1$^+$ cells in bone marrow exhibit the highest clonogenic potential [48], assessment of the number of colonies showed that LNGFR^{Low+}THY-1^{High+} cells in dental pulp have a significantly higher colony-forming potential than LNGFR$^+$THY-1$^+$ cells [50]. LNGFR^{Low+}THY-1^{High+} cells are uniformly small and have a spindle-shaped (MSC-like) morphology (Fig. 1d). The cell population considered to be DPSCs comprises two cell types, and it seems that purity can be increased by selecting one of these. However, a LNGFR^{Low+}THY-1^{High+} cell population was not observed in FACS profiles of human BMMSCs stained with anti-LNGFR and anti-THY-1 antibodies [48]. The discrepancy of the expression pattern of cell surface markers between dental pulp tissue and bone marrow tissue may be due to differences in the origin of the cells. Dental pulp tissue is thought to be

derived from migrating neural crest cells, whereas bone marrow tissue originates from the mesoderm and neural crest [51, 52]. During development, neural crest cells from the dorsal neural tube migrate to various locations and divide into four main functional domains, namely, the cranial neural crest, the trunk neural crest, the vagal and sacral neural crest, and the cardiac neural crest. Neural crest cells differentiate into a vast range of cells, including neurons and glial cells of the peripheral nervous system, smooth muscle cells, bone, and cartilage cells. Each distinct cell type responds to specific migration and differentiation signals to generate the appropriate cells and tissues [53]. Therefore, the phenotypes and biological properties of each cell type may differ.

Biological properties of stem cells from dental pulp

DPSCs and SHEDs have a high proliferation rate and a multilineage differentiation capability, including osteogenic, chondrogenic, adipogenic, neurogenic, and myogenic potentials [3–5]. Osteogenic differentiation of DPSCs is easily induced in vitro by adding dexamethasone, ascorbic acid, and β-glycerophosphate to culture medium supplemented with fetal bovine serum [54, 55]. DPSCs express bone markers such as alkaline phosphatase, type 1 collagen, osteocalcin, and osteonectin under osteogenic induction [3, 56]. DPSCs have a faster population doubling time and a higher mineralization potential than BMMSCs [6, 7]. SHEDs have a higher proliferation rate and a higher capability for osteogenic differentiation than BMMSCs and even DPSCs [4, 57]. Overall, DPSCs and SHEDs are more suitable than BMMSCs for mineralized tissue regeneration. In our study, prospectively isolated LNGFR^{Low+}THY-1^{High+} DPSCs showed a high clonogenic potential and a multipotent differentiation capability for mesenchymal lineages (Fig. 2a). The adipogenic, osteogenic, and chondrogenic capacities of LNGFR^{Low+}THY-1^{High+} cells were higher than those of LNGFR$^+$THY-1$^+$ cells (Fig. 2a, b) [50]. Interestingly, the proliferation rates of LNGFR^{Low+}THY-1^{High+} cells and LNGFR$^+$THY-1$^+$ cells did not significantly differ at early passages. Therefore, cultured hDPSCs isolated from crude dental pulp cells contain two cell types that originate from LNGFR^{Low+}THY-1^{High+} and LNGFR$^+$THY-1$^+$ cells. High LNGFR expression may inhibit differentiation of hDPSCs into osteoblasts and adipocytes [38], while low LNGFR expression might maintain the stemness of hDPSCs in the dental pulp microenvironment. THY-1$^+$ dental pulp cells localized in the sub-odontoblastic layer can differentiate into hard tissue-forming cells and may thus provide a source of odontoblastic cells [58]. THY-1$^+$ human adipose-derived stromal cells show osteogenic potential in vitro and significantly increase bone formation in a calvarial defect model [59]. THY-1$^+$ cells in other

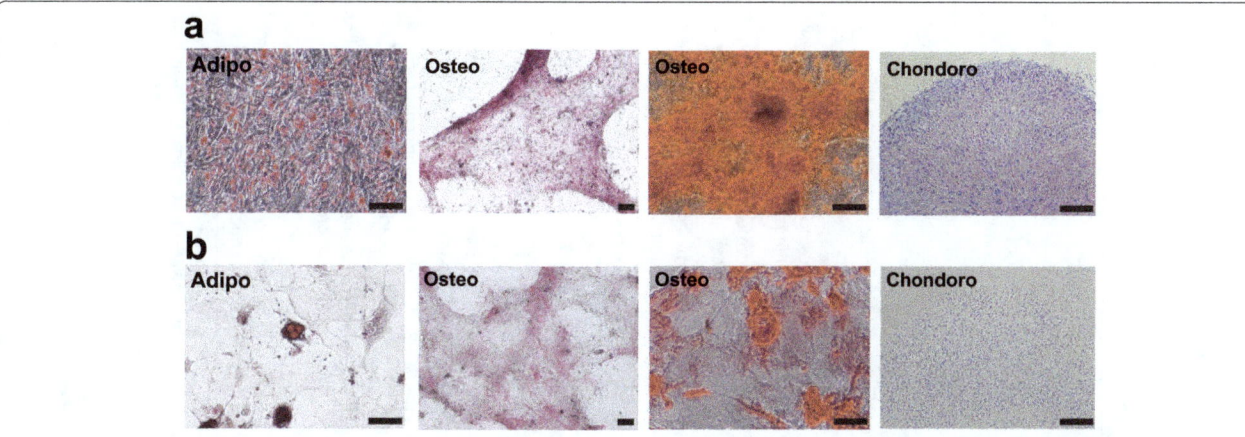

Fig. 2 a Adipogenic (Adipo), osteogenic (Osteo), and chondorogenic (Chondro) differentiation of LNGFR^{Low+}THY-1^{High+} cells. *Scale bars* = 100 μm.
b Adipogenic (Adipo), osteogenic (Osteo), and chondorogenic (Chondro) differentiation of LNGFR^{+}THY-1^{+} cells. *Scale bars* = 100 μm

tissues also show a high proliferative capacity and osteogenic potential [60, 61]. These reports suggest that THY-1 is important to isolate stem cell-like cells with a potent mineralization potential. LNGFR^{Low+}THY-1^{High+} DPSCs display a high proliferation rate and a long-term survival using a transillumination procedure such as cranial windows when transplanted into cranial defects of immunodeficient mice [50]. Therefore, LNGFR^{Low+}THY-1$^{High\ +}$ cells can increase the cell viability in cell transplantation, and this is considered to be advantage for differentiation into osteoblasts and secretion of each growth factor to promote bone morphogenesis. For successful tissue engineering, formation of blood vessels toward the transplanted tissue is required for transportation of oxygen and nutrients to the transplanted cells. When transplanted, stem cells such as DPSCs promote angiogenesis for bone regeneration in the maxillofacial region. DPSCs have a paracrine effect by stimulating the formation of blood vessels in the host tissue through secretion of angiogenic factors [62–68]. Furthermore, DPSCs and SHEDs may have stronger immunomodulatory properties and high anti-apoptotic activity [69–76]. Thus, DPSCs and SHEDs could also have potential for clinical applications in autologous stem cell transplantation for bone regenerative therapy.

Studies of bone regeneration in the cranio-maxillofacial region using stem cells from dental pulp

There are many studies of bone regeneration using DPSCs and SHEDs in the cranio-maxillofacial region in vivo because these cells have high osteogenic potential (Table 2). Several studies reported that transplantation of expanded DPSCs and SHEDs with scaffolds, such as fibroin, collagen membrane, and hydroxyapatite/tricalcium phosphate ceramic particles, repairs critical-size cranial bone defects of mice and rats [8, 77, 78]. Yamada et al. demonstrated that cell-based therapy using stem cells derived from deciduous teeth and dental pulp of puppies together with platelet-rich plasma can induce new bone formation in critical-size mandibular bone defects [79]. Ito et al. demonstrated that the high osteogenic ability of DPSCs contributes to the osseointegration of dental implants [80]. Alkaisi et al. reported that SHEDs can enhance bone consolidation in a rabbit mandibular distraction model [81]. A study of a large animal model showed that stem cells from deciduous teeth of miniature pigs regenerate bone to repair critical-size swine mandible bone defects [82]. In terms of clinical applications of DPSCs in humans, a biocomplex constructed from DPSCs and a collagen sponge scaffold was reported to be useful for bone tissue repair in human mandibular bone defects after extraction of third molars [83]. However, these cells might have been contaminated by non-regenerative cells with a poor bone-formation ability because these studies did not use purified cells.

Several studies investigated bone formation using hDPSCs purified by MACS for the repair of bone defects. Pisciotta et al. reported that STRO-1^{+} hDPSCs cultured in human serum-containing medium repair critical-size parietal bone defects in immunocompromised rats [84]. Giuliani et al. reported that CD34^{+} hDPSCs together with a collagen sponge regenerate compact bone with uniform vascularization after tooth extraction [85]. Ricco et al. reported that CD34^{+}c-kit $^{+}$STRO-1^{+} hDPSCs with fibroin scaffolds induce mature bone formation and repair critical-size bone defects in immunocompromised rats [86].

In our study, LNGFR^{Low+}THY-1^{High+} and LNGFR^{+}THY-1^{+} cells prospectively isolated by FACS were transplanted into critical-sized calvarial defects to evaluate their therapeutic potential [50]. LNGFR^{Low+}THY-1^{High+} hDPSCs exhibit long-term survival and osteoblastic differentiation in immunohistochemical analyses. Microcomputed tomography-guided morphometric analysis showed that

Table 2 Studies of bone regeneration by stem cells from dental pulp in the cranio-maxillofacial region in vivo

Authors and year		Targeted site	Cell source	Selection	Host	Scaffolds	Results
de Mendonca et al. [78]	2008	Cranial bone defect	Human DPSCs	–	Rat	Collagen membrane	Induction of mature bone formation
Seo et al. [8]	2008	Critical-size calvarial bone defect	Human SHEDs	–	Mouse	HA/TCP	Repair of defects and substantial bone formation
Zheng et al. [82]	2009	Orofacial bone defects	Stem cells from porcine (miniature pig) deciduous teeth	–	Miniature pig	β-TCP	More efficient regeneration of critical-size mandibular bone defects
d'Aquino et al. [83]	2009	Alveolar bone defect after extraction of impacted third molars	Human DPSCs	–	Human	Collagen sponge	Complete restoration of bone defects
Ito et al. [80]	2011	Osseointegration of dental implants	Canine DPSCs	–	Dog	PRP	High osteogenic potential to assist dental implant integration
Yamada et al. [79]	2011	Mandibular bone defect	Canine DPSCs and stem cells from deciduous teeth	–	Dog	PRP	Well-formed mature bone using both cell lines
Liu et al. [55]	2011	Critical-size alveolar bone defect	Rabbit DPSCs	–	Rabbit	rhBMP2 + nHAC/PL	Early mineralization and excellent bone formation
Ricco et al. [86]	2012	Critical-size cranial bone defect	Human DPSCs	$CD34^+c\text{-}Kit^+STRO\text{-}1^+$ (MACS)	Rat	Fibroin scaffolds	Mature bone formation and defect correction
Pisciotta et al. [84]	2012	Critical-size parietal bone defect	Human DPSCs	$STRO\text{-}1^+$ (MACS)	Rat	Collagen constructs	Restoration of critical parietal bone defects
Alkaisi et al. [81]	2013	Distracted area of mandibular bone	Human SHEDs	–	Rabbit	–	Enhancement of the bone consolidation period in mandibular distraction osteogenesis
Annibali et al. [77]	2013	Critical-size calvarial bone defect	Human DPSCs/PeSCs	–	Mouse	Porcine collagen + GDPB, β-TCP, Aga/nHA	β-TCP alone is more effective than β-TCP seeded with DPSCs/PeSCs
Giuliani et al. [85]	2013	Mandibular bone defect after tooth extraction	Human DPSCs	$CD34^+$ (MACS)	Human	Collagen sponge	Regeneration of compact-type bone with uniform vascularization
Yasui et al. [50]	2016	Critical-size calvarial bone defect	Human DPSCs	$LNGFR^{Low+}/THY\text{-}1^{High+}$ (FACS)	Mouse	Collagen membrane	$LNGFR^{Low+}/THY\text{-}1^{High+}$ DPSCs promote new bone formation to repair critical-size calvarial defects

Aga/nHA a sponge of agarose and nanohydroxyapatite, DPSCs dental pulp stem/progenitor cells, FACS fluorescence-activated cell sorting, GDPB granular deproteinized bovine bone, HA hydroxyapatite, LNGFR low-affinity nerve growth factor, MACS magnetic-activated cell sorting, nHAC/PLA nanohydroxyapatite/collagen/poly(L-lactide), PeSCs periosteal stem cells, PRP platelet-rich plasma, rhBMP-2 recombinant human bone morphogenetic protein 2, SHEDs stem cells from human exfoliated deciduous teeth, TCP tricalcium phosphate, THY-1 thymocyte antigen 1

LNGFR^{Low+}THY-1^{High+} cells induce the highest level of bone regeneration after transplantation into calvarial defects. The bone-formation potential of LNGFR^{Low}$^+$THY-1^{High+} cells is markedly higher than that of LNGFR$^+$THY-1$^+$ cells. Therefore, traditionally cultured DPSCs isolated from crude dental pulp cells are considered to comprise two cell types, namely, highly osteogenic cells and lowly osteogenic cells. We believe that enrichment of regenerative cells will lead to successful bone regenerative therapy through high levels of engraftment, survival, and proliferation post-transplantation.

Conclusions

Considering clinical applications for bone regeneration, cell-based therapy using DPSCs requires a prolonged period of culture to obtain a sufficient number of cells for transplantation because only a small number of DPSCs can be obtained from a single tooth. Therefore, it is important to stabilize the quality and quantity of transplanted cells by ensuring they have high proliferative and osteogenic capabilities. Cultured DPSCs isolated from crude dental pulp cells are considered to comprise two cell types: regenerative and non-regenerative cells. Hence, isolation of the optimal cell population for bone regeneration is important for regenerative therapy. There is a pressing need to identify selective markers of DPSCs with high osteogenic potential. LNGFR and THY-1 can be used to prospectively isolate a pure population of DPSCs from human dental pulp by FACS. However, purification of DPSCs using these markers is still insufficient compared with that of BMMSCs. Consequently, it is necessary to further enhance their purity by using additional markers. Furthermore, specific markers of other easily obtained dental stem cells should be identified to acquire a cell source for cranio-maxillofacial bone regeneration in a future study because DPSCs cannot be obtained from non-vital teeth.

Abbreviations
BMMSCs: Stem cells from bone marrow; CM: Conditioned media; DPSCs: Dental pulp stem cells/progenitor cells; FACS: Fluorescence-activated cell sorting; hDPSCs: Human dental pulp stem cells/progenitor cells; LNGFR: Low-affinity nerve growth factor; MACS: Magnetic-activated cell sorting; MSCs: Mesenchymal stem cells; NCSCs: Neural crest stem cells; SHEDs: Stem cells from human exfoliated deciduous teeth; SP: Side population; THY-1: Thymocyte antigen 1

Acknowledgements
We thank our colleagues, laboratory members, and collaborators for their excellent experimental assistance and discussions.

Funding
This work was supported by Japanese Society for the Promotion of Science (JSPS) KAKENHI grants (Grant Nos. 23792293, 25861895, and 16 K11656) to T.Y.

Authors' contributions
All authors have read and approved the final manuscript.

Competing interests
H.O. is the Editor-in-Chief of this journal and a member of the Scientific Advisory Board of SanBio Co., Ltd (Tokyo, Japan). Y. Matsuzaki concurrently is a director of PuREC, Co., Ltd (Shimane, Japan). The other authors declare that they have no competing of interest.

Author details
[1]Department of Dentistry and Oral Surgery, Keio University School of Medicine, 35 Shinanomachi, Shinjuku-ku, Tokyo 160-8582, Japan. [2]Department of Physiology, Keio University School of Medicine, 35 Shinanomachi, Shinjuku-ku, Tokyo 160-8582, Japan. [3]Department of Dentistry and Oral Surgery, Kawasaki Municipal Kawasaki Hospital, 12-1 Shinkawadori, Kawasaki-ku, Kawasaki, Kanagawa 210-0013, Japan. [4]Department of Biochemistry and Biophysics, Graduate School of Health Care Sciences, Tokyo Medical and Dental University, 1-5-45 Yushima Bunkyo-ku, Tokyo 113-8510, Japan. [5]Department of Cancer Biology, Faculty of Medicine, Shimane University, 89-1 Enya-cho, Izumo, Shimane 693-8501, Japan.

References
1. Liu H, Gronthos S, Shi S. Dental pulp stem cells. Methods Enzymol. 2006;419:99–113.
2. Batouli S, Miura M, Brahim J, Tsutsui TW, Fisher LW, Gronthos S, Robey PG, Shi S. Comparison of stem-cell-mediated osteogenesis and dentinogenesis. J Dent Res. 2003;82:976–81.
3. Gronthos S, Mankani M, Brahim J, Robey PG, Shi S. Postnatal human dental pulp stem cells (DPSCs) in vitro and in vivo. Proc Natl Acad Sci U S A. 2000;97:13625–30.
4. Miura M, Gronthos S, Zhao M, Lu B, Fisher LW, Robey PG, et al. SHED: stem cells from human exfoliated deciduous teeth. Proc Natl Acad Sci U S A. 2003;100:5807–12.
5. Huang GT, Gronthos S, Shi S. Mesenchymal stem cells derived from dental tissues vs. those from other sources: their biology and role in regenerative medicine. J Dent Res. 2009;88:792–806.
6. Alge DL, Zhou D, Adams LL, Wyss BK, Shadday MD, Woods EJ, et al. Donor-matched comparison of dental pulp stem cells and bone marrow-derived mesenchymal stem cells in a rat model. J Tissue Eng Regen Med. 2010;4:73–81.
7. Jensen J, Tvedesoe C, Rolfing JH, Foldager CB, Lysdahl H, Kraft DC, et al. Dental pulp-derived stromal cells exhibit a higher osteogenic potency than bone marrow-derived stromal cells in vitro and in a porcine critical-size bone defect model. SICOT J. 2016;2:16.
8. Seo BM, Sonoyama W, Yamaza T, Coppe C, Kikuiri T, Akiyama K, et al. SHED repair critical-size calvarial defects in mice. Oral Dis. 2008;14:428–34.
9. d'Aquino R, Graziano A, Sampaolesi M, Laino G, Pirozzi G, De Rosa A, et al. Human postnatal dental pulp cells co-differentiate into osteoblasts and endotheliocytes: a pivotal synergy leading to adult bone tissue formation. Cell Death Differ. 2007;14:1162–71.
10. Yu J, He H, Tang C, Zhang G, Li Y, Wang R, et al. Differentiation potential of STRO-1+ dental pulp stem cells changes during cell passaging. BMC Cell Biol. 2010;11:32.
11. Cannon TY, Strub GM, Yawn RJ, Day TA. Oromandibular reconstruction. Clin Anat. 2012;25:108–19.
12. Yamada H, Nakaoka K, Sonoyama T, Kumagai K, Ikawa T, Shigeta Y, et al. Clinical usefulness of mandibular reconstruction using custom-made titanium mesh tray and autogenous particulate cancellous bone and marrow harvested from tibia and/or ilia. J Craniofac Surg. 2016;27:586–92.
13. Nkenke E, Neukam FW. Autogenous bone harvesting and grafting in advanced jaw resorption: morbidity, resorption and implant survival. Eur J Oral Implantol. 2014;7(Suppl 2):S203–217.
14. Wu J, Li B, Lin X. Histological outcomes of sinus augmentation for dental implants with calcium phosphate or deproteinized bovine

bone: a systematic review and meta-analysis. Int J Oral Maxillofac Surg. 2016;45:1471–7.

15. Petite H, Viateau V, Bensaid W, Meunier A, de Pollak C, Bourguignon M, et al. Tissue-engineered bone regeneration. Nat Biotechnol. 2000;18:959–63.

16. Zhao J, Hu J, Wang S, Sun X, Xia L, Zhang X, et al. Combination of beta-TCP and BMP-2 gene-modified bMSCs to heal critical size mandibular defects in rats. Oral Dis. 2010;16:46–54.

17. Xia L, Xu Y, Chang Q, Sun X, Zeng D, Zhang W, et al. Maxillary sinus floor elevation using BMP-2 and Nell-1 gene-modified bone marrow stromal cells and TCP in rabbits. Calcif Tissue Int. 2011;89:53–64.

18. Zhang D, Chu F, Yang Y, Xia L, Zeng D, Uludag H, et al. Orthodontic tooth movement in alveolar cleft repaired with a tissue engineering bone: an experimental study in dogs. Tissue Eng Part A. 2011;17:1313–25.

19. Ueda M, Yamada Y, Kagami H, Hibi H. Injectable bone applied for ridge augmentation and dental implant placement: human progress study. Implant Dent. 2008;17:82–90.

20. Rajan A, Eubanks E, Edwards S, Aronovich S, Travan S, Rudek I, et al. Optimized cell survival and seeding efficiency for craniofacial tissue engineering using clinical stem cell therapy. Stem Cells Transl Med. 2014;3:1495–503.

21. Sonoyama W, Liu Y, Yamaza T, Tuan RS, Wang S, Shi S, et al. Characterization of the apical papilla and its residing stem cells from human immature permanent teeth: a pilot study. J Endod. 2008;34:166–71.

22. Kato T, Hattori K, Deguchi T, Katsube Y, Matsumoto T, Ohgushi H, et al. Osteogenic potential of rat stromal cells derived from periodontal ligament. J Tissue Eng Regen Med. 2011;5:798–805.

23. Honda MJ, Imaizumi M, Suzuki H, Ohshima S, Tsuchiya S, Satomura K. Stem cells isolated from human dental follicles have osteogenic potential. Oral Surg Oral Med Oral Pathol Oral Radiol Endod. 2011;111:700–8.

24. Shi S, Gronthos S. Perivascular niche of postnatal mesenchymal stem cells in human bone marrow and dental pulp. J Bone Miner Res. 2003; 18:696–704.

25. Yang X, van den Dolder J, Walboomers XF, Zhang W, Bian Z, Fan M, et al. The odontogenic potential of STRO-1 sorted rat dental pulp stem cells in vitro. J Tissue Eng Regen Med. 2007;1:66–73.

26. Yang X, Zhang W, van den Dolder J, Walboomers XF, Bian Z, Fan M, et al. Multilineage potential of STRO-1+ rat dental pulp cells in vitro. J Tissue Eng Regen Med. 2007;1:128–35.

27. Laino G, Carinci F, Graziano A, d'Aquino R, Lanza V, De Rosa A, et al. In vitro bone production using stem cells derived from human dental pulp. J Craniofac Surg. 2006;17:511–5.

28. Pisciotta A, Carnevale G, Meloni S, Riccio M, De Biasi S, Gibellini L, et al. Human Dental pulp stem cells (hDPSCs): isolation, enrichment and comparative differentiation of two sub-populations. BMC Dev Biol. 2015;15:14.

29. Gandia C, Arminan A, Garcia-Verdugo JM, Lledo E, Ruiz A, Minana MD, et al. Human dental pulp stem cells improve left ventricular function, induce angiogenesis, and reduce infarct size in rats with acute myocardial infarction. Stem Cells. 2008;26:638–45.

30. Honda MJ, Nakashima F, Satomura K, Shinohara Y, Tsuchiya S, Watanabe N, et al. Side population cells expressing ABCG2 in human adult dental pulp tissue. Int Endod J. 2007;40:949–58.

31. Iohara K, Zheng L, Ito M, Tomokiyo A, Matsushita K, Nakashima M. Side population cells isolated from porcine dental pulp tissue with self-renewal and multipotency for dentinogenesis, chondrogenesis, adipogenesis, and neurogenesis. Stem Cells. 2006;24:2493–503.

32. Matsuzaki Y, Kinjo K, Mulligan RC, Okano H. Unexpectedly efficient homing capacity of purified murine hematopoietic stem cells. Immunity. 2004;20:87–93.

33. Iohara K, Imabayashi K, Ishizaka R, Watanabe A, Nabekura J, Ito M, et al. Complete pulp regeneration after pulpectomy by transplantation of CD105+ stem cells with stromal cell-derived factor-1. Tissue Eng Part A. 2011;17:1911–20.

34. Iohara K, Zheng L, Wake H, Ito M, Nabekura J, Wakita H, et al. A novel stem cell source for vasculogenesis in ischemia: subfraction of side population cells from dental pulp. Stem Cells. 2008;26:2408–18.

35. Iohara K, Zheng L, Ito M, Ishizaka R, Nakamura H, Into T, et al. Regeneration of dental pulp after pulpotomy by transplantation of CD31(–)/CD146(–) side population cells from a canine tooth. Regen Med. 2009;4:377–85.

36. Kerkis I, Kerkis A, Dozortsev D, Stukart-Parsons GC, Gomes Massironi SM, Pereira LV, et al. Isolation and characterization of a population of immature dental pulp stem cells expressing OCT-4 and other embryonic stem cell markers. Cells Tissues Organs. 2006;184:105–16.

37. Kawanabe N, Fukushima H, Ishihara Y, Yanagita T, Kurosaka H, Yamashiro T. Isolation and characterization of SSEA-4-positive subpopulation of human deciduous dental pulp cells. Clin Oral Investig. 2015;19:363–71.

38. Mikami Y, Ishii Y, Watanabe N, Shirakawa T, Suzuki S, Irie S, et al. CD271/p75(NTR) inhibits the differentiation of mesenchymal stem cells into osteogenic, adipogenic, chondrogenic, and myogenic lineages. Stem Cells Dev. 2011;20:901–13.

39. Waddington RJ, Youde SJ, Lee CP, Sloan AJ. Isolation of distinct progenitor stem cell populations from dental pulp. Cells Tissues Organs. 2009;189:268–74.

40. Morrison SJ, White PM, Zock C, Anderson DJ. Prospective identification, isolation by flow cytometry, and in vivo self-renewal of multipotent mammalian neural crest stem cells. Cell. 1999;96:737–49.

41. Chai Y, Jiang X, Ito Y, Bringas Jr P, Han J, Rowitch DH, et al. Fate of the mammalian cranial neural crest during tooth and mandibular morphogenesis. Development. 2000;127:1671–9.

42. Deng MJ, Jin Y, Shi JN, Lu HB, Liu Y, He DW, et al. Multilineage differentiation of ectomesenchymal cells isolated from the first branchial arch. Tissue Eng. 2004;10:1597–606.

43. Xing Y, Nie X, Chen G, Wen X, Li G, Zhou X, et al. Comparison of P75 NTR-positive and -negative etcomesenchymal stem cell odontogenic differentiation through epithelial-mesenchymal interaction. Cell Prolif. 2016;49:185–94.

44. Pan W, Kremer KL, Kaidonis X, Ludlow VE, Rogers ML, Xie J, et al. Characterization of p75 neurotrophin receptor expression in human dental pulp stem cells. Int J Dev Neurosci. 2016;53:90–8.

45. Al-Zer H, Apel C, Heiland M, Friedrich RE, Jung O, Kroeger N, et al. Enrichment and schwann cell differentiation of neural crest-derived dental pulp stem cells. In Vivo. 2015;29:319–26.

46. Kaukua N, Shahidi MK, Konstantinidou C, Dyachuk V, Kaucka M, Furlan A, et al. Glial origin of mesenchymal stem cells in a tooth model system. Nature. 2014;513:551–4.

47. Ouchi T, Morikawa S, Shibata S, Fukuda K, Okuno H, Fujimura T, et al. LNGFR + THY1+ human pluripotent stem cell-derived neural crest-like cells have the potential to develop into mesenchymal stem cells. Differentiation. 2016;92:270–80.

48. Mabuchi Y, Morikawa S, Harada S, Niibe K, Suzuki S, Renault-Mihara F, et al. LNGFR(+)THY-1(+)VCAM-1(hi+) cells reveal functionally distinct subpopulations in mesenchymal stem cells. Stem Cell Rep. 2013;1:152–65.

49. Ogata Y, Mabuchi Y, Yoshida M, Suto EG, Suzuki N, Muneta T, et al. Purified human synovium mesenchymal stem cells as a good resource for cartilage regeneration. PLoS One. 2015;10:e0129096.

50. Yasui T, Mabuchi Y, Toriumi H, Ebine T, Niibe K, Houlihan DD, et al. Purified human dental pulp stem cells promote osteogenic regeneration. J Dent Res. 2016;95:206–14.

51. Janebodin K, Horst OV, Ieronimakis N, Balasundaram G, Reesukumal K, Pratumvinit B, et al. Isolation and characterization of neural crest-derived stem cells from dental pulp of neonatal mice. PLoS One. 2011;6:e27526.

52. Morikawa S, Mabuchi Y, Niibe K, Suzuki S, Nagoshi N, Sunabori T, et al. Development of mesenchymal stem cells partially originate from the neural crest. Biochem Biophys Res Commun. 2009;379:1114–9.

53. Bhatt S, Diaz R, Trainor PA: signals and switches in mammalian neural crest cell differentiation. Cold Spring Harb Perspect Biol. 2013;5. doi:10.1101/cshperspect.a008326.

54. Langenbach F, Handschel J. Effects of dexamethasone, ascorbic acid and beta-glycerophosphate on the osteogenic differentiation of stem cells in vitro. Stem Cell Res Ther. 2013;4:117.

55. Liu HC, E LL, Wang DS, Su F, Wu X, Shi ZP, et al. Reconstruction of alveolar bone defects using bone morphogenetic protein 2 mediated rabbit dental pulp stem cells seeded on nano-hydroxyapatite/collagen/poly(L-lactide). Tissue Eng Part A. 2011;17:2417–33.

56. Yamada Y, Nakamura S, Ito K, Sugito T, Yoshimi R, Nagasaka T, et al. A feasibility of useful cell-based therapy by bone regeneration with deciduous tooth stem cells, dental pulp stem cells, or bone-marrow-derived mesenchymal stem cells for clinical study using tissue engineering technology. Tissue Eng Part A. 2010;16:1891–900.

57. Wang X, Sha XJ, Li GH, Yang FS, Ji K, Wen LY, et al. Comparative characterization of stem cells from human exfoliated deciduous teeth and dental pulp stem cells. Arch Oral Biol. 2012;57:1231–40.

58. Hosoya A, Hiraga T, Ninomiya T, Yukita A, Yoshiba K, Yoshiba N, et al. Thy-1-positive cells in the subodontoblastic layer possess high potential to differentiate into hard tissue-forming cells. Histochem Cell Biol. 2012; 137:733–42.

59. Chung MT, Liu C, Hyun JS, Lo DD, Montoro DT, Hasegawa M, et al. CD90 (Thy-1)-positive selection enhances osteogenic capacity of human adipose-derived stromal cells. Tissue Eng Part A. 2013;19:989–97.

60. Kim YK, Nakata H, Yamamoto M, Miyasaka M, Kasugai S, Kuroda S. Osteogenic potential of mouse periosteum-derived cells sorted for CD90 in vitro and in vivo. Stem Cells Transl Med. 2016;5:227–34.

61. Nakamura H, Yukita A, Ninomiya T, Hosoya A, Hiraga T, Ozawa H. Localization of Thy-1-positive cells in the perichondrium during endochondral ossification. J Histochem Cytochem. 2010;58:455–62.

62. Bronckaers A, Hilkens P, Fanton Y, Struys T, Gervois P, Politis C, et al. Angiogenic properties of human dental pulp stem cells. PLoS ONE. 2013;8:e71104.

63. Nakashima M, Iohara K, Sugiyama M. Human dental pulp stem cells with highly angiogenic and neurogenic potential for possible use in pulp regeneration. Cytokine Growth Factor Rev. 2009;20:435–40.

64. Aranha AM, Zhang Z, Neiva KG, Costa CA, Hebling J, Nor JE. Hypoxia enhances the angiogenic potential of human dental pulp cells. J Endod. 2010;36:1633–7.

65. Matsushita K, Motani R, Sakuta T, Yamaguchi N, Koga T, Matsuo K, et al. The role of vascular endothelial growth factor in human dental pulp cells: induction of chemotaxis, proliferation, and differentiation and activation of the AP-1-dependent signaling pathway. J Dent Res. 2000;79:1596–603.

66. Tran-Hung L, Laurent P, Camps J, About I. Quantification of angiogenic growth factors released by human dental cells after injury. Arch Oral Biol. 2008;53:9–13.

67. Tran-Hung L, Mathieu S, About I. Role of human pulp fibroblasts in angiogenesis. J Dent Res. 2006;85:819–23.

68. Hilkens P, Fanton Y, Martens W, Gervois P, Struys T, Politis C, et al. Pro-angiogenic impact of dental stem cells in vitro and in vivo. Stem Cell Res. 2014;12:778–90.

69. Pierdomenico L, Bonsi L, Calvitti M, Rondelli D, Arpinati M, Chirumbolo G, et al. Multipotent mesenchymal stem cells with immunosuppressive activity can be easily isolated from dental pulp. Transplantation. 2005;80:836–42.

70. Zhao Y, Wang L, Jin Y, Shi S. Fas ligand regulates the immunomodulatory properties of dental pulp stem cells. J Dent Res. 2012;91:948–54.

71. Yamaza T, Kentaro A, Chen C, Liu Y, Shi Y, Gronthos S, et al. Immunomodulatory properties of stem cells from human exfoliated deciduous teeth. Stem Cell Res Ther. 2010;1:5.

72. Omi M, Hata M, Nakamura N, Miyabe M, Kobayashi Y, Kamiya H, et al. Transplantation of dental pulp stem cells suppressed inflammation in sciatic nerves by promoting macrophage polarization towards anti-inflammation phenotypes and ameliorated diabetic polyneuropathy. J Diabetes Investig. 2016;7:485–96.

73. Sakai K, Yamamoto A, Matsubara K, Nakamura S, Naruse M, Yamagata M, et al. Human dental pulp-derived stem cells promote locomotor recovery after complete transection of the rat spinal cord by multiple neuro-regenerative mechanisms. J Clin Invest. 2012;122:80–90.

74. Demircan PC, Sariboyaci AE, Unal ZS, Gacar G, Subasi C, Karaoz E. Immunoregulatory effects of human dental pulp-derived stem cells on T cells: comparison of transwell co-culture and mixed lymphocyte reaction systems. Cytotherapy. 2011;13:1205–20.

75. Yamaguchi S, Shibata R, Yamamoto N, Nishikawa M, Hibi H, Tanigawa T, et al. Dental pulp-derived stem cell conditioned medium reduces cardiac injury following ischemia-reperfusion. Sci Rep. 2015;5:16295.

76. Matsubara K, Matsushita Y, Sakai K, Kano F, Kondo M, Noda M, et al. Secreted ectodomain of sialic acid-binding Ig-like lectin-9 and monocyte chemoattractant protein-1 promote recovery after rat spinal cord injury by altering macrophage polarity. J Neurosci. 2015;35:2452–64.

77. Annibali S, Cicconetti A, Cristalli MP, Giordano G, Trisi P, Pilloni A, et al. A comparative morphometric analysis of biodegradable scaffolds as carriers for dental pulp and periosteal stem cells in a model of bone regeneration. J Craniofac Surg. 2013;24:866–71.

78. de Mendonca Costa A, Bueno DF, Martins MT, Kerkis I, Kerkis A, Fanganiello RD, et al. Reconstruction of large cranial defects in nonimmunosuppressed experimental design with human dental pulp stem cells. J Craniofac Surg. 2008;19:204–10.

79. Yamada Y, Ito K, Nakamura S, Ueda M, Nagasaka T. Promising cell-based therapy for bone regeneration using stem cells from deciduous teeth, dental pulp, and bone marrow. Cell Transplant. 2011;20:1003–13.

80. Ito K, Yamada Y, Nakamura S, Ueda M. Osteogenic potential of effective bone engineering using dental pulp stem cells, bone marrow stem cells, and periosteal cells for osseointegration of dental implants. Int J Oral Maxillofac Implants. 2011;26:947–54.

81. Alkaisi A, Ismail AR, Mutum SS, Ahmad ZA, Masudi S, Abd Razak NH. Transplantation of human dental pulp stem cells: enhance bone consolidation in mandibular distraction osteogenesis. J Oral Maxillofac Surg. 2013;71(10):1758.e1–13.

82. Zheng Y, Liu Y, Zhang CM, Zhang HY, Li WH, Shi S, et al. Stem cells from deciduous tooth repair mandibular defect in swine. J Dent Res. 2009;88:249–54.

83. d'Aquino R, De Rosa A, Lanza V, Tirino V, Laino L, Graziano A, et al. Human mandible bone defect repair by the grafting of dental pulp stem/progenitor cells and collagen sponge biocomplexes. Eur Cell Mater. 2009;18:75–83.

84. Pisciotta A, Riccio M, Carnevale G, Beretti F, Gibellini L, Maraldi T, et al. Human serum promotes osteogenic differentiation of human dental pulp stem cells in vitro and in vivo. PLoS One. 2012;7:e50542.

85. Giuliani A, Manescu A, Langer M, Rustichelli F, Desiderio V, Paino F, et al. Three years after transplants in human mandibles, histological and in-line holotomography revealed that stem cells regenerated a compact rather than a spongy bone: biological and clinical implications. Stem Cells Transl Med. 2013;2:316–24.

86. Riccio M, Maraldi T, Pisciotta A, La Sala GB, Ferrari A, Bruzzesi G, et al. Fibroin scaffold repairs critical-size bone defects in vivo supported by human amniotic fluid and dental pulp stem cells. Tissue Eng Part A. 2012;18:1006–13.

87. Riccio M, Resca E, Maraldi T, Pisciotta A, Ferrari A, Bruzzesi G, et al. Human dental pulp stem cells produce mineralized matrix in 2D and 3D cultures. Eur J Histochem. 2010;54:e46.

13

RANKL system in vascular and valve calcification with aging

Ryo Kawakami[1,2], Hironori Nakagami[3*], Takahisa Noma[1], Koji Ohmori[1], Masakazu Kohno[1] and Ryuichi Morishita[2]

Abstract

Vascular and cardiac valve calcification is associated with cardiovascular mortality in the general population. Increasing clinical and experimental evidence suggests that inflammation accelerates the progression of calcification, which has molecules in common with bone metabolism. For example, osteopontin (OPN), osteoprotegerin (OPG), receptor activator of the nuclear factor κB ligand (RANKL), and alkaline phosphatase (ALP) are proposed to play central roles in the calcification or demineralization of atherosclerotic lesions and the calcification of cardiac valves. Abnormalities in the balance of these proteins may lead to perturbations in vascular/valve calcification. "How to prevent calcification" is a common task based on conventional data; however, several pathological findings indicate that heavily calcified plaques are stable, which may not lead to coronary events. Vulnerable plaques tend to be either noncalcified or only mildly or moderately calcified. "How to treat calcification," which depends on the details of the specific patient, thus remains a difficult challenge. In addition to the detection of calcification, characterization as well as quantification of it is necessary for optimal treatment of this pathology in the future.

Keywords: Vascular calcification, Cardiac valve calcification, Osteoporosis, RANK, RANKL, OPG, VICs, ECs, VSMCs

Background

The saying "a man is as old as his arteries" (a person grows old with their blood vessels), which William Osler quoted to describe the association between blood vessels and anti-aging in 1898 [1], remains relevant for many researchers and clinicians who are studying the central concepts of anti-aging. We have realized the importance of these words with the arrival of gluttony and the aging of our society over the past 100 years. For many decades, vascular and cardiac valve calcification has been regarded as consequences of aging. Studies now confirm that vascular and valvular calcification is an actively regulated process and shares many features with bone development and metabolism. Here, we focus on the molecular mechanism underlying the calcification of the aorta and cardiac valves and propose an answer to the question of "how to treat calcification".

Bone metabolism and aortic calcification with aging

Aortic calcification is an aging marker during the progression of atherosclerosis. Many studies have reported that aortic calcification and cardiovascular events are highly related in the elderly. This has been demonstrated with the development of recent diagnostic imaging systems. Rodondi et al. prospectively investigated the prognoses of patients aged more than 65 years with vascular calcification for 13 years to determine whether aortic calcification is a risk factor of cardiovascular disease [2]. Patients with aortic calcification were more likely to die of any cause (47 vs. 27 %, $P < 0.001$) and cardiovascular-specific causes (18 vs. 11 %, $P < 0.001$) during follow-up than those without aortic calcification. In analyses adjusted for age and cardiovascular risk factors, aortic calcification was associated with an increased rate of all-cause mortality (hazard ratio (HR), 1.37; 95 % confidence interval (CI), 1.15–1.64) [2]. Okuno et al. followed 515 hemodialysis patients, of whom 291 patients (56.5 %) had abdominal aortic calcification (AAC) [3]. During a mean follow-up of 51 months, there were 103 all-cause deaths, of which 41 were from cardiovascular diseases. Of patients with and without AAC, 27.8 and 9.8 % died, respectively (11.6 and 3.1 % from cardiovascular

* Correspondence: nakagami@gts.med.osaka-u.ac.jp
[3]Department of Health Development and Medicine, Graduate School of Medicine, Osaka University, 2-2 Yamada-oka, Suita 565-0871, Osaka, Japan
Full list of author information is available at the end of the article

diseases, respectively). Additionally, using multivariate Cox proportional hazards analysis, the presence of AAC was significantly associated with increased all-cause mortality (HR, 2.07; 95 % CI, 1.21–3.56) and increased cardiovascular mortality (HR, 2.39; 95 % CI, 1.01–5.66) after adjustment for age, hemodialysis duration, diabetes, serum albumin level, and C-reactive protein level. These epidemiologic studies suggest that aortic calcification may be a risk factor as well as a complication.

Vascular calcification and osteoporosis are common age-related processes and are associated with adverse clinical outcomes, including ischemic cardiac events, claudication, and mortality. Vascular calcification was previously considered passive and degenerative, but it is now recognized as a pathobiological process sharing many features with embryonic bone formation. Importantly, several bone matrix proteins are expressed in calcified arteries, which indicate that the cellular and molecular mechanisms of arterial calcification are similar to those of bone metabolism. Bostrom et al. demonstrated the expression of osteogenic differentiation factor bone morphogenetic protein-2 (BMP-2) in calcified human plaques and blood vessel tissue constitutive cells, such as endothelial cells (ECs), vascular smooth muscle cells (VSMCs), and macrophages, in vascular calcification. Furthermore, it was shown that

VSMCs could be differentiated into osteoblast-like cells by stimulation with BMP-2 [4]. Both bone metabolic disorder and vascular calcification are degenerative diseases that are common in the elderly population, and they are frequently observed in the same individuals. The constancy of mineral metabolism is maintained by the active balance of osteoblasts and osteoclasts in bone tissue; however, the contribution of osteoclast-like cells to aortic calcification is not yet well understood. Thus, the mineralization processes in bone metabolism and those in vascular calcification may be somewhat different.

The RANKL system in vascular and valve calcification

To address the unexplored mechanisms for this phenomenon, we focused on the receptor activator of nuclear factor κB (RANK), the RANK ligand (RANKL), and osteoprotegerin (OPG) from the tumor necrosis factor (TNF)-related family, which is associated with this mechanism. RANKL is highly expressed by T cells in lymphoid tissues and osteoblast/stromal cells in trabecular bone, particularly in areas undergoing active bone remodeling or inflammatory osteolysis [5]. In the bone, RANKL binds as a homotrimer to RANK on the surface of monocyte/macrophage lineage cells, and RANKL expression by osteoblasts/stromal cells is essential, together with permissive macrophage colony-stimulating

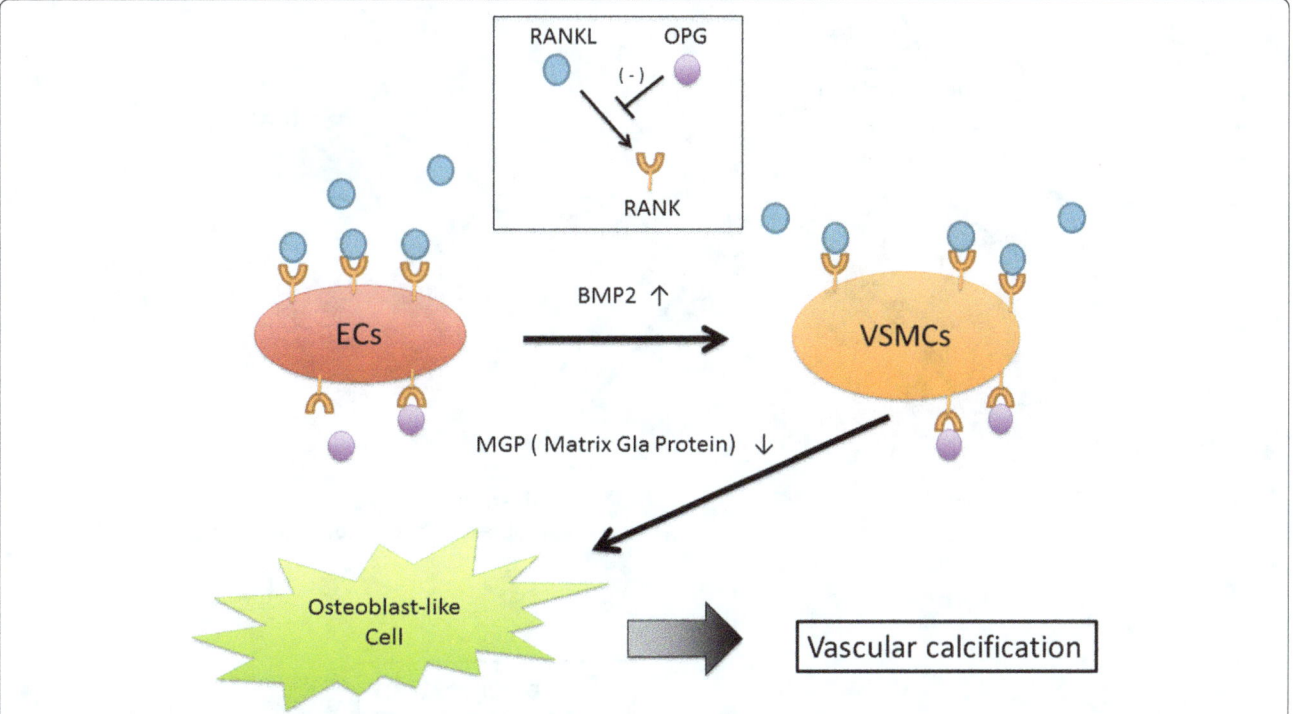

Fig. 1 Scheme of vascular calcification through the RANK/RANKL/OPG axis. In vascular cells, RANK is expressed in both ECs and smooth muscle cells (VSMCs), and RANKL is primarily expressed in VSMCs. RANKL directly stimulates osteogenic differentiation of VSMCs via a decrease in MGP and indirectly promotes osteogenesis via BMP2, which is part of the TGF-β superfamily, from ECs. Promoting osteogenic differentiation by RANKL in VSMCs leads to synthesis of bone proteins and matrix calcification within the arterial vessel

factor (M-CSF) levels, for the complete development of osteoclasts from monocytic precursors under normal or pathological conditions [5]. RANKL activities are blocked by OPG, which functions as a decoy receptor to prevent RANKL/RANK interactions and inhibits osteoclast formation. Interestingly, we demonstrated that the expression of RANKL/RANK/OPG was upregulated in calcified arteries and that RANKL accelerated differentiation of human smooth muscle cells into osteoblast-like cells (Fig. 1). In a human study, serum OPG levels were positively associated with vascular calcification [6]. The diverse actions of RANKL in the bone and the aorta may be the clues to understanding mineralization during aortic calcification.

Aortic valve calcification and stenosis are major medical problems facing an aging society. Calcification of the aortic valve gets increasingly common and occurs in conjunction with high mortality in the setting of advanced age, congestive heart failure, and end-stage renal disease, in which mechanical stress interacts with metabolic and inflammatory disturbances. The identification of osteoblast-like and osteoclast-like cells in human tissue has led to a major paradigm shift in this field. Although valve calcification was considered a passive, degenerative, and untreatable disorder of "wear and tear" unrelated to atherosclerosis, it is now recognized

as a disease that is regulated similarly to atherosclerotic calcification, which is promoted by systemic and local inflammatory milieu, characteristic of metabolic syndrome, and type 2 diabetes. Ectopic mineralization of the aortic valve involves several immunological reactions. Accumulating evidence suggests that fibrocalcific remodeling of the aortic valve is associated with activation of the NF-κB pathway and that the expression of TNF-α and IL-6 are increased in mineralized human aortic valves. These activators of the canonical NF-κB pathway promote an osteogenic process, as well as the mineralization of valve interstitial cells (VICs), the main cellular component of the aortic valve.

The RANKL/OPG axis may also regulate aortic valve calcification. Bucay et al. reported that OPG-deficient mice developed osteoporosis and valve calcification [7]. Kaden et al. showed that RANKL was present in human stenotic aortic valves, but not in normal valves. Conversely, OPG expression was higher in normal valves than in stenotic valves [8]. OPG-positive cells were specifically decreased in areas of focal calcification. Moreover, RANKL increased matrix calcification and ALP activity and facilitated the osteoblast transcription factor runx2 in cultured human aortic valve myofibroblasts (Fig. 2). In contrast, Weiss et al. demonstrated

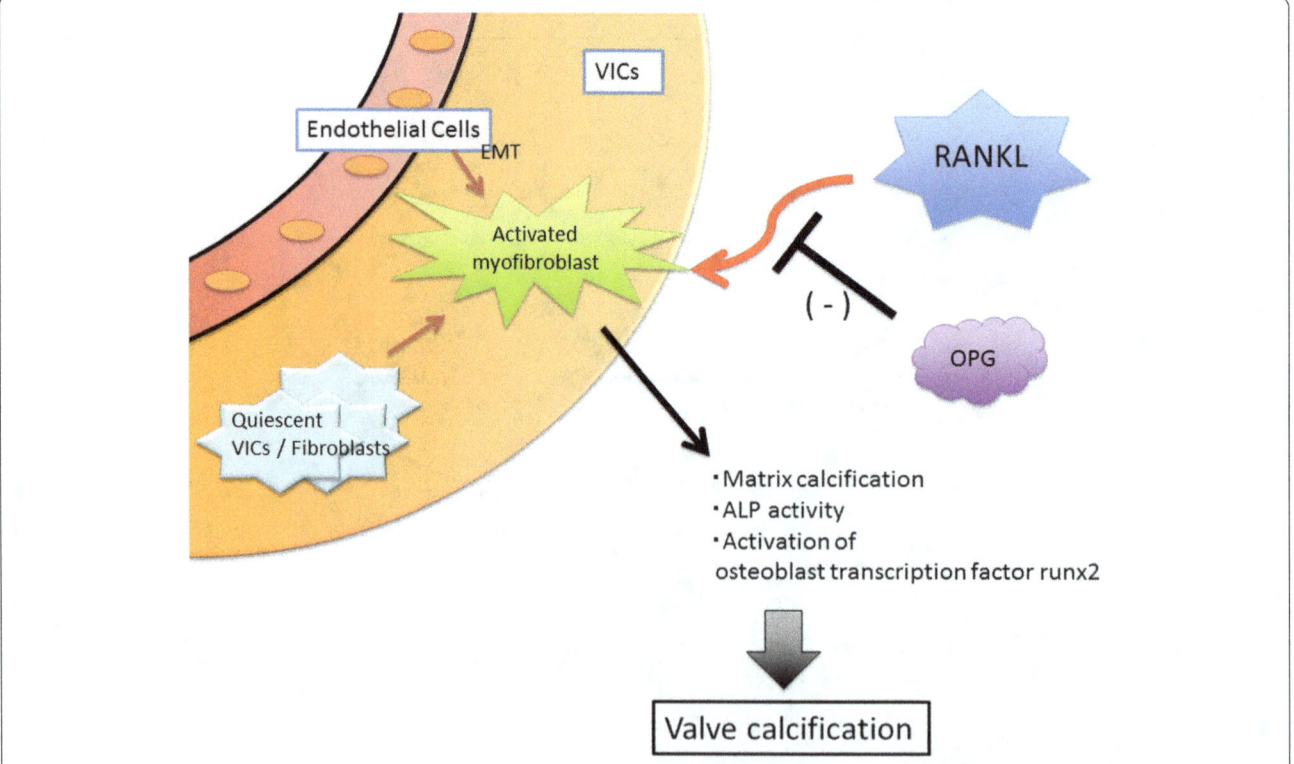

Fig. 2 Potential origin of cells that contribute to valve calcification and fibrosis. Valve interstitial cells (VICs) are the main cellular component of the aortic valve. In interstitial cells, activated myofibroblasts are likely to arise from either quiescent VICs or a subpopulation of endothelial cells that undergo endothelial to mesenchymal transformation (EMT). RANKL increased the matrix calcification, ALP activity, and activation of the osteoblast transcription factor runx2 in cultured human aortic valve myofibroblasts. OPG prevents the interaction of RANKL with its receptor, RANK

that in low-density lipoprotein receptor (LDLR)-deficient ApoB-100 mice fed a high fat diet, the administration of OPG reduced valve calcification through the inhibition of osteogenic transformation but did not prevent valve fibrosis or lipid deposition, suggesting a specific effect of OPG on calcification [9]. These observations suggest that RANKL/OPG may regulate valve calcification both directly and indirectly through regulation of the inflammatory response.

Therapeutic strategy for calcification

Vascular and valve calcification is an important diagnostic and therapeutic target for the diagnosis and treatment in an aging society. Many studies have reported that vascular and valve calcification is highly associated with mortality. Coronary artery calcium (CAC) has a strong predictive value for incident cardiovascular disease (CVD) events. The Agatston score, the standard CAC score, is weighted upward for greater calcium density. Criqui et al. conducted a multicenter, prospective observational Multi-Ethnic Study of Atherosclerosis (MESA) study at six US field centers with 3398 men and women aged 45 to 84 years [10]. During a median of 7.6 years of follow-up, CAC volume scores showed an independent association with incident coronary heart

disease (CHD), with a HR of 1.81 (95 % CI, 1.47–2.23) per standard deviation (SD = 1.6) increase and an absolute risk increase of 6.1 per 1000 person-years, and with CVD, with HR of 1.68 (95 % CI, 1.42–1.98) per SD increase and an absolute risk increase of 7.9 per 1000 person-years. As it progresses, valve calcification can lead to more severe stenosis or regurgitation. Therefore, it is a prognostic factor for cardiovascular mortality. Because the development of calcification should be prevented, several therapeutic drugs to suppress calcified process have recently been described. Allison et al. examined the relationship between estrogen therapy and coronary artery calcium in a randomized clinical trial [11]. They performed computed tomography of the heart in 1064 postmenopausal women who were 50 to 79 years of age at randomization and had undergone hysterectomy. Coronary artery calcium (or Agatston) scores were measured to evaluate calcification. After a mean of 7.4 years of treatment and an additional 1.3 years to be performed (8.7 years after randomization), the mean coronary artery calcium score was lower among women receiving estrogen than among those receiving placebo (83.1 vs. 123.1, $P = 0.02$ by rank test).

As described above, these observations suggest that RANKL signaling may play a permissive role in the

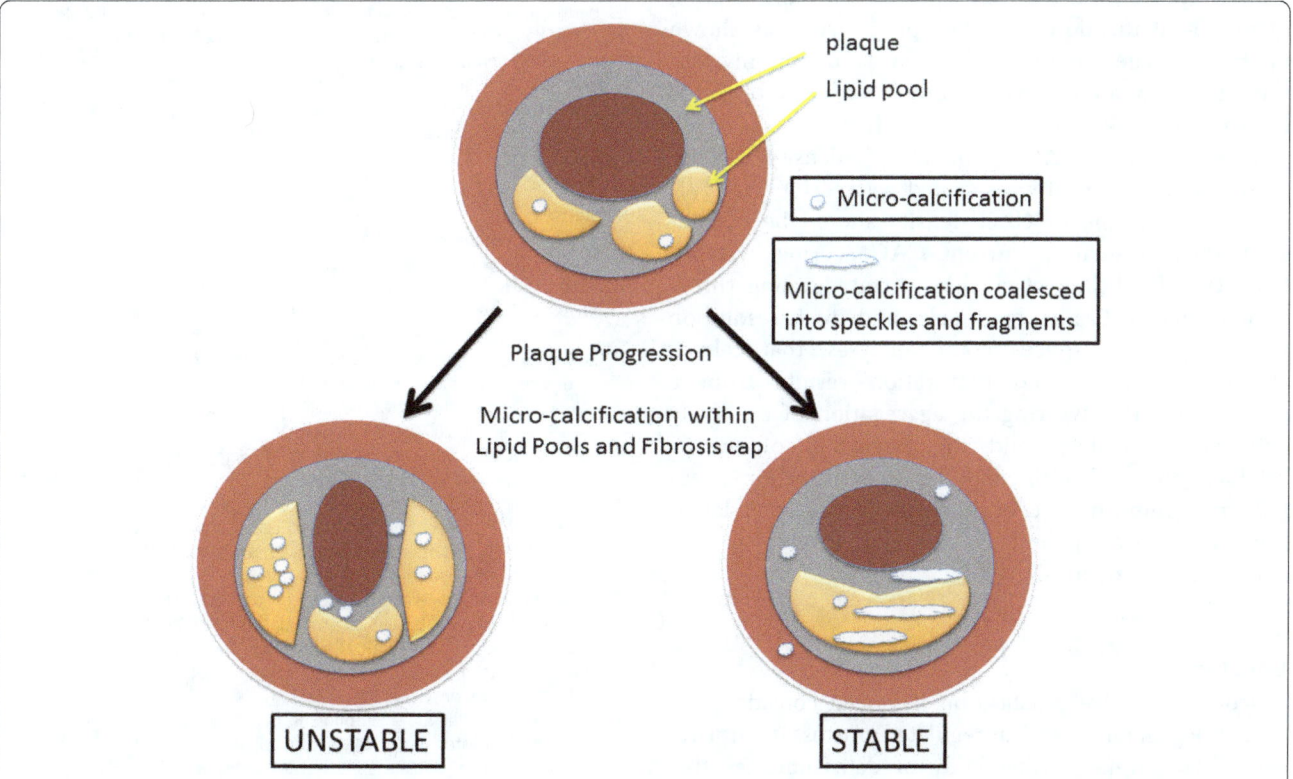

Fig. 3 Scheme of plaque calcification. Natural plaque progression involves lipid-pool expansion coupled with micro-calcifications within lipid pools. Micro-calcifications are also commonly found within an overlying fibrous cap. If these micro-calcifications coalesce into speckles and fragments during therapy or atheroma progression, vessel wall stresses may decrease significantly, contributing to plaque stability

development of calcific aortic valve disease. Therefore, vascular and valve calcification has strong relationships with immunity, and both innate and adaptive immunity play a role in the development of calcification. As discussed above, estrogen therapy may have anti-calcific effects. In addition, denosumab, an anti-RANKL monoclonal antibody that is also used for the treatment of osteoporosis, may also exert anti-calcific effects. However, because these therapies have complex biological actions possibly causing side effects, their uses in the prevention of calcification is limited.

We have discussed "how to prevent calcification," but "how to treat preexisting calcification" remains unclear. We hypothesized that calcification volume itself is responsible to the increased incidence of CVD events. This hypothesis is supported by the observation that CAC volume was positively and independently associated with CHD and CVD risk. Conversely, recent data suggest that increased plaque calcium density may be protective against CVD. Criqui et al. also reported that CAC density scores showed an independent inverse association with CHD, with an HR of 0.73 (95 % CI, 0.58–0.91) per SD (SD = 0.7) increase and an absolute risk decrease of 2.0 per 1000 person-years, as well as CVD, with an HR of 0.71 (95 % CI, 0.60–0.85) per SD increase and an absolute risk decrease 3.4 per 1000 person years [10]. Moreover, Puri et al. reported the contribution of micro-calcification to plaque progression, as shown in Fig. 3. The micro-calcification is commonly observed within an overlying fibrous cap and tends to increase the risk of plaque rupture [12].

At any level of CAC volume, CAC density was inversely and significantly associated with CHD and CVD risk [10]. The role of CAC density should be considered when evaluating current CAC scoring systems. Recently, Hutcheson et al. demonstrated, using three-dimensional collagen hydrogels and high-resolution microscopic and spectroscopic analyses, that calcific mineral formation and maturation results from a series of events involving the aggregation of calcifying extracellular vesicles and the formation of micro-calcifications and ultimately large calcification areas [13]. It is important to evaluate the treatment adaptation of calcification both in vitro and in vivo by utilizing these modalities.

Conclusions

Vascular and valve calcification has been considered as purely degenerative and unregulated processes until recently. However, growing body of data indicates that there are multiple causes of vascular and valve calcification, including inflammatory, metabolic, genetic, and epigenetic mechanisms, which cross-talk each other in a complicated manner. Although it is important to prevent vascular and valve calcification, it is also important to optimize the therapeutic strategy according to the defined characteristics of present calcification.

Abbreviations
AAC: abdominal aortic calcification; BMP-2: bone morphogenetic protein-2; CAC: coronary artery calcium; CHD: coronary heart disease; CI: 95 % confidence interval; CVD: cardiovascular disease; ECs: endothelial cells; HR: hazard ratio; M-CSF: macrophage colony-stimulating factor; OPG: osteoprotegerin; RANK: receptor activator of nuclear factor κB; RANKL: RANK ligand; TNF: tumor necrosis factor; VICs: valve interstitial cells; VSMCs: vascular smooth muscle cells.

Funding
This work was partially supported by a Grant-in-Aid for Scientific Research from the Ministry of Education, Culture, Sports, Science and Technology.

Authors' contributions
RK and HN wrote the paper. TN, KO, MK, and RM discussed and agreed with the manuscript. All the authors discussed and agreed on the submission of the manuscript.

Competing interests
The Department of Clinical Gene Therapy is financially supported by AnGes MG, Novartis, Shionogi, Boeringher, and Rohto. The Division of Vascular Medicine and Epigenetics is financially supported by AnGes MG and Daicel. R.M. is a founder and stockholder of AnGes MG and a former board member.

Author details
[1]Department of Cardiorenal and Cerebrovascular Medicine, Faculty of Medicine, Kagawa University, Kagawa 761-0793, Japan. [2]Department of Clinical Gene Therapy, Graduate School of Medicine, Osaka University, Kagawa 565-0871, Japan. [3]Department of Health Development and Medicine, Graduate School of Medicine, Osaka University, 2-2 Yamada-oka, Suita 565-0871, Osaka, Japan.

References
1. Osler W. The principles and practice of medicine. 3rd edition. New York, London: D. Appleton and company; 1898.
2. Rodondi N, Taylor BC, Bauer DC, Lui LY, Vogt MT, Fink HA, et al. Association between aortic calcification and total and cardiovascular mortality in older women. J Intern Med. 2007;261:238–44.
3. Okuno S, Ishimura E, Kitatani K, Fujino Y, Kohno K, Maeno Y, et al. Presence of abdominal aortic calcification is significantly associated with all-cause and cardiovascular mortality in maintenance hemodialysis patients. Am J Kidney Dis. 2007;49:417–25.
4. Bostrom K, Watson KE, Horn S, Wortham C, Herman IM, Demer LL. Bone morphogenetic protein expression in human atherosclerotic lesions. J Clin Invest. 1993;91:1800–9.
5. Collin-Osdoby P. Regulation of vascular calcification by osteoclast regulatory factors RANKL and osteoprotegerin. Circ Res. 2004;95:1046–57.
6. Kosaku N, Takashi A, Keiko U, Shigeru O, Takashi T, Wako Y. Serum osteoprotegerin levels and the extent of vascular calcification in haemodialysis patients. Nephrol Dial Transplant. 2004;19:1886–9.
7. Bucay N, Sarosi I, Dunstan CR, Morony S, Tarpley J, Capparelli C, et al. Osteoprotegerin-deficient mice develop early onset osteoporosis and arterial calcification. Genes Dev. 1998;12:1260–8.
8. Kaden JJ, Bickelhaupt S, Grobholz R, Haase KK, Sarikoc A, Kilic R, et al. Receptor activator of nuclear factor kappaB ligand and osteoprotegerin regulate aortic valve calcification. J Mol Cell Cardiol. 2004;36:57–66.
9. Weiss RM, Lund DD, Chu Y, Brooks RM, Zimmerman KA, El Accaoui R, et al. Osteoprotegerin inhibits aortic valve calcification and preserves valve function in hypercholesterolemic mice. PLoS One. 2013;8:e65201.

10. Criqui MH, Denenberg JO, Ix JH, McClelland RL, Wassel CL, Rifkin DE, et al. Calcium density of coronary artery plaque and risk of incident cardiovascular events. JAMA. 2014;311:271–8.

11. Allison MA, Manson JE, Langer RD, Carr JJ, Rossouw JE, Pettinger MB, et al. Oophorectomy, hormone therapy, and subclinical coronary artery disease in women with hysterectomy: the Women's Health Initiative coronary artery calcium study. Menopause. 2008;15:639–47.

12. Puri R, Nicholls SJ, Shao M, Kataoka Y, Uno K, Kapadia SR, et al. Impact of statins on serial coronary calcification during atheroma progression and regression. J Am Coll Cardiol. 2015;65:1273–82.

13. Hutcheson JD, Goettsch C, Bertazzo S, Maldonado N, Ruiz JL, Goh W, et al. Genesis and growth of extracellular-vesicle-derived microcalcification in atherosclerotic plaques. Nat Mater. 2016;15:335–43.

14

Dysfunctional immunoproteasomes in autoinflammatory diseases

Hideki Arimochi, Yuki Sasaki, Akiko Kitamura and Koji Yasutomo[*]

Abstract

Recent progress in DNA sequencing technology has made it possible to identify specific genetic mutations in familial disorders. For example, autoinflammatory syndromes are caused by mutations in gene coding for immunoproteasomes. These diseases include Japanese autoinflammatory syndrome with lipodystrophy, Nakajo-Nishimura syndrome, joint contractures, muscular atrophy, microcytic anemia, panniculitis-associated lipodystrophy syndrome, and chronic atypical neutrophilic dermatosis with lipodystrophy and elevated temperature syndrome. Causal mutations of these syndromes are present in gene coding for subunits of the immunoproteasome. Importantly, a genetically modified mouse that lacks the catalytic subunit of immunoproteasomes does not always develop an autoinflammatory syndrome. Analysis of causal gene mutations, assessment of patients' phenotypic changes, and appropriate animal models will be indispensable for clarifying the underlying mechanisms responsible for the development of autoinflammatory syndromes and establishing curative approaches.

Keywords: Autoinflammation, Genetics, Immunoproteasomes

Background

Inflammation is caused by a variety of factors including endogenous abnormalities, infection, and toxins and involved in immune-mediated disorders including autoimmune or autoinflammatory disorders. Autoimmune disorders are caused by hyper-reactivity of the immune system against self-derived antigens [1, 2]. On the other hand, recent studies have uncovered other types of inflammatory pathologies termed "autoinflammation" that are induced by activation of innate immune cells without apparent infection or autoimmune responses. Autoinflammatory syndromes are hereditary diseases and mainly caused by a mutation of a single gene that codes for a component of NACHT, LRR, and PYD domain-containing protein (NLRP) inflammasomes, cytosolic DNA danger sensing machinery, cytokine receptors, and immunoproteasomes [3–5]. However, the causal gene mutations are unclear and/or involve multiple mutations in some cases.

We and the other groups have reported an autoinflammatory syndrome in which the gene for proteasome subunit beta-type 8 (*PSMB8*) has been altered [6–9]. The

mutation causes dysfunction of the immunoproteasomes, resulting in the accumulation of ubiquitin-coupled proteins. Although it is now clear that the dysregulation of immunoproteasomes causes an autoinflammatory syndrome, the molecular mechanism of the inflammatory response is unclear. Here, we discuss the recent progress in the genetic analysis of autoinflammatory syndromes caused by dysfunctional immunoproteasomes.

Main text
Proteasomes and immunoproteasomes
The proteasome is a multi-subunit protease complex that degrades ubiquitinated proteins in the cytosol for rapid turnover [10, 11]. The 26S standard proteasome is composed of a 19S and 20S proteasome unit. The 20S proteasome is formed by the 14 α subunits and the 14 β subunits, in which β1 (coded by the *PSMB6* gene), β2 (coded by *PSMB7* gene), and β5 (coded by *PSMB5* gene) subunits possess protease activities. The standard proteasome is present in most eukaryotic cells, and the thymoproteasome is a specific proteasome found in the thymus [12]. The immunoproteasome is a special proteasome composed of β1i (coded by *PSMB9*), β2i (coded by *PSMB10*), and β5i (coded by *PSMB8*) subunits instead of the β1, β2, and β5 subunits of the standard proteasome,

* Correspondence: yasutomo@tokushima-u.ac.jp
Department of Immunology and Parasitology, Graduate School of Medicine, Tokushima University, 3-18-15 Kuramoto, Tokushima 770-8503, Japan

respectively. The immunoproteasome-specific β subunits are induced by interferon-γ stimulation. The β5i subunit possesses strong chymotrypsin-like activity, and β1i and β2i subunits have caspase and trypsin-like activities, respectively [13]. The immunoproteasome efficiently generates peptides presented by MHC class I and degradation of oxidized proteins to maintain cellular homeostasis [14].

Autoinflammatory syndromes with proteasome dysfunction

Autoinflammatory diseases resulting from dysfunctional proteasomes are termed "proteasome-associated autoinflammatory syndromes" (PRAAS) [15]. PRAAS include Japanese autoinflammatory syndrome with lipodystrophy (JASL) [7], Nakajo-Nishimura syndrome (NNS) [8], joint contractures, muscular atrophy, microcytic anemia, panniculitis-associated lipodystrophy (JMP) syndrome [6], and chronic atypical neutrophilic dermatosis with lipodystrophy and elevated temperature (CANDLE) syndrome [9] (Fig. 1).

JASL is characterized by recurrent fever, nodular erythema, high CRP levels, and hypergammaglobulinemia together with a loss of adipose tissue in the upper part of the body. Three JASL patients from 2 consanguineous families showed high fever and severe inflammation, although they did not possess autoantibodies or an immunocompromised constitution [7]. Patients with the JMP syndrome were found in two family lines in Mexico and Portugal. They showed hepatosplenomegaly; macrosomia; lipodystrophy of face, arms, and chest; sclerodermic skin with erythematous lesions; microcytic anemia with higher serum levels of interferon-γ, IL-8, and IL-6; and hypergammaglobulinemia [6]. NNS is a wasting disease seen early in life and it has been found only in the Japanese population [8]. The patients show elongated and thickened fingers, periodic high fever, nodular erythema, lipomuscular atrophy with joint contractures, myositis, and hypergammaglobulinemia. Cell extracts prepared from the patients indicated that three immunoproteasome-related protease activities were below

normal compared with healthy controls. CANDLE syndrome patients have been found in Jewish, Spanish, Caucasian, and Hispanic populations. They also show recurrent fevers; delayed physical development; hypochromic or normocytic anemia; progressive lipodystrophy; joint pain; and increased acute phase reactants with variable clinical features, including skin hyperpigmentation, spot alopecia, and polytrichia [9].

Causal mutations leading to JASL and other autoinflammatory syndromes with dysfunctional proteasomes

In a search for the causal mutation of JASL, we used SNP homozygosity mapping, linking analysis, and exome analysis [7]. We identified a specific mutation of the *PSMB8* gene present in chromosome 6 in patients from 2 distinct Japanese families. This mutation was homozygous with a transversion of guanine to adenine with an amino acid change from glycine to valine at a position of 197 (p.G197V) of the PSMB8 protein. The original amino acid has been conserved across animal species, suggesting an important role of this amino acid in the maintenance of form and function of the protein.

NNS, JMP, and CANDLE syndromes are also caused by mutations in the *PSMB8* gene, although different regions are involved [6, 8, 9]. Agarwal et al. found a homozygous missense mutation of C to T at position 224 (c.C224T) in the *PSMB8* gene, resulting in a p.T75M change in JMP patients [6]. Arima et al. reported that the causal mutation of NNS is a p.G201V mutation in *PSMB8* exon 5 [8] and Liu and co-workers described one patient with the CANDLE syndrome who possessed a homozygous nonsense mutation at position 405 resulting in a C to A change with a protein truncation. Four others were homozygous and two others had a heterozygous missense mutation at c.C224T. In a Caucasian patient, no mutation in the *PSMB8* gene was found [9]. Recently, new mutations related to the CANDLE syndrome were identified in the *PSMA3* gene coding α7, *PSMB4* coding β7, and *PSMB9* coding β1i as well as *PSMB8* and proteasome

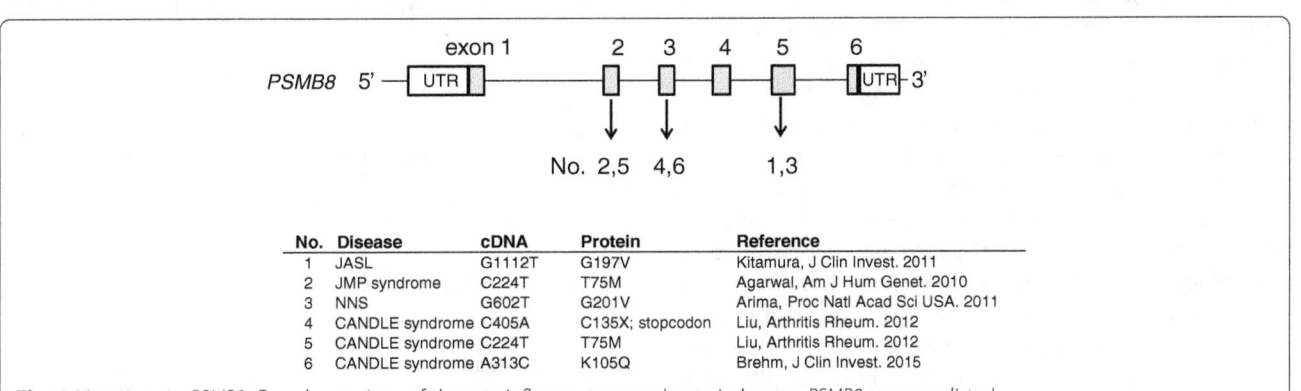

No.	Disease	cDNA	Protein	Reference
1	JASL	G1112T	G197V	Kitamura, J Clin Invest. 2011
2	JMP syndrome	C224T	T75M	Agarwal, Am J Hum Genet. 2010
3	NNS	G602T	G201V	Arima, Proc Natl Acad Sci USA. 2011
4	CANDLE syndrome	C405A	C135X; stopcodon	Liu, Arthritis Rheum. 2012
5	CANDLE syndrome	C224T	T75M	Liu, Arthritis Rheum. 2012
6	CANDLE syndrome	A313C	K105Q	Brehm, J Clin Invest. 2015

Fig. 1 Mutations in *PSMB8*. Causal mutations of the autoinflammatory syndrome in human *PSMB8* gene are listed

maturation protein (POMP) genes from 8 patients [16]. One patient had two heterozygous PSMB4 gene mutations that were c.G(-9)A. in the 5′ UTR and a 9-bp inframe deletion caused p.D212_V214del. Other PSMB4 mutations were heterozygous variants c.44insG/p.P16Sfs*45 found in a Jamaican patient and a monoallelic nonsense mutation c.C666A/p.Y222X found in an Irish patient. The mutations in PSMA3 found in two unrelated patients were heterozygous 3-bp in-frame deletions (c.696_698delAAG/ p.R233del) and c.T(404+2)G/p.H111Ffs*10 at the splicing site. The mutation in PSMB9 was a missense substitution (c.G494A) and affected a conserved amino acid residue (p.G165D). A newly identified PSMB8 mutation was a heterozygous missense mutation of c.A313C/p.K105Q in an Irish patient. A mutation in the POMP gene of a Palestinian patient was a heterozygous frameshift mutation, c.344_345insTTTGA/p.E115Dfs*20. Another mutation in the PSMB8 gene resulted in a p.Q49K change that was found in patients of juvenile rheumatoid arthritis that had some clinical features similar to NNS [17].

Effects of PSMB8 protein abnormality on cellular physiology and animal disease models

Mutations found in the PSMB8 gene from autoinflammatory syndrome patients can affect the PSMB8 protein and immunoproteasome functions. The G201V mutation found in NNS patients affects both the proteolytic activity of β5i and the assembly of the immunoproteasome. These conclusions are based on the observation that an accumulation of immature 20S proteasome precursors was found in NNS cells [7]. Immortalized lymphoblasts derived from a JMP patient showed reduced chymotrypsin-like activity without an effect on trypsin-like or caspase-like activity. Brehm et al. described hematopoietic and non-hematopoietic cells derived from CANDLE patients who had different types of mutations, including those leading to abnormal protein expression, protein folding, proteasome assembly, proteasome activity, and strong type 1 IFN expression [16]. Immortalized transformed B cells from a JASL patient showed lower expression of PSMB8 at the mRNA and protein levels, and the activities of caspase-like, trypsin-like, and chymotrypsin-like proteases in cell extracts were decreased compared with healthy control samples [7]. The reduced expression of mature PSMB8 protein was also confirmed in the skin of a JASL patient. Immature proteasomes were increased in JASL cells, indicating that the immunoproteasome assembly was defective in the mutant cells. Consistent with these data, ubiquitinated proteins were increased in cell extracts of transformed cells and the skin of a JASL patient. IL-6 expression in the skin of the patient and cells carrying mutant PSMB8 proteins were increased via p38 MAP kinase signaling [7]. Kasagi et al. also reported serum IL-6

levels in JASL patients were higher than those of healthy controls [18].

PSMB8 knockout mice grow normally and no spontaneous inflammation is observed, unlike patients with dysfunctional proteasome syndromes. Seifert et al. reported that β5i-deficient mice showed symptoms of experimental allergic encephalomyelitis [14]. However, it has been reported that PSMB8 deletion or treatment with its specific inhibitor suppresses autoreactive immune responses in murine models of arthritis, diabetes [19], experimental colitis [20], Hashimoto's thyroiditis [21], and lupus-like disease [22]. These suppressive effects may relate to the ability of β5i-deficient or specific inhibitor-treated cells to diminish Th1, Th2, and Th17 differentiation and enhance regulatory T cell differentiation [23]. The production of IL-23 by activated monocytes and IFN-γ and IL-2 by activated T cells is also blocked by treatment of the cells with a selective inhibitor of β5i [24]. Therefore, to determine how missense mutations in PSMB8 cause inflammatory responses in human, it will be necessary to establish mice that harbor a mutation in the PSMB8 gene.

Conclusions

Improvements in genotyping efficiency, sequencing technology, and statistical methodology have made it possible for researchers to identify specific gene mutations associated with autoinflammatory syndromes. Some mutations and polymorphisms connected to dysregulated proteasome syndromes have been reported, but the functional consequences of genetic variations are not fully understood. To increase our understanding of the pathophysiology of these diseases, basic and advanced studies with tissues from patients and genetically modified animals will be required to determine how the mutations affect cellular physiology and proteasome function. Analysis of causal gene mutations, the subsequent phenotypic changes in autoinflammatory syndrome patients, and establishment of a proper animal model for these diseases will be indispensable to clarify the mechanisms of autoinflammatory syndrome development and to develop cures for these diseases.

Acknowledgements
We thank Mrs C. Miyamoto for her editorial assistance. This work is supported by AMED-CREST (KY).

Funding
The studies are supported by AMED-CREST.

Authors' contributions
HA, YS, AK, and KY wrote the review. All authors read and approved the final manuscript.

Competing interests

The authors declare that they have no competing interests.

References

1. van Kempen TS, Wenink MH, Leijten EF, Radstake TR, Boes M. Perception of self: distinguishing autoimmunity from autoinflammation. Nat Rev Rheumatol. 2015;11(8):483–92.
2. Sakaguchi S, Miyara M, Costantino CM, Hafler DA. FOXP3+ regulatory T cells in the human immune system. Nat Rev Immunol. 2010;10(7):490–500.
3. Goldbach-Mansky R, Kastner DL. Autoinflammation: the prominent role of IL-1 in monogenic autoinflammatory diseases and implications for common illnesses. J Allergy Clin Immunol. 2009;124(6):1141–9. quiz 1150–1141.
4. Aksentijevich I, Kastner DL. Genetics of monogenic autoinflammatory diseases: past successes, future challenges. Nat Rev Rheumatol. 2011;7(8):469–78.
5. Park H, Bourla AB, Kastner DL, Colbert RA, Siegel RM. Lighting the fires within: the cell biology of autoinflammatory diseases. Nat Rev Immunol. 2012;12(8):570–80.
6. Agarwal AK, Xing C, DeMartino GN, Mizrachi D, Hernandez MD, Sousa AB, et al. PSMB8 encoding the beta5i proteasome subunit is mutated in joint contractures, muscle atrophy, microcytic anemia, and panniculitis-induced lipodystrophy syndrome. Am J Hum Genet. 2010;87(6):866–72.
7. Kitamura A, Maekawa Y, Uehara H, Izumi K, Kawachi I, Nishizawa M, et al. A mutation in the immunoproteasome subunit PSMB8 causes autoinflammation and lipodystrophy in humans. J Clin Invest. 2011;121(10):4150–60.
8. Arima K, Kinoshita A, Mishima H, Kanazawa N, Kaneko T, Mizushima T, et al. Proteasome assembly defect due to a proteasome subunit beta type 8 (PSMB8) mutation causes the autoinflammatory disorder, Nakajo-Nishimura syndrome. Proc Natl Acad Sci U S A. 2011;108(36):14914–9.
9. Liu Y, Ramot Y, Torrelo A, Paller AS, Si N, Babay S, et al. Mutations in proteasome subunit beta type 8 cause chronic atypical neutrophilic dermatosis with lipodystrophy and elevated temperature with evidence of genetic and phenotypic heterogeneity. Arthritis Rheum. 2012;64(3):895–907.
10. Kimura Y, Tanaka K. Regulatory mechanisms involved in the control of ubiquitin homeostasis. J Biochem. 2010;147(6):793–8.
11. Geng F, Wenzel S, Tansey WP. Ubiquitin and proteasomes in transcription. Annu Rev Biochem. 2012;81:177–201.
12. Murata S, Sasaki K, Kishimoto T, Niwa S, Hayashi H, Takahama Y, et al. Regulation of CD8+ T cell development by thymus-specific proteasomes. Science. 2007;316(5829):1349–53.
13. Murata S, Yashiroda H, Tanaka K. Molecular mechanisms of proteasome assembly. Nat Rev Mol Cell Biol. 2009;10(2):104–15.
14. Seifert U, Bialy LP, Ebstein F, Bech-Otschir D, Voigt A, Schroter F, et al. Immunoproteasomes preserve protein homeostasis upon interferon-induced oxidative stress. Cell. 2010;142(4):613–24.
15. McDermott A, Jacks J, Kessler M, Emanuel PD, Gao L. Proteasome-associated autoinflammatory syndromes: advances in pathogeneses, clinical presentations, diagnosis, and management. Int J Dermatol. 2015;54(2):121–9.
16. Brehm A, Liu Y, Sheikh A, Marrero B, Omoyinmi E, Zhou Q, et al. Additive loss-of-function proteasome subunit mutations in CANDLE/PRAAS patients promote type I IFN production. J Clin Invest. 2015;125(11):4196–211.
17. Prahalad S, Kingsbury DJ, Griffin TA, Cooper BL, Glass DN, Maksymowych WP, et al. Polymorphism in the MHC-encoded LMP7 gene: association with JRA without functional significance for immunoproteasome assembly. J Rheumatol. 2001;28(10):2320–5.
18. Kasagi S, Kawano S, Nakazawa T, Sugino H, Koshiba M, Ichinose K, et al. A case of periodic-fever-syndrome-like disorder with lipodystrophy, myositis, and autoimmune abnormalities. Mod Rheumatol. 2008;18(2):203–7.
19. Basler M, Mundt S, Muchamuel T, Moll C, Jiang J, Groettrup M, et al. Inhibition of the immunoproteasome ameliorates experimental autoimmune encephalomyelitis. EMBO Mol Med. 2014;6(2):226–38.
20. Basler M, Dajee M, Moll C, Groettrup M, Kirk CJ. Prevention of experimental colitis by a selective inhibitor of the immunoproteasome. J Immunol. 2010;185(1):634–41.
21. Nagayama Y, Nakahara M, Shimamura M, Horie I, Arima K, Abiru N. Prophylactic and therapeutic efficacies of a selective inhibitor of the immunoproteasome for Hashimoto's thyroiditis, but not for Graves' hyperthyroidism, in mice. Clin Exp Immunol. 2012;168(3):268–73.
22. Ichikawa HT, Conley T, Muchamuel T, Jiang J, Lee S, Owen T, et al. Beneficial effect of novel proteasome inhibitors in murine lupus via dual inhibition of type I interferon and autoantibody-secreting cells. Arthritis Rheum. 2012;64(2):493–503.
23. Kalim KW, Basler M, Kirk CJ, Groettrup M. Immunoproteasome subunit LMP7 deficiency and inhibition suppresses Th1 and Th17 but enhances regulatory T cell differentiation. J Immunol. 2012;189(8):4182–93.
24. Muchamuel T, Basler M, Aujay MA, Suzuki E, Kalim KW, Lauer C, et al. A selective inhibitor of the immunoproteasome subunit LMP7 blocks cytokine production and attenuates progression of experimental arthritis. Nat Med. 2009;15(7):781–7.

15

Quantitative assessment of angiogenesis and pericyte coverage in human cell-derived vascular sprouts

Jan Eglinger[1,2,3]* (iD), Haiko Karsjens[1,2] and Eckhard Lammert[1,2]*

Abstract

Background: Pericytes, surrounding the endothelium, fulfill diverse functions that are crucial for vascular homeostasis. The loss of pericytes is associated with pathologies, such as diabetic retinopathy and Alzheimer's disease. Thus, there exists a need for an experimental system that combines pharmacologic manipulation and quantification of pericyte coverage during sprouting angiogenesis. Here, we describe an in vitro angiogenesis assay that develops lumenized vascular sprouts composed of endothelial cells enveloped by pericytes, with the additional ability to comparatively screen the effect of multiple small molecules simultaneously. For automated analysis, we also present an ImageJ plugin tool we developed to quantify sprout morphology and pericyte coverage.

Methods: Human umbilical vein endothelial cells and human brain vascular pericytes were coated on microcarrier beads and embedded in fibrin gels in a 96-well plate to form lumenized vascular sprouts. After treatment with pharmacologic compounds, sprouts were fixed, stained, and imaged via optical z-sections over the area of each well. The maximum intensity projections of these images were stitched together to form montages of the wells, and those montages were processed and analyzed.

Results: Vascular sprouts formed within 4–12 days and contained a patent lumen surrounded by a layer of human endothelial cells and pericytes. Using our workflow and image analysis, pericyte coverage after treatment with various compounds was successfully quantified.

Conclusions: Here we present a robust in vitro assay using primary human vascular cells that allows researchers to analyze the effects of multiple compounds on sprouting angiogenesis and pericyte coverage. Our ImageJ plugin offers automated evaluation across multiple different vascular parameters, such as sprout length, cell density, branch points, and pericyte coverage.

Keywords: Angiogenesis, Pericytes, Sprouting, Image analysis, Morphometry

Background

Sprouting angiogenesis, the formation of new capillary branches from pre-existing blood vessels or lymphatic vessels, is required to build functional vascular networks, and altered sprouting angiogenesis is involved in many diseases [1].

Sprouting is induced by activation of endothelial cells (ECs) via growth factors such as vascular endothelial growth factor (VEGF), platelet-derived growth factor (PDGF), placental growth factor (PlGF), and hypoxia-inducible factor (HIF)-1α [2]. Activated ECs proliferate, extend into the surrounding tissue [3], and recruit pericytes to attach to the outer wall of the newly formed vessels [4]. The presence of pericytes on mature capillaries is required for stabilization of the endothelium and for regulation of blood flow, as observed in the blood–brain barrier [5, 6]. Pericytes are in close contact with ECs, as they extend long cytoplasmic processes across several ECs to encircle the EC-derived vascular tubes. Moreover, they share a basement membrane and physically interact via numerous contacts such as for example peg-socket junctions, adhesion plaques, or gap junctions [7]. Dysfunctional interplay between pericytes and

* Correspondence: jan.eglinger@fmi.ch; lammert@uni-duesseldorf.de
[1]Institute of Metabolic Physiology, Heinrich-Heine University, Düsseldorf, Germany

the endothelium is frequently the cause or consequence of many diseases [8–10], resulting in increased vascular permeability and defective vessel maturation, which promote vessel leakage and inflammation [11]. Cancer cells, for instance, can induce detachment of pericytes from quiescent vasculature, thereby activating ECs to sprout into the surrounding tissue [12]. Pericyte detachment is also one of the first pathological hallmarks during diabetic retinopathy. The disease begins with a thickening of the vascular basement membrane, followed by a loss of pericytes and an increase in vascular permeability [13]. Ultimately, neovascularization causes hemorrhaging and vision loss [14]. On the contrary, after stroke, pericytes constrict around capillaries to decrease blood flow. When these pericytes die, the blood–brain barrier is disrupted, leading to progressive neuronal damage [15].

It is hypothesized that pericytes also play a regulatory role during angiogenesis [11, 16]. Our aim was to develop a method to assess pericyte coverage during sprouting angiogenesis in a defined human cellular system. We modified a sprouting assay that involves ECs and was previously used in a number of recent publications [17–19]. Nakatsu et al. described an optimized angiogenesis assay that leads to vascular sprouts with a defined lumen. This assay uses fibrin as an extracellular matrix and is characterized by the formation of vascular sprouts that harbor patent multi-cellular lumens and a basement membrane [20]. The sprouts undergo many critical steps that occur in vivo during angiogenesis. In order to mimic the in vivo vasculature as accurately as possible, we have modified their protocol to include human vascular pericytes [7]. After co-culturing ECs and pericytes, we verified that sprouts have lumens and that pericytes attach to the outer wall of vascular sprouts. Further, we adapted the original method for use in multi-well plates in order to simultaneously test and compare multiple treatments under reproducible conditions. Finally, for consistent analysis of sprout morphology and pericyte coverage, we developed an ImageJ plugin that measures sprout number, length and width, as well as cell density and pericyte coverage of vascular sprouts. While similar tools were published for standardized quantification of other angiogenesis assays, such as "Angiotool" for the quantification of retinal vascular networks [21], or "Aqual" for the aortic ring assay [22], no such standardized tool was previously available for the bead sprouting assay. Using our optimized analysis workflow, we tested more than 40 compounds for their biological effects on sprout morphology and pericyte coverage.

Here, we describe a standardized procedure of the bead sprouting assay using human umbilical vein ECs (HUVECs) and human brain vascular pericytes (HBVPs). To ensure comparability between experimental repetitions

as well as between different researchers performing the experiments, we developed, using the plugin tool described below, a standardized automated quantitative analysis of developing angiogenic sprouts covered with pericytes.

Methods

Cell culture

We used HUVEC (Lonza) up to passage 6 [23], HBVP (ScienCell) were used up to passage 4, and Detroit-551 human skin fibroblasts (HSF; ATCC) up to passage 20. For experimental reproducibility, primary cells were used up to the passage number recommended by the respective supplier (Lonza, ScienCell, ATCC), as primary cells lose their identity and responsiveness to angiogenic stimuli at higher passages [23]. Cells were cultured in endothelial growth medium (EGM-2; Lonza) at least 24 h prior to starting the sprouting assay.

Sprouting assay

A detailed step-by-step protocol for the sprouting assay is available in Additional files 1, 2 and 3. The procedure is based on a sprouting assay reported previously [17–19] that we extended to include pericytes and be adaptable for culture in a 96-well plate. In short, dextran-coated Cytodex-3 microcarrier beads (GE Healthcare) were incubated with HUVEC and HBVP in EGM-2 (Lonza) overnight. We found an endothelial-to-pericyte ratio of 10:1 to yield optimal pericyte coverage of developing sprouts in accordance with cell ratios found in tissues varying between 1:1 and 10:1 [7, 24]. Cell-coated beads were then embedded into fibrin gels by adding 90 μl beads in PBS (200 beads/ml) with 2.5 mg/ml fibrinogen (Sigma-Aldrich) to 8-μl thrombin (0.625 U/ml, Sigma-Aldrich) per well in a 96- well plate (μclear, Greiner Bio-One). The gels were overlaid with human skin fibroblasts at 1000 cells per well. As previously published, the cross-talk between ECs and fibroblasts, but not their direct contact, was shown to be required for the formation of stable lumenized sprouts [17]. Two hundred microliters of EGM-2 were subsequently added to each well. Plates were incubated at 37 °C, 5% CO_2, and medium was changed every other day. After 6 days, when lumenized sprouts were observed, treatment was started by adding compounds at the respective concentrations to each well. Medium and compounds were changed every other day. The frequency of changing medium and compounds was chosen based on preliminary experiments that showed a significant decrease in sprout number and length upon treatment with the VEGFR inhibitor SU5416.

Phalloidin staining

For assays containing ECs only, fibrin gels were fixed overnight using 4% paraformaldehyde in PBS. Subsequently, gels were washed with PBS, blocked with PBS containing 0.2% Triton X-100 and 1% BSA, and stained with Alexa Fluor-488-conjugated phalloidin and DAPI (for timing and details, see protocol in Additional file 3). After three washes (10 min in PBS), the plate containing the gels was imaged as described below.

Immunostaining

Fibrin gels containing EC/pericyte sprouts were fixed using 4% paraformaldehyde in PBS. Subsequently, gels were washed with PBS, blocked with PBS containing 3% Triton X-100 and 1% BSA, incubated with primary antibodies (rabbit polyclonal anti-human Erg-1/2/3, Santa Cruz; mouse monoclonal anti-human NG2, Abcam) for at least 60 h, washed with PBS, and stained with secondary antibodies (Alexa Fluor 488 donkey anti-mouse IgG, Life Technologies; Cy3 AffiniPure donkey anti-rabbit IgG, Jackson ImmunoResearch), as well as Alexa Fluor 647-conjugated phalloidin and DAPI for at least 40 h (for timing and details, see protocol in Additional file 3). After three washes (PBS), the plate containing the gels was imaged as described below.

Microscopy

We used an inverted microscope (Zeiss Axio Observer.Z1) with an automated stage to acquire multi-tile z-stacks (10-μm intervals) of stained sprouts, using a Zeiss 10×/NA0.45 objective lens. Both a Zeiss ApoTome system equipped with Colibri LED light source, as well as a Zeiss LSM 710 confocal microscope system were used for imaging. Images were acquired in grid positions and subsequently stitched using the Grid/Collection stitching plugin in Fiji [25], resulting in a continuous image coverage of 70% of each well (3 × 3 mm).

Image analysis

Images were analyzed using the Fiji distribution of ImageJ [26] at version ImageJ 2.0.0-rc-15/1.49k; Java 1.6.0_65 (available as a Life-Line Version from https://imagej.net/Downloads). We developed a plugin for sprout analysis that is available from the *Angiogenesis* update site within ImageJ and is maintained to work with the newest version of Fiji (see https://imagej.net/Following_an_update_site for instructions how to install the plugin in Fiji). Documentation for our plugin is available at https://imagej.net/Sprout_Morphology. For each z-stack acquired, the maximum intensity projection (MIP) was created (see Additional file 4) and processed using our plugin. For each 96-well plate, representative MIPs were used to adjust analysis parameters to improve image clarity across the entire dataset. Using the provided script (see Additional file 5), the plugin was then run on every continuous image to consistently analyze the entire dataset.

Statistical analysis

The results of the sprout analysis were normalized to either a PBS control or a DMSO control, depending on the solvent used to reconstitute each treatment compound (see Additional file 6: Table S1). Within one assay, the values for repeated conditions in separate wells were weighted according to the number of beads in each well. Significant increase or decrease of each measurement parameter at each treatment condition was determined using a one-sample t test.

Results
Lumen formation and pericyte coverage in multi-cellular sprouts

To assess vascular lumen formation within endothelial cell (EC)-derived vascular sprouts with and without pericytes, we seeded HUVEC in the presence or absence of HBVP onto microcarrier beads that subsequently were embedded into fibrin gels. In Fig. 1, a summary of the experimental design is shown, which can be performed in either 96-well plates to screen compounds (Fig. 1a, left side) or in glass-bottom dishes for staining with various different antibodies (Fig. 1a, right side). A timeline of the assay and the structure of a typical vascular sprout derived from human ECs and pericytes is also shown (Fig. 1b, c).

After an incubation of either 2 (with pericytes) or 4 days (without pericytes), the first sprouts formed a patent vascular lumen detectable by bright field transmission light microscopy (Fig. 2a). After fixation and staining of the F-actin cytoskeleton by fluorescently labeled phalloidin, a lumen was also detected in optical cross-sections of confocal z-stacks (Fig. 2b). Vascular sprouts were composed of multiple cells connected through VE-cadherin positive junctions and surrounded by a vascular basement membrane containing laminin (Fig. 2c). Pericytes aligned to the abluminal side of the vascular sprouts (Fig. 2d, e).

Quantitative measurement of sprout morphology and pericyte coverage

We developed a plugin for ImageJ to measure parameters of sprout morphology (Fig. 3). For image analysis with our plugin, MIPs of sprout images were created. The adjustment of analysis parameters was performed on a selected subset of images representative of the variability within the whole dataset. We adjusted the measurement parameters for each of the analysis steps (Fig. 3a–c), including the number of beads (Fig. 3d–f), number of vascular sprouts (Fig. 3g–i), total number of nuclei (Fig. 3j–l), and area covered with pericytes (Fig. 3m–p). The MIPs of whole well images from 96-well plates or single beads in glass-bottom dishes were analyzed using the ImageJ plugin we developed.

An example of the produced image-based quantitation is shown in Fig. 4. Starting with the original input image (Fig. 4a), our plugin detects the bead

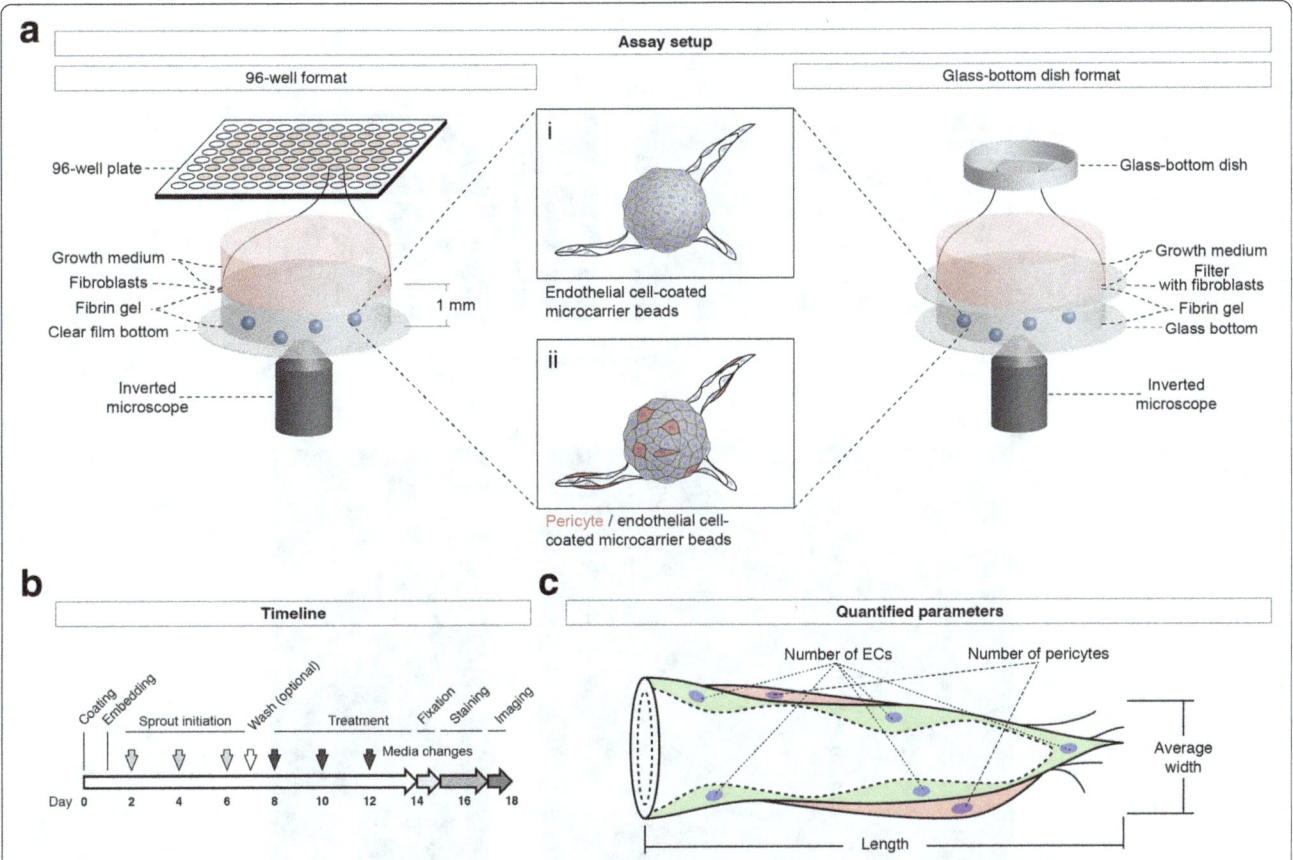

Fig. 1 Setup and workflow of the EC/pericyte sprouting assay. **a** Schematic drawing of the assay setup: A 1:10 co-culture of pericytes (*red*) and endothelial cells are coated on microcarrier beads (centre) that are then embedded into fibrin gels in each of the inner 60 wells of a 96-well plate (*left*). Alternatively, cell-coated beads are embedded into fibrin gels in a glass-bottom culture dish (*right*). The fibrin gels are subsequently covered with a layer of fibroblast cells (*left*), which can also be placed onto filters (*right*) to facilitate removal and subsequent staining. Developing sprouts are cultured in growth medium containing the desired treatment, and they can be imaged using an inverted microscope. **b** Timeline of the assay procedure: after coating ECs or ECs/pericytes on microcarrier beads and embedding them in fibrin gels, sprouts are grown for up to 6 days, optionally supplied with 10-μM vanadate to accelerate sprout growth; after removal of vanadate by washing with growth medium, treatment with test compounds or growth factors can be pursued for another 6 days; for image analysis, sprouts are fixed, stained, and imaged using an inverted microscope. **c** Schematic representation of a sprout containing ECs (*green*) and pericytes (*red*), indicating the quantified sprout parameters

(Fig. 4b) and the sprouts connected to it (Fig. 4c). The intensity of immunostaining against NG2, a pericyte marker, is used to segment pericyte area in the image (Fig. 4d). The presence or absence of Erg-1/2/3 staining is used to classify DAPI-positive cell nuclei into EC and pericyte-derived nuclei (Fig. 4e–g). For length measurements, the morphological skeleton of the sprouts is generated (Fig. 4h). The segmentation results are then used to measure morphological parameters of vascular sprouts, such as sprout number, length and width, as well as cell density, the ratio between ECs and pericytes, and the area of pericyte coverage (Fig. 4m).

Assessment of small molecule modifiers of angiogenesis identifies specific modulators of pericyte coverage

Using our analysis workflow, we tested more than 40 compounds on their effect on sprout morphology and pericyte coverage (Additional file 6: Table S1). We

selected in particular those compounds that target pathways reported to modulate angiogenesis (e.g., SU5416, a potent inhibitor of VEGFR-2 [27]; PDGFR inhibitors [10]; Y27632, a Rho kinase inhibitor [28]; a γ-secretase inhibitor (Notch signaling) [29]; and modulators of cAMP signaling [30]) in order to come up with a set of molecules to be used in a proof-of-concept study. The results are summarized in Additional file 7: Table S2 and Additional file 8: Table S3. In sprouts consisting of only ECs, we identified compounds that significantly decreased (11 compounds) or increased (6 compounds) sprout number ($p < 0.05$) with at least one of the concentrations used (Additional file 7: Table S2). Using a cut-off value of $p < 0.01$ (to reduce the chance of finding false positives), the number of compounds considered significantly decreasing or increasing sprout number was 6 and 3, respectively. Similarly, sprout length was significantly decreased with 12 (with $p < 0.01$, 5) compounds

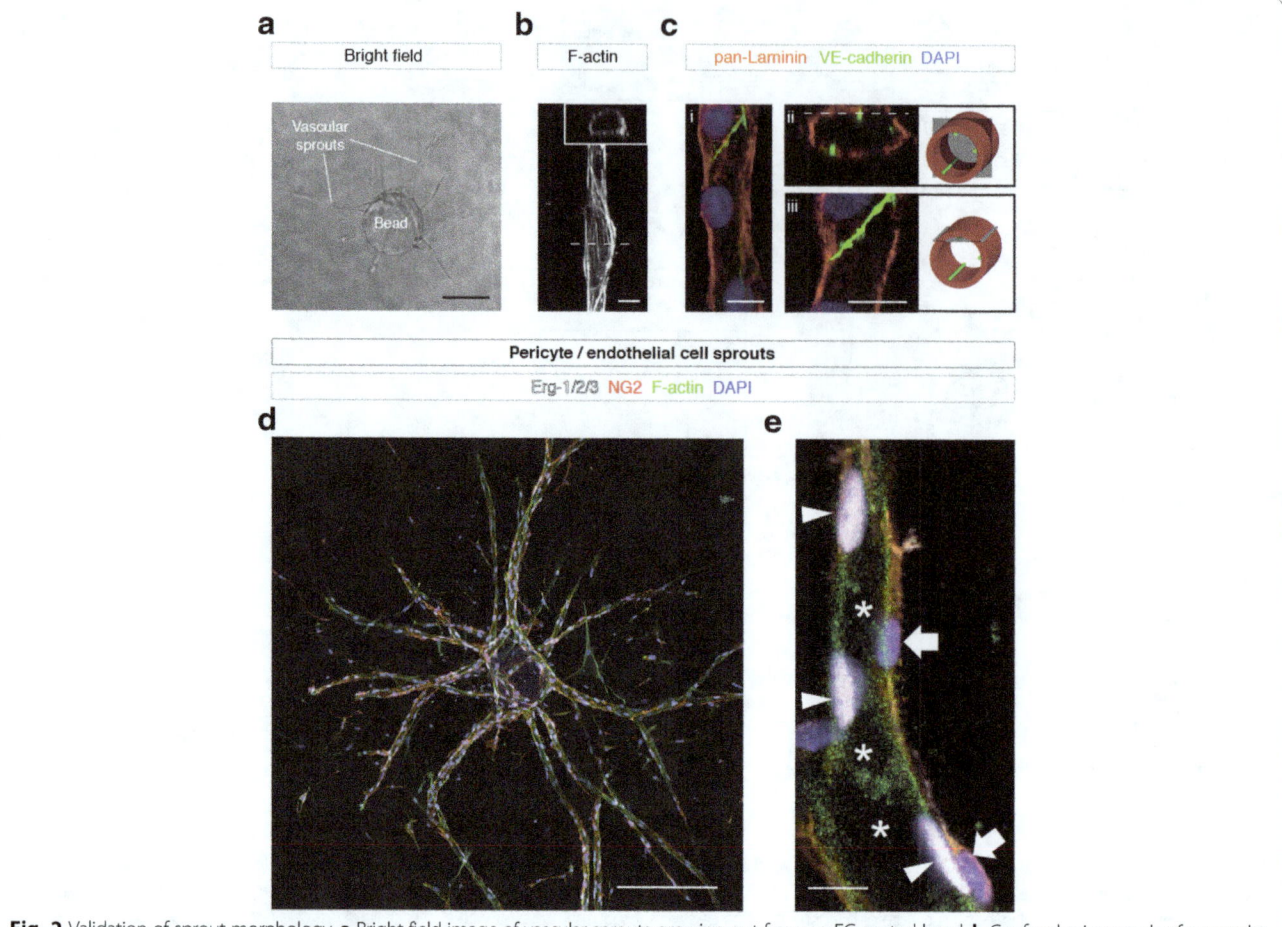

Fig. 2 Validation of sprout morphology. **a** Bright field image of vascular sprouts growing out from an EC-coated bead. **b** Confocal micrograph of a vascular sprout stained for F-actin; a patent lumen is seen on an optical cross-section (*inset*). **c** Confocal micrographs of a vascular sprout stained for laminin (*red*), VE-cadherin (*green*), and nuclei (DAPI, *blue*); maximum intensity projection (*i*), optical cross-section (*ii*), and optical longitudinal section (*iii*); 3D configuration of the optical sections is depicted in simplified illustrations (*right*). **d**, **e** Confocal micrographs of human pericyte/EC-derived vascular sprouts stained for endothelial nuclei (Erg-1/2/3, *white*), pericytes (NG2, *red*), F-actin (phalloidin, *green*), and nuclei (DAPI, *blue*); maximum intensity projection showing a bead with connected sprouts (**d**), optical longitudinal section of a single sprout (**e**), showing the vascular lumen (*asterisks*), EC nuclei (*arrowheads*), and pericyte nuclei (*block arrows*). Scale bars, **a** 200 μm; **b**, **c** 10 μm; **d** 200 μm; **e** 10 μm

and increased with 3 compounds (with $p < 0.01$, 1). In the presence of pericytes, none of the compounds decreased the number of sprouts significantly with the concentrations used, and only 3 compounds significantly increased sprout number (with $p < 0.01$, 0; Additional file 8: Table S3). Sprout length was significantly decreased with 8 (with $p < 0.01$, 3) compounds and significantly increased with 2 (with $p < 0.01$, 0) compounds.

For EC-only sprouts, we measured sprout width and cell density as additional parameters. We found that 8 out of 41 compounds specifically and significantly ($p < 0.05$) change sprout width and/or cell density without affecting sprout number or length (Additional file 7: Table S2). Similarly, we found that 12 out of 42 compounds specifically changed pericyte coverage in human EC/pericyte-derived vascular sprouts (Additional file 8: Table S3).

Discussion

The bead sprouting angiogenesis assay in its original form as described by Nakatsu et al. has been used in a number of publications to test the specific effects of agents (e.g., siRNAs, antibodies, chemical inhibitors) on angiogenesis, and to complement results from in vivo experiments [31–34]. However, until now, this assay has not included the important influence of pericytes on vascular sprout formation. We believe that the presented assay compares favorably with prior uses of published assays, since the co-culture of pericytes and ECs better mimics the in vivo vascular system. In addition, the three-dimensional bead angiogenic sprouting assay has been used with other cell types than HUVEC such as human lung ECs [35] and human lymphatic ECs [36].

The bead sprouting assay experimental design has several advantages over many comparable in vitro methods,

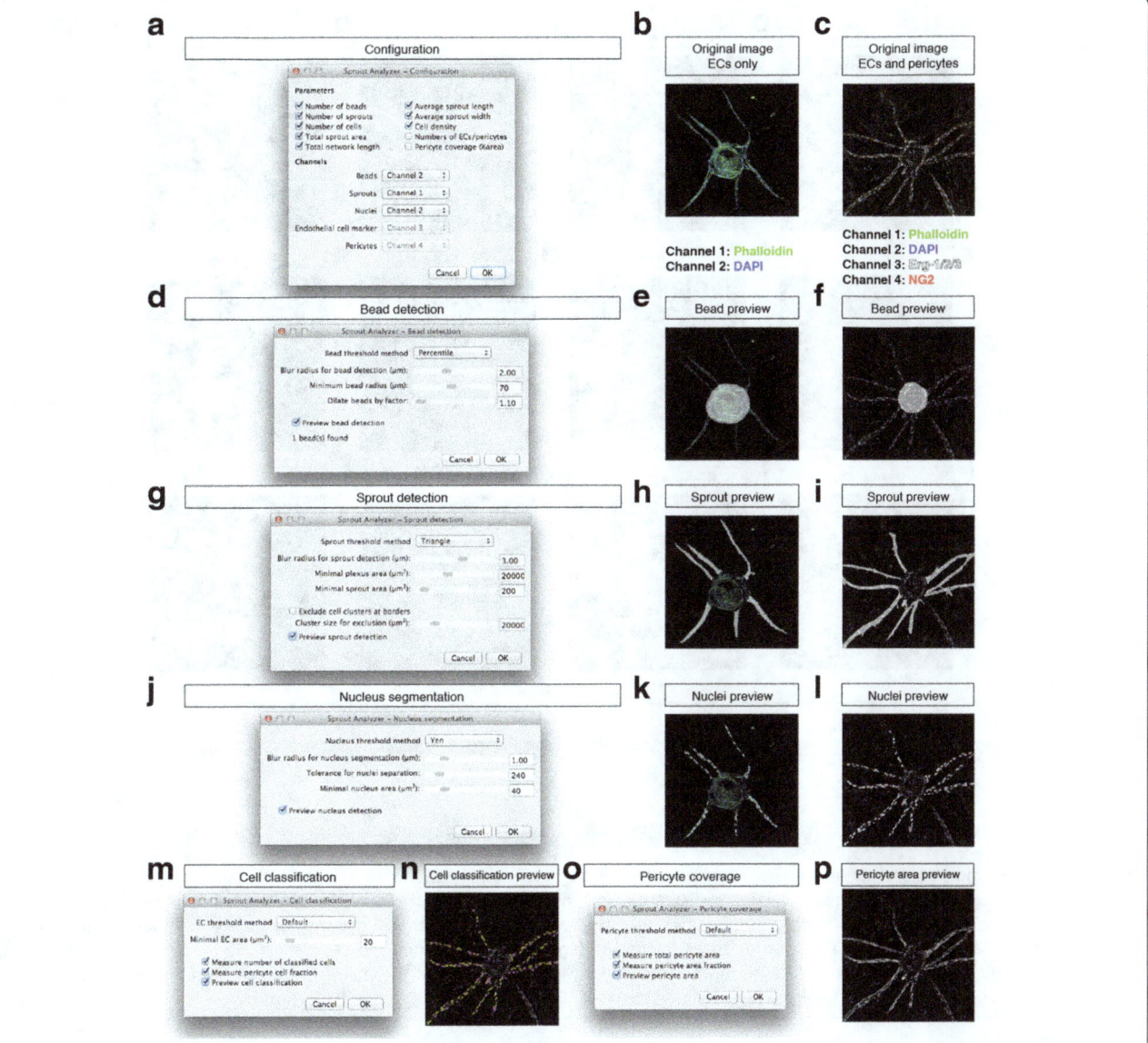

Fig. 3 Configuration of the *Sprout Analyzer* plugin. **a** Dialog to configure output measurement parameters and to define input configuration, i.e., which image channel contains which staining information. **b** Example image showing a microcarrier bead with vascular sprouts stained for F-actin using phalloidin-AF488 (*green*) and nuclei using DAPI (*blue*). **c** Example image with EC/pericyte-derived sprouts stained for F-actin using phalloidin-AF488 (*green*), nuclei using DAPI (*blue*), EC nuclei using an anti-Erg-1/2/3 antibody (*white*), and pericytes using an anti-NG2 antibody (*red*). **d** Dialog to configure bead detection; when the preview checkbox is activated, a bead mask image (*white*) is overlaid onto the image (**e** and **f** for the original images in **b** and **c**, respectively). **g** Dialog to configure sprout detection; when the preview checkbox is activated, a sprout mask image (*white*) is overlaid onto the image (**h**, **i**). **j** Dialog to configure nucleus detection; when the preview checkbox is activated, a nucleus mask image (*white*) is overlaid onto the image (**k**, **l**). **m** Dialog to configure cell classification; when the preview checkbox is activated, a preview showing ECs (*yellow*) and pericytes (*magenta*) is overlaid onto the image (**n**). **o** Dialog to configure pericyte coverage measurement; when the preview checkbox is activated, a pericyte area mask image (*white*) is overlaid onto the image (**p**). For detailed instructions, see protocol in Additional file 3, Additional file 1: Video S1, and Additional file 2: Video S2

namely, a defined cellular composition including ECs and pericytes. Based on a reproducible 3D environment, the assay produces multi-cellular lumenized sprouts that possess an abluminal basement membrane [20].

The assay reproduces the cellular mechanisms necessary to form lumenized tubes, in contrast to assays that focus solely on EC migration [37]. The new ImageJ

plugin allows for straightforward quantification of pericyte coverage in addition to sprout morphology (see Additional file 2: Video S2). Future applications of this assay will benefit from the detailed quantitative analysis provided by our toolkit. Admittedly, a limitation of the assay is the absence of blood flow. However, methods providing a blood flow require a more complex setup,

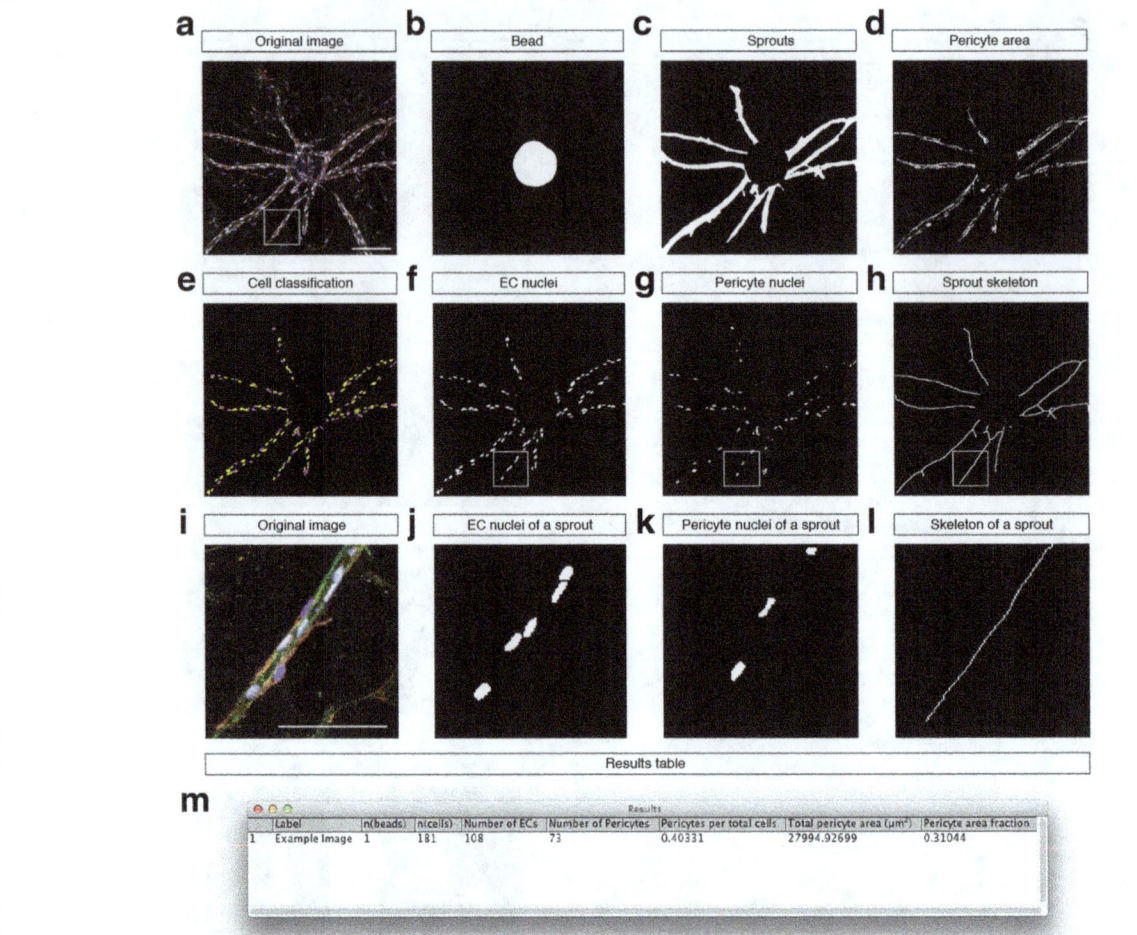

Fig. 4 Automated multi-parametric image analysis of sprouting angiogenesis with pericytes. **a** Confocal micrograph (maximum intensity projection) showing a bead with sprouts stained for F-actin (*green*), nuclei (*blue*), endothelial nuclei (*white*), and pericytes (*red*). **b–d** Result images showing segmentation results (*white*): segmented bead (**b**), total sprout area (**c**) and pericyte area (**d**). **e** Cell classification result showing endothelial nuclei (*yellow*) and pericyte nuclei (*magenta*). **f–g** Result images from the cell classification showing EC nuclei (**f**) and pericyte nuclei (**g**). **h** Sprout skeleton for length measurements. **i–l** Magnified details of the marked region in (**a**, **f–h**). **m** Result table shown after running our plugin on the example image shown in **a**. Scale bars, **a–h** 200 μm; **i–l** 100 μm

thereby limiting the sample size. A detailed comparison of assays highlighting their respective features is shown in Additional file 9: Table S4.

With the addition of pericytes, this sprouting angiogenesis assay is useful to measure effects of different compounds on pericyte coverage. In our assay, we often observed vascular sprouts with leading ECs and pericytes in close vicinity to the endothelium, covering the abluminal side of sprouts with long cellular protrusions (Fig. 4i–l). The observed sprout morphology is characteristic of pericyte-covered sprouting capillaries in vivo [6, 7, 10].

Within our test compounds, the number of compounds that decreased sprout number and length was higher than those that increased these two parameters. On an evolutionary-optimized cellular mechanism like angiogenesis, it is not surprising to find more inhibiting than

activating factors. In addition, we observed that the presence of pericytes on the vessel walls stabilized vascular sprouts; in the EC/pericyte sprouts, fewer compounds were able to decrease sprout number, although they were used at the same concentrations in both experiments.

It should be noted that our sprouting assay, while recapitulating the in vivo morphology of pericyte-wrapped sprouts, suffers from the natural biological variability present in primary human cells. A careful analysis of its statistical power should therefore be performed when designing larger studies using this assay to draw meaningful conclusions. Our proof-of-concept study is limited by its small sample size, since no robotic platform for high-throughput screening was used. However, when comparing groups of compounds with shared properties, we observed similar behaviors. For example, we observed that compounds regulating intracellular cyclic adenosine monophosphate (cAMP) levels or activating protein kinase A (i.e., 6-Bnz, Forskolin, IBMX, Sp-cAMPS) tended to increase sprout width in our assay (see Additional file 7: Table S2). In addition, the assay setup also allows measuring the number of branch points per sprout, in particular when sprouts are given enough time to form branched networks and a larger sample size is used. Therefore, we also added an option to measure the number of branch points in our plugin (Additional file 10: Figure S1), based on the "Analyze Skeleton" plugin included in Fiji [38].

The ImageJ plugin we developed provides a comprehensive quantification of morphological parameters in vascular sprouts. By providing an analysis specific to the bead sprouting assay, it helps researchers using this assay to get useful measurements, while still offering flexibility in the choice of parameters as well as the possibility of adaptations, as its source code is fully available.

Conclusions

Our methodology allows for quantitative assessment of morphology and pericyte coverage in vascular sprouts developed from human endothelial cells and human pericytes in vitro. We were also able to observe some of the expected effects of anti-angiogenic substances, such as those of VEGF and PDGF receptor inhibitors. The in vitro bead sprouting angiogenesis assay with pericytes therefore represents a novel, helpful addition to various in vivo experiments. Our plugin for ImageJ allows to quantify the results of this assay and is a novel and freely available quantification tool in the field of digital pathology.

Additional files

Additional file 1: Movie introducing the bead sprouting assay and our software analysis.
Additional file 2: Movie demonstrating the analysis of human EC/pericyte-derived vascular sprouts.
Additional file 3: Step-by-step protocol for the pericyte sprouting assay. This protocol contains several options of performing the bead sprouting assay, e.g., with or without pericytes, in a glass-bottom dish or a 96-well plate format, and with different stainings.
Additional file 4: ImageJ macro to create maximum intensity projections. ImageJ macro (ijm) format; open the file using ImageJ, e.g., by dragging onto the ImageJ main window.
Additional file 5: ImageJ macro to process image folders. ImageJ macro (ijm) format; open the file using ImageJ, e.g., by dragging onto the ImageJ main window.
Additional file 6: Table S1. List of compounds and concentrations used. The compounds were used at two concentrations, indicated in the columns $10 \times IC_{50}$ and $100 \times IC_{50}$, respectively. The values were chosen according to published values for the half maximal inhibitory concentrations of the inhibitors with respect to their target molecules in vitro or in accordance with literature using the respective compounds in a similar assay setup. Literature references for each compound are listed in the reference column.
Additional file 7: Table S2. Results of a pilot screen for EC-derived vascular sprouts. Changes considered significant with a cut-off p value of $p < 0.05$ (two-sided one-sample t test compared to solvent control) are colored in red and green to indicate decrease and increase compared to controls, respectively. $N = 3$ assays with 8 wells per compound each.

Additional file 8: Table S3. Results of a pilot screen for EC/pericyte-derived vascular sprouts. Changes considered significant with a cut-off p value of $p < 0.05$ (two-sided one-sample t test compared to solvent control) are colored in red and green to indicate decrease and increase compared to controls, respectively. $N = 3$ assays with 8 wells per compound each.
Additional file 9: Table S4. Comparison of in vitro and ex vivo assays. Comparison of in vitro and ex vivo assays to study sprouting angiogenesis, EC migration, and pericyte coverage. The method presented here is highlighted in green. Symbols used are the following: +, possible/present; −, not possible/not present; n.s., not shown.
Additional file 10: Figure S1. Quantification of branching level. (a) Confocal micrograph (maximum intensity projection) of a sprouting vascular plexus growing from four microcarrier beads, stained for F-actin (green) and nuclei (red). (b) Result image showing bead (dark grey) and sprout (light grey) segmentation. (c) Result image showing the sprout skeletons; branch points have been highlighted in red. (d) The option to measure branching level (red box) is available in the configuration dialog. (e) Result table reporting the average number of branch points per sprout (avg n(branch points), red box).

Abbreviations
EC: Endothelial cell; EGM-2: Endothelial growth medium-2; HBVP: Human brain vascular pericytes; HIF-1α: Hypoxia-inducible factor 1α; HSF: Human skin fibroblasts; HUVEC: Human umbilical vein endothelial cells; MIP: Maximum intensity projection; PDGF: Platelet-derived growth factor; PlGF: Placental growth factor; VEGF: Vascular endothelial growth factor

Acknowledgements
We thank the members of the Institute of Metabolic Physiology for helpful comments, in particular to M. Kelly-Goss for her helpful suggestions.

Funding
This work was supported by the German Center for Diabetes Research (DZD e.V.), the Federal Ministry of Health, and the Ministry for Innovation, Science and Research of North Rhine-Westphalia.

Authors' contributions
JE performed the assay experiments, prepared the figures, performed the statistics, programmed the ImageJ plugin, and wrote the manuscript. HK optimized the immunostaining procedure for 96-well plates. EL supervised JE and HK during their Ph.D. theses, provided advice, and wrote the manuscript together with JE. All authors read and approved the final manuscript.

Competing interests
The authors declare that they have no competing interests.

Author details
[1]Institute of Metabolic Physiology, Heinrich-Heine University, Düsseldorf, Germany. [2]Institute for Beta Cell Biology, Leibniz Center for Diabetes Research, German Diabetes Center (DDZ), Düsseldorf, Germany. [3]Current address: Friedrich Miescher Institute for Biomedical Research, Basel, Switzerland.

References
1. Potente M, Gerhardt H, Carmeliet P. Basic and therapeutic aspects of angiogenesis. Cell. 2011;146(6):873–87. doi:10.1016/j.cell.2011.08.039.
2. Conway EM, Collen D, Carmeliet P. Molecular mechanisms of blood vessel growth. Cardiovasc Res. 2001;49(3):507–21.
3. Gerhardt H, Betsholtz C. How do endothelial cells orientate? EXS. 2005;94:3–15.

4. Herbert SP, Stainier DY. Molecular control of endothelial cell behaviour during blood vessel morphogenesis. Nat Rev Mol Cell Biol. 2011;12(9):551–64. doi:10.1038/nrm3176.

5. Armulik A, Genove G, Mae M, Nisancioglu MH, Wallgard E, Niaudet C, et al. Pericytes regulate the blood-brain barrier. Nature. 2010;468(7323):557–61. doi:10.1038/nature09522.

6. Mishra A, O'Farrell FM, Reynell C, Hamilton NB, Hall CN, Attwell D. Imaging pericytes and capillary diameter in brain slices and isolated retinae. Nat Protoc. 2014;9(2):323–36. doi:10.1038/nprot.2014.019.

7. Armulik A, Genové G, Betsholtz C. Pericytes: developmental, physiological, and pathological perspectives, problems, and promises. Dev Cell. 2011;21:193–215. doi:10.1016/j.devcel.2011.07.001.

8. Hammes HP, Lin J, Wagner P, Feng Y, Vom Hagen F, Krzizok T, et al. Angiopoietin-2 causes pericyte dropout in the normal retina: evidence for involvement in diabetic retinopathy. Diabetes. 2004;53:1104–10. doi:10.2337/diabetes.53.4.1104.

9. Pfister F, Feng Y, Hagen F, Hoffmann S, Molema G, Hillebrands JL, Shani M, Deutsch U, Hammes HP. Pericyte migration: a novel mechanism of pericyte loss in experimental diabetic retinopathy. Diabetes. 2008;57:2495–502. doi:10.2337/db08-0325.

10. Armulik A, Abramsson A, Betsholtz C. Endothelial/pericyte interactions. Circ Res. 2005;97:512–23. doi:10.1161/01.RES.0000182903.16652.d7.

11. Gerhardt H, Betsholtz C. Endothelial-pericyte interactions in angiogenesis. Cell Tissue Res. 2003;314(1):15–23. doi:10.1007/s00441-003-0745-x.

12. Raza A, Franklin MJ, Dudek AZ. Pericytes and vessel maturation during tumor angiogenesis and metastasis. Am J Hematol. 2010;85:593–8. doi:10.1002/ajh.21745.

13. Beltramo E, Porta M. Pericyte loss in diabetic retinopathy: mechanisms and consequences. Curr Med Chem. 2013;20(26):3218–25.

14. Hammes HP, Feng Y, Pfister F, Brownlee M. Diabetic retinopathy: targeting vasoregression. Diabetes. 2011;60:9–16. doi:10.2337/db10-0454.

15. Hall CN, Reynell C, Gesslein B, Hamilton NB, Mishra A, Sutherland B, et al. Capillary pericytes regulate cerebral blood flow in health and disease. Nature. 2014;508:55–60. doi:10.1038/nature13165.

16. Ribatti D, Nico B, Crivellato E. The role of pericytes in angiogenesis. Int J Dev Biol. 2011;55(3):261–8. doi:10.1387/ijdb.103167dr.

17. Nakatsu MN, Sainson RC, Aoto JN, Taylor KL, Aitkenhead M, Perez-del-Pulgar S, et al. Angiogenic sprouting and capillary lumen formation modeled by human umbilical vein endothelial cells (HUVEC) in fibrin gels: the role of fibroblasts and Angiopoietin-1. Microvasc Res. 2003;66(2):102–12.

18. Nakatsu MN, Davis J, Hughes CC. Optimized fibrin gel bead assay for the study of angiogenesis. J Vis Exp. 2007;3:186. doi:10.3791/186.

19. Nakatsu MN, Hughes CC. An optimized three-dimensional in vitro model for the analysis of angiogenesis. Methods Enzymol. 2008;443:65–82. doi:10.1016/S0076-6879(08)02004-1.

20. Nikolova G, Strilic B, Lammert E. The vascular niche and its basement membrane. Trends Cell Biol. 2007;17(1):19–25. doi:10.1016/j.tcb.2006.11.005.

21. Zudaire E, Gambardella L, Kurcz C, Vermeren S. A computational tool for quantitative analysis of vascular networks. PLoS One. 2011;6(11):e27385. doi:10.1371/journal.pone.0027385.

22. Boettcher M, Gloe T, de Wit C. Semiautomatic quantification of angiogenesis. J Surg Res. 2010;162(1):132–9. doi:10.1016/j.jss.2008.12.009.

23. Bouis D, Hospers GA, Meijer C, Molema G, Mulder NH. Endothelium in vitro: a review of human vascular endothelial cell lines for blood vessel-related research. Angiogenesis. 2001;4(2):91–102.

24. Shepro D, Morel NM. Pericyte physiology. FASEB J. 1993;7(11):1031–8.

25. Preibisch S, Saalfeld S, Tomancak P. Globally optimal stitching of tiled 3D microscopic image acquisitions. Bioinformatics. 2009;25(11):1463–5. doi:10.1093/bioinformatics/btp184.

26. Schindelin J, Arganda-Carreras I, Frise E, Kaynig V, Longair M, Pietzsch T, et al. Fiji: an open-source platform for biological-image analysis. Nat Methods. 2012;9(7):676–82. doi:10.1038/nmeth.2019.

27. Mendel DB, Schreck RE, West DC, Li G, Strawn LM, Tanciongco SS, Vasile S, Shawver LK, Cherrington JM. The angiogenesis inhibitor SU5416 has long-lasting effects on vascular endothelial growth factor receptor phosphorylation and function. Clin Cancer Res. 2000;6:4848–58.

28. Strilic B, Kucera T, Eglinger J, Hughes MR, McNagny KM, Tsukita S, et al. The molecular basis of vascular lumen formation in the developing mouse aorta. Dev Cell. 2009;17(4):505–15. doi:10.1016/j.devcel.2009.08.011.

29. Schulz B, Pruessmeyer J, Maretzky T, Ludwig A, Blobel CP, Saftig P, et al. ADAM10 regulates endothelial permeability and T-Cell transmigration by proteolysis of vascular endothelial cadherin. Circ Res. 2008;102(10):1192–201. doi:10.1161/CIRCRESAHA.107.169805.

30. Namkoong S, Kim CK, Cho YL, Kim JH, Lee H, Ha KS, et al. Forskolin increases angiogenesis through the coordinated cross-talk of PKA-dependent VEGF expression and Epac-mediated PI3K/Akt/eNOS signaling. Cell Signal. 2009;21:906–15. doi:10.1016/j.cellsig.2009.01.038.

31. Strilic B, Eglinger J, Krieg M, Zeeb M, Axnick J, Babal P, et al. Electrostatic cell-surface repulsion initiates lumen formation in developing blood vessels. Curr Biol. 2010;20(22):2003–9. doi:10.1016/j.cub.2010.09.061.

32. Kachgal S, Putnam AJ. Mesenchymal stem cells from adipose and bone marrow promote angiogenesis via distinct cytokine and protease expression mechanisms. Angiogenesis. 2011;14(1):47–59. doi:10.1007/s10456-010-9194-9.

33. van Meeteren LA, Thorikay M, Bergqvist S, Pardali E, Stampino CG, Hu-Lowe D, et al. Anti-human activin receptor-like kinase 1 (ALK1) antibody attenuates bone morphogenetic protein 9 (BMP9)-induced ALK1 signaling and interferes with endothelial cell sprouting. J Biol Chem. 2012;287(22):18551–61. doi:10.1074/jbc.M111.338103.

34. Wilson CW, Parker LH, Hall CJ, Smyczek T, Mak J, Crow A, et al. Rasip1 regulates vertebrate vascular endothelial junction stability through Epac1-Rap1 signaling. Blood. 2013;122(22):3678–90. doi:10.1182/blood-2013-02-483156.

35. Wimmer R, Cseh B, Maier B, Scherrer K, Baccarini M. Angiogenic sprouting requires the fine tuning of endothelial cell cohesion by the Raf-1/Rok-alpha complex. Dev Cell. 2012;22(1):158–71. doi:10.1016/j.devcel.2011.11.012.

36. Zheng W, Tammela T, Yamamoto M, Anisimov A, Holopainen T, Kaijalainen S, et al. Notch restricts lymphatic vessel sprouting induced by vascular endothelial growth factor. Blood. 2011;118(4):1154–62. doi:10.1182/blood-2010-11-317800.

37. Liang CC, Park AY, Guan JL. In vitro scratch assay: a convenient and inexpensive method for analysis of cell migration in vitro. Nat Protoc. 2007;2(2):329–33. doi:10.1038/nprot.2007.30.

38. Arganda-Carreras I, Fernandez-Gonzalez R, Munoz-Barrutia A, Ortiz-De-Solorzano C. 3D reconstruction of histological sections: application to mammary gland tissue. Microsc Res Tech. 2010;73(11):1019–29. doi:10.1002/jemt.20829.

16

Metabolic regulation by secreted phospholipase A$_2$

Hiroyasu Sato[1], Yoshitaka Taketomi[1] and Makoto Murakami[1,2]*

Abstract

Within the phospholipase A$_2$ (PLA$_2$) superfamily that hydrolyzes phospholipids to yield fatty acids and lysophospholipids, the secreted PLA$_2$ (sPLA$_2$) enzymes comprise the largest family that contains 11 isoforms in mammals. Individual sPLA$_2$s exhibit unique distributions and specific enzymatic properties, suggesting their distinct biological roles. While sPLA$_2$s have long been implicated in inflammation and atherosclerosis, it has become evident that they are involved in diverse biological events through lipid mediator-dependent or mediator-independent processes in a given microenvironment. In recent years, new biological aspects of sPLA$_2$s have been revealed using their transgenic and knockout mouse models in combination with mass spectrometric lipidomics to unveil their target substrates and products in vivo. In this review, we summarize our current knowledge of the roles of sPLA$_2$s in metabolic disorders including obesity, hepatic steatosis, diabetes, insulin resistance, and adipose tissue inflammation.

Keywords: Fatty acid, Lipoprotein, Obesity, Phospholipid, Phospholipase A$_2$

Background

Phospholipase A$_2$ (PLA$_2$) is a group of enzymes that hydrolyze phospholipids to yield fatty acids and lysophospholipids (Fig. 1). In general, this reaction is best known as the initial, rate-limiting step of arachidonate metabolism leading to the production of bioactive lipid mediators including prostaglandins and leukotrienes. The mammalian genome encodes more than 30 PLA$_2$s or related enzymes, among which the secreted phospholipase A$_2$ (sPLA$_2$) family consists of low molecular mass and Ca^{2+}-requiring enzymes with a conserved His-Asp catalytic dyad and includes 11 isoforms (IB, IIA, IIC, IID, IIE, IIF, III, V, X, XIIA, and XIIB) [1–5]. Beyond cytosolic PLA$_2$ (cPLA$_2\alpha$; group IVA PLA$_2$) whose regulatory roles in arachidonate metabolism have been well documented [6], the biological roles of sPLA$_2$s remained a mystery for more than two decades. Recent studies using mice that have been gene manipulated for sPLA$_2$s have begun to reveal their distinct and unique roles in various biological events [7–14]. The current understanding of the in vivo functions of sPLA$_2$s has been summarized in several reviews [1–5].

* Correspondence: murakami-mk@igakuken.or.jp
[1]Lipid Metabolism Project, The Tokyo Metropolitan Institute of Medical Science, 2-1-6 Kamikitazawa, Setagaya-ku, Tokyo 156-8506, Japan
[2]AMED-CREST, Japan Agency for Medical Research and Development, Tokyo 100-0004, Japan

Historically, sPLA$_2$s have long been implicated in inflammation and atherosclerosis. This idea stems from the observations that sPLA$_2$-IIA, a prototypic "inflammatory sPLA$_2$," is induced during inflammation [15] and that hydrolysis of low-density lipoprotein (LDL) by sPLA$_2$s gives rise to pro-atherogenic LDL, which promotes macrophage foam cell formation in vitro [16, 17]. Indeed, subsequent genetic and pharmacological approaches support the pro-inflammatory or atherosclerotic roles of sPLA$_2$s [10–14]. However, the regulatory roles of sPLA$_2$s in metabolic disorders including obesity and insulin resistance have not yet been fully elucidated. Recently, it has become clear that several sPLA$_2$s are expressed in the adipose tissue or gastrointestinal (GI) tract and have variable influences on systemic metabolic states [18–20]. Here, we will make an overview of the novel biological roles of sPLA$_2$s and the lipid pathways underlying metabolic regulation, as revealed by sophisticated knockout and lipidomics techniques.

sPLA$_2$-V, a "metabolic sPLA$_2$"

Metabolic syndrome is increasing at an explosive rate worldwide due to a pandemic of obesity associated with diabetes, insulin resistance, non-alcoholic fatty liver disease, and hyperlipidemia [21]. The mechanisms connecting obesity to insulin resistance include an elevated level

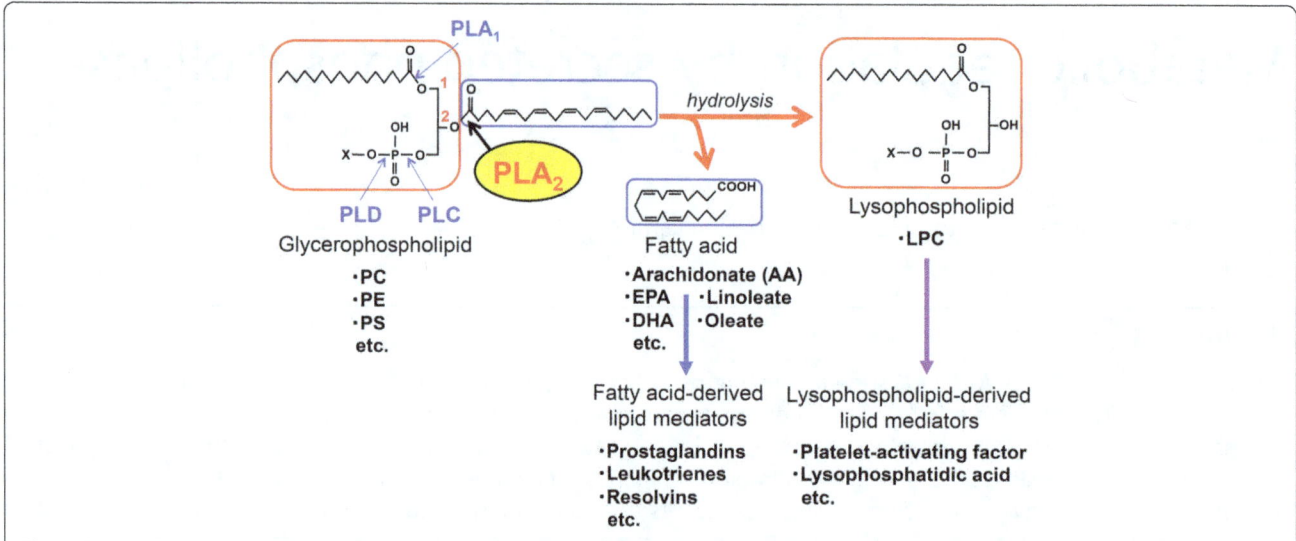

Fig. 1 PLA$_2$ reaction. PLA$_2$ hydrolyzes the *sn*-2 position of glycerophospholipids to yield fatty acids (typically unsaturated) and lysophospholipids. Phospholipases A$_1$, C, and D (PLA$_1$, PLC, and PLD, respectively) cleave other ester bonds in the glycerophospholipid molecule. Unsaturated fatty acids and lysophospholipids are further metabolized to a variety of lipid mediators

of circulating lipids, ectopic lipid deposition leading to lipotoxicity, and chronic inflammation in metabolically active tissues [22]. Obesity arises through the dysregulations of intracellular lipid metabolism or extracellular lipid partitioning among tissues, and the perturbation of intracellular/extracellular lipases variably and often profoundly affect obesity and insulin resistance [23–26]. For instance, lipoprotein lipase is an obesity susceptibility factor showing an inverse relationship between its activity and obesity-related traits in humans [23]. The imbalanced accumulation of LDL in favor of high-density lipoprotein (HDL) is a critical risk factor not only for atherosclerosis but also for insulin intolerance [27]. As lipoprotein particles are shielded by phospholipids, aberrant lipoprotein phospholipid metabolism could also influence lipid partitioning and thereby obesity.

Among the sPLA$_2$ isoforms, sPLA$_2$-V potently hydrolyzes phospholipids in lipoproteins (LDL > HDL) in vitro [17]. However, studies using *Pla2g5*$^{-/-}$ mice have failed to demonstrate the participation of sPLA$_2$-V in LDL metabolism in atherosclerosis models [11, 28]. Except for studies using sPLA$_2$-overexpressing transgenic mice [17, 29, 30], no reports have firmly established whether endogenous sPLA$_2$s affect lipoprotein metabolism in vivo. In a microarray search for unique lipase-related genes whose expressions are associated with obesity, we recently found that sPLA$_2$-V (and sPLA$_2$-IIE; see below) is robustly induced in adipocytes of obese mice [18]. This sPLA$_2$-V induction is dependent on adipogenesis plus endoplasmic reticulum (ER) stress. Because of this property plus the fact that sPLA$_2$-V is constitutively expressed at relatively high levels in several metabolic tissues such as the heart and skeletal muscle, we refer to sPLA$_2$-V as a "metabolic sPLA$_2$."

Notably, when fed a high-fat diet (HFD), *Pla2g5*$^{-/-}$ mice display hyperlipidemia with higher plasma levels of LDL, increased obesity and hepatic steatosis, and lower insulin sensitivity [18]. Furthermore, the adipose tissues in *Pla2g5*$^{-/-}$ mice show a greater infiltration of M1 macrophages and a higher expression of pro-inflammatory cytokines. Thus, sPLA$_2$-V plays anti-obesity and anti-inflammatory roles in the context of metabolic disorders. Lipidomics have revealed that sPLA$_2$-V secreted from hypertrophic adipocytes preferentially hydrolyzes phosphatidylcholine (PC) in fat-overladen LDL to release unsaturated fatty acids (e.g., oleate and linoleate) in vivo [18]. As such, the increased LDL lipid levels in *Pla2g5*$^{-/-}$ mice could impact on adipocyte hypertrophy and the fatty liver. Furthermore, in accordance with the alterations in LDL phospholipids, the levels of free oleate and linoleate are lower in the adipose tissue of HFD-fed *Pla2g5*$^{-/-}$ mice than in that of WT mice. These unsaturated fatty acids released by sPLA$_2$-V dampen the M1 macrophage polarization by saturated fatty acids (e.g., palmitate) likely through the attenuation of ER stress. This mechanism fits with the view that sPLA$_2$-V has an apparent, even if not strict, substrate preference for PC bearing a fatty acid with a low degree of unsaturation.

It remains obscure whether the sPLA$_2$-V action would depend on the production of ω6 arachidonic acid-derived eicosanoids (e.g., prostaglandins and leukotrienes) or ω3 polyunsaturated fatty acid (e.g., eicosapentaenoic acid and docosahexaenoic acid)-derived pro-resolving lipid mediators (e.g., resolvins and protectins), since the adipose tissue levels of these fatty acid metabolites were not affected by *Pla2g5* deficiency. Rather, sPLA$_2$-V contributes to controlling the quality of the lipids, i.e., the balance between saturated (detrimental) and unsaturated (beneficial) fatty acids, in adipose tissue microenvironments, providing a novel insight into the sPLA$_2$ action beyond lipid mediators. Together, these results reveal a functional link between lipoprotein metabolism and anti-inflammation for this particular sPLA$_2$ and provide a rationale for the long-standing issue of the physiological importance of lipoprotein hydrolysis by this extracellular enzyme family (Fig. 2).

Another intriguing feature of sPLA$_2$-V is that it is a "Th2/M2-prone sPLA$_2$," allowing a shift in the immune balance toward the Th2/M2 status. Apart from the crucial role of adipocyte- rather than macrophage-derived sPLA$_2$-V in obesity, the *Pla2g5* expression in macrophages is markedly induced by the M2-skewing Th2 cytokines IL-4 and IL-13 and the *Pla2g5* ablation decreases the Th2-mediated immune responses [18, 31]. In vitro, exogenous sPLA$_2$-V is capable of facilitating the M2 polarization of macrophages probably through augmenting the prostaglandin E$_2$ production [18]. Furthermore, in human macrophages, sPLA$_2$-V induced by IL-4 promotes phagocytosis through the production of lysophosphatidylethanolamine [32]. Given the increased incidence of metabolic disorders resulting from the genetic ablation of Th2 or M2 inducers (e.g., *Il4*, *Il13*, *Il33*, *Stat6*, or *Pparg*) [33], the decreased whole-body Th2/M2 status resulting from *Pla2g5* deficiency may also contribute to the exacerbation of obesity-associated inflammation. This notion also accords with the observations that *Pla2g5$^{-/-}$* mice are protected from asthma (Th2 dependent) [31], while suffering from more severe fungal infection (Th1 dependent) or arthritis (Th17 dependent) [10, 34], where the Th2 immunity counteracts the Th1/Th17-based inflammations. Thus, the fact that sPLA$_2$-V acts as a Th2/M2-prone sPLA$_2$ can account for the pro- versus anti-inflammatory actions of this enzyme in distinct immunopathological settings (Fig. 3).

Notably, in humans, *Pla2g5* gene polymorphisms correlate with the LDL levels in subjects with type 2 diabetes or obesity [35, 36]. The in vitro sPLA$_2$-V susceptibility of LDL from patients with type 2 diabetes is greater than that of LDL from healthy controls [37]. Moreover, the *Pla2g5* expression in the human visceral adipose tissue inversely correlates with LDL plasma levels [18]. These results imply a human relevance for the metabolic role of sPLA$_2$-V.

sPLA$_2$-IIE, another "metabolic sPLA$_2$"

We also found that sPLA$_2$-IIE, which remained a functionally orphan sPLA$_2$ for more than a decade, acts as another "metabolic" sPLA$_2$ that is induced in hypertrophic adipocytes [18]. An adipogenic stimulus is sufficient for induction of sPLA$_2$-IIE in adipocytes. *Pla2g2e$^{-/-}$* mice are modestly protected from diet-induced obesity, hepatic steatosis, and hyperlipidemia. In contrast to sPLA$_2$-V, which hydrolyzes PC in LDL to selectively release oleate and linoleate (see above), sPLA$_2$-IIE preferentially hydrolyzes minor lipoprotein phospholipids, phosphatidylserine (PS), and phosphatidylethanolamine (PE), with no apparent fatty acid selectivity. As such, sPLA$_2$-IIE alters the lipid composition of lipoproteins, thereby moderately affecting the lipid accumulation in the adipose tissue and liver.

Although the molecular mechanism that links lipoprotein PS/PE hydrolysis with obesity still remains unclear, this study revealed for the first time the importance of

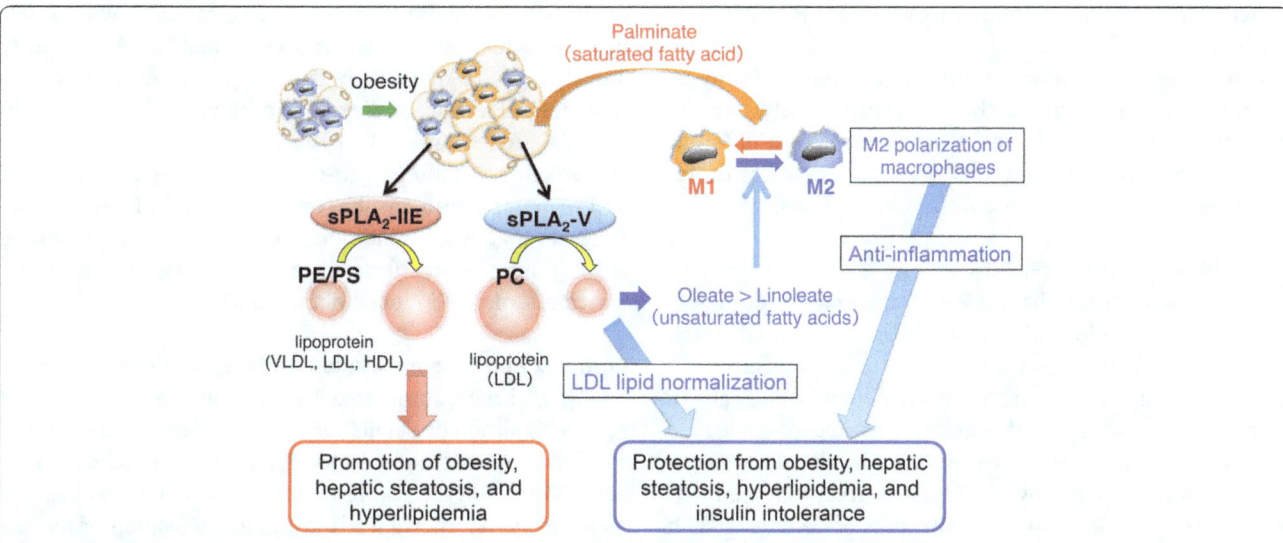

Fig. 2 Metabolic regulation by "metabolic sPLA$_2$s." During obesity, two sPLA$_2$s (IIE and V) are induced in hypertrophic adipocytes. sPLA$_2$-IIE hydrolyzes PE and PS in lipoproteins (VLDL, LDL, and HDL) and facilitates fat accumulation into the peripheral tissues. sPLA$_2$-V hydrolyzes PC in LDL to release oleate and linoleate, which counteracts the palmitate-induced M1 polarization of macrophages and thereby sequesters adipose tissue inflammation [18]

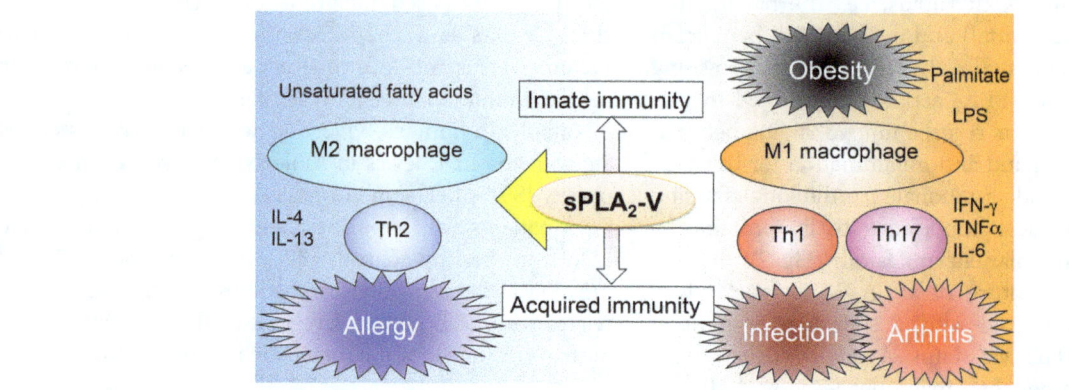

Fig. 3 Immune balance regulation by sPLA$_2$-V. sPLA$_2$-V is induced in the M2 macrophages and Th2 cells by IL-4 or IL-13 and promotes Th2/M2-dominant immunity such as asthma [31, 32]. Conversely, sPLA$_2$-V plays protective roles in Th1- or Th17-type immune responses including obesity, infection, and arthritis [10, 18, 34]

these minor lipoprotein phospholipids in metabolic regulation. As the increase of the negative charges in lipoproteins by oxidative modification renders the particles smaller, the increase of the anionic phospholipids (e.g., PS) in lipoproteins by the absence of sPLA$_2$-IIE may also afford a similar effect. Alternatively, lysophosphatidylethanolamine or lysophosphatidylserine produced by sPLA$_2$-IIE might have some metabolic effects, a possibility that awaits future studies. Collectively, these results underscore the physiological relevance of lipoprotein hydrolysis by distinct sPLA$_2$s and highlight the importance of "metabolic sPLA$_2$s" as the integrated regulators of metabolic responses (Fig. 2).

On the other hand, another study has recently reported that $Pla2g2e^{-/-}$ mice accumulate more epididymal fat as they age [38]. During adipogenesis, the genetic deletion or siRNA knockdown of sPLA$_2$-IIE increases the triglyceride in adipocytes, while its overexpression or exogenous addition facilitates lipolysis. Although the reason for the discrepancy between the two studies is unclear, it might have arisen from different experimental conditions (HFD versus chow diets or female versus male mice) in different animal facilities.

sPLA$_2$-IB, a "digestive sPLA$_2$"
Systemic lipid metabolism is often affected by the digestion and absorption of dietary lipids in the GI tract. sPLA$_2$-IB is synthesized by pancreatic acinar cells, and after secretion as a zymogen into pancreatic juice, an N-terminal propeptide of the inactive zymogen is cleaved by trypsin to yield an active enzyme in the duodenum. The hydrolysis of PC by sPLA$_2$-IB is greatly accelerated in the presence of a low concentration of detergent such as deoxycholate [39]. This property appears to be physiologically important since the digestion of dietary phospholipids by sPLA$_2$-IB occurs in the presence of bile acid in the GI tract.

$Pla2g1b^{-/-}$ mice show resistance to obesity, lower plasma insulin and leptin levels, and improved glucose tolerance when fed a high-fat/carbohydrate diet [40]. These phenotypes of $Pla2g1b^{-/-}$ mice are most likely due to a marked reduction in the hydrolysis of dietary and biliary PC and thereby in the production and absorption of lysophosphatidylcholine (LPC) in the GI tract. The increased intestinal absorption of LPC promotes postprandial hyperglycemia by inhibiting the glucose uptake by the liver and muscle, and accordingly, the absence of sPLA$_2$-IB reduces the postprandial LPC levels, leading to improved insulin sensitivity and hepatic fatty acid oxidation [41, 42]. It is noteworthy that $Pla2g1b^{-/-}$ mice on a $Ldlr^{-/-}$ background are protected from body weight gain and atherosclerosis in response to a hypercaloric diet [43] and that the oral administration of the sPLA$_2$ inhibitor methyl indoxam along with a diabetogenic diet effectively suppresses diet-induced obesity and diabetes in mice likely through the prevention of the intestinal digestion of dietary and biliary PC by sPLA$_2$-IB [44]. In further support of these observations, pancreatic acinar cell-specific $Pla2g1b$-transgenic mice develop more severe obesity and insulin resistance [45]. These results suggest that the inhibition of sPLA$_2$-IB, a "digestive sPLA$_2$," may be an effective oral therapeutic option for the treatment of diet-induced obesity and diabetes.

Complex and enigmatic roles of sPLA$_2$-X in metabolism
Lastly, we briefly summarize the possible metabolic roles of sPLA$_2$-X, although details remain uncertain because of the fact that conflicting results have been obtained. Like sPLA$_2$-IB, sPLA$_2$-X also has an N-terminal propeptide, and its proteolytic removal leads to the full activation of the enzyme. A series of studies have provided some insights into the functional link of sPLA$_2$-X-released polyunsaturated fatty acids to lipid-sensing nuclear receptor signaling. Macrophages from $Pla2g10^{-/-}$ mice show an increased

expression of the cholesterol efflux transporters ABCA1 and ABCG1, and this effect appears to be dependent on the suppression of the liver X receptor (LXR) by sPLA$_2$-X-released polyunsaturated fatty acids [46]. Moreover, the increased cholesterol content of the lipid rafts in $Pla2g10^{-/-}$ macrophages leads to significant reduction of endotoxin-induced inflammation [47]. The sPLA$_2$-X-dependent suppression of LXR can also occur in the adipose tissue, where $Pla2g10$ deficiency facilitates adipogenesis and obesity [48], and in the adrenal glands, where its deficiency promotes corticosteroidogenesis through the activation of steroidogenic acute regulatory protein [49]. In the latter case, pro-sPLA$_2$-X is proteolytically processed to a mature, active form by the protein convertases furin and PCSK6, which are induced by the adrenocorticotropic hormone, in adrenal cells [50]. However, as far as we have been able to examine, the $Pla2g10$ expression in mouse macrophages and the adipose tissue is very low, arguing against the above observations. Rather, we prefer the idea that sPLA$_2$-X might be expressed in a limited subset of these cells or supplied from proximal or distal cells in a paracrine manner.

On the other hand, we have shown that sPLA$_2$-X is expressed abundantly in GI-lining cells and participates in phospholipid digestion [19]. Accordingly, $Pla2g10^{-/-}$ mice display a reduced age-associated adiposity and improved insulin sensitivity in the skeletal muscle, likely through a mechanism reminiscent of that in $Pla2g1b^{-/-}$ mice. Thus, the two "digestive sPLA$_2$s" (IB and X) may spatiotemporally control the hydrolysis of dietary and biliary phospholipids and thereby the absorption of their hydrolytic products, depending on the quantity and quality of the dietary and biliary fat input. As in the case of $Pla2g2e^{-/-}$ mice (see above), the opposite phenotypes of $Pla2g10^{-/-}$ mice observed in different studies might have been due to differences in the experimental models or housing conditions employed, and further studies will be necessary to clarify more definitively the roles and mechanistic actions of sPLA$_2$-X in metabolism.

It has been recently reported that the glucose-stimulated insulin secretion by islet β cells is augmented in $Pla2g10^{-/-}$ mice, underscoring a novel metabolic role of sPLA$_2$-X [51]. Mechanistically, sPLA$_2$-X negatively regulates insulin secretion by augmenting the cyclooxygenase-2-dependent prostaglandin E$_2$ production. In this scenario, targeting sPLA$_2$-X may be an effective therapeutic option for enhancing β cell function in the treatment of diabetes.

Conclusions

It is now obvious that at least four sPLA$_2$s are involved in metabolic regulation through distinct mechanisms, as summarized below. sPLA$_2$-V is induced in hypertrophic adipocytes by obesity-associated ER stress and hydrolyzes PC in hyperlipidemic LDL to facilitate the skewing of macrophages from M1 to M2 subsets, thereby conferring protection from adipose tissue inflammation, insulin resistance, obesity, hepatic steatosis, and hyperlipidemia. The saturated fatty acids supplied abundantly from adipocytes trigger the M1 polarization of macrophages, which is counterregulated by the sPLA$_2$-V-driven unsaturated fatty acids from LDL. sPLA$_2$-IIE is induced in adipocytes in accordance with adipogenesis and hydrolyzes PE and PS in lipoproteins, eventually promoting fat storage in the adipose tissue and liver. sPLA$_2$-IB, a pancreatic sPLA$_2$ that is secreted into the GI lumen, hydrolyzes dietary and biliary phospholipids to promote lipid digestion and absorption, which is associated with obesity and hepatic insulin resistance. sPLA$_2$-X variably affects metabolism possibly through the production of polyunsaturated fatty acids that modify the LXR signaling in the adipose tissue, through the digestion of the dietary and biliary phospholipids in the gut, or through the generation of prostaglandin E$_2$ that suppresses insulin secretion in the pancreatic islet. In addition, sPLA$_2$-IIA is abundantly expressed in the human and rat adipose tissues in obesity and the pharmacological inhibition of this isoform attenuates the adipose tissue inflammation in rats [18, 52]. It remains possible that other sPLA$_2$ isoforms may also participate in metabolic regulation, and this issue is now under investigation. Together, these studies have brought about a paradigm shift toward a better understanding of the biological roles of this extracellular lipolytic enzyme family as coordinators of metabolism.

Competing interests
The authors declare that they have no competing interests.

Authors' contributions
HS, YT, and MM wrote this review. All authors read and approved the final manuscript.

Acknowledgments
We thank Dr. A. Kumoanogoh (University of Osaka, Japan) for providing an opportunity to write this manuscript.

Funding
This work was supported by a grant-in-aid for scientific research from the Ministry of Education, Science, Culture, Sports and Technology of Japan and AMED-CREST from the Japan Agency for Medical Research and Development.

References
1. Lambeau G, Gelb MH. Biochemistry and physiology of mammalian secreted phospholipases A$_2$. Annu Rev Biochem. 2008;77:495–520.
2. Murakami M, Taketomi Y, Girard C, Yamamoto K, Lambeau G. Emerging roles of secreted phospholipase A$_2$ enzymes: lessons from transgenic and knockout mice. Biochimie. 2010;92:561–82.
3. Dennis EA, Cao J, Hsu YH, Magrioti V, Kokotos G. Phospholipase A$_2$ enzymes: physical structure, biological function, disease implication, chemical inhibition, and therapeutic intervention. Chem Rev. 2011;111:6130–85.
4. Murakami M, Taketomi Y, Miki Y, Sato H, Hirabayashi T, Yamamoto K. Recent progress in phospholipase A$_2$ research: from cells to animals to humans. Prog Lipid Res. 2011;50:152–92.
5. Murakami M, Sato H, Miki Y, Yamamoto K, Taketomi Y. A new era of secreted phospholipase A$_2$. J Lipid Res. 2015;56:1248–61.

6. Uozumi N, Kume K, Nagase T, Nakatani N, Ishii S, Tashiro F, et al. Role of cytosolic phospholipase A_2 in allergic response and parturition. Nature. 1997;390:618–22.

7. Taketomi Y, Ueno N, Kojima T, Sato H, Murase R, Yamamoto K, et al. Mast cell maturation is driven via a group III phospholipase A_2-prostaglandin D_2-DP1 receptor paracrine axis. Nat Immunol. 2013;14:554–63.

8. Sato H, Taketomi Y, Isogai Y, Miki Y, Yamamoto K, Masuda S, et al. Group III secreted phospholipase A_2 regulates epididymal sperm maturation and fertility in mice. J Clin Invest. 2010;120:1400–14.

9. Yamamoto K, Taketomi Y, Isogai Y, Miki Y, Sato H, Masuda S, et al. Hair follicular expression and function of group X secreted phospholipase A_2 in mouse skin. J Biol Chem. 2011;286:11616–31.

10. Boilard E, Lai Y, Larabee K, Balestrieri B, Ghomashchi F, Fujioka D, et al. A novel anti-inflammatory role for secretory phospholipase A_2 in immune complex-mediated arthritis. EMBO Mol Med. 2010;2:172–87.

11. Bostrom MA, Boyanovsky BB, Jordan CT, Wadsworth MP, Taatjes DJ, de Beer FC, et al. Group V secretory phospholipase A_2 promotes atherosclerosis: evidence from genetically altered mice. Arterioscler Thromb Vasc Biol. 2007;27:600–6.

12. Henderson Jr WR, Chi EY, Bollinger JG, Tien YT, Ye X, Castelli L, et al. Importance of group X-secreted phospholipase A_2 in allergen-induced airway inflammation and remodeling in a mouse asthma model. J Exp Med. 2007;204:865–77.

13. Muñoz NM, Meliton AY, Arm JP, Bonventre JV, Cho W, Leff AR. Deletion of secretory group V phospholipase A_2 attenuates cell migration and airway hyperresponsiveness in immunosensitized mice. J Immunol. 2007;179:4800–7.

14. Yamamoto K, Miki Y, Sato M, Taketomi Y, Nishito Y, Taya C, et al. The role of group IIF-secreted phospholipase A2 in epidermal homeostasis and hyperplasia. J Exp Med. 2015;212:1901–19.

15. Seilhamer JJ, Pruzanski W, Vadas P, Plant S, Miller JA, Kloss J, et al. Cloning and recombinant expression of phospholipase A_2 present in rheumatoid arthritic synovial fluid. J Biol Chem. 1989;264:5335–8.

16. Hanasaki K, Yamada K, Yamamoto S, Ishimoto Y, Saiga A, Ono T, et al. Potent modification of low density lipoprotein by group X secretory phospholipase A_2 is linked to macrophage foam cell formation. J Biol Chem. 2002;277:29116–24.

17. Sato H, Kato R, Isogai Y, Saka S, Ohtsuki M, Taketomi Y, et al. Analyses of group III secreted phospholipase A_2 transgenic mice reveal potential participation of this enzyme in plasma lipoprotein modification, macrophage foam cell formation, and atherosclerosis. J Biol Chem. 2008;283:33483–97.

18. Sato H, Taketomi Y, Ushida A, Isogai Y, Kojima T, Hirabayashi T, et al. The adipocyte-inducible secreted phospholipases PLA2G5 and PLA2G2E play distinct roles in obesity. Cell Metab. 2014;20:119–32.

19. Sato H, Isogai Y, Masuda S, Taketomi Y, Miki Y, Kamei D, et al. Physiological roles of group X-secreted phospholipase A_2 in reproduction, gastrointestinal phospholipid digestion, and neuronal function. J Biol Chem. 2011;286:11632–48.

20. Hui DY. Phospholipase A_2 enzymes in metabolic and cardiovascular diseases. Curr Opin Lipidol. 2012;23:235–40.

21. Despres JP, Lemieux I. Abdominal obesity and metabolic syndrome. Nature. 2006;444:881–7.

22. Hotamisligil GS. Inflammation and metabolic disorders. Nature. 2006;444:860–7.

23. Chen Y, Zhu J, Lum PY, Yang X, Pinto S, MacNeil DJ, et al. Variations in DNA elucidate molecular networks that cause disease. Nature. 2008;452:429–35.

24. Chiu HK, Qian K, Ogimoto K, Morton GJ, Wisse BE, Agrawal N, et al. Mice lacking hepatic lipase are lean and protected against diet-induced obesity and hepatic steatosis. Endocrinology. 2010;151:993–1001.

25. Haemmerle G, Lass A, Zimmermann R, Gorkiewicz G, Meyer C, Rozman J, et al. Defective lipolysis and altered energy metabolism in mice lacking adipose triglyceride lipase. Science. 2006;312:734–7.

26. Wang H, Knaub LA, Jensen DR, Young Jung D, Hong EG, Ko HJ, et al. Skeletal muscle-specific deletion of lipoprotein lipase enhances insulin signaling in skeletal muscle but causes insulin resistance in liver and other tissues. Diabetes. 2009;58:116–24.

27. Avramoglu RK, Basciano H, Adeli K. Lipid and lipoprotein dysregulation in insulin resistant states. Clin Chim Acta. 2006;368:1–19.

28. Boyanovsky B, Zack M, Forrest K, Webb NR. The capacity of group V $sPLA_2$ to increase atherogenicity of ApoE$^{-/-}$ and LDLR$^{-/-}$ mouse LDL in vitro predicts its atherogenic role in vivo. Arterioscler Thromb Vasc Biol. 2009;29:532–8.

29. Ivandic B, Castellani LW, Wang XP, Qiao JH, Mehrabian M, Navab M, et al. Role of group II secretory phospholipase A_2 in atherosclerosis: 1. Increased atherogenesis and altered lipoproteins in transgenic mice expressing group IIa phospholipase A_2. Arterioscler Thromb Vasc Biol. 1999;19:1284–90.

30. Yamamoto K, Isogai Y, Sato H, Taketomi Y, Murakami M. Secreted phospholipase A_2, lipoprotein hydrolysis, and atherosclerosis: integration with lipidomics. Anal Bioanal Chem. 2011;400:1829–42.

31. Ohta S, Imamura M, Xing W, Boyce JA, Balestrieri B. Group V secretory phospholipase A_2 is involved in macrophage activation and is sufficient for macrophage effector functions in allergic pulmonary inflammation. J Immunol. 2013;190:5927–38.

32. Rubio JM, Rodríguez JP, Gil-de-Gómez L, Guijas C, Balboa MA, Balsinde J. Group V secreted phospholipase A_2 is upregulated by IL-4 in human macrophages and mediates phagocytosis via hydrolysis of ethanolamine phospholipids. J Immunol. 2015;194:3327–39.

33. Odegaard JI, Chawla A. The immune system as a sensor of the metabolic state. Immunity. 2013;38:644–54.

34. Balestrieri B, Maekawa A, Xing W, Gelb MH, Katz HR, Arm JP. Group V secretory phospholipase A_2 modulates phagosome maturation and regulates the innate immune response against Candida albicans. J Immunol. 2009;182:4891–8.

35. Sergouniotis PI, Davidson AE, Mackay DS, Lenassi E, Li Z, Robson AG, et al. Biallelic mutations in PLA2G5, encoding group V phospholipase A_2, cause benign fleck retina. Am J Hum Genet. 2011;89:782–91.

36. Wootton PT, Arora NL, Drenos F, Thompson SR, Cooper JA, Stephens JW, et al. Tagging SNP haplotype analysis of the secretory PLA$_2$-V gene, PLA2G5, shows strong association with LDL and oxLDL levels, suggesting functional distinction from sPLA$_2$-IIA: results from the UDACS study. Hum Mol Genet. 2007;16:1437–44.

37. Pettersson C, Fogelstrand L, Rosengren B, Stahlman S, Hurt-Camejo E, Fagerberg B, et al. Increased lipolysis by secretory phospholipase A_2 group V of lipoproteins in diabetic dyslipidaemia. J Intern Med. 2008;264:155–65.

38. Zhi H, Qu L, Wu F, Chen L, Tao J. Group IIE secretory phospholipase A_2 regulates lipolysis in adipocytes. Obesity (Silver Spring). 2015;23:760–8.

39. Jain MK, Egmond MR, Verheij HM, Apitz-Castro R, Dijkman R, De Haas GH. Interaction of phospholipase A_2 and phospholipid bilayers. Biochim Biophys Acta. 1982;688:341–8.

40. Huggins KW, Boileau AC, Hui DY. Protection against diet-induced obesity and obesity-related insulin resistance in Group 1B PLA$_2$-deficient mice. Am J Physiol Endocrinol Metab. 2002;283:E994–E1001.

41. Labonté ED, Kirby RJ, Schildmeyer NM, Cannon AM, Huggins KW, Hui DY. Group 1B phospholipase A_2-mediated lysophospholipid absorption directly contributes to postprandial hyperglycemia. Diabetes. 2006;55:935–41.

42. Labonté ED, Pfluger PT, Cash JG, Kuhel DG, Roja JC, Magness DP, et al. Postprandial lysophospholipid suppresses hepatic fatty acid oxidation: the molecular link between group 1B phospholipase A_2 and diet-induced obesity. FASEB J. 2010;24:2516–24.

43. Hollie NI, Konaniah ES, Goodin C, Hui DY. Group 1B phospholipase A_2 inactivation suppresses atherosclerosis and metabolic diseases in LDL receptor-deficient mice. Atherosclerosis. 2014;234:377–80.

44. Hui DY, Cope MJ, Labonté ED, Chang HT, Shao J, Goka E, et al. The phospholipase A_2 inhibitor methyl indoxam suppresses diet-induced obesity and glucose intolerance in mice. Br J Pharmacol. 2009;157:1263–9.

45. Cash JG, Kuhel DG, Goodin C, Hui DY. Pancreatic acinar cell-specific overexpression of group 1B phospholipase A_2 exacerbates diet-induced obesity and insulin resistance in mice. Int J Obes (Lond). 2011;35:877–81.

46. Shridas P, Bailey WM, Gizard F, Oslund RC, Gelb MH, Bruemmer D, et al. Group X secretory phospholipase A_2 negatively regulates ABCA1 and ABCG1 expression and cholesterol efflux in macrophages. Arterioscler Thromb Vasc Biol. 2010;30:2014–21.

47. Shridas P, Bailey WM, Talbott KR, Oslund RC, Gelb MH, Webb NR. Group X secretory phospholipase A_2 enhances TLR4 signaling in macrophages. J Immunol. 2011;187:482–9.

48. Li X, Shridas P, Forrest K, Bailey W, Webb NR. Group X secretory phospholipase A_2 negatively regulates adipogenesis in murine models. FASEB J. 2010;24:4313–24.

49. Shridas P, Bailey WM, Boyanovsky BB, Oslund RC, Gelb MH, Webb NR. Group X secretory phospholipase A_2 regulates the expression of steroidogenic acute regulatory protein (StAR) in mouse adrenal glands. J Biol Chem. 2010;285:20031–9.

50. Layne JD, Shridas P, Webb NR. Ectopically expressed pro-group X secretory phospholipase A_2 is proteolytically activated in mouse adrenal cells by furin-like proprotein convertases: implications for the regulation of adrenal steroidogenesis. J Biol Chem. 2015;290:7851–60.

51. Shridas P, Zahoor L, Forrest KJ, Layne JD, Webb NR. Group X secretory phospholipase A_2 regulates insulin secretion through a cyclooxygenase-2-dependent mechanism. J Biol Chem. 2014;289(40):27410–7.

52. Iyer A, Lim J, Poudyal H, Reid RC, Suen JY, Webster J, et al. An inhibitor of phospholipase A_2 group IIA modulates adipocyte signaling and protects against diet-induced metabolic syndrome in rats. Diabetes. 2012;61:2320–9.

17

Applications of reconstituted inflammasomes in a cell-free system to drug discovery and elucidation of the pathogenesis of autoinflammatory diseases

Naoe Kaneko[1], Tomoyuki Iwasaki[1], Yuki Ito[1], Hiroyuki Takeda[2], Tatsuya Sawasaki[3], Shinnosuke Morikawa[1], Naoko Nakano[1], Mie Kurata[1] and Junya Masumoto[1]* ⓘ

Abstract

The inflammasome, typically consisting of a Nod-like receptor, apoptosis-associated speck-like protein, and pro-caspase-1, has recently been identified as a huge intracellular complex, which plays a crucial role in interleukin-1 maturation or specific physiological functions. Two Nod-like receptors, such as nucleotide-binding oligomerization domains-containing protein (Nod)1 and Nod2, interact with the receptor-interacting protein serine-threonine kinase (RIPK)2 accompanied by Iκ-B kinase (IKK) complexes to construct the nodosome, leading to nuclear factor (NF)-κB activation. The aberrant activation of inflammasomes or nodosomes causes autoinflammatory diseases. Therefore, inflammasomes may be attractive targets to treat autoinflammatory diseases. Our aim is to develop reconstituted inflammasomes in a cell-free system to discover specific molecular-target drugs and elucidate the molecular pathogenesis of autoinflammatory diseases. In this review, we describe reconstituted inflammasomes in a cell-free system.

Keywords: Cell-free, Interleukin-1β, Inflammasome

Background

Inflammasomes have recently been identified as expanding intracellular complexes that play important roles not only in innate immunity but also in maintaining specific physiological functions [1–3]. The aberrant activation of inflammasomes is thought to be linked to various diseases, including inflammatory diseases, degenerative diseases, and tumors [4, 5]. Therefore, inflammasomes may be attractive targets to treat these diseases. Autoinflammatory diseases are known to be caused by genetic mutations of inflammasome components [6–9]. Thus, we aim to develop reconstituted inflammasomes in a cell-free system in order to identify specific molecular-target drugs and elucidate the molecular pathogenesis of autoinflammatory diseases. In this review, we briefly describe the functions of several inflammasomes and related diseases, and reconstituted inflammasomes in a cell-free system.

* Correspondence: masumoto@m.ehime-u.ac.jp
[1]Department of Pathology, Ehime University Graduate School of Medicine and Proteo-Science Center, Shitsukawa 454, Toon 791-0295, Ehime, Japan
Full list of author information is available at the end of the article

General functions of inflammasomes and related diseases

The inflammasomes have been known as interleukin (IL)-1β processing platforms [10, 11]. There are several well-characterized inflammasomes: NACHT, LRR (NLR), and PYD domain-containing protein (NLRP)1 inflammasome [11], NLRP3 inflammasome [12], absent in melanoma (AIM)2 inflammasome [13–16], NLR and CARD domain-containing protein (NLRC)4 inflammasome [17], and pyrin inflammasome [18]. The inflammasome typically consists of an intracellular pathogen pattern-recognition receptor, an adaptor protein apoptosis-associated speck-like protein containing a caspase recruitment domain (ASC), and pro-caspase-1.

The NLRP1 inflammasome was the first described inflammasome to be described [11]. It has been reported to be activated by muramyl dipeptide (MDP), anthrax lethal toxins, and related to neuronal diseases [19].

The NLRP3 inflammasome is a prototype inflammasome, activated by various pathogen-associated molecular pattern molecules (PAMPs) and damage-associated molecular pattern molecules (DAMPs) [20]. NLRP3-activated PAMPs have been reported to include bacterium-derived pore-forming toxins, lethal toxins, flagellin/rod proteins, MDP, RNA, DNA, virus-derived RNA, M2 protein, fungus-derived β-glucans, hypha mannan, zymosan, and protozoon-derived hemozoin [21]. NLRP3-activated DAMPs include self-derived ATP, cholesterol crystals, monosodium urate (MSU) crystals, calcium pyrophosphate dihydrate (CPPD) crystals, glucose, β-amyloid, hyaluronic acid, and environment-derived alum, asbestos, silica, alloy particles, UV radiation, and skin irritants [21].

A single amino acid mutation in NLRP3 results in enhanced inflammasome activation, termed cryopyrin-associated periodic syndrome (CAPS), including familial cold autoinflammatory syndrome (FCAS), Muckle–Wells syndrome (MWS), and neonatal-onset multisystem inflammatory disease (NOMID)/chronic infantile neurologic, cutaneous, and arthritis (CINCA) syndrome, which leads to greater IL-1β secretion without DAMPs or PAMPs [22–27].

The AIM2 inflammasome consists of AIM2, ASC, and pro-caspase-1. AIM2 was originally identified as an interferon-gamma inducible gene product consisting of an N-terminal pyrin domain (PYD) and C-terminal hematopoietic interferon-inducible nuclear proteins with a 200-amino acid repeat (HIN-200) domain. AIM2 is differentially expressed following the suppression of the tumorigenic phenotype in a malignant melanoma cell line [28], and it subsequently acts as a sensor for cytoplasmic DNA, which forms an inflammasome with the ligand and ASC to activate caspase-1 [13–16]. The inappropriate recognition of cytoplasmic self-DNA by AIM2 contributes to the development of psoriasis, dermatitis, arthritis, and other autoimmune and inflammatory diseases [29].

The NLRC4 inflammasome consists of NLRC4, ASC, and pro-caspase-1. Since the protein-binding motif of NLRC4 is CARD instead of the PYD, NLRC4 interacts with ASC as well as pro-caspase-1 through their CARD. NLRC4 constitutes an inflammasome, which is required for the recognition of bacterial flagellin [30, 31]. Several mutations in the nucleotide-binding domain of NLRC4 cause autoinflammatory diseases, early-onset recurrent fever flares, and macrophage activation syndrome (MAS) [32–34].

Pyrin has been identified as a causative gene of the *MEFV* product of familial Mediterranean fever (FMF), an autosomal recessive inherited autoinflammatory syndrome [35]. Pyrin not only regulates several inflammasomes [36–38] but also constructs an inflammasome with ASC and pro-caspase-1, upon recognizing some pathogens [18, 39, 40]. Thus, FMF patients with some pyrin mutations are thought to show autosomal dominant inheritance [41–43].

General functions of the nodosomes and related diseases

Nod1 and Nod2, both of which are involved in host recognition of small molecules, activate NF-κB in response to sensing the component of peptidoglycan [44–47]. NF-κB activation in Nod1 and Nod2 depends on RIPK2 and IKK machinery [48]. The core ligand structure of Nod2 is *N*-Acetyl muramyl-L-alanyl-D-isoglutamine hydrate, also known as MDP, of which the structure is common in bacteria. The ligand for Nod1 is a dipeptide designated as D-glutamyl-*meso*-diaminopimelic acid (*i*E-DAP), with the structure being derived from a subgroup of bacteria [44–47].

Functional activation by genetic mutations of Nod2 is associated with autoinflammatory diseases, Blau syndrome (BS), and early-onset sarcoidosis (EOS), which are characteristics of systemic granulomatous diseases [49]. However, genetic and functional defects of Nod2 are associated with susceptibility to Crohn's disease, an inflammatory bowel disease. There is no known Nod1-related autoinflammatory disease, but associations between SNPs in NOD1 and several immune-related diseases, such as inflammatory bowel disease, atopic eczema, asthma, and rheumatoid arthritis have been reported [50–53].

Wheat germ cell-free protein synthesis for inflammasomes

To construct reconstituted inflammasomes in a cell-free system, we employed the wheat germ cell-free protein synthesis system rather than *Escherichia coli* expression system [54]. When we identified ASC a central adaptor protein of inflammasomes, ASC was discovered in the Triton X-100-insoluble fraction of promyelocytic leukemia cell line HL-60 cells [55], and it was difficult to synthesize recombinant NLRP3 protein using *E. coli* expression due to its solubility. On the other hand, the wheat germ cell-free protein synthesis has numerous advantages, such as low cost, ease of availability in large amounts, low endogenous incorporation, and the capacity to synthesize high-molecular-weight proteins [54]. In addition, it is suitable for the expression of eukaryotic proteins because it is eukaryotic system [55].

Reconstituted AIM2 inflammasome in a cell-free system

First, we describe an AIM2 inflammasome in a cell-free system as a prototype [56] because the AIM2 inflammasome has been well-characterized, and its ligand was reported to be present in poly-deoxyadenylic-deoxythymidylic acid, poly(dA:dT). The direct interaction between AIM2 and poly(dA:dT) was elucidated using the amplified luminescent proximity homogeneous assay (Alpha) [14]. In addition, activation of the AIM2 inflammasome has been reported to be related to various diseases [57–62], and it is thought to be an attractive drug target for diseases.

Our reconstituted AIM2 inflammasome basically consists of AIM2 and ASC, and it is considered sufficient for drug and ligand discovery as it assembles without pro-caspase-1 or any other components [56].

To synthesize the AIM2 inflammasome, PCR products for AIM2 and ASC were inserted into a Gateway™ pDONR™221 Vector (pDONR221) (Life Technologies, Carlsbad, CA, USA) using Gateway™ BP Clonase™ II Enzyme mix (Life Technologies, Carlsbad, CA, USA) to generate entry clones. The AIM2 entry clone pDONR221-AIM2 was inserted into pEU-E01-GW-bls-STOP for cell-free protein expression. The ASC entry clones pDONR221-ASC and pDONR221-ASC-PYD were inserted into pEU-E01-FLAG-GW-STOP using the Gateway™ LR Clonase™ II Enzyme mix (Life Technologies, Carlsbad, CA, USA). The constructed plasmids were used to synthesize specific proteins with the WEPRO1240 Expression Kit (Cell-Free, Inc., Matsuyama, Japan) [56].

In our AIM2 inflammasome, proximity between AIM2 and ASC is detected by the Alpha using the combination of protein-A-conjugated Alpha acceptor beads for FLAG-tagged proteins and streptavidin-conjugated Alpha donor beads for biotinylated proteins (Fig. 1).

The AIM2 inflammasome in a cell-free system assembles with its previously reported ligand poly(dA:dT), and the interaction between AIM2 and ASC was disrupted by anti-human ASC mAb, and previously reported inhibitors CRID3 and glycyrrhizin. Thus, our reconstituted AIM2 inflammasome in a cell-free system is useful for investigating novel ligands and drug discovery [56].

Reconstituted NLRP3 inflammasome in a cell-free system

When AIM2 is replaced by NLRP3, we can easily develop the NLRP3 inflammasome in a cell-free system.

There are so many mutations in NLRP3 that causes of autoinflammatory diseases including CAPS, and NLRP3 involve various inflammasomopathies. Thus, the reconstituted NLRP3 inflammasome in a cell-free system will be a useful tool for investigating inflammasomopathies and drug discovery. In this context, we are going to develop reconstituted NLRP3 inflammasome in a cell-free system.

Reconstituted Nod2 nodosome in a cell-free system

The autoinflammatory disease Blau syndrome (BS)/ early-onset sarcoidosis (EOS) is caused by a point mutation of Nod2 [49]. Therefore, the Nod2 nodosome may be an attractive drug target for the treatment of BS/EOS. We aimed to develop a reconstituted protein–protein interaction assay system between wild-type Nod2 and the BS/EOS-associated mutants of Nod2 and RIPK2 in a cell-free system, called the reconstituted Nod2 nodosome in a cell-free system [63].

The plasmids vector pDONR221-Nod2 and BS/EOS-associated mutants, pDONR221-Nod2-R334W and pDONR221-Nod2-N670K, were constructed. pDONR 221-RIPK2 and pDONR221-RIPK2-CARD were also constructed. Then, the proteins Nod2-WT-Btn, Nod2-R334W-Btn, Nod2-N670K-Btn, FLAG-RIPK2 and FLAG-RIPK2-CARD were synthesized using the wheat germ cell-free system in the same way as AIM2.

In our Nod2 nodosome, proximity between Nod2 and RIPK2 is basically detected by Alpha using the combination of protein-A-conjugated Alpha acceptor beads for FLAG-tagged proteins and streptavidin-conjugated Alpha donor beads for biotinylated proteins. The Nod2 nodosome in a cell-free system assembles with its previously reported ligand MDP. The Nod2 nodosomes with BS/EOS-associated mutations Nod2-R334W and Nod2-N670K were more sensitive to MDP than Nod2-WT. Therefore, we think that our Nod2 nodosome in a cell-free

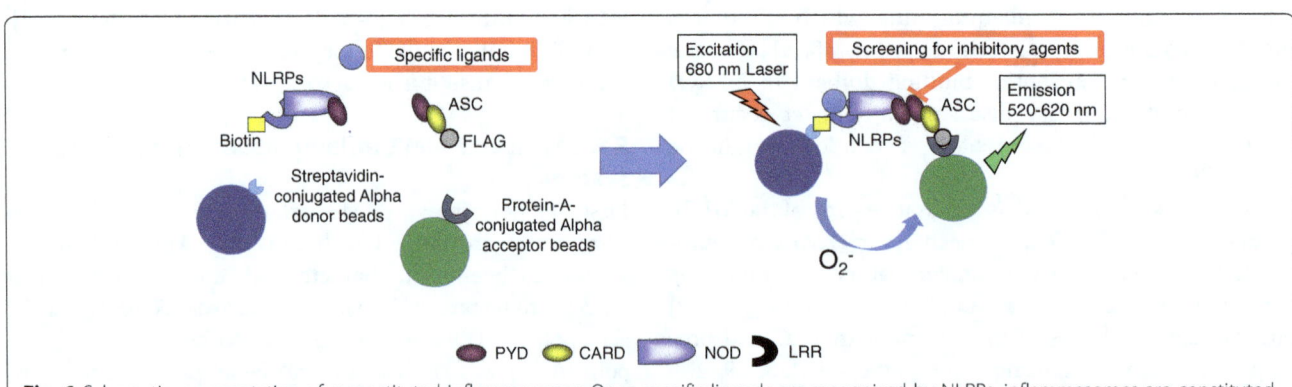

Fig. 1 Schematic representation of reconstituted inflammasomes. Once specific ligands are recognized by NLRPs, inflammasomes are constituted. Then, chemical energy of reactive oxygen from donor beads is transferred to acceptor beads and a signal is detected

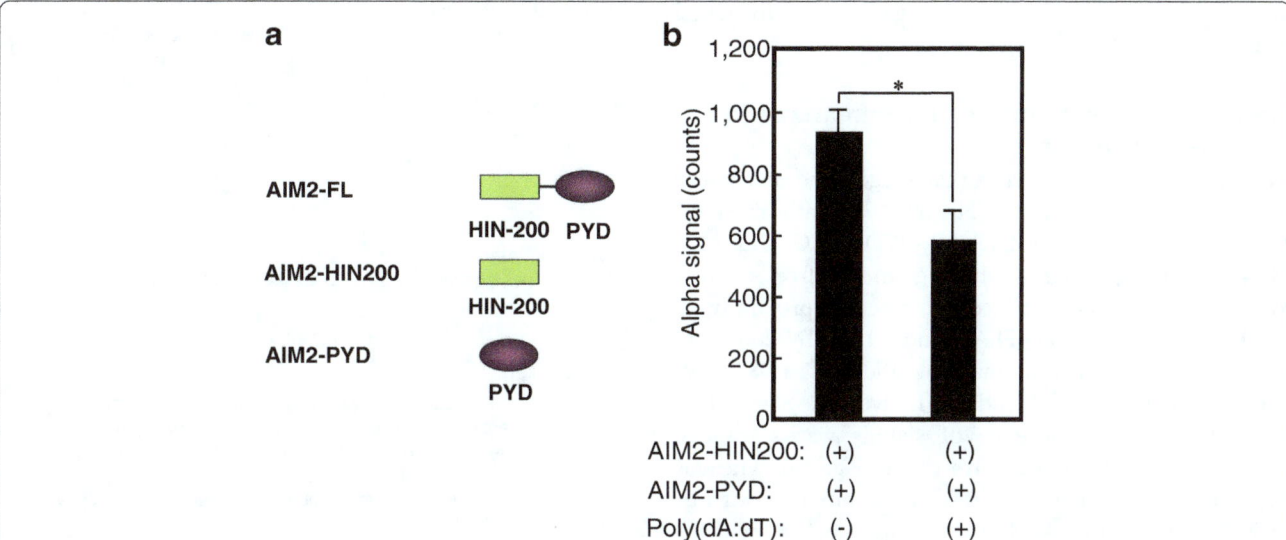

Fig. 2 poly(dA:dT) reduces the amplified luminescent proximity signal between the PYD domain of AIM2 and the HIN-200 domain of AIM2. A schematic representation of full-length AIM2 (AIM2-FL) and its truncated proteins, the HIN200 domain of AIM2 (AIM2-HIN200) and PYD domain of AIM2 (AIM2-PYD). We synthesized two truncated forms of AIM2, AIM2-PYD-FLAG and AIM-HIN-200-Biotin, using a wheat germ cell-free synthesis system (**a**). Synthetic protein–protein interactions were detected by the amplified luminescent proximity homogeneous assay (Alpha). A total of 100 ng of each protein indicated was incubated with 5 μg/mL anti-FLAG mAb M2, 16.67 μg/mL protein-A-conjugated Alpha acceptor beads (PerkinElmer, Waltham, MA, USA), and 16.67 μg/mL streptavidin-conjugated Alpha donor beads (PerkinElmer, Waltham, MA, USA) for 24 h with or without 5 mg/mL poly(dA:dT) (Invivogen, San Diego, CA, USA). Responses (counts) were measured using EnSpire™ Multimode Plate Reader (PerkinElmer, Waltham, MA, USA). The results are given as means ± standard deviation from triplicate wells. *Asterisk* indicates significance ($p < 0.01$) (**b**)

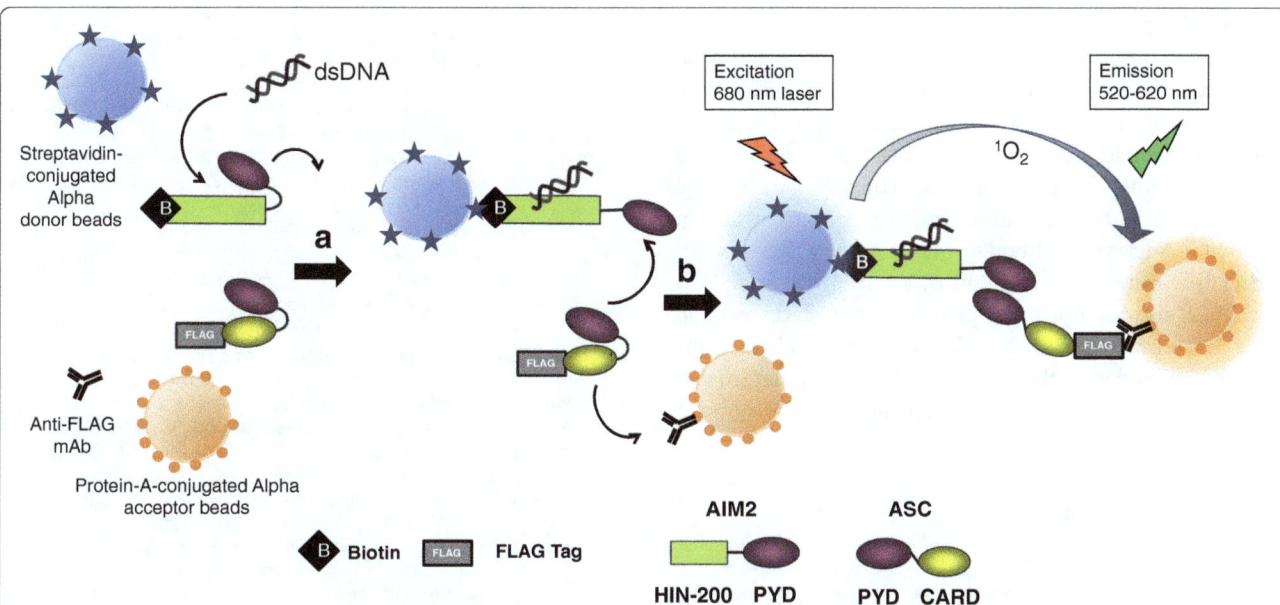

Fig. 3 A possible mechanism of AIM2 inflammasome in a cell-free system. The PYD domain of AIM2 interacts with the HIN-200 domain of AIM2 loosely upon being incubated with no materials. Once a specific ligand poly(dA:dT) stringently interacts with the HIN-200 domain of AIM2 and streptavidin-conjugated donor beads, then the PYD domain of AIM2 apart from the HIN-200 domain of AIM2 opens to interact with the PYD domain of ASC (**a**). Since the PYD domain of ASC loosely interacts with the CARD domain of ASC, the interaction between the PYD domain of AIM2 and PYD domain of ASC is thought to open the CARD domain of ASC, which will lead to interaction with protein A-conjugated acceptor beads (**b**)

system can be a useful tool for investigating the pathogenesis of BS/EOS and drug discovery [63].

How does the reconstituted inflammasome in a cell-free system work?

We show representative data that suggest the mechanism of how this system works (Fig. 2). We synthesized two truncated forms of AIM2, AIM2-PYD-FLAG and AIM-HIN-200-Biotin, using a wheat germ cell-free synthesis system (Fig. 2a). The amplified luminescence proximity signal between AIM2-PYD-FLAG and AIM-HIN-200-Biotin was 940.0 ± 100.5 with no materials and 626.7 ± 98.7 upon incubation with poly(dA:dT) (Invivogen, San Diego, CA, USA). The difference of signals was significant ($p = 0.000917$) using Student's t test (Fig. 2b). The data suggest that the PYD domain of AIM2 interacts with the HIN-200 domain of AIM2 loosely upon being incubated with no materials. Once the specific ligand poly(dA:dT) stringently interacts with the HIN-200 domain of AIM2, then the PYD domain of AIM2 apart from the HIN-200 domain of AIM2 is open to interact with the PYD domain of ASC. Since the PYD domain of ASC has been reported to loosely interact with the CARD domain of ASC [64], the interaction between the PYD domain of AIM2 and PYD domain of ASC is thought to open the CARD domain of ASC, which will lead to interaction with protein A-conjugated acceptor beads in the cell-free system (Fig. 3), or downstream CARD domain of caspase-1 in cells.

Conclusions

Various inflammasomes are thought to play important roles in the maintenance of the homeostasis of cells, tissues, and organs. Excess inflammasome signaling caused by genetic mutations or pathogens may contribute to known or unknown autoinflammatory diseases. Thus, inflammasomes are expected to become attractive targets to treat autoinflammatory diseases. Although our cell-free system is limited in that only an initial event of assembly between ASC or RIPK2 and an upstream protein is detected, reconstituted inflammasomes in a cell-free system will be useful tools for investigating the pathogenesis of autoinflammatory diseases and discovery of their therapeutics.

Acknowledgements
Not applicable.

Funding
This work was supported by the Platform for Drug Discovery, Informatics and Structural Life Science from the Ministry of Education, Culture, Sports, Science and Technology, Japan (H.T., T.S., and J.M.), the Center for Clinical and Translational Research of Kyushu University (J.M.), and a Grant-in-Aid for translational research toward the clarification of autoinflammatory mechanisms by familial Mediterranean fever (FMF). Inflammasome based on the Mediterranean fever (*MEFV*) gene analysis 26310301 from The Ministry of Health, Labour and Welfare, Japan (J.M.), and Grants-in-Aid for Scientific Research (JSPS KAKENHI grant numbers 26293232 26305024 and 17H04656) from The Ministry of Education, Culture, Sports, Science and Technology, Japan (J.M.).

Authors' contributions
The manuscript was written by all authors. Briefly, NK described about AIM2, TI described about Nod2, YI described about NLRP3. HT and TS synthesized proteins and described about wheat germ cell-free protein synthesis. SM, NN, MK drew figures. NK and JM described about inflammasome-related diseases and organized them. All authors read and approved the final manuscript.

Competing interests
All authors declare that they have no competing interests.

Author details
[1]Department of Pathology, Ehime University Graduate School of Medicine and Proteo-Science Center, Shitsukawa 454, Toon 791-0295, Ehime, Japan. [2]Divison of Proteo-Drug-Discovery Sciences, Ehime University Proteo-Science Center, Bunkyocho 3, Matsuyama 790-8577, Ehime, Japan. [3]Division of Cell-free Sciences, Ehime University Proteo-Science Center, Bunkyocho 3, Matsuyama 790-8577, Ehime, Japan.

References
1. Martinon F, Mayor A, Tschopp J. The inflammasomes: guardians of the body. Annu Rev Immunol. 2009;27:229–65.
2. Alnemri ES. Sensing cytoplasmic danger signals by the inflammasome. J Clin Immunol. 2010;30(4):512–9.
3. Franchi L, Eigenbrod T, Muñoz-Planillo R, Nuñez G. The inflammasome: a caspase-1-activation platform that regulates immune responses and disease pathogenesis. Nat Immunol. 2009;10(3):241–7.
4. Masters SL, Simon A, Aksentijevich I, Kastner DL. Horror autoinflammaticus: the molecular pathophysiology of autoinflammatory disease (*). Annu Rev Immunol. 2009;27:621–68.
5. Chen GY, Núñez G. Inflammasomes in intestinal inflammation and cancer. Gastroenterology. 2011;141(6):1986–99.
6. McDermott MF, Aksentijevich I, Galon J, McDermott EM, Ogunkolade BW, Centola M, Mansfield E, Gadina M, Karenko L, Pettersson T, McCarthy J, Frucht DM, Aringer M, Torosyan Y, Teppo AM, Wilson M, Karaarslan HM, Wan Y, Todd I, Wood G, Schlimgen R, Kumarajeewa TR, Cooper SM, Vella JP, Amos CI, Mulley J, Quane KA, Molloy MG, Ranki A, Powell RJ, Hitman GA, O'Shea JJ, Kastner DL. Germline mutations in the extracellular domains of the 55 kDa TNF receptor, TNFR1, define a family of dominantly inherited autoinflammatory syndromes. Cell. 1999;97(1):133–44.
7. Kastner DL, Aksentijevich I, Goldbach-Mansky R. Autoinflammatory disease reloaded: a clinical perspective. Cell. 2010;140(6):784–90.
8. Ombrello MJ, Kastner DL. Autoinflammation in 2010: expanding clinical spectrum and broadening therapeutic horizons. Nat Rev Rheumatol. 2011;7(2):82–4.
9. Pathak S, McDermott MF, Savic S. Autoinflammatory diseases: update on classification diagnosis and management. J Clin Pathol. 2017;70(1):1–8.
10. Srinivasula SM, Poyet JL, Razmara M, Datta P, Zhang Z, Alnemri ES. The PYRIN-CARD protein ASC is an activating adaptor for caspase-1. J Biol Chem. 2002;277(24):21119–22.
11. Martinon F, Burns K, Tschopp J. The inflammasome: a molecular platform triggering activation of inflammatory caspases and processing of proIL-β. Mol Cell. 2002;10(2):417–26.
12. Agostini L, Martinon F, Burns K, McDermott MF, Hawkins PN, Tschopp J. NALP3 forms an IL-1β-processing inflammasome with increased activity in Muckle-Wells autoinflammatory disorder. Immunity. 2004;20(3):319–25.
13. Roberts TL, Idris A, Dunn JA, Kelly GM, Burnton CM, Hodgson S, Hardy LL, Garceau V, Sweet MJ, Ross IL, Hume DA, Stacey KJ. HIN-200 proteins regulate caspase activation in response to foreign cytoplasmic DNA. Science. 2009;323(5917):1057–60.
14. Hornung V, Ablasser A, Charrel-Dennis M, Bauernfeind F, Horvath G, Caffrey DR, Latz E, Fitzgerald KA. AIM2 recognizes cytosolic dsDNA and forms a caspase-1-activating inflammasome with ASC. Nature. 2009;458(7237):514–8.
15. Fernandes-Alnemri T, Yu JW, Datta P, Wu J, Alnemri ES. AIM2 activates the inflammasome and cell death in response to cytoplasmic DNA. Nature. 2009;458(7237):509–13.
16. Bürckstümmer T, Baumann C, Blüml S, Dixit E, Dürnberger G, Jahn H, Planyavsky M, Bilban M, Colinge J, Bennett KL, Superti-Furga G. An

orthogonal proteomic-genomic screen identifies AIM2 as a cytoplasmic DNA sensor for the inflammasome. Nat Immunol. 2009;10(3):266–72.

17. Mariathasan S, Newton K, Monack DM, Vucic D, French DM, Lee WP, Roose-Girma M, Erickson S, Dixit VM. Differential activation of the inflammasome by caspase-1 adaptors ASC and Ipaf. Nature. 2004;430(6996):213–8.

18. Yu JW, Wu J, Zhang Z, Datta P, Ibrahimi I, Taniguchi S, Sagara J, Fernandes-Alnemri T, Alnemri ES. Cryopyrin and pyrin activate caspase-1, but not NF-κB, via ASC oligomerization. Cell Death Differ. 2006;13(2):236–49.

19. Walsh JG, Muruve DA, Power C. Inflammasomes in the CNS. Nat Rev Neurosci. 2014;15(2):84–97.

20. Latz E, Xiao TS, Stutz A. Activation and regulation of the inflammasomes. Nat Rev Immunol. 2013;13(6):397–411.

21. Davis BK, Wen H, Ting JP. The inflammasome NLRs in immunity, inflammation, and associated diseases. Annu Rev Immunol. 2011;29:707–35.

22. Hoffman HM, Mueller JL, Broide DH, Wanderer AA, Kolodner RD. Mutation of a new gene encoding a putative pyrin-like protein causes familial cold autoinflammatory syndrome and Muckle-Wells syndrome. Nat Genet. 2001;29(3):301–5.

23. Aksentijevich I, Nowak M, Mallah M, Chae JJ, Watford WT, Hofmann SR, Stein L, Russo R, Goldsmith D, Dent P, Rosenberg HF, Austin F, Remmers EF, Balow Jr JE, Rosenzweig S, Komarow H, Shoham NG, Wood G, Jones J, Mangra N, Carrero H, Adams BS, Moore TL, Schikler K, Hoffman H, Lovell DJ, Lipnick R, Barron K, O'Shea JJ, Kastner DL, Goldbach-Mansky R. De novo CIAS1 mutations, cytokine activation, and evidence for genetic heterogeneity in patients with neonatal-onset multisystem inflammatory disease (NOMID): a new member of the expanding family of pyrin-associated autoinflammatory diseases. Arthritis Rheum. 2002;46(12):3340–8.

24. Feldmann J, Prieur AM, Quartier P, Berquin P, Certain S, Cortis E, Teillac-Hamel D, Fischer A, de Saint Basile G. Chronic infantile neurological cutaneous and articular syndrome is caused by mutations in CIAS1, a gene highly expressed in polymorphonuclear cells and chondrocytes. Am J Hum Genet. 2002;71(1):198–203.

25. Goldbach-Mansky R, Dailey NJ, Canna SW, Gelabert A, Jones J, Rubin BI, Kim HJ, Brewer C, Zalewski C, Wiggs E, Hill S, Turner ML, Karp BI, Aksentijevich I, Pucino F, Penzak SR, Haverkamp MH, Stein L, Adams BS, Moore TL, Fuhlbrigge RC, Shaham B, Jarvis JN, O'Neil K, Vehe RK, Beitz LO, Gardner G, Hannan WP, Warren RW, Horn W, Cole JL, Paul SM, Hawkins PN, Pham TH, Snyder C, Wesley RA, Hoffmann SC, Holland SM, Butman JA, Kastner DL. Neonatal-onset multisystem inflammatory disease responsive to interleukin-1β inhibition. N Engl J Med. 2006;355(6):581–92.

26. Gattorno M, Tassi S, Carta S, Delfino L, Ferlito F, Pelagatti MA, D'Osualdo A, Buoncompagni A, Alpigiani MG, Alessio M, Martini A, Rubartelli A. Pattern of interleukin-1β secretion in response to lipopolysaccharide and ATP before and after interleukin-1 blockade in patients with CIAS1 mutations. Arthritis Rheum. 2007;56(9):3138–48.

27. Hoffman HM, Brydges SD. Genetic and molecular basis of inflammasome-mediated disease. J Biol Chem. 2011;286(13):10889–96.

28. DeYoung KL, Ray ME, Su YA, Anzick SL, Johnstone RW, Trapani JA, Meltzer PS, Trent JM. Cloning a novel member of the human interferon-inducible gene family associated with control of tumorigenicity in a model of human melanoma. Oncogene. 1997;15(4):453–7.

29. Man SM, Karki R, Kanneganti TD. AIM2 inflammasome in infection, cancer, and autoimmunity: role in DNA sensing, inflammation, and innate immunity. Eur J Immunol. 2016;46(2):269–80.

30. Miao EA, Alpuche-Aranda CM, Dors M, Clark AE, Bader MW, Miller SI, Aderem A. Cytoplasmic flagellin activates caspase-1 and secretion of interleukin 1beta via Ipaf. Nat Immunol. 2006;7(6):569–75.

31. Franchi L, Amer A, Body-Malapel M, Kanneganti TD, Ozören N, Jagirdar R, Inohara N, Vandenabeele P, Bertin J, Coyle A, Grant EP, Núñez G. Cytosolic flagellin requires Ipaf for activation of caspase-1 and interleukin 1beta in salmonella-infected macrophages. Nat Immunol. 2006;7(6):576–82.

32. Romberg N, Al Moussawi K, Nelson-Williams C, Stiegler AL, Loring E, Choi M, Overton J, Meffre E, Khokha MK, Huttner AJ, West B, Podoltsev NA, Boggon TJ, Kazmierczak BI, Lifton RP. Mutation of NLRC4 causes a syndrome of enterocolitis and autoinflammation. Nat Genet. 2014;46(10):1135–9.

33. Canna SW, de Jesus AA, Gouni S, Brooks SR, Marrero B, Liu Y, DiMattia MA, Zaal KJ, Sanchez GA, Kim H, Chapelle D, Plass N, Huang Y, Villarino AV, Biancotto A, Fleisher TA, Duncan JA, O'Shea JJ, Benseler S, Grom A, Deng Z, Laxer RM, Goldbach-Mansky R. An activating NLRC4 inflammasome mutation causes autoinflammation with recurrent macrophage activation syndrome. Nat Genet. 2014;46(10):1140–6.

34. Kitamura A, Sasaki Y, Abe T, Kano H, Yasutomo K. An inherited mutation in NLRC4 causes autoinflammation in human and mice. J Exp Med. 2014;211(12):2385–96.

35. The International FMF Consortium. Ancient missense mutations in a new member of the RoRet gene family are likely to cause familial Mediterranean fever. The International FMF Consortium Cell. 1997;90(4):797–807.

36. Dowds TA, Masumoto J, Chen FF, Ogura Y, Inohara N, Núñez G. Regulation of cryopyrin/Pypaf1 signaling by pyrin, the familial Mediterranean fever gene product. Biochem Biophys Res Commun. 2003;302(3):575–80.

37. Masumoto J, Dowds TA, Schaner P, Chen FF, Ogura Y, Li M, Zhu L, Katsuyama T, Sagara J, Taniguchi S, Gumucio DL, Núñez G, Inohara N. ASC is an activating adaptor for NF-kappa B and caspase-8-dependent apoptosis. Biochem Biophys Res Commun. 2003;303(1):69–73.

38. Papin S, Cuenin S, Agostini L, Martinon F, Werner S, Beer HD, Grütter C, Grütter M, Tschopp J. The SPRY domain of Pyrin, mutated in familial Mediterranean fever patients, interacts with inflammasome components and inhibits proIL-1β processing. Cell Death Differ. 2007;14(8):1457–66.

39. Mansfield E, Chae JJ, Komarow HD, Brotz TM, Frucht DM, Aksentijevich I, Kastner DL. The familial Mediterranean fever protein, pyrin, associates with microtubules and colocalizes with actin filaments. Blood. 2001;98(3):851–9.

40. Kim ML, Chae JJ, Park YH, De Nardo D, Stirzaker RA, Ko HJ, Tye H, Cengia L, DiRago L, Metcalf D, Roberts AW, Kastner DL, Lew AM, Lyras D, Kile BT, Croker BA, Masters SL. Aberrant actin depolymerization triggers the pyrin inflammasome and autoinflammatory disease that is dependent on IL-18, not IL-1β. J Exp Med. 2015;212(6):927–38.

41. Fukushima Y, Obara K, Hirata H, Sugiyama K, Fukuda T, Takabe K. Three Japanese patients (mother and two children) with familial Mediterranean fever associated with compound heterozygosity for L110P/E148Q/M694I and an autosomal true dominant inheritance pattern. Asian Pac J Allergy Immunol. 2013;31(4):325–9.

42. Stoffels M, Szperl A, Simon A, Netea MG, Plantinga TS, van Deuren M, Kamphuis S, Lachmann HJ, Cuppen E, Kloosterman WP, Frenkel J, van Diemen CC, Wijmenga C, van Gijn M, van der Meer JW. MEFV mutations affecting pyrin amino acid 577 cause autosomal dominant autoinflammatory disease. Ann Rheum Dis. 2014;73(2):455–61.

43. Marzano A, Damiani G, Ceccherini I, Berti E, Gattorno M, Cugno M. Autoinflammation in pyoderma gangrenosum and its syndromic form PASH. Br J Dermatol. 2016. doi:10.1111/bjd.15226 [Epub ahead of print].

44. Chamaillard M, Hashimoto M, Horie Y, Masumoto J, Qiu S, Saab L, Ogura Y, Kawasaki A, Fukase K, Kusumoto S, Valvano MA, Foster SJ, Mak TW, Núñez G, Inohara N. An essential role for NOD1 in host recognition of bacterial peptidoglycan containing diaminopimelic acid. Nat Immunol. 2003;4(7):702–7.

45. Girardin SE, Boneca IG, Carneiro LA, Antignac A, Jéhanno M, Viala J, Tedin K, Taha MK, Labigne A, Zähringer U, Coyle AJ, DiStefano PS, Bertin J, Sansonetti PJ, Philpott DJ. Nod1 detects a unique muropeptide from gram-negative bacterial peptidoglycan. Science. 2003;300(5625):1584–7.

46. Inohara N, Ogura Y, Fontalba A, Gutierrez O, Pons F, Crespo J, Fukase K, Inamura S, Kusumoto S, Hashimoto M, Foster SJ, Moran AP, Fernandez-Luna JL, Nuñez G. Host recognition of bacterial muramyl dipeptide mediated through NOD2. Implications for Crohn's disease. J Biol Chem. 2003;278(8):5509–12.

47. Girardin SE, Boneca IG, Viala J, Chamaillard M, Labigne A, Thomas G, Philpott DJ, Sansonetti PJ. Nod2 is a general sensor of peptidoglycan through muramyl dipeptide (MDP) detection. J Biol Chem. 2003;278(11):8869–72.

48. Kobayashi K, Inohara N, Hernandez LD, Galán JE, Núñez G, Janeway CA, Medzhitov R, Flavell RA. RIPK2/Rip2/CARDIAK mediates signalling for receptors of the innate and adaptive immune systems. Nature. 2002;416(6877):194–9.

49. Miceli-Richard C, Lesage S, Rybojad M, Prieur AM, Manouvrier-Hanu S, Häfner R, Chamaillard M, Zouali H, Thomas G, Hugot JP. CARD15 mutations in Blau syndrome. Nat Genet. 2001;29(1):19–20.

50. McGovern DP, Hysi P, Ahmad T, van Heel DA, Moffatt MF, Carey A, Cookson WO, Jewell DP. Association between a complex insertion/deletion polymorphism in NOD1 (CARD4) and susceptibility to inflammatory bowel disease. Hum Mol Genet. 2005;14(10):1245–50.

51. Weidinger S, Klopp N, Rummler L, Wagenpfeil S, Novak N, Baurecht HJ, Groer W, Darsow U, Heinrich J, Gauger A, Schafer T, Jakob T, Behrendt H, Wichmann HE, Ring J, Illig T. Association of NOD1 polymorphisms with atopic eczema and related phenotypes. J Allergy Clin Immunol. 2005;116(1):177–84.

52. Hysi P, Kabesch M, Moffatt MF, Schedel M, Carr D, Zhang Y, Boardman B, von Mutius E, Weiland SK, Leupold W, Fritzsch C, Klopp N, Musk AW, James A,

Nunez G, Inohara N, Cookson WO. NOD1 variation, immunoglobulin E and asthma. Hum Mol Genet. 2005;14(7):935–41.

53. Plantinga TS, Fransen J, Knevel R, Netea MG, Zwerina J, Helsen MM, van der Meer JW, van Riel PL, Schett G, van der Helm-van Mil AH, van den Berg WB, Joosten LA. Role of NOD1 polymorphism in susceptibility and clinical progression of rheumatoid arthritis. Rheumatology (Oxford). 2013;52(5):806–14.

54. Madin K, Sawasaki T, Ogasawara T, Endo Y. A highly efficient and robust cell-free protein synthesis system prepared from wheat embryos: plants apparently contain a suicide system directed at ribosomes. Proc Natl Acad Sci U S A. 2000;97(2):559–64.

55. Masumoto J, Taniguchi S, Ayukawa K, Sarvotham H, Kishino T, Niikawa N, Hidaka E, Katsuyama T, Higuchi T, Sagara J. ASC, a novel 22-kDa protein, aggregates during apoptosis of human promyelocytic leukemia HL-60 cells. J Biol Chem. 1999;274(48):33835–8.

56. Kaneko N, Ito Y, Iwasaki T, Takeda H, Sawasaki T, Migita K, Agematsu K, Kawakami A, Morikawa S, Mokuda S, Kurata M, Masumoto J. Reconstituted AIM2 inflammasome in cell-free system. J Immunol Methods. 2015;426:76–81.

57. Dombrowski Y, Peric M, Koglin S, Kammerbauer C, Göss C, Anz D, Simanski M, Gläser R, Harder J, Hornung V, Gallo RL, Ruzicka T, Besch R, Schauber J. Cytosolic DNA triggers inflammasome activation in keratinocytes in psoriatic lesions. Sci Transl Med. 2011;3(82):82ra38.

58. Javierre BM, Fernandez AF, Richter J, Al-Shahrour F, Martin-Subero JI, Rodriguez-Ubreva J, Berdasco M, Fraga MF, O'Hanlon TP, Rider LG, Jacinto FV, Lopez-Longo FJ, Dopazo J, Forn M, Peinado MA, Carreño L, Sawalha AH, Harley JB, Siebert R, Esteller M, Miller FW, Ballestar E. Changes in the pattern of DNA methylation associate with twin discordance in systemic lupus erythematosus. Genome Res. 2010;20(2):170–9.

59. Dihlmann S, Erhart P, Mehrabi A, Nickkholgh A, Lasitschka F, Böckler D, Hakimi M. Increased expression and activation of absent in melanoma 2 inflammasome components in lymphocytic infiltrates of abdominal aortic aneurysms. Mol Med. 2014;20:230–7.

60. Zhen J, Zhang L, Pan J, Ma S, Yu X, Li X, Chen S, Du W. AIM2 mediates inflammation-associated renal damage in hepatitis B virus-associated glomerulonephritis by regulating caspase-1, IL-1β, and IL-18. Mediators Inflamm. 2014;2014:190860.

61. Dihlmann S, Tao S, Echterdiek F, Herpel E, Jansen L, Chang-Claude J, Brenner H, Hoffmeister M, Kloor M. Lack of absent in melanoma 2 (AIM2) expression in tumor cells is closely associated with poor survival in colorectal cancer patients. Int J Cancer. 2014;135(10):2387–96.

62. Ponomareva L, Liu H, Duan X, Dickerson E, Shen H, Panchanathan R, Choubey D. AIM2, an IFN-inducible cytosolic DNA sensor, in the development of benign prostate hyperplasia and prostate cancer. Mol Cancer Res. 2013;11(10):1193–202.

63. Iwasaki T, Kaneko N, Ito Y, Takeda H, Sawasaki T, Heike T, Migita K, Agematsu K, Kawakami A, Morikawa S, Mokuda S, Kurata M, Masumoto J. Nod2-nodosome in a cell-free system: implications in pathogenesis and drug discovery for Blau syndrome and early-onset sarcoidosis. ScientificWorldJournal. 2016;2016:2597376.

64. Masumoto J, Taniguchi S, Sagara J. Pyrin N-terminal homology domain- and caspase recruitment domain-dependent oligomerization of ASC. Biochem Biophys Res Commun. 2001;280(3):652–5.

18

Considerations in hiPSC-derived cartilage for articular cartilage repair

Akihiro Yamashita[1], Yoshihiro Tamamura[1], Miho Morioka[1], Peter Karagiannis[2], Nobuyuki Shima[1] and Noriyuki Tsumaki[1*]

Abstract

Background: A lack of cell or tissue sources hampers regenerative medicine for articular cartilage damage.

Main text: We review and discuss the possible use of pluripotent stem cells as a new source for future clinical use. Human induced pluripotent stem cells (hiPSCs) have several advantages over human embryonic stem cells (hESCs). Methods for the generation of chondrocytes and cartilage from hiPSCs have been developed. To reduce the cost of this regenerative medicine, allogeneic transplantation is preferable. hiPSC-derived cartilage shows low immunogenicity like native cartilage, because the cartilage is avascular and chondrocytes are segregated by the extracellular matrix. In addition, we consider our experience with the aberrant deposition of lipofuscin or melanin on cartilage during the chondrogenic differentiation of hiPSCs.

Short conclusion: Cartilage generated from allogeneic hiPSC-derived cartilage can be used to repair articular cartilage damage.

Keywords: Chondrocytes, Articular cartilage, Regeneration, Induced pluripotent stem cells, Transplantation

Background

Articular cartilage covers the ends of bones and composes joints, providing lubrication between opposing bones during joint motion. Cartilage is avascular and consists of chondrocytes embedded in abundant extracellular matrix (ECM), in which collagen fibrils form three-dimensional (3D) networks that provide scaffolding for proteoglycan. One function of cartilage ECM is to confer mechanical properties to cartilage tissue in order to sustain smooth joint motion. Chondrocytes and cartilage ECM have a mutually dependent relationship: Chondrocytes produce and maintain ECM, and ECM is necessary for the chondrocytes to sustain their chondrocytic property including the production of cartilage ECM. This mutual relationship is indispensable for the homeostasis of cartilage. Cartilage, when damaged through trauma, has only limited capacity for repair, probably because the damage causes a loss of cartilage ECM, disrupting the chondrocytic environment. The continued use of joints with damaged cartilage and poor repair capacity gradually expands the damaged area on the joint surface, resulting in debilitating conditions such as osteoarthritis.

Current regenerative treatments for articular cartilage damage

Microfracture is the preferred treatment when the size of the articular cartilage defect is relatively small (less than 2–4 cm^2). In this treatment, the damaged area of the cartilage is removed to create a defect, and small holes are made through the subchondral bone, which allows bone marrow cells to fill the defect. However, the resulting repair tissue made by the bone marrow cells is fibrous, which is not as functional as articular cartilage. Mosaicplasty is another preferred treatment for small defects. Here, multiple autologous cylindrical osteochondral grafts are harvested from the periphery of the articular surface and implanted into the damaged area. Mosaicplasty has the advantage of transplanting viable hyaline-like cartilage. Nevertheless, this technique is restricted by the availability of harvestable autologous graft and by the donor-site morbidity [1]. For larger articular cartilage defects, autologous chondrocyte transplantation (ACI) is preferred. Here, a small piece of cartilage is harvested from the periphery of the articular surface and subjected to treatment for the isolation of its

* Correspondence: ntsumaki@cira.kyoto-u.ac.jp
[1]Cell Induction and Regulation Field, Department of Clinical Application, Center for iPS Cell Research and Application, Kyoto University, Kyoto, Japan
Full list of author information is available at the end of the article

chondrocytes. These chondrocytes are then expanded in monolayer culture and transplanted into the damaged area [2]. Although ACI provides good clinical results, it has limitations. The isolation of chondrocytes from cartilage ECM in culture causes a loss of the chondrocytic property and results in the conversion of the chondrocytes to fibroblastic cells [3–5]. Thus, the repaired tissue includes fibrous tissue, which has inferior joint function compared with articular cartilage [6]. Further, the transplanted cells constitute only a limited portion of the repaired tissue, while the remainder is composed of host cells. In fact, the benefit of the transplanted cells may partly come from the secretion of factors that stimulate the host cells, i.e., trophic effects. In addition to the physiology of the repair, another demerit of ACI is that patients are burdened with sacrificing donor sites and two-stage surgery.

Mesenchymal stem cells (MSCs) are alternative cell sources for cartilage repair. MSCs can be obtained from the bone marrow, adipose tissue, and synovium. Although MSCs have an ability to be differentiated toward chondrocytes, this ability tends to be lost after expansion [7]. Evidence that transplanted MSC-derived chondrocytes constitute repaired cartilage in vivo is scant, and, like ACI, the effects of the transplanted MSCs are considered trophic, in which secreted factors from the MSCs stimulate host cells to repair the tissue [8–10].

Because the repair mechanism of ACI and MSC transplantation involves trophic factors that act on host cells, microfracture is often employed with these methods to provide host cells from the bone marrow. However, whatever the stimulation, there is a limitation in the quality of the repair tissue so long the treatment depends on host cells for the creation of repair tissue.

The transplantation of allogeneic cartilage could resolve the scarcity of cells and the poor chondrocytic property of the transplants. Allogeneic cartilage transplantation is distinct from ACI or MSC transplantation in that the transplants are not mere cells, but actual cartilage tissue that can constitute most of the repair. Cartilage is considered immunoprivileged tissue [11, 12] because it lacks vasculature and because chondrocytes are embedded in the ECM, protecting the cells from immunological reactions. Indeed, allogeneic cartilage harvested from juveniles [12–16] have been transplanted successfully to treat defects. However, the lack of donors, the heterogeneous quality of the cartilage, and the risk of disease transmission are all limitations associated with allogeneic sources.

Chondrocytes and cartilage generated from pluripotent stem cells as a source for regenerative medicine

The scarcity of allogeneic sources could potentially be resolved with human pluripotent stem cells (hPSCs) such as human embryonic stem cells (hESCs) [17] and human induced pluripotent stem cells (hiPSCs) [18]. ESCs and

iPSCs share characteristic properties, such as pluripotency and self-renewal, and can be maintained in identical culture conditions. However, they differ in their preparation: ESCs are acquired from inner cell mass of embryos, while iPSCs are somatic cells, such as skin cells or blood cells, that have been reprogrammed to the pluripotent state by the introduction of specific factors [19]. Methods for the differentiation of both cells toward chondrocytes have been developed and are interchangeable. Because hESCs and hiPSCs can be expanded almost infinitely due to their self-renewal capacity, a large number of chondrocytes can be prepared. In fact, it is now possible to generate enough chondrocytes of good quality for regenerative medicine at the experimental level, although several issues must be resolved before translating these experimental findings to the clinic.

Autologous vs. allogeneic transplantation

One advantage of hiPSCs over hESCs is that their creation does not involve the destruction of an embryo, thus avoiding certain ethical controversies. Another merit is that hiPSCs can be made from the patient's own cells, permitting the possibility of autologous transplants [20]. However, the preparation of patient-iPSCs and subsequent differentiation under good manufacturing practice (GMP) guidelines is costly. To reduce the cost and to provide treatment to a large population, a bank of allogeneic clinical GMP grade hiPSC lines is being established [21, 22]. To reduce the risk of immune rejection during the transplantation of tissues generated from allogeneic hiPSCs, this iPSC library is prepared from donors homozygous for major HLA types. It is much easier to prepare homozygous HLA hiPSCs than hESCs, because it is easier to find individuals who bear homozygous HLA types and are willing to donate their somatic cells for iPSC generation compared with embryos for ESC generation. It is estimated that a bank of 1, 50, and 140 cell lines homozygous for major HLA types from Japan would respectively match 17, 73, and 90% of the population [22].

As explained above, cartilage is considered to have low immunogenicity, and the transplantation of allogeneic cartilage has been performed in a large number of patients without matching for HLA types and without the administration of immunosuppressive drugs. The transplantation of allogeneic, particulated juvenile articular cartilage has given good clinical results [14], although the long-term clinical outcome remains to be investigated. Cartilage can be generated from hiPSCs by making hiPSC-derived chondrocytes that produce and deposit ECM around themselves in 3D culture [23, 24]. The avascular structure of cartilage and ECM produced from the chondrocytes prevent a recipient's immune cells from contacting the chondrocytes in the transplanted hiPSC-derived cartilage. Mixed lymphocyte reaction assays have shown that hiPSC-derived cartilage has the low immunogenicity of human cartilage [25].

Moreover, hiPSC-derived chondrocytes are more similar to juvenile chondrocytes than to adult chondrocytes, and it has been reported that cartilage from juveniles have more anabolic activity and are less antigenic than those from adults [12, 16, 26]. These findings imply that cartilage prepared from a single allogeneic hiPSC or hESC clone could be used for all patients, which would standardize the quality and lower the cost of this regenerative medicine.

Generation of cartilage from hiPSCs

The basic principle in currently available protocols for the chondrogenic differentiation of PSCs is to direct cell fate to chondrocytic lineage and to eliminate non-chondrocytic cells [20, 27–29]. To realize this scheme, the composition of the culture medium and supplements, including growth factors such as TGF-β, BMP, WNT, and FGF; the cell density; and the coating of the dishes on which the cells are grown must be considered.

We previously developed a method to generate cartilage from hiPSCs [23, 24]. hiPSCs in adhesion culture were initially differentiated into mesendodermal cells in the presence of WNT and Activin. Then, the cells were differentiated into chondrocytes in chondrogenic medium containing TGF-β, BMP-2, and GDF-5. The resulting chondrocytes were subsequently transferred into 3D suspension culture in which the chondrocytes secreted and accumulated cartilage ECM around themselves to create cartilaginous tissues that look like white particles of 2–3 mm diameter (Fig. 1a, b). Histological analysis of each particle showed that the particles consisted of central cartilaginous tissue and were surrounded by membranous tissue (Fig. 1c). This structure may correspond to cartilage surrounded by perichondrium. Although the observation periods are limited, transplantation of the hiPSC-derived cartilage into articular cartilage defects in immunodeficient rats and immunosuppressed mini-pigs showed that the transplanted cartilage survived and had potential for integration into native cartilage [24]. These results suggest that hiPSC-derived cartilage can be used to repair articular cartilage damage.

Aberrant deposition of lipofuscin or melanin during chondrogenic differentiation of hiPSCs

Protocols for chondrogenic differentiation should be robust and produce cartilage of high quality. However, it

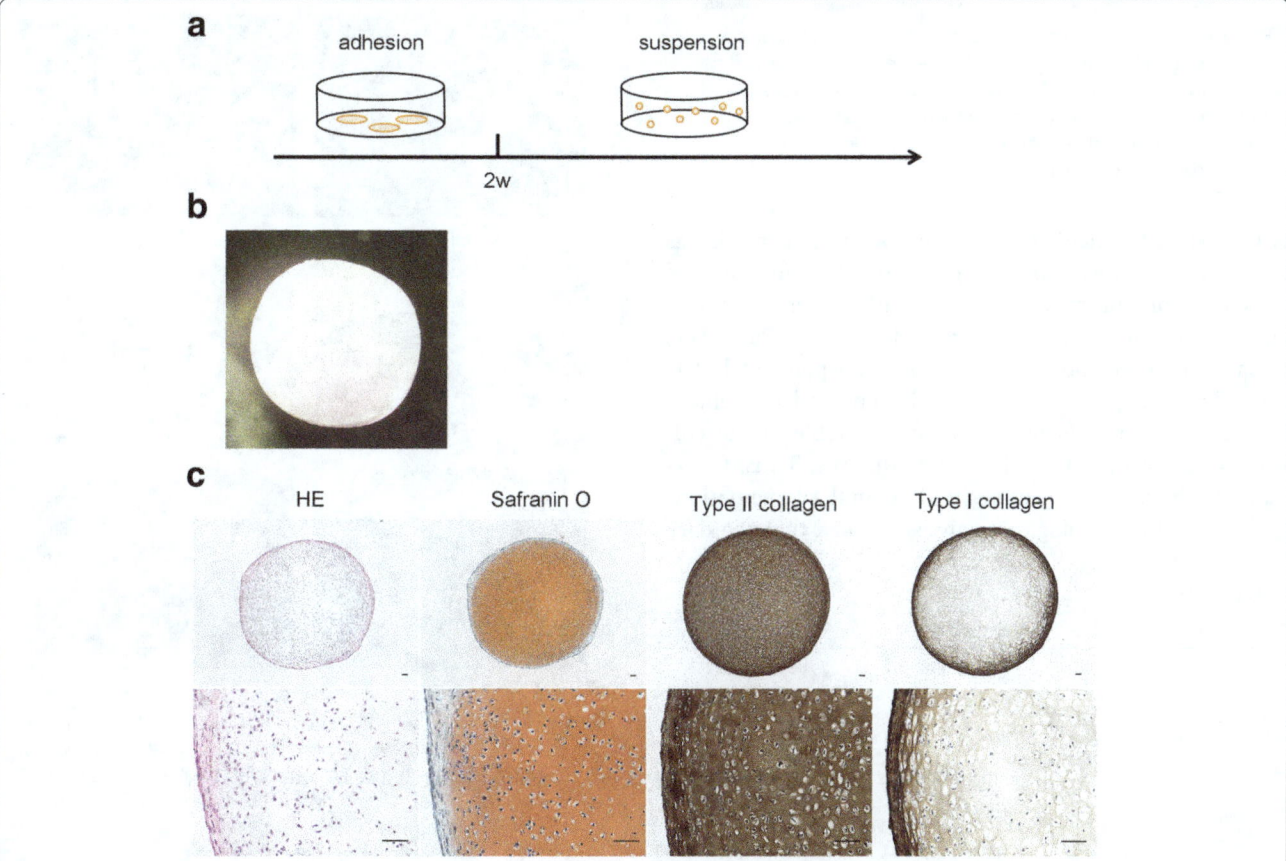

Fig. 1 Generation of cartilaginous particles from hiPSCs. **a** Scheme of the chondrogenic differentiation of hiPSCs. **b** Image of a hiPSC-derived cartilaginous particle at 12 weeks. **c** Histological analysis of the hiPSC-derived cartilaginous particle at 12 weeks. Semiserial sections were stained with hematoxylin-eosin and safranin O-fast green-iron hematoxylin and immunostained with anti-type II collagen antibodies and anti-type I collagen antibodies. Bars, 50 μm.

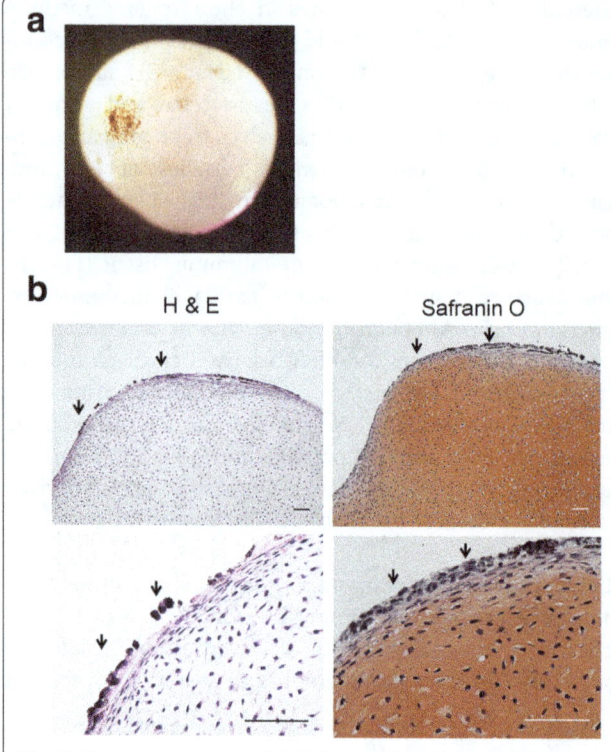

Fig. 2 Aberrant emergence of dark dots on the surface of hiPSC-derived cartilaginous particles. **a** Image of a hiPSC-derived cartilaginous particle with dark dots at 12 weeks. **b** Histological analysis of the hiPSC-derived cartilaginous particle in **a**. Semiserial sections were stained with hematoxylin-eosin and safranin O-fast green-iron hematoxylin. Arrows indicate dark dots. Bars, 50 μm.

is known in the field that culture does not always go as expected. As an example, we have observed unexplained dark dots on the surface of some hiPSC-derived cartilaginous particles on rare occasion (Fig. 2a). This phenomenon was observed in several independent hiPSC lines. The presence of malaria pathogens and formalin is known to cause artificial dark pigments (Table 1), but culture conditions are free of these substances. Thus, to explain these dots, we investigated natural pigmentations (Table 1) [30]. Histological analysis revealed that the dark

Table 1 Pigments

Source	Pigment type	Color
Hematogenous	Hemoglobin	Red to brown
	Hemosiderin	Yellow to brown
	Bile	Yellow to brown
	Porphyrin	Dark brown
Non-hematogenous	Melanin	Brown to black
	Chromaffin	Dark brown
	Lipofuscin	Yellow to brown
Artifact	Malaria	Dark brown
	Formalin	Dark brown

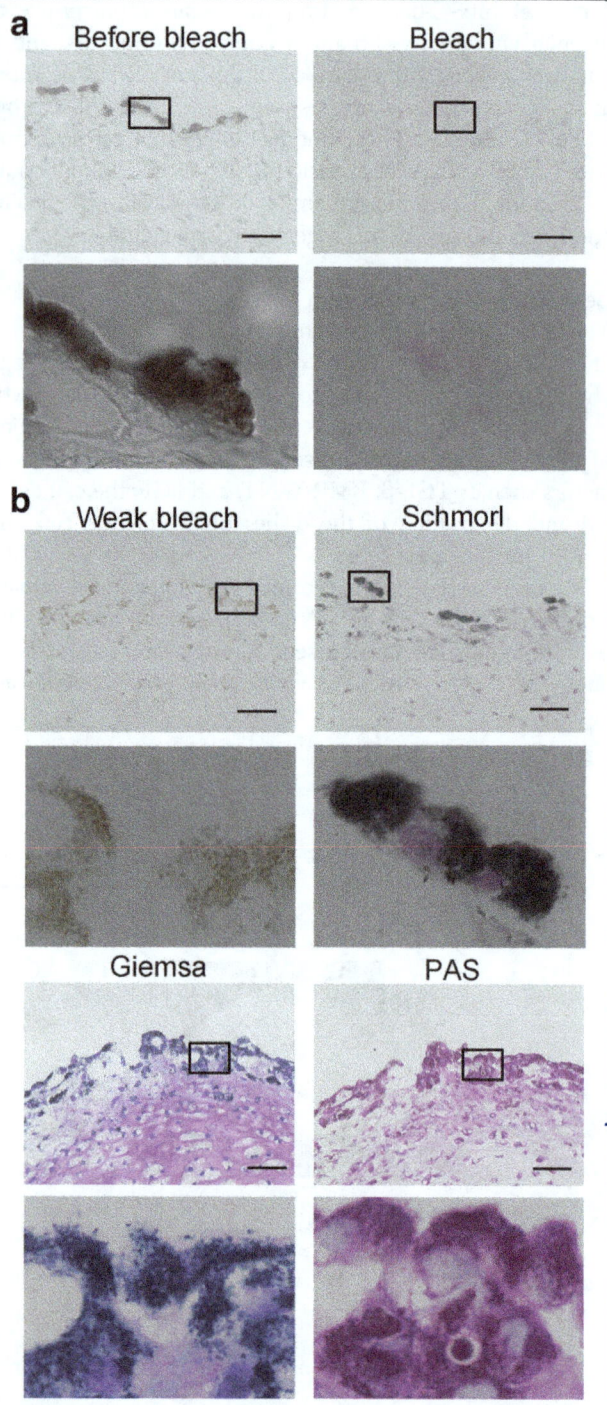

Fig. 3 Analysis of dark dots on hiPSC-derived cartilaginous particles. Histological analysis of a hiPSC-derived cartilaginous particle with dark dots at 12 weeks. **a** Sections were bleached and counterstained with kernechtrot. **b** Sections were initially bleached weakly and subjected to PAS staining, Giemsa staining, and Schmorl's reaction. Bars, 50 μm. Boxed regions are magnified in the images below.

dots resided in the cytoplasm of cells located on the surface of the particles (Fig. 2b). The dark dots lost color after bleaching by treatment with potassium permanganate, suggesting they are not hematogenous pigments, which are resistant to bleaching [31] (Fig. 3a). Among non-hematogenous pigments, melanin, chromaffin, and lipofuscin look dark and are sensitive to bleach [32, 33]. These three pigments can be discriminated by reactions to PAS staining, Schmorl's reaction, and Giemsa staining (Table 2) [32–35]. Further investigation found that the dark dots were positively stained with Schmorl [34]. Giemsa staining indicated dark blue [35], but we could not rule out that it indicated dark green (Fig. 3b). The area stained by PAS overlapped the dark dots, although not completely. Based on these findings, we considered the dark dots on the surface of hiPSC-derived cartilage to be either lipofuscin or possibly melanin. Either case could compromise the use of these particles for regenerative medicine.

Lipofuscin is a cross-linked aggregate that consists of oxidized proteins and lipids and is resistant to cellular proteolytic systems [36, 37]. Lipofuscin is insoluble and is not exocytosed by cells such that it resides in the cytosol. Lipofuscin is found in postmitotic cells in various tissues and organs and has two sources. One is damaged mitochondria caused by a malfunction of the mitochondrial repair system due to aging and/or excess amounts of reactive oxygen species (ROS). The other is damaged proteins, such as oxidized proteins and unfolded proteins that cross-link in the cytosol. Normally, these damaged particles are taken up by lysosomes and degraded. A failure in this degradation leads to the damaged mitochondria and proteins within the lysosomes cross-linking and binding more particles, such as lipids, to produce lipofuscin. Lipofuscin enters the cytosol if the lysosomes rupture. There, lipofuscin may disturb cell function and consume both lysosomal enzyme capacity and lysosomal space, further reducing lysosomal degradation capacity. Furthermore, it may have a chemically reactive surface that can disturb cellular metabolism. Lipofuscin has been reported to accumulate in natural cartilage [38]. Although the effects of lipofuscin on cartilage metabolism are unknown, culture conditions that produce no lipofuscin should be used for repairing cartilage damage.

The mechanism by which dark dots aberrantly form during the chondrogenic differentiation of hiPSCs remains to be elucidated. We found the dark dots reproducibly appeared when we increased cell density during the differentiation of hiPSCs toward chondrocytes. Consistently, dark dots did not appear when the differentiation protocol was done without cell overgrowth. It has been reported that lipofuscin forms in the chondrogenic micromass culture of chick limb bud mesenchymal cells when they are treated with agents that increase the generation of OH(.) radicals [39]. Whether the generation of OH(.) radicals contributes to the dark dots seen with cell overgrowth during the chondrogenic differentiation of hiPSCs remains to be determined.

On the other hand, if the dark dots are due to the presence of melanin, then it is likely that a differentiated subpopulation took the melanocyte fate. It is unknown whether here too cell densities could have an effect. The contamination of melanocytes in the hiPSC-derived cartilage would inevitably compromise the repair process after transplantation because this subpopulation does not have chondrogenic function. Whichever causes the dark dots (lipofuscin or melanin), cartilage particles generated from iPSCs should avoid their presence when considering the repair of articular cartilage damage.

Conclusions

Cartilage is a tissue that consists of chondrocytes and ECM, which are mutually dependent. The healing mechanisms by cell transplantation such as ACI or MSC transplantation into articular cartilage defects may depend on trophic effects, whereas the transplantation of cartilage tissue can produce repair tissue of good quality. hiPSCs promise a new generation of cartilage therapy. Cartilage tissue can be produced by the differentiation of hiPSCs into chondrocytes followed by transferring the cells into 3D suspension culture in which the chondrocytes secrete and accumulate surrounding cartilage ECM. hiPSC-derived cartilage has low immunogenicity like natural cartilage and can be transplanted in an allogeneic manner for the treatment of articular cartilage damage. The differentiation of iPSCs to cartilage should be tightly controlled to avoid the presence of non-cartilaginous elements such as lipofuscin or melanin.

Table 2 Pigments and staining methods

Staining	Non-hematogenous pigment			Hematogenous pigment
	Lipofuscin	Melanin	Chromaffin	
Bleach	Sensitive	Sensitive	Weakly sensitive	Resistant
PAS	Positive	Negative	Negative	Negative
Giemsa	Ortho-chromasia (dark blue)	Meta-chromasia (dark green)	Meta-chromasia (red purple)	
Schmorl's reaction	Positive	Positive	Weakly positive	
Berlin blue	Negative	Negative	Negative	Positive (hemosiderin)

Methods

Chondrogenic differentiation of hiPSCs

Cartilaginous particles were generated from hiPSCs as described previously [24] with modification. hiPSCs-derived cartilaginous particles generated 12 weeks after the start of the differentiation were used.

Histological analysis

hiPSC-derived cartilaginous particles were fixed with 4% paraformaldehyde, processed, and embedded in paraffin. Semiserial sections were stained with hematoxylin-eosin and safranin O-fast green-iron hematoxylin and immuno-stained with anti-type II collagen antibody and goat anti-type I collagen antibody, as described previously [24].

Semiserial sections were bleached with 0.25% potassium permanganate (Nacalai) for 1 h, then with 2% oxalic acid for 2 min, and finally counterstained with kernechtrot (Muto pure chemicals).

For Schmorl's reaction, PAS staining, and Giemsa staining, semiserial sections were initially weakly bleached with 0.25% potassium permanganate (Nacalai) for 3 min and 2% oxalic acid for 2 min. The sections were subjected to Schmorl's reaction by being stained with ferric chloride (Wako) and counterstained with kernechtrot. The sections were subjected to PAS staining by being treated with Schiff's reagent (Wako) for 10 min and counterstained with hematoxylin. Finally, the sections were subjected to Giemsa staining by being stained with Giemsa stain solution composed of Giemsa (Merck), methanol, and sodium carbonate (Nacalai) for 3 h.

Acknowledgements

We thank Nobuyuki Yajima and Osamu Kusuoka for assistance and helpful discussions. This study was supported in part by Scientific Research Grant No. 15H02561 (to N.T.) and No. 18H02923 (to N.T.) from MEXT, and the Practical Research Project for Rare/Intractable Diseases (step 0) Grant No. 17ek0109215h0001 (to N.T.), Centers for Clinical Application Research on Specific Disease/Organ (type B) Grant No. 17bm0304004h0005 (to N.T.), Core Center for iPS Cell Research Grant No. 17bm0104001h0005 (to N.T.), and the Acceleration Program for Intractable Diseases Research utilizing Disease-specific iPS cells Grant No. 17bm0804006h0001 (to N.T.).

Authors contributions

All authors contributed to the writing of the manuscript. All authors consented to publication. All authors read and approved the final manuscript.

Competing interests

The authors declare that they have no competing interests.

Author details

[1]Cell Induction and Regulation Field, Department of Clinical Application, Center for iPS Cell Research and Application, Kyoto University, Kyoto, Japan. [2]International Public Communications Office, Center for iPS Cell Research and Application, Kyoto University, Kyoto, Japan.

References

1. Andrade R, Vasta S, Pereira R, Pereira H, Papalia R, Karahan M, Oliveira JM, Reis RL, Espregueira-Mendes J. Knee donor-site morbidity after mosaicplasty—a systematic review. J Exp Orthop. 2016;3(1):31.
2. Brittberg M, Lindahl A, Nilsson A, Ohlsson C, Isaksson O, Peterson L. Treatment of deep cartilage defects in the knee with autologous chondrocyte transplantation. N Engl J Med. 1994;331(14):889–95.
3. Ma B, Leijten JC, Wu L, Kip M, van Blitterswijk CA, Post JN, Karperien M. Gene expression profiling of dedifferentiated human articular chondrocytes in monolayer culture. Osteoarthr Cartil. 2013;21(4):599–603.
4. von der Mark K, Gauss V, von der Mark H, Müller P. Relationship between cell shape and type of collagen synthesised as chondrocytes lose their cartilage phenotype in culture. Nature. 1977;267:531–2.
5. Benya PD, Padilla SR, Nimni ME. Independent regulation of collagen types by chondrocytes during the loss of differentiated function in culture. Cell. 1978;15:1313–21.
6. Nixon AJ, Begum L, Mohammed HO, Huibregtse B, O'Callaghan MM, Matthews GL. Autologous chondrocyte implantation drives early chondrogenesis and organized repair in extensive full- and partial-thickness cartilage defects in an equine model. J Orthop Res. 2011;29:1121–30.
7. Ho AD, Wagner W, Franke W. Heterogeneity of mesenchymal stromal cell preparations. Cytotherapy. 2008;10(4):320–30.
8. Ansboro S, Roelofs AJ, De Bari C. Mesenchymal stem cells for the management of rheumatoid arthritis: immune modulation, repair or both? Curr Opin Rheumatol. 2017;29(2):201–7.
9. Caplan AI. Adult mesenchymal stem cells: when, where, and how. Stem Cells Int. 2015;2015:628767.
10. Caplan AI. MSCs: the sentinel and safe-guards of injury. J Cell Physiol. 2016; 231(7):1413–6.
11. Chesterman PJ, Smith AU. Homotransplantation of articular cartilage and isolated chondrocytes. An experimental study in rabbits. J Bone Joint Surg Br. 1968;50(1):184–97.
12. Adkisson HD, Milliman C, Zhang X, Mauch K, Maziarz RT, Streeter PR. Immune evasion by neocartilage-derived chondrocytes: implications for biologic repair of joint articular cartilage. Stem Cell Res. 2010;4(1):57–68.
13. Erdmann J. ISTO technologies aims to rescue damaged joints. Chem Biol. 2011;18(3):275–6.
14. Farr J, Tabet SK, Margerrison E, Cole BJ. Clinical, radiographic, and histological outcomes after cartilage repair with particulated juvenile articular cartilage: a 2-year prospective study. Am J Sports Med. 2014; 42(6):1417–25.
15. Tompkins M. DeNovo NT allograft. Oper Tech Sports Med. 2013;21:82–9.
16. HDt A, Martin JA, Amendola RL, Milliman C, Mauch KA, Katwal AB, Seyedin M, Amendola A, Streeter PR, Buckwalter JA. The potential of human allogeneic juvenile chondrocytes for restoration of articular cartilage. Am J Sports Med. 2010;38(7):1324–33.
17. Thomson JA, Itskovitz-Eldor J, Shapiro SS, Waknitz MA, Swiergiel JJ, Marshall VS, Jones JM. Embryonic stem cell lines derived from human blastocysts. Science. 1998;282(5391):1145–7.
18. Takahashi K, Tanabe K, Ohnuki M, Narita M, Ichisaka T, Tomoda K, Yamanaka S. Induction of pluripotent stem cells from adult human fibroblasts by defined factors. Cell. 2007;131(5):861–72.
19. Takahashi K, Yamanaka S. Induction of pluripotent stem cells from mouse embryonic and adult fibroblast cultures by defined factors. Cell. 2006;126(4): 663–76.
20. Tsumaki N, Okada M, Yamashita A. iPS cell technologies and cartilage regeneration. Bone. 2015;70:48–54.
21. Turner M, Leslie S, Martin NG, Peschanski M, Rao M, Taylor CJ, Trounson A, Turner D, Yamanaka S, Wilmut I. Toward the development of a global induced pluripotent stem cell library. Cell Stem Cell. 2013;13(4):382–4.

22. Okita K, Matsumura Y, Sato Y, Okada A, Morizane A, Okamoto S, Hong H, Nakagawa M, Tanabe K, Tezuka K-i, et al. A more efficient method to generate integration-free human iPS cells. Nat Methods. 2011;8(5):409–12.

23. Yamashita A, Morioka M, Kishi H, Kimura T, Yahara Y, Okada M, Fujita K, Sawai H, Ikegawa S, Tsumaki N. Statin treatment rescues FGFR3 skeletal dysplasia phenotypes. Nature. 2014;513(7519):507-11.

24. Yamashita A, Morioka M, Yahara Y, Okada M, Kobayashi T, Kuriyama S, Matsuda S, Tsumaki N. Generation of scaffoldless hyaline cartilaginous tissue from human iPSCs. Stem Cell Reports. 2015;4(3):404–18.

25. Kimura T, Yamashita A, Ozono K, Tsumaki N. Limited immunogenicity of human induced pluripotent stem cell-derived cartilages. Tissue Eng Part A. 2016;22(23–24):1367–75.

26. Lee J, Smeriglio P, Chu CR, Bhutani N. Human iPSC-derived chondrocytes mimic juvenile chondrocyte function for the dual advantage of increased proliferation and resistance to IL-1beta. Stem Cell Res Ther. 2017;8(1):244.

27. Driessen BJH, Logie C, Vonk LA. Cellular reprogramming for clinical cartilage repair. Cell Biol Toxicol. 2017;33(4):329–49.

28. Oldershaw RA. Cell sources for the regeneration of articular cartilage: the past, the horizon and the future. Int J Exp Pathol. 2012;93:389–400.

29. Liu H, Yang L, Yu FF, Wang S, Wu C, Qu C, Lammi MJ, Guo X. The potential of induced pluripotent stem cells as a tool to study skeletal dysplasias and cartilage-related pathologic conditions. Osteoarthr Cartil. 2017;25(5):616–24.

30. Suvarna KS, Layton C, Bancroft JD. Pigments and minerals, Bancroft's Theory and Practice of Histological Techniques, Eighth edn: ELSEVIER; 2019.

31. McManus JFA, Mowry RW. Staining methods, histologic and histochemical. New York: Hoeber; 1960.

32. Senba M. Staining properties of melanin and lipofuscin pigments. Am J Clin Pathol. 1986;86(4):556–7.

33. Coupland RE, Heath ID. Chromaffin cells, mast cells and melanin. I. The granular cells of the skin. J Endocrinol. 1961;22:59–69.

34. Goldfischer S, Bernstein J. Lipofuscin (aging) pigment granules of the newborn human liver. J Cell Biol. 1969;42(1):253–61.

35. Pinkus H, Hunter R. Simplified acid orcein and Giemsa technique for routine staining of skin sections. Arch Dermatol. 1960;82:699–700.

36. Jung T, Bader N, Grune T. Lipofuscin: formation, distribution, and metabolic consequences. Ann N Y Acad Sci. 2007;1119:97–111.

37. Terman A, Brunk UT. Lipofuscin: mechanisms of formation and increase with age. APMIS. 1998;106(2):265–76.

38. Matsumoto K, Ishimaru D, Ogawa H, Akiyama H. Black colouration of the knee articular cartilage after spontaneously recurrent haemarthrosis. Case Rep Orthop. 2016;2016:1238392.

39. Zsupan I, Hadhazy C, Nagy V, Jeney F, Nagy I. The effect of OH(.) radicals generated by Fenton reaction on the growth and cartilage differentiation in limb bud cell culture. J Submicrosc Cytol. 1987;19(3):445–54.

19

Recent advances in the treatment of skin involvement in systemic sclerosis

Yoshihide Asano

Abstract

Skin fibrosis is a devastating clinical condition commonly seen in skin-restricted and systemic disorders. The goal of skin fibrosis treatment is the restoration of abnormally activated dermal fibroblasts producing the excessive amount of extracellular matrix, which is generally a final consequence of the complex disease process including the activation of vascular and immune systems. Among various skin fibrotic conditions, the molecular mechanisms underlying dermal fibroblast activation have been mostly well studied in systemic sclerosis (SSc). SSc is a multisystem autoimmune and vascular disease resulting in extensive fibrosis of the skin and various internal organs. Since SSc pathogenesis is believed to include all the critical components regulating tissue fibrosis, the studies on anti-fibrotic drugs against SSc provide us much useful information regarding the strategy for the treatment of various skin fibrotic conditions. In the recent decade, as is the case with other autoimmune and inflammatory diseases, the molecular targeting therapy with monoclonal antibody has been clinically well examined in SSc. Promising clinical outcomes are so far reported in tocilizumab (an anti-IL-6 receptor antibody), rituximab (an anti-CD20 antibody), and fresolimumab (an anti-TGF-β antibody). The analysis of gene expression profiles in skin lesions of SSc patients treated with tocilizumab or fresolimumab revealed a critical role of monocyte-macrophage lineage cells in the development of skin fibrosis and the involvement of IL-6 and TGF-β in the activation of those cells. Considering that B cells modulate the differentiation and activation of macrophages, favorable clinical outcomes of rituximab treatment imply the central role of B cell/monocyte-macrophage lineage cell axis in the pathogenesis of SSc. This scenario may be applicable at least partly to other skin fibrotic conditions. In this review article, the currently available data on these drugs are summarized and the future directions are discussed.

Background

Skin fibrosis is a devastating clinical condition resulting in severe disability and seriously affecting morbidity, which commonly occurs in skin-restricted and systemic disorders, including systemic sclerosis (SSc), localized scleroderma, and chronic graft-versus-host disease. It is widely accepted that constitutively activated dermal fibroblasts play a crucial role in the development and maintenance of skin fibrosis through the production of excessive amount of extracelluar matrix, but anti-fibrotic therapies targeting those cells generally elicit a limited effect on this pathological condition. In a sense, this is plausible because fibroblasts manifest a pro-fibrotic phenotype as a final consequence of the complex disease process consisting of complicated cell-cell interactions and networks of soluble factors. For instance, the fibrotic skin condition is generally related to T helper (Th)2/Th17-skewed immune polarization [1, 2], M2 macrophage differentiation [3], increased infiltration of plasmacytoid dendritic cells [4], increased endothelial intercellular adhesion molecule-1 expression [5], endothelial-to-mesenchymal transition [6], epithelial cell activation [7], and/or adipocyte-myofibroblast transdifferentiation [8]. In particular, autoimmunity and/or inflammation seem to play a central role because corticosteroids and/or immunosuppressants are effective for most of the skin fibrotic disorders even though clinical outcomes are variable in individual cases. Therefore, immune cells and several key molecules are the critical targets to interfere with the complex disease process underlying skin fibrosis. The molecular targeting therapy has recently caught much attention to achieve this goal and also would be helpful to further understand the

Correspondence: yasano-tky@umin.ac.jp
Department of Dermatology, Graduate School of Medicine, University of Tokyo, 7-3-1 Hongo, Bunkyo-ku, Tokyo 113-8655, Japan

pathogenesis of this clinical entity when favorable outcomes are obtained.

Among skin fibrotic conditions, the molecular mechanisms resulting in dermal fibroblast activation have been mostly well studied in SSc. SSc is characterized by extensive dermal fibrosis following aberrant activation of immune and vascular systems, in which all the critical components regulating tissue fibrosis are included [9, 10]. Therefore, the studies on anti-fibrotic drugs against SSc provide us much useful information regarding the strategy for the treatment of various skin fibrotic conditions. In the recent decade, as is the case with other autoimmune and inflammatory diseases, the molecular targeting therapy with monoclonal antibody has been clinically well examined in SSc. Promising clinical outcomes have been reported in tocilizumab (an anti-interleukin-6 (IL-6) receptor antibody), rituximab (an anti-CD20 antibody), and fresolimumab (an anti-transforming growth factor (TGF)-β antibody). In this review article, the currently available data on these drugs are summarized and the future directions are discussed.

Tocilizumab

The role of IL-6 in SSc

Increasing evidence suggests a critical contribution of IL-6 to the development of tissue fibrosis and vasculopathy as well as inflammation associated with SSc. First, IL-6 is much more abundantly expressed in various types of cells, including dermal fibroblasts, dermal microvascular endothelial cells, inflammatory cells, and keratinocytes, of SSc lesional skin than in those cells of healthy control skin [11]. Consistently, the phosphorylation of signal transducer and activator of transcription 3 (STAT3), which is induced by the activation of IL-6 receptor/gp130 complex, is broadly detectable in various cell types, most remarkably in dermal microvascular endothelial cells, of SSc lesional skin irrespective of disease subtypes and disease duration, while totally absent or marginal in any cell types of healthy control skin [12]. More importantly, the elevation of serum IL-6 levels is associated with poor prognosis of this disease [11]. In in vitro studies SSc dermal fibroblasts seem to be activated by IL-6 in autocrine/paracrine manners [11, 13], and the activation of endothelial IL-6/STAT3 axis induces proliferation, migration, vascular instability, and endothelial-to-mesenchymal transition [14], all of which are characteristically seen in SSc endothelial cells [10]. With respect to the immunological aspect, IL-6 promotes the differentiation of Th2 cells and that of Th17 cells together with TGF-β [15], possibly contributing to the predominance of Th2 and Th17 cytokine production in SSc lesional skin [16]. These evidence strongly imply the possibility that tocilizumab modifies all the three

cardinal pathological features of SSc, namely, inflammation, vasculopathy, and tissue fibrosis.

The effect of tocilizumab on SSc

Truly supporting the contribution of IL-6 signaling to SSc development, a favorable clinical effect of tocilizumab on skin sclerosis has been reported. Following two case series [17, 18], the detailed results of the faSScinate study (phase II trial of tocilizumab for SSc) was documented in 2016 [19]. After 24-week administration of tocilizumab (162 mg per each subcutaneous weekly injection), skin score estimated by Two-Gene SSc Skin Biomarker was significantly improved in diffuse cutaneous SSc (dcSSc) patients, who had disease duration of <5 years and IL-6-related inflammatory features (the elevation of C-reactive protein, erythrocyte sedimentation rate, or platelet count), compared with the placebo group. Based on this favorable clinical outcome, the global phase III trial is currently under the way with the larger number of SSc patients.

Another important finding in the faSScinate study was the alteration of gene expression profile in SSc lesional skin after the administration of tocilizumab [20]. The DNA microarray analysis with skin biopsy samples taken before and 24 weeks after the initial injection revealed that tocilizumab suppresses a cluster of genes related to M2 macrophages, suggesting a critical role of M2 macrophages in the development of skin fibrosis and a critical contribution of IL-6 to this process in SSc. M2 macrophages are derived from monocyte-macrophage lineage cells, which also provide a precursor of pro-angiogenic hematopoietic cells and fibrocytes [21, 22]. Indeed, in parallel with the reduction of skin sclerosis, the restoration of abnormal nailfold capillary changes and the healing of refractory digital ulcers were also reported after the administration of tocilizumab [12, 18]. Therefore, the target of tocilizumab treatment is at least partially the monocyte-macrophage lineage cells contributing to inflammatory, vascular, and fibrotic manifestations of SSc.

Rituximab

The role of B cells in SSc

As represented by the SSc-specific sequential disease process, autoimmunity precedes the development of vasculopathy and tissue fibrosis, suggesting that aberrantly activated immune system plays a central role in the pathogenesis of SSc. At this moment, the direct role of SSc-related antinuclear antibodies, such as antibodies against topoisomerase I, centromere, and RNA polymerase III antigens, still remains unknown, but the close association of these antibodies with clinical manifestations suggests that altered B cell phenotypes possibly correlate with the central abnormality driving the progression of this disease through the genetic and epigenetic mechanisms shared with other cell types and/or the complex interaction with other immune and non-immune cells.

A critical role of aberrantly activated B cells has been implicated in the development of SSc-like features in murine animal models. Relevant to the elevated expression of CD19, a critical activator, in SSc B cells, *Cd19* transgenic mice exhibit hypergammaglobulinemia and autoantibody production due to the abnormal activation of B cells [23]. Tight-skin mice show hypodermal fibrosis, hypergammaglobulinemia, and positivity of antinuclear antibody and anti-topoisomerase I antibody, but both CD19 loss and B cell depletion by anti-CD20 antibody result in the reduction of these abnormalities [24, 25]. Supporting these findings, it is generally accepted that in addition to antibody production, B cells play multifaceted roles in immune system, such as cytokine production, antigen presentation, macrophage differentiation and activation, and lymphoid tissue development [26]. Consistently, B cell depletion therapy broadly affects disease processes of autoimmune diseases, such as rheumatoid arthritis, systemic lupus erythematosus, antinuetrophil cytoplasmic antibody-associated vasculitis, dermatomyositis/polymyositis, and primary Sjögren's syndrome as well as SSc [27].

The effect of rituximab on SSc

In the first pilot study by Lafyatis et al. [28], 15 dcSSc patients with disease duration of <18 months were administered rituximab (1000 mg, twice, 2 weeks apart). In skin biopsy samples, the decrease in the number of myofibroblasts and skin-infiltrating B cells was evident at week 24 despite no significant change of modified Rodnan total skin thickness score (mRSS). In another pilot study reported by Smith et al. [29], 8 cases of dcSSc with disease duration of <4 years were administered rituximab (1000 mg, twice, 2 weeks apart) together with 100 mg methylprednisolone at each infusion. mRSS was significantly improved at week 24 compared with the baseline. Skin biopsy specimens taken at week 12 revealed the decrease in collage deposition and the number of myofibroblasts and skin-infiltrating B cells compared with those taken at the baseline. As a common finding in these two studies, no significant effect was detected on pulmonary function test results.

On the other hand, Daoussis et al. [30] performed a randomized controlled study of rituximab on 14 dcSSc patients, in which 8 patients were treated with two cycles of rituximab at baseline and week 24 (each cycle consisted of 4 weekly infusions (375 mg/m^2)) and 6 patients received standard treatment alone. A year after the initiation of treatment, a significant reduction of mRSS was seen in the rituximab group, while not in the control group. More importantly, both of %FVC (forced vital capacity) and %DLco (diffusion capacity of the lungs for carbon monoxide) were significantly improved in the rituximab group, while no significant changes were seen in the control group. Similar favorable efficacy was reported in a nested case-control study using the European Scleroderma Trial and Research (EUSTAR) database [31]. In 63 SSc patients treated with rituximab, mRSS was significantly improved compared with closely matched control patient group. As well, %FVC was stabilized in the rituximab group, while not in the placebo group. Similar clinical effects of rituximab were recently reported by Daoussis et al. [32] in 51 SSc patients with interstitial lung disease (ILD). These three studies documented a potential disease-modifying effect of rituximab on skin fibrosis and ILD of SSc.

There is another report by Bosello et al. [33] regarding the long-term effect of rituximab in 20 SSc patients treated with rituximab (1000 mg, twice, 2 weeks apart). mRSS was significantly improved at 6 months and thereafter. As for ILD, among six patients with %FVC of <80%, %FVC was significantly improved from 64.3 to 71.0% at 1 year but decreased to 65.7% at the last follow-up period (mean follow-up of 48.5 +/− 20.4 months). The analysis of laboratory data displayed the recovery of B cells between 6 and 12 months, no change of serum IgG and IgA levels throughout the follow-up period, and a significant decrease in serum IgM levels at 6 months and thereafter. In some patients, relapse of skin sclerosis was attenuated by readministration of rituximab.

In addition, there are several case reports or case series in which calcinosis, digital ulcers, or arterial stiffness were improved by rituximab therapy [34–36]. Taken together, B cell depletion therapy is potentially able to modify the three cardinal pathological features of SSc, namely, fibrosis, vasculopathy, and autoimmunity. These results suggest that B cells are involved in the activation of vascular and fibrotic processes in addition to the activation of immune system in SSc.

Fresolimumab
The role of TGF-β in SSc

TGF-β is a key growth factor regulating the activation status of dermal fibroblasts in SSc [37]. Although the expression pattern of TGF-β in the lesional skin of SSc is still controversial, TGF-β expression levels generally seem to be higher in patients with early and active disease, but weak or undetectable in patients with established skin fibrosis. So far, the expression profile of the three isoforms of TGF-β is generally understood as follows: (i) all the three isoforms of TGF-β are detectable in the extracellular matrix and (ii) the expression of TGF-β1 and TGF-β2 is most prominent around dermal vessels and is associated with perivascular infiltrating mononuclear cells [38–40]. Given that TGF-β action is determined by the state of activation and differentiation of the target cells and the presence and concentration of other cytokines and growth factors, TGF-β potentially promotes inflammation by recruiting leukocytes through the regulation of cell adhesion molecules and the creation of chemokine gradient, by activating leukocytes, and by inducing various pro-inflammatory cytokines and other mediators in early stage of SSc. In sclerotic stage, SSc dermal fibroblasts are constitutively activated with the pro-fibrotic phenotype quite similar to that of normal fibroblasts treated with TGF-β1 even though the expression of TGF-β is weak or undetectable in the skin [41]. This observation suggests that once activated, SSc fibroblasts establish a self activation system at least partially via autocrine TGF-β signaling. The increased expression of latent TGF-β receptors, including integrin αVβ3, αVβ5, and thrombospondin-1, contribute to this process in SSc dermal fibroblasts [42–46]. These receptors recruit and activate latent TGF-β on the cell surface and efficiently increase the concentration of active TGF-β around SSc fibroblasts. Therefore, dermal fibroblasts may be constitutively activated by autocrine TGF-β in SSc lesional skin. Thus, TGF-β is a promising therapeutic target of this disease.

The effect of anti-TGF-β antibody on SSc

A decade ago, the phase I and II clinical trials of metelimumab, a neutralizing antibody against TGF-β1, were conducted [47]. Forty-five dcSSc patients with disease duration of <18 months and moderate mRSS were treated with metelimumab (0.5, 5, or 10 mg/kg, intravenously, four infusions, 6 weeks apart) or placebo. Six months after the first infusion, no beneficial effect of metelimumab on skin sclerosis was observed. Taken it into account that all the three isoforms of TGF-β, especially TGF-β1 and TGF-β2, are highly expressed in the lesional skin of early and active SSc, the blockade of TGB-β1 alone seems to be insufficient to attenuate skin fibrosis of SSc. Indeed, all the three isoforms bind to the same receptors and exert similar biological effects on the proliferation, differentiation, and development of various cell types, and immune system. Therefore, the antibody blocking all the three isoforms was generated after this clinical trial.

In 2015, the result of phase II clinical trial of fresolimumab, a neutralizing antibody against TGF-β1, β2, and β3, was reported [48]. SSc patients with disease duration of <2 years and mRSS of equal or more than 15, who were on a stable dose of 10 mg/day or less of prednisone and no other immunosuppressants, were enrolled. Fifteen patients were treated with fresolimumab (twice [1 mg/kg], 4 weeks apart for 7 cases and once [5 mg/kg] for 8 cases), in which a case was withdrawn at week 4,

and 4 cases were additionally treated with immunosuppressants during the safety follow-up period (one patient at week 9 and three patients at week 11). mRSS was significantly improved in both groups at week 11 and 17 compared with the baseline, while exacerbated at week 24. Consistently, in the analysis of gene expression profile in skin lesions, mRNA levels of the *THBS1* and *COMP* genes, which is included in 4 gene biomarkers [49], were decreased and reversed in parallel with the resolution and exacerbation of skin sclerosis, respectively. In addition, *CTGF*, *SERPINE1*, and *COL10A1* mRNA levels correlated with mRSS. Also, mRNA levels of the *CD14*, *CD163*, and *MS4A4A* genes, markers of monocyte-macrophage lineage cells, correlated with mRSS. Consistent with these results, the number of myofibroblasts was decreased after the treatment, though the thickness of the dermis was not changed.

As for the tolerability, bleeding and anemia were reported. Two cases experienced bleeding from gastric antral vascular ectasia which required blood transfusion. Bleeding from the gingiva, nose, and conjunctiva was also reported, and 10 out of 15 cases showed more than 10% decrease in hemoglobin levels during the study period. One patient died due to heart failure with severe cardiac fibrosis, though skin fibrosis was rapidly improved after receiving one dose of fresolimumab (5 mg).

This study firstly provided clear evidence that TGF-β is truly involved in the development of skin fibrosis in SSc and the blockade of all the three isoforms of TGF-β can be a therapeutic strategy for skin sclerosis. In parallel with the decreased extracellular matrix production, monocyte-macrophage lineage-related gene expression was reduced, suggesting that TGF-β is involved in the skin infiltration of monocyte-macrophage lineage cells which play a critical part in the development of skin fibrosis as well as vasculopathy [21, 22].

Conclusions

Although the detailed molecular mechanism leading to extensive tissue fibrosis still remains largely unknown in SSc, the favorable clinical outcomes of tocilizumab, rituximab, and fresolimuab provide us useful information to speculate the role of the key molecules and cells in its developmental process. The inactivation of monocyte-macrophage lineage cells in parallel of skin fibrosis resolution, which is commonly seen in SSc patients treated with tocilizumab and fresolimumab, strongly suggest the crucial role of monocyte-macrophage lineage cells and the involvement of IL-6 and TGF-β in the activation of those cells during the fibrotic process of this disease. Monocyte-macrophage lineage cells provide precursors of pro-angiogenic hematopoietic cells, the altered phenotype of which is associated with the development of SSc vasculopathy [21]. The restoration of nailfold vascular abnormalities by tocilizumab treatment supports a broad spectrum of roles of monocyte-macrophage lineage cells in SSc pathogenesis [12]. Considering that B cells modulate the differentiation and activation of macrophages [26, 50], B cell depletion therapy possibly acts on the pathological process targeted by tocilizumab and fresolimumab, namely, monocyte-macrophage lineage cells. At this moment, this is still just a hypothesis based on clinical outcomes, but further studies on the B cell/monocyte-macrophage lineage cell axis would shed new light on the molecular mechanism of tissue fibrosis in SSc, as well as other skin fibrotic disorders.

Abbreviations

DLco: Diffusion capacity of the lungs for carbon monoxide; FVC: Forced vital capacity; IL-6: Interleukin-6; ILD: Interstitial lung disease; mRSS: Modified Rodnan total skin thickness score; SSc: Systemic sclerosis; STAT3: Signal transducer and activator of transcription 3; TGF: Transforming growth factor; Th: T helper

Competing interests

The author declares no competing interests.

References

1. Matsushita T, Hasegawa M, Hamaguchi Y, Takehara K, Sato S. Longitudinal analysis of serum cytokine concentrations in systemic sclerosis: association of interleukin 12 elevation with spontaneous regression of skin sclerosis. J Rheumatol. 2006;33:275–84.

2. Murata M, Fujimoto M, Matsushita T, Hamaguchi Y, Hasegawa M, Takehara K, et al. Clinical association of serum interleukin-17 levels in systemic sclerosis: is systemic sclerosis a Th17 disease? J Dermatol Sci. 2008;50:240–2.

3. Higashi-Kuwata N, Jinnin M, Makino T, Fukushima S, Inoue Y, Muchemwa FC, et al. Characterization of monocyte/macrophage subsets in the skin and peripheral blood derived from patients with systemic sclerosis. Arthritis Res Ther. 2010;12:R128.

4. Duan H, Fleming J, Pritchard DK, Amon LM, Xue J, Arnett HA, et al. Combined analysis of monocyte and lymphocyte messenger RNA expression with serum protein profiles in patients with scleroderma. Arthritis Rheum. 2008;58:1465–74.

5. Gruschwitz MS, Vieth G. Up-regulation of class II major histocompatibility complex and intercellular adhesion molecule 1 expression on scleroderma fibroblasts and endothelial cells by interferon-gamma and tumor necrosis factor alpha in the early disease stage. Arthritis Rheum. 1997;40:540–50.

6. Jimenez SA. Role of endothelial to mesenchymal transition in the pathogenesis of the vascular alterations in systemic sclerosis. ISRN Rheumatol. 2013;2013:835948.

7. Takahashi T, Asano Y, Sugawara K, Yamashita T, Nakamura K, Saigusa R, et al. Epithelial Fli1 deficiency drives systemic autoimmunity and fibrosis: possible roles in scleroderma. J Exp Med. in press doi: 10.1084/jem.20160247.

8. Marangoni RG, Korman BD, Wei J, Wood TA, Graham LV, Whitfield ML, et al. Myofibroblasts in murine cutaneous fibrosis originate from adiponectin-positive intradermal progenitors. Arthritis Rheumatol. 2015;67:1062–73.

9. Denton CP. Systemic sclerosis: from pathogenesis to targeted therapy. Clin Exp Rheumatol. 2015;33(4 Suppl 92):S3–7.

10. Asano Y, Sato S. Vasculopathy in scleroderma. Semin Immunopathol. 2015;37:489–500.

11. Khan K, Xu S, Nihtyanova S, Derrett-Smith E, Abraham D, Denton CP, et al. Clinical and pathological significance of interleukin 6 overexpression in systemic sclerosis. Ann Rheum Dis. 2012;71:1235–42.

12. Taniguchi T, Asano Y, Fukasawa T, Yoshizaki A, Sato S. Critical contribution of the interleukin-6/signal transducer and activator of transcription 3 axis to vasculopathy associated with systemic sclerosis. J Dermatol. in press doi: 10.1111/1346-8138.13827.

13. Garbers C, Aparicio-Siegmund S, Rose-John S. The IL-6/gp130/STAT3

14. Magrini E, Cavallaro U, Bianchi F. Microarray profiling of L1-overexpressing endothelial cells reveals STAT3 activation via IL-6/IL-6Rα axis. Genom Data. 2015;4:137–9.

15. Dienz O, Rincon M. The effects of IL-6 on CD4 T cell responses. Clin Immunol. 2009;130:27–33.

16. Nakashima T, Jinnin M, Yamane K, Honda N, Kajihara I, Makino T, et al. Impaired IL-17 signaling pathway contributes to the increased collagen expression in scleroderma fibroblasts. J Immunol. 2012;188:3573–83.

17. Shima Y, Kuwahara Y, Murota H, Kitaba S, Kawai M, Hirano T, et al. The skin of patients with systemic sclerosis softened during the treatment with anti-IL-6 receptor antibody tocilizumab. Rheumatology (Oxford). 2010;49:2408–12.

18. Fernandes das Neves M, Oliveira S, Amaral MC, Delgado Alves J. Treatment of systemic sclerosis with tocilizumab. Rheumatology (Oxford). 2015;54:371–2.

19. Khanna D, Denton CP, Jahreis A, van Laar JM, Frech TM, Anderson ME, et al. Safety and efficacy of subcutaneous tocilizumab in adults with systemic sclerosis (faSScinate): a phase 2, randomised, controlled trial. Lancet. 2016;387:2630–40.

20. Tsou PS, Rabquer BJ, Ohara RA, Stinson WA, Campbell PL, Amin MA, et al. Scleroderma dermal microvascular endothelial cells exhibit defective response to pro-angiogenic chemokines. Rheumatology (Oxford). 2016;55:745–54.

21. Yamaguchi Y, Kuwana M. Proangiogenic hematopoietic cells of monocytic origin: roles in vascular regeneration and pathogenic processes of systemic sclerosis. Histol Histopathol. 2013;28:175–83.

22. Tourkina E, Bonner M, Oates J, Hofbauer A, Richard M, Znoyko S, et al. Altered monocyte and fibrocyte phenotype and function in scleroderma interstitial lung disease: reversal by caveolin-1 scaffolding domain peptide. Fibrogenesis Tissue Repair. 2011;4:15.

23. Sato S, Hasegawa M, Fujimoto M, Tedder TF, Takehara K. Quantitative genetic variation in CD19 expression correlates with autoimmunity. J Immunol. 2000;165:6635–43.

24. Saito E, Fujimoto M, Hasegawa M, Komura K, Hamaguchi Y, Kaburagi Y, et al. CD19-dependent B lymphocyte signaling thresholds influence skin fibrosis and autoimmunity in the tight-skin mouse. J Clin Invest. 2002;109:1453–62.

25. Hasegawa M, Hamaguchi Y, Yanaba K, Bouaziz JD, Uchida J, Fujimoto M, et al. B-lymphocyte depletion reduces skin fibrosis and autoimmunity in the tight-skin mouse model for systemic sclerosis. Am J Pathol. 2006;169:954–66.

26. Yoshizaki A. B lymphocytes in systemic sclerosis: abnormalities and therapeutic targets. J Dermatol. 2016;43:39–45.

27. Faurschou M, Jayne DR. Anti-B cell antibody therapies for inflammatory rheumatic diseases. Annu Rev Med. 2014;65:263–78.

28. Lafyatis R, Kissin E, York M, Farina G, Viger K, Fritzler MJ, et al. B cell depletion with rituximab in patients with diffuse cutaneous systemic sclerosis. Arthritis Rheum. 2009;60:578–83.

29. Smith V, Van Praet JT, Vandooren B, Van der Cruyssen B, Naeyaert JM, Decuman S, et al. Rituximab in diffuse cutaneous systemic sclerosis: an open-label clinical and histopathological study. Ann Rheum Dis. 2010;69:193–7.

30. Daoussis D, Liossis SN, Tsamandas AC, Kalogeropoulou C, Kazantzi A, Sirinian C, et al. Experience with rituximab in scleroderma: results from a 1-year, proof-of-principle study. Rheumatology (Oxford). 2010;49:271–80.

31. Jordan S, Distler JH, Maurer B, Huscher D, van Laar JM, Allanore Y, et al. Effects and safety of rituximab in systemic sclerosis: an analysis from the European Scleroderma Trial and Research (EUSTAR) group. Ann Rheum Dis. 2015;74:1188–94.

32. Daoussis D, Melissaropoulos K, Sakellaropoulos G, Antonopoulos I, Markatseli TE, Simopoulou T, et al. A multicenter, open-label, comparative study of B-cell depletion therapy with Rituximab for systemic sclerosis-associated interstitial lung disease. Semin Arthritis Rheum. in press doi: 10.1016/j.semarthrit.2016.10.003.

33. Bosello SL, De Luca G, Rucco M, Berardi G, Falcione M, Danza FM, et al. Long-term efficacy of B cell depletion therapy on lung and skin involvement in diffuse systemic sclerosis. Semin Arthritis Rheum. 2015;44:428–36.

34. Daoussis D, Antonopoulos I, Liossis SN, Yiannopoulos G, Andonopoulos AP. Treatment of systemic sclerosis-associated calcinosis: a case report of

rituximab-induced regression of CREST-related calcinosis and review of the literature. Semin Arthritis Rheum. 2012;41:822–9.

35. Khor CG, Chen XL, Lin TS, Lu CH, Hsieh SC. Rituximab for refractory digital infarcts and ulcers in systemic sclerosis. Clin Rheumatol. 2014;33:1019–20.

36. Maslyanskiy AL, Lapin SV, Kolesova EP, Penin IN, Cheshuina MD, Feist E, et al. Effects of rituximab therapy on elastic properties of vascular wall in patients with progressive systemic sclerosis. Clin Exp Rheumatol. 2014;32(6 Suppl 86):S-228.

37. Varga J, Pasche B. Transforming growth factor beta as a therapeutic target in systemic sclerosis. Nat Rev Rheumatol. 2009;5:200–6.

38. Gruschwitz M, Müller PU, Sepp N, Hofer E, Fontana A, Wick G. Transcription and expression of transforming growth factor type β in the skin of progressive systemic sclerosis: a mediator of fibrosis? J Invest Dermatol. 1990;94:197–203.

39. Querfeld C, Eckes B, Huerkamp C, Krieg T, Sollberg S. Expression of TGF-β1, -β2 and -β3 in localized and systemic scleroderma. J Dermatol Sci. 1999;21:13–22.

40. Kulozik M, Hogg A, Lankat-Buttgereit B, Krieg T. Co-localization of transforming growth factor β2 with α1(I) procollagen mRNA in tissue sections of patients with systemic sclerosis. J Clin Invest. 1990;86:917–22.

41. Asano Y, Ihn H, Yamane K, Kubo M, Tamaki K. Impaired Smad7-Smurf-mediated negative regulation of TGF-β signaling in scleroderma fibroblasts. J Clin Invest. 2004;113:253–64.

42. Asano Y, Ihn H, Yamane K, Jinnin M, Mimura Y, Tamaki K. Increased expression of integrin αVβ3 contributes to the establishment of autocrine TGF-β signaling in scleroderma fibroblasts. J Immunol. 2005;175:7708–18.

43. Asano Y, Ihn H, Yamane K, Kubo M, Tamaki K. Increased expression levels of integrin αVβ5 on scleroderma fibroblasts. Am J Pathol. 2004;164:1275–92.

44. Asano Y, Ihn H, Yamane K, Jinnin M, Mimura Y, Tamaki K. Involvement of αVβ5 integrin-mediated activation of latent transforming growth factor β1 in autocrine transforming growth factor β signaling in systemic sclerosis fibroblasts. Arthritis Rheum. 2005;52:2897–905.

45. Asano Y, Ihn H, Yamane K, Jinnin M, Tamaki K. Increased expression of integrin αVβ5 induces the myofibroblastic differentiation of dermal fibroblasts. Am J Pathol. 2006;168:499–510.

46. Mimura Y, Ihn H, Jinnin M, Asano Y, Yamane K, Tamaki K. Constitutive thrombospondin-1 overexpression contributes to autocrine transforming growth factor-β signaling in cultured scleroderma fibroblasts. Am J Pathol. 2005;166:1451–63.

47. Denton CP, Merkel PA, Furst DE, Khanna D, Emery P, Hsu VM, et al. Recombinant human anti-transforming growth factor β1 antibody therapy in systemic sclerosis: a multicenter, randomized, placebo-controlled phase I/II trial of CAT-192. Arthritis Rheum. 2007;56:323–33.

48. Rice LM, Padilla CM, McLaughlin SR, Mathes A, Ziemek J, Goummih S, et al. Fresolimumab treatment decreases biomarkers and improves clinical symptoms in systemic sclerosis patients. J Clin Invest. 2015;125:2795–807.

49. Farina G, Lafyatis D, Lemaire R, Lafyatis R. A four-gene biomarker predicts skin disease in patients with diffuse cutaneous systemic sclerosis. Arthritis Rheum. 2010;62:580–8.

50. Castiglione F, Tieri P, Palma A, Jarrah AS. Statistical ensemble of gene regulatory networks of macrophage differentiation. BMC Bioinform. 2016;17 Suppl 19:506.

20

Periodontal Infectogenomics

Gurjeet Kaur, Vishakha Grover, Nandini Bhaskar, Rose Kanwaljeet Kaur and Ashish Jain[*]

Abstract

Periodontal diseases are chronic infectious disease in which the pathogenic bacteria initiate the host immune response leading to the destruction of tooth supporting tissue and eventually result in the tooth loss. It has multifactorial etiological factors including local, systemic, environmental and genetic factors. The effect of genetic factors on periodontal disease is already under extensive research and has explained the role of polymorphisms of immune mediators affecting disease response. The role genetic factors in pathogens colonisation is emerged as a new field of research as "infectogenomics". It is a rapidly evolving and high-priority research area now days. It further elaborates the role of genetic factors in disease pathogenesis and help in the treatment, control and early prevention of infection. The aim of this review is to summarise the contemporary evidence available in the field of periodontal infectogenomics to draw some valuable conclusions to further elaborate its role in disease pathogenesis and its application in the clinical practice. This will open up opportunity for more extensive research in this field.

Keywords: Infectogenomics, Genetics, Microbes, Periodontitis, Bacterial species, Invasion, Proliferation

Background

Periodontal disease is a highly prevalent, multifactorial, chronic inflammatory disease of periodontium eventually leading to destruction of supportive tissues of teeth and tooth loss. The interaction between microbes present in dental plaque and host immune response is a major determinant of progression and clinical manifestations of periodontal disease [1, 2]. However, there are multitude of factors like systemic, environmental and genetic which directly or indirectly influence this association at multiple levels [3, 4]. It has been seen that individuals harbouring almost equivalent local etiological factors could represent the diverse disease severity. These observations lead to the idea of some unrecognised components of the host genetic constitution or the environment which was responsible for differences in their susceptibility of disease [5, 6]. The disease susceptibility is determined by immune response of the body as applies to periodontal disease, which is largely determined by genetic or epigenetic factors [6, 7]. The effects of these factors have been extensively studied over the last 20 years using different study designs. This has resulted in a significant paradigm shift in the aetiology of periodontal disease with the increased emphasis on host and its genetic constitution as modifiers of the bacterially induced disease and for increased risk of disease occurrence and severity.

A huge published literature is available regarding genetic analysis using candidate gene and human leukocyte antigen (HLA) markers for periodontitis among which the polymorphism studies of genes coding for cytokines have received the most attention [7]. Lot of investigations have been conducted to identify specific gene polymorphisms associated with risk for periodontal diseases. No specific single gene polymorphism could be defined, owing to polygenic nature of disease [6].

The altered immune response due to these gene polymorphisms affects the microbial composition present in periodontal environment. Humans are considered supra-organisms consisting of trillions of symbiotic, commensal and pathogenic bacteria [8, 9]. The oral cavity contains over 1000 different microorganisms including 700 different species with as many as 19,000 different bacterial phylotypes which are mostly commensal in nature [3, 8]. A myriad of host factors is responsible for the development of composition of oral microbiome, its role in oral health and disease which further shows subject to subject variation [8, 10]. Many polymorphisms affecting the immune response have been linked to periodontal disease which indirectly may have an impact on the quantity and quality of microbial colonisation [3].

---

[*] Correspondence: ashish@justice.com
Department of Periodontology, Dr Harvansh Singh Judge Institute of Dental Sciences and Hospital, Panjab University, Sector-25, Chandigarh, India

This has led to a novel concept in aetiology of periodontal disease i.e. "infectogenomics".

The concept of infectogenomics

Infectogenomics was first defined by Kellam and Weiss (2006) as the study of interaction between host genetic variations and colonisation by pathogenic microbes [11]. This term is in line with the word pharmacogenetics in which the appearance of a disease or symptom following exposure to an infectious agent can be regarded as an unusual side effect just like an adverse reaction to a drug [11]. With the alteration in the host genotype, these adverse reactions can be severe in one person as compared to the other.

The concept for infectogenomics states that the genetic defects in the recognition and response pathways of the host to identify microbial pathogens predispose to either altered microbial colonisation or misrecognition of normal microbiota leading to dysbiosis and appearance of infectious disease [9]. This hypothesis of association between host genomic adaptations and microbiome is well studied in many systemic disease conditions. A specific disease endemic to a particular population is known to cause certain genetic mutations as a result of this selective disease susceptibility and renders the population in subsequent generations resistant in due course of time. The classical example of this concept of selective pressure is studied in malaria endemic areas where the modifications in the human haemoglobin genes make this population resistant to malaria [12, 13]. Such mechanisms strongly support the concept of genetics linking disease susceptibility. Converse to this the concept of infectogenomics which suggests the reverse relationship that certain genetic constitutions are particularly susceptible to the disease and this is mediated by the selective pressure in terms of microbial colonisation or proliferation [3, 14, 15].

The genomic adaptations of the host can have effect either on the pathogen invasion or on pathogen proliferation [3, 9]. After the invasion of pathogens in the human body, the interaction between the pattern recognition receptors (PRRs) and the pathogen associated molecular patterns (PAMPs) generate cellular signalling against microbes. Any mutation or modifications in the PRR genes may thus result in either its altered expression or affect its ability to recognise microbial constituents effecting invasion of pathogens in the host [9]. A well documented association is between the CCR5-Δ32 deletion allele and human immunodeficiency virus (HIV) resistance. CCR5 chemokine receptor is used by HIV strains to gain entry into immune system cells. So, CCR5-Δ32 deletion allele provided almost complete resistance against HIV-1 in homozygous state and partial resistance with slower disease progression in heterozygous state [16–18]. It was hypothesised that this modification in the

genetic constitution arose in high risk population due to selective pressure from bubonic plague or small pox [17]. Next step in the pathogenesis is the proliferation of the pathogens that trigger immune-pathological reactions which determines the severity and progression of infectious disease. Inflammation being a central mechanism in many chronic human diseases, any alteration in immune regulatory genes may affect the disease pathogenesis. Selective genetic variations may result in skewing the microbial composition toward more pathological microbes or alters the host response for developing resistance for a particular pathogen [9]. This mechanism is well documented as conferring resistance to malaria in subjects with haemoglobin S (HbS) variant in malaria endemic population [12, 13]. In the individuals presenting with HbS homozygous traits the presence of *Plasmodium falciparum* causes the red cells to rupture, thus inhibits its proliferation or colonisation [19]. Converse to this is a well studied association between the cystic fibrosis and *Pseudomonas aeruginosa* infection in which the ΔF508 mutation in cystic fibrosis transmembrane conductance regulator (CFTR) gene lead to hypersusceptibility to chronic lung infection due to alterations in pH, ion concentrations and formation of dehydrated airway surface layer which contributes to increased proliferation of *Pseudomonas aeruginosa* [20, 21]. Other examples are protective role of T-helper cells type 2 (Th2) immune responses against Schistosomiasis [12], polygenic susceptibility to tuberculosis [22] and protection against chronic viral hepatitis [23]. However, in case of extensively studied inflammatory bowel disease the genetic mutations have affect on both the pathogen invasion and proliferation; explains the bidirectional relationship of the microbiome interactions with host genetics as between altered host immune function and altered bacterial community functions, features or by-products [15, 24]. So, these medical evidences provide us with some clear patterns of associations emerging in the field of infectogenomics.

Periodontal infectogenomics

With the advancement in the research it has been seen that the most prevalent chronic periodontitis being multifactorial also entails a dysbiotic oral microbial shift and a deregulated host inflammatory response resulting in progressive periodontal tissue destruction [10, 25]. Earlier the main focus for the genetic analyses was the association of periodontal disease with altered immune response taking into consideration some candidate genes related to immune pathways. In the past 15 years a lot of research work is mainly focused on this new concept of periodontal infectogenomics which will potentially help to better understand the pathogenesis of periodontal disease.

Genetic factors affecting periodontal pathogen invasion

In periodontal environment, microbes causing infection must have the ability to attach to the tissue surface, to multiply, to compete against other microbial species and to defend against host responses [3, 9]. One of the key systems for immune surveillance is complement system which links the innate and the adaptive arms of the host immune response [26, 27]. In monogenic Ehler Danlos Syndrome the alterations in C1R or C1S genes encoding for complement 1 subunits C1r and C1s has been documented as a link between connective tissue pathology with classical complement pathway [28]. Integrative gene prioritisation method has listed C3 among the top 21 most promising candidate genes involved in periodontitis (Polygenic condition) [26, 29]. Animal model investigations have indicated that complement is involved in both the dysbiotic transformation and the inflammatory response that leads to destruction of periodontal tissue. Similar findings have been reported in human clinical and histological studies [26]. In Hong Kong Chinese population single nucleotide polymorphism of C5 (rs17611) with genotype AG and the haplotype CGCA containing rs1035029, rs17611, rs25681 and rs992670 has been found to be significantly more prevalent in periodontitis patients than in healthy controls [27, 30]. Only the MBL2 homozygote (O/O) variant type, a secreted pattern-recognition molecule in the cascade of lectin pathway, could provoke the virulence of *A. actinomycetemcomitans* with no difference found between *P. gingivalis* and/or inflammatory markers in saliva and periodontal tissue destruction in study subject [31].

The mutations in few pattern recognition receptors including toll like receptors (TLRs), NOD-like receptors (NLRs), formyl peptide recptors and Fc receptors have been studied so far to express the alteration or the misrecognition of microbial constituents resulting in altered response to microbes. The effect of genetic polymorphisms in these receptors is mainly expressed as their response characteristics at the protein and mRNA level after exposure to various cytokines and microbes. The *CD14* -260CT + TT genotype is found to have higher frequencies of red complex bacteria i.e. *Porphyromonas gingivalis*, *Treponema denticola* and *Tannerella forsythia* particularly in renal transplant patients with cyclosporine A induced gingival overgrowth which is associated with high interleukin-1β (IL-1β) levels [32]. The altered immune response due to immunosuppressive medication and disruption of normal symbiotic relation can be plausible explanation for these findings. In contrast, the CD14 -159TT variant has found to have a protective role in periodontitis patients by reducing subgingival colonisation of *Prevotella intermedia* [33]. In the healthy individuals the mutant type of *TLR 4* (Asp299Gly heterozygote) has been appeared less responsive to

Porphyromonas gingivalis than wild type TLR4(normal) [34]. But no association has been seen with TLR4 polymorphisms (Asp299Gly and Thr399Ile) in periodontitis patients in relation to subgingival occurrence of periodontopathogens [33]. Similarly, TLR 2 polymorphism (−16,934 T/A) in both healthy and periodontitis patients has shown no association [35]. In Czech population, the TLR-9 haplotype -1486 T/− 1237 T/+2848A has been found to increase the susceptibility of chronic periodontitis but without affecting the subgingival colonisation of bacteria [35]. Another, extensively studied receptor is *Fc receptors* only in two alleles i.e. *FcγRII* and *FcγRIII* types. FcγRIIa131H/H genotype has been found to be hyperreactive phenotype of the polymorphonuclear neutrophils (PMNs), which release more bioactive molecules in response to periodontal pathogens and aggravate the periodontal destruction [36, 37]. In contrary to this the FcγRIIb-nt645 + 25AA genotype has been seen to be linked with more severe periodontitis in Japanese population, due to suppression of humoral response against periodontopathic [38, 39]. Similarly, inefficient phagocytosis of bacteria by neutrophils in FcγRIIIb-NA2 subjects is responsible for an increased levels of bacteria in gingival crevice leading to high risk of periodontitis [40]. Most of the investigations were documented in chronic periodontitis, only a single polymorphism studied in relation to aggressive periodontitis is nt324 A/A FcαRI polymorphism. It exhibited similarly a decreased phagocytosis of periodontopathic bacteria *Porphyromonas gingivalis* in Japanese population [41]. This body of literature revealed that functional differences in the activity of immune cells possibly lead to inter individual differences in the subgingival colonisation of periodontal pathogens and the development of periodontitis.

Genetic factors affecting periodontal pathogen proliferation/ clearance

The recognition of invaded periodontopathogens leads to the activation of immune regulatory mechanisms which is deterministic for the onset and progression of periodontal disease. It was hypothesised that alteration in the genetic constitution of components of immune regulatory mechanism can alter the subgingival environment for the proliferation of microbes in both healthy and diseased state of periodontium.

Chronic periodontitis

The polymorphisms in the cluster of *IL-1* gene have been the most extensively studied polymorphism as to explore the link of periodontal disease pathogenesis. Infact, a genetic susceptibility kit based on IL-1β polymorphisms has been commercialised. But apart from the direct effect on host defence mechanisms, indirect bearing of the polymorphisms on periodontal microbes also has been documented. The subjects with IL-1A(+ 4845) and IL-1B(+ 3954) genotype have exhibited higher mean counts of subgingival species belonging to red and orange complexes like *Tannerella forsythia, Treponema denticola, Fusobacterium nucleatum* subspecies, *Fusobacterium periodonticum, Campylobacter gracilis, Campylobacter showae, Streptococcus constellatu, Streptococcus intermedius, Streptococcus gordonii* and 3 *Capnocytophaga* species in sites with increasing pocket depth [42]. In contrast, the Caucasian subjects with this single nucleotide polymorphisms (SNPs) presenting periodontitis has demonstrated negative association with the subgingival colonisation of microbes [43–46]. But individually IL-1β + 3954 genotype had exhibited higher prevalence of *Porphyromonas gingivalis, Tannerella forsythia* and *Treponema denticola* species in subgingival sites and higher expression of IL-1β mRNA [47]. So, additively both can affect the potential outcome of periodontal disease. In a group of subjects with periodontitis with IL-1A-889 and IL-1B + 3953 genotype the total count of red complex (*Porphyromonas gingivalis, Tannerella forsythia* and *Treponema denticola*), orange complex (*Fusobacterium nucleatum, Peptostreptococcus micros, Prevotella intermedia, Campylobacter rectus*) bacteria and of *Campylobacter rectus* has been found to be 3-fold and 2-fold higher than the negative genotype subjects [48]. So, IL-1 genotype is considered as a nonmandatory but a contributable risk factor for periodontal disease progression and no definitive conclusions could be drawn on the effect of this genotype on the individual subject's overall mean bacterial load or of their colonisation by specific bacterial clusters. However, allelic forms of same gene polymorphism differentially affect the colonisation of same pathogens. As Caucasian individuals with *IL-2* -330,166 TT:TT genotype has presented with a positive association for the subgingival presence of *Porphyromonas gingivalis* and bacteria of the red complex, but individually subjects with interleukin-2166 TT genotype have been more oftenly infected with *Porphyromonas gingivalis* and bacteria of the red complex whereas a decreased occurrence of *Porphyromonas gingivalis* and bacteria of the red complex found in interleukin-2 -330 TG-positive subjects with a decrease in the odds ratio for chronic periodontitis (odds ratio = 0.394) whereas IL2 -166TT and haplotype IL-2 -330,166 TT:TT associated with an increase in odds ratio (odds ratio = 2.82 or 2.97) [49]. Such kind of observations can pave pathway for the use of gene polymorphisms and their haplotype combination as a putative prognostic factors for chronic periodontitis. The level of periodontopathogens *Porphyromonas gingivalis, Tannerella forsythia* and *Treponema denticola* has been found to be higher in Caucasians with chronic periodontitis carrying *IL-4* haplotype with *Treponema denticola* detected in higher counts at diseased sites [50]. This was attributed that the gene polymorphisms alter the immune

response against pathogens either by promoting the proinflammatory cytokine production or by suppression of anti-inflammatory function. So, the alteration in a single gene can influence the various cytokines by altering dominated arm of immune response as seen for the levels of IL-4 and IL-13 which are influenced by IL-4 receptor complex specially the *IL-4RA Q551R* and associated with diseases such as the Hyper-IgE syndrome, Atopic dermatitis, Asthma, Systemic lupus erythematosus (SLE), Sjörgren syndrom, Systemic scleroderma, and Cutaneous mastocytosis, where an allergic or autoimmune pathogenesis is assumed [51]. At the same time, this alteration in the immune response have an impact on pathogen colonisation with QR + RR polymorphism of IL-4RA Q551R found to be associated with increased presence of *Tannerella forsythia* in same population [52]. The polymorphism have either enhanced the signal transduction inducing a Th2 dominated response which was ineffective against periodontopathogens or decreased signal transduction with a dominated Th1 type of immune response [52]. So, the altered immune response could cause destructive disease even at lower bacterial loads via influencing response to bacteria rather than their counts. As analysed in the diseased sites of AGT/TTC patients of *IL8* gene polymorphisms – 845 T/C, – 738 T/C, –251A/T, + 396 T/G and + 781C/T, a higher levels of *Porphyromonas gingivalis, Tannerella forsythia, Treponema denticola* and red complex have been detected as compared to the patients with ATC/TTC genotype presenting similar clinical parameters suggesting the more destructive inflammatory response even after a lower microbial challenge in patients with ATC/TTC genotype [53]. Similarly, the level of pathogens has been found to be higher in the patients without IL-8 haplotype than with the haplotype patients at the diseased site [54]. In Caucasian patients presenting IL-8 + 781CC genotype with chronic periodontitis the destructive frequency of *Tannerella forsythia* was much less explaining the more destructive immune response [55]. However, in relation to *IL-10*, a multifunctional anti inflammatory cytokine, the subjects positive for ACC, ATA and ACA/ATA have been associated with decreased prevalence of *Prevotella intermedia* as compared to GCC/GCC positive subjects [56]. The genetic constitution was associated with low IL-10 production which is responsible for high local immune response against *Prevotella intermedia* implicated in severe periodontal tissue destruction [56]. Most of polymorphisms analysed in relation to chronic periodontitis have an impact mainly on pathogens belonging to red or orange complexes. However, a strong association has been seen with *Aggregatibacter actinomycetemcomitans* in *IL-6* -174GG genotype subjects considering all subject and tooth related factors [57]. The periodontal pathogen colonisation was found to be unaffected by *IL-12* genotype polymorphisms where as *IFN-γ* 874 AA carriers have been documented for decreased odds ratio for the presence of *Aggregatibacter actinomycetemcomitans* in the oral cavity. Moreover, IFN-γ 874TA predisposed to infection with *Prevotella intermedia* in a group of Caucasian subjects presenting with all disease states [58]. IL-12 and IFN-γ are known to bear a significant application as the maintenance of balance between the Th1 and Th2 type of immune responses. IFN-γ 874 AA genotype carriers primarily activate Th2 cells, as a low producer IFN-γ, only few Th1 cells are also activated, making a more pronounced humoral immune response more effective against *Aggregatibacter actinomycetemcomitans*. Conversely, in subjects who expressed the genotype IFN-γ 874 TA, an intermediate IFN-γ production was associated with an unbalanced Th1/Th2 immune response against *Prevotella intermedia* [58]. There was found to be negatively associated relationship of IFN-γ polymorphisms with the periodontal pathogen colonisation in healthy and chronic periodontitis group in Czech population [59].

Many other cytokines gene polymorphisms like tumour necrosis factor-α (TNF-α), HLA- II, nuclear factor kappa β (NF-κβ), Vitamin D receptor, T bet, MMP8, Apolipoprotein E, peroxisome proliferator activated receptor gamma (PPARγ) involved in periodontal disease pathogenesis are also studied in context with periodontal infectogenomics. Only TNF-α -308GG/−238GG haplotype showed more frequent presence of *Prevotella intermedia* in Caucasians [60]. Similar findings have been reported in coronary heart patients with severe periodontitis in carriers positive for AG + AA genotype and A-allele of TNF-α -308G > A with a risk of 1.4 fold [61]. However, no differences have been found in the frequency or in the load of the periodontopathogens investigated in the different TNFA − 308 genotype groups [62]. The TBX21 -1993 T/C polymorphism of key transcription factor T-bet also found to be involved in the impact of Th1 responses but no association has been documented with load of red complex bacteria [63]. Similarly, no association with the subgingival occurrence of pathogens has been found for Taq1 polymorphisms of vitamin D receptor [64], MMP8 -799C/T and + 17C/G variants [65], polymorphisms of Apolipoprotein E [66] and PPARγPro12Ala polymorphism [67]. To delineate further, more well designed and controlled studies are needed to explore the associations between microbes and host genetic constitution.

Aggressive periodontitis

The most extensively studied polymorphism is of *IL-6* gene especially in subjects with aggressive periodontitis. IL-6 -174G genotype has been found to be associated with *Aggregatibacter actinomycetemcomitans* in generalised aggressive periodontitis patients and with both *Aggregatibacter actinomycetemcomitans* and *Porphyromonas gingivalis*

in IL-6 -174GG and IL-6 -6106AA polymorphisms [68, 69]. A survey of Indian population on the IL-6 -174 polymorphism presented that in addition to *Aggregatibacter actinomycetemcomitans* another bacteria *Capnocytophaga sputigena* belonging to the green complex found in increased counts in periodontal pockets [70]. The haplotype – 174 G, – 572 C, – 1363 G, – 1480 C, and – 6106 A alleles have been reported to be associated with higher detection of *Aggregatibacter actinomycetemcomitans* whereas haplotype – 174 C, – 572 C, – 1363 T, – 1480 G, and – 6106 A alleles have supposedly protective function toward *Aggregatibacter actinomycetemcomitans* colonisation [69]. So, these findings to some extent confirm the hypothesis that complex interactions between the microbiota and host genome can affect the susceptibility to aggressive periodontitis. Such strong association can be explained as mainly due to faster hyperinflammatory immune response and stimulation of the overgrowth of some particular component of opportunistic organisms making the IL-6 hyperproducer individuals prone to increased risk for periodontal tissue destruction. A rare group of Caucasian population with *IL-1α* rs1800587, *IL-1β* rs1143634 genotype and composite genotype (rs1800587_rs1143634), a significant association of genetic variants and the twofold higher risk of subgingival occurrence of *Aggregatibacter actinomycetemcomitans* have been proved [71]. Further, *IL-8* -251TT genotype subjects also presented with the increased odds ratio for presence of *Aggregatibacter actinomycetemcomitans* in same population [55]. However, longitudinal investigations failed to confirm the role of this host- bacterium interplay in pathogenesis of aggressive periodontitis and its relation to IL-1 composite genotype [72]. In Japanese population, the gene polymorphisms of more frequent 5′ flanking region of *IL12RB2* has been associated with higher serum IgG titres against periodontal bacteria *Aggregatibacter actinomycetemcomitans*, *Capnocytophaga ochracea*, *Eikenella corrodens*, *Fusobacterium nucliatum* [73]. This explained the skewing of immune response toward Th2 responses with higher production of immunoglobulins after infection with periodontal bacteria in carrier group. Major histocompatibility complex-II (*MHC-II*) gene polymorphisms in same population presented with a suggestive hypothesis that the determination of the location of atypical BamHI restriction site in the HLA-DQB1 gene might be useful for determining a tendency toward high susceptibility to localised aggressive periodontitis with *Tannerella Forsythia* infection [74]. The *NF-κβ*-94del/del genotype has also presented with positive association to aggressive periodontitis and with the subgingival occurrence of *Aggregatibacter actinomycetemcomitans* in Caucasians [75].

In response to Periodonatal therapy

In Caucasian subjects with IL-1A + 4845/ IL-1B-3954 genotype undergoing supportive periodontal therapy, it has been suggested that a lower bacterial load is required in IL-1 gene positive subjects to develop the same level of periodontitis as in IL-1 gene–negative subjects as analysed from the bacterial load at different sites [76]. However, the periodontal therapy has been found to be equally effective and efficient to reduce the counts of periodontopathogens irrespective of their genetic background [50]. Therefore, the response to periodontal therapy has been found independent of the genetic profile of individual.

Other periodontal conditions

In order to study the impact of the genetic constitution on implants, a retrospective study in subjects with IL-1α – 889 and IL-1β + 3953 polymorphisms has been reported to be associated with higher implant loss in synergism with the smoking but without any alteration in microbial colonisation [77].

Among the rare conditions, the IL-10 SNPs has been analysed in renal transplant patients with cyclosporine-A induced gingival overgrowth in a Chinese population and found to be associated with the higher prevalence of *Porphyromonas gingivalis* and *Treponema denticola* especially in subjects with ATA haplotype [78]. So, the low IL-10 expression amplifies the local inflammatory response contributing to development of gingival overgrowth which favours the overgrowth of periodontal pathogens mainly *Porphyromonas gingivalis* and *Treponema denticola*.

A hypothesis has been made to explain the role of infectogenomics in perio- systemic relationship mainly in type 2 diabetes mellitus in association with IL-1 genotype polymorphisms and suggested that dental plaque remains the major contributory factor to progressive periodontitis with periodontal interleukin-1 gene polymorphisms and differences in oral microbiota seem to play only a subordinate role [79].

Through the discrete result from all the studies are difficult to be drawn and the mechanisms yet to explain further. However, the possible biological explanations have been put forth in literature as [42, 45]:

a) The cytokines might directly affect the growth and/ or virulence activity of bacterial species.

b) Indirect mechanism considers that an increased inflammatory response to a given microbial challenge occurs due to an over-production of cytokines. An increased gingival crevice fluid flow in response to inflammation might foster increased levels of subgingival species, particularly species of the red and orange complexes. So, increased levels of these species in turn may affect the local tissues leading to increased inflammation and pocket formation.

c) Both the overall lower serum antibody levels and specific titers against selected bacteria have responsible for their colonisation.

Genome wide association studies in context of periodontal Infectogenomics

The concept of periodontal infectogenomics has been investigated in genome wide association studies (GWAS) also in addition to cross sectional or case control study designs. Among participants of the Atherosclerosis Risk in Communities (ARIC) longitudinal cohort investigation (The ARIC Investigators, 1989) did not reveal a significant genome wide signals but suggested that 13 loci, including KCNK1, FBXO38, UHRF2, IL33, RUNX2, TRPS1, CAMTA1, and VAMP3, provide an evidence of association for red and orange complex microbiota except *Aggregatibacter actinomycetemcomitans* [2]. These results are further carried forward in another genome association study using MAGENTA (meta-analysis gene set enrichment of variant associations) approach to obtain gene-centric and gene set association results. The statistically significant association has been found for 6 genes; 4 with severe chronic periodontitis (*NIN, ABHD12B, WHAMM, AP3B2*) and 2 with high periodontal pathogen colonisation (red complex – *KCNK1, Porphyromonas gingivalis* – *DAB2IP*). The top gene sets included have been: for severe chronic periodontitis - endoplasmic reticulum membrane, cytochrome P450, microsome and oxidation reduction; for moderate chronic periodontitis - regulation of gene expression, zinc ion binding, BMP signalling pathway and ruffle; for periodontal pathogen colonisation-circadian clock system for red complex, G alpha Z signalling events for orange complex, KEGG mismatch repair for *Aggregatibacter actinomycetemcomitans* and protein binding for *Porphyromonas gingivalis* [25]. Thus, highlighted genes in previously identified loci and new candidate genes for explaining possible pathways associated with chronic periodontitis.

Recently genome wide association of chronic periodontitis is conducted by supplementing clinical data with biological intermediates of microbial burden and local inflammatory response with the formation of periodontal complex traits (PCTs). PCT1 has been characterised by a uniformly high pathogen load (Socransky trait), PCT4 with a mixed infection community whereas PCT3 and PCT5 have been dominated by *Aggregatibacter actinomycetemcomitans* and *Porphyromonas gingivalis*, respectively [10]. The genome-wide significant signals have been detected as mentioned in Table 1.

These highlighted loci mainly include genes associated with immune response and epithelial barrier function which enhance the disease susceptibility in the presence of a dysbiotic microbial structure [10]. However, these loci have not been associated with clinically defined disease

Table 1 Genome wide significant signals and the closest gene associated

Locus	SNP	Closest gene
PCT1 (Socransky Trait)		
16q11.2	rs1156327	CLEC19A (C-type lectin domain family 19 member A)
14q21	rs3811273	TRA (Transfer gene)
12q14	rs17184007	GGTA2P (Glycoprotein, Alpha- Galactosyltransferase 2 Pseudogene)
13q32.3	rs9557237	TM9SF2 (Transmembrane 9 Superfamily Member 2)
1q12	rs1633266	IFI16 (Interferon, Gamma-Inducible Protein 16)
3q12	rs17718700	RBMS3 (RNA Binding Motif Single Stranded Interacting Protein 3)
PCT3 (Aa Trait)		
4p15.33	rs4074082	C1QTNF7 (C1q and tumour necrosis factor-related protein 7)
8q24.3	rs9772881	TSNARE (T-SNARE Domain Containing)
PCT4 (Mixed Infection)		
7q21.1	rs10232172	HPVC1 (Human Papillomavirus (type 18) E5 Central Sequence Like 1)
PCT5(Pg Trait)		
12q14	rs7135417	SLC15A4 (Solute Carrier Family 15 Member 4)
11q14	rs6488099	PKP2 (plakophilin 2)
15q24	Rs904310	SNRPN (Small Nuclear Ribonucleoprotein Polypeptide N)

which raises the possibility that these PCTs may be genetically tractable endophenotypes that nevertheless have little relevance to disease defined with clinical criteria alone. This has been suggested that the six PCTs, although having overlapping clinical presentations, may actually reflect six different conditions with distinct genetic risk profiles that may be discoverable only in the context of specific patterns of microbial dysbiosis and inflammatory response [10]. These new findings provide a logical sub-classification of disease based upon genetic and microbial-inflammatory signatures that warrants further validation.

Recently, a systematic review has been conducted on the periodontal infectogenomics included a total of 43 studies consisted of candidate genes and the above mentioned genome wide analyses and given a conclusion that there is no evidence yet that neither IL- 1 genetic polymorphisms nor any other investigated genetic polymorphisms are associated with presence and counts of subgingival microbiota. This is because of the heterogeneity and complexity of the study, case control study approach, small sample sizes and risk of bias analysis [80].

Summary

To summarise, the host genotype may affect the colonisation pattern of subgingival species has been extensively discussed in the past few years. Nibali L et al. have reported that IL-6 hyperproducers (IL-6-174GG genotype subjects) show consistent association with *Aggregatibacter actinomycetemcomitans* detection in several independent studies in different populations. However, majority of the investigations of IL-1 and TNF-α polymorphisms have

primarily reported association with subgingival colonisation of red and orange complex bacteria, but failed to give conclusive statements due to heterogeneity. The haplotypes of IL-4, IL-8 and IL-10 polymorphisms also has been associated with microbial colonisation. Other investigations about candidate genes vis IL-2, IL-12, IFN-γ, HLA class II, NF-κβ, vitamin D receptor, MMP-8, T-bet, apolipoprotein E and PPARγ polymorphisms had not documented any significant association with the pathogen colonisation. The findings from the published literature emphasises that in IL-2, IFN-γ, HLA class II and NF-κβ genotype needs further exploration of this association. Specifically, genotypes affecting pathogen detection receptors viz. CD14 260 CT + TT genotype has showed association with the red complex bacterias. MBL2 homozygote variant is found to be the only studied complement component suggesting the possibility to provoke the virulence of A. actinomycetemcomitans and Fcγ receptors reported the hyperactive phenotype of PMNs affecting the PMN function mainly phagocytosis and oxidative burst, resulting in severe microbial effect on periodontal tissue. Some of the polymorphisms associated with enhancement in special periodontal conditions as in case of gingival overgrowth subjects, the CD14 260 and IL-10 haplotype have been associated with the microbial colonisation of red complex bacteria. Since GWAS have been recently introduced in study of Periodontology, the evidence needs further exploration to define some conclusive association. So, the contemporary evidence available to explain the concept of periodontal imfectogenomics is complied as shown in Table 2.

Table 2 Summary of contemporary evidence related to periodontal infectogenomics

Authors	Study Design	Ethnicity	Number Of Patients	Clinical Groups	Analysed Gene Polymorphisms	Analysed Microbes	Associations
Complement System (MBL)							
Liukkonen A et al. 2017 [31]	CS	Finnish Study Population	222	Generalised Periodontitis, Localised Periodontitis, Periodontitis free	MBL2 (allele D, allele B, allele C) Grouped as: wild-type A/A, heterozygote A/O homozygote O/O	Aa P. gingivalis	MBL2 homozygote variant (O/O) type could provoke the virulence of Aa
TLR							
Kinane DF et al. 2006 [34]	In vitro	–	HGECs from healthy gingival tissues from 6 healthy subjects	Two HGECs from subjects heterozygous for the TLR4 polymorphism and four with the wild-type TLR4.	TLR4 Asp299Gly and Thr399Ile (Mutant type) TLR4 normal (Wild type)	P. gingivalis	Wild type TLR4 (Normal) appears more responsive to P.gingivalis than the mutant type
Holla LI et al. 2010 [35]	CC	Caucasian	481	CP and H	TLR2 2408G/A, i.e. Arg753Gln and -16934A/T TLR9-1486C/T, -1237C/T and 12848A/G	Aa P. gingivalis P. intermedia T. forsythia T. denticola P. micros F. nucleatum	Not significant
CD14							
Schulz S et al. 2008 [33]	CC	Caucasian	213	AgP, CP and H	CD14 -159C > T, TLR4 Asp299Gly, Thr399Ile	P. gingivalis P. intermedia T. forsythia Aa T. denticola	CD14 -159TT genotype + patients: < P. intermedia detection
Gong Y et al. 2013 [32]	CS	–	204	Renal transplant patients with and without cyclosporine A induced gingival overgrowth	CD14-260C > T	P. gingivalis P. intermedia T. forsythia Aa T. denticola	Gingival overgrowth patients with CD14-260 CT + TT: > detection of P. gingivalis, T. forsythia,T. denticola and red complex.
FcR							
Kobayashi T et al. 2000 [81]	CC	Japanese	33	CP and H	FcγRIIIb-NA1 and FcγRIIIb-NA2	P.gingivalis	CP patients with both FcγRIIIb-NA1/NA1 and FcγRIIIb-NA2/NA2 genotypes: lower stimulation index for IgG1- and IgG3-mediated phagocytosis in PMNs
Kaneko S et al. 2004 [41]	CC	Japanese and Caucasian	185	AgP	FcαRI nt324 A → G	P. gingivalis	FcαRI nt324 A/A in AgP: decreased phagocytosis of P. gingivalis
Wolf DL et al. 2006 [36]	CC	Caucasian	205	CP and H	FcγRIIIb NA1/NA2, FcγIIa 131R/H	19 bacterial stains	Not significant

Table 2 Summary of contemporary evidence related to periodontal infectogenomics (*Continued*)

Authors	Study Design	Ethnicity	Number Of Patients	Clinical Groups	Analysed Gene Polymorphisms	Analysed Microbes	Associations
Nicu EA et al. 2007 [37]	CS	Mixed	98	CP	FcγRIIa131H/R	Aa	In CP patients with FcγRIIa (H/H): increased phagocytosis, degraulation and elastase release after stimulation with Aa
Wang Y et al. 2012 [38]	CC	Japanese	119	CP and H (females post delivery)	FcγRIIbnt645 + 25A/G, FcγRIIb-nt646-184A/ G,FcγRIIb-1232 T,FcγRIIa-R131H,FcγRIIIaV158F,Fc-γRIIIb-NA1/NA2	P. gingivalis P. intermedia Aa	Not significant
Sugita N et al. 2012 [39]	CS	Japanese	32	CP and H	FcγRIIb-nt645 + 25A/G	P.gingivalis	FcγRIIb-nt645 + 25AA genotype: < IgG4 levels produced against P. gingivalis sonicate and IgG2 produced against the P. gingivalis 40-kDa outer membrane protein (OMP)
IL-1							
Socransky SS et al. 2000 [42]	CS	–	108	CP	IL-1A + 4845 and IL-1B + 3954	40 taxa	IL-1genotype + subjects: > counts of T. forsythia, T. denticola, F.nucleatum, F. periodonticum, Campylobacter gracilis, C. showae, Streptococcus constellatus. Streptococcus intermedius, Streptococcus gordonii and 3 Capnocytophage species
Cullinan MP et al. 2001 [43]	L	Caucasian	295	CP	IL-1a + 4845 and IL-1B + 3954	Aa P. gingivalis P. intermedia	Not significant
Papapanou PN et al. 2001 [45]	CC	Caucasian	205	CP and H	IL-1A + 4845 and IL-1B + 3953	19 bacterial stains	Not significant
Jansson H et al. 2005 [77]	L	–	22	Patients with dental implants	IL-1α-889 and IL-1β + 3953	P. gingivalis P. nigrescens Aa	Not significant
Kowalski J et al. 2006 [48]	CS	–	16	CP	IL-1A-889 and IL-1B + 3953	P. gingivalis P. intermedia T. forsythia Aa T. denticola F. nucleatum E. corrodens P. micros C. rectus	IL-1 genotype + subjects: Higher total count of C. Rectus, red complex and orange complex bacteria IL-1genotype - subjects: Higher mean titre of P. intermedia

Table 2 Summary of contemporary evidence related to periodontal infectogenomics (Continued)

Authors	Study Design	Ethnicity	Number Of Patients	Clinical Groups	Analysed Gene Polymorphisms	Analysed Microbes	Associations
Agerbaek MR et al. 2006 [76]	CS	Caucasian	151	CP in supportive periodontal therapy	IL-1A + 4845 and IL-1B-3954	40 taxa	IL-1 genotype negative subjects: > total bacteria load and > levels of Aa, E. nodatum, P. gingivalis, Streptococcus anginosus
Kratka Z et al. 2007 [72]	L	–	20	AgP	IL-1A -889C/T and IL-1B +3953C/T	P. gingivalis, P. intermedia, T. forsythia, Aa, T. denticola	Not significant
Ferreira SB et al. 2008 [47]	CC	Mixed	292	CP and H	IL-1β 3954	P. gingivalis, T. forsythia, Aa, T. denticola	Not significant
Gonçalves L de S et al. 2009 [46]	CC	Mixed	105	CP and H (Grouped into HIV on HARRT and non HIV)	IL-1A + 4845 and IL-1B +3954	33 bacterial species	Not significant
Schulz S et al. 2011 [71]	CC	Caucasian	248	AgP, CP and H	IL1α(rs180058),IL-1β (rs16944, rs1143634), IL-1R (rs2234650), and IL-1RA (rs315952)	P. gingivalis, P. intermedia, T. forsythia, Aa, T. denticola	IL-1α rs1800587, Il-1β rs 1,143,634 and composite genotype: > Aa detection in AgP group
Cantore S et al. 2014 [44]	CC	Italian Caucasian	195	H and CP	IL-1α + 4845 and IL-1β +3954	Subgingival species	Not significant
Deppe H et al. 2015 [79]	Prospective	Caucasian	104	Type 2 diabetes mellitus patients and healthy controls	IL-1A, IL-1B and IL-1RN	Red, orange, green, yellow and purple complexes	Not significant
IL-2							
Reichert S et al. 2009 [49]	CC	Caucasian	200	AgP, CP and H	IL-2 -330 T/G and 166 G/T	P. gingivalis, P. intermedia, T. forsythia, Aa, T. denticola	IL-2-330, 166 TT-TT haplotype and 166TT: > detection of P. gingivalis and red complex IL-2 -330 TG: < P. gingivalis and red complex
IL-4							
Reichert S et al. 2011 [52]	CC	Caucasian	243	AgP, CP and H	IL-4RA Q551R	P. gingivalis, P. intermedia, T. forsythia, Aa, T. denticola	QR + RR polymorphism: Presence of T. forsythia
Finoti LS et al. 2013 [50]	CC	Caucasian	39	CP and H	IL-4 -590C/T, +33C/T and VNTR	P. gingivalis, T. forsythia, T. denticola	IL-4 TCI/CCI haplotype in CP: higher levels of P. gingivalis, T. forsythia, T. denticola
	CC	–	62	CP and H		P. gingivalis	

Table 2 Summary of contemporary evidence related to periodontal infectogenomics (Continued)

Authors	Study Design	Ethnicity	Number Of Patients	Clinical Groups	Analysed Gene Polymorphisms	Analysed Microbes	Associations
Bartova J et al. 2014 [51]					IL-4 -590c/T and intron 3 VNTR	P. intermedia, T. forsythia, Aa	IL-4 -590CC and 11 of IL-4 VNTR: T. forsythia stimulates production of cytokines TNFα, IL-6, IL-10, IFNγ, IL-10, and IL-1β while P. intermedia affects the in vitro production of IL-6 and IL-10 CP.
IL-6							
Nibali L et al. 2007 [68]	CS	Mixed	45	AgP	IL-6 -174, Fcα, FcγRIIa, FcγRIIb, FcγRIIIa, FcγRIIIb, FPR, TNF and VDR	Aa, P. gingivalis, T. forsythia	IL-6 -174GG and Fcγ haplotypes: >Aa detection
Nibali L et al. 2008 [69]	CS	Mixed	107	AgP and CP	IL-1A -889, IL-1B -511, +3954 IL-6 -174, -572, -1363, -1480, -6106, TLR4-299,-399, TNFα -308	Aa, P. gingivalis, T. forsythia	IL-6 -6106 AA and IL-6 haplotypes (-174G, -572C, -1363G, -1480C, -6106A): > detection of Aa
Nibali L et al. 2010 [57]	CS	Mixed	40	CP	IL-6 -174G > C	Aa, P. gingivalis	IL-6 -174GG: >Aa detection
Nibali L et al. 2011 [70]	CS	Indian	251	H and with periodontal disease	IL-6 -174, -572, -1363, -6106 and -1480	40 taxa	IL-6 -174GG: > counts of Aa and detection and counts of C. Sputigena
Nibali L et al. 2013 [82]	L	Caucasian	12	AgP	IL-6 -1363, -1480	Aa	IL6 haplotype: >counts of Aa before and after treatment
IL-8							
Linhartova PB et al. 2013 [55]	CC	Caucasian	492	AgP, CP and H	IL-8 -845C/T, -251A/T, +396 G/T and +781C/T	P. gingivalis, P. intermedia, T. forsythia, Aa, T. denticola, F. nucleatum, P. micros	IL8 -251 T in AgP: > A. actinomycetemcomitans detection CC genotype of IL8 +781 T/C variant in CP: < T. forsythia detection In non-periodontitis subjects with T allele of IL8 +396G/T variant or TT genotype: <F. nucleatum detection.
Finoti LS et al. 2013 [54]	CS	Mixed	65	CP and H	IL-8 ATC/TTC	P. gingivalis, T. forsythia, T. denticola	Not significant
Finoti LS et al. 2013 [53]	CS	Mixed	30	CP and H	IL-8 ATC/TTC and AGT/TTC haplotype	P. gingivalis, T. forsythia, T. denticola	The diseased sites of AGT/TTC patients: harbour higher levels of P. gingivalis, T. denticola, T. forsythia, and red complex

Table 2 Summary of contemporary evidence related to periodontal infectogenomics *(Continued)*

Authors	Study Design	Ethnicity	Number Of Patients	Clinical Groups	Analysed Gene Polymorphisms	Analysed Microbes	Associations
IL-10							
Reichert S et al. 2008 [56]	CC	Caucasian	93	AgP, CP and H	IL-10 -1082G > A, -819C > T and -590C > A	P. gingivalis, P. intermedia, T. forsythia, Aa, T. denticola	IL-10 ACC, ATA and ACC/ATA haplotypes: < P. intermedia detection. IL-10 GCC/GCC haplotype: > P. intermedia detection
Luo Y et al. 2013 [78]	CS	Chinese	202	Renal transplant patients with and without cyclosporine A induced gingival overgrowth	IL-10 -1082, −819 and −592	P. gingivalis, P. intermedia, T. forsythia, Aa, T. denticola	Gingival overgrowth patients with ATA haplotype: higher detection and count of P. gingivalis and T. denticola
IFN-γ & IL-12							
Takeuchi-Hatanaka K et al., 2008 [73]	CS	Japanese	110	AgP, severe CP, mild CP and H	5' flanking region of IL12RB2	P. gingivalis, P. intermedia, T. forsythia, Aa, T. denticola, F. nucleatum, E. corrodens	Higher serum IgG titres against periodontopathic bacteria in patients with variant alleles
Reichert S et al. 2008 [58]	CC	Caucasian	198	AgP, CP and H	IFN-γ 874 T/A, IL-12 1188A/C	P. gingivalis, P. intermedia, T. forsythia, Aa, T. denticola	IFN-γ 874AA: < detection of Aa. IFN-γ 874TA: > detection of P. intermedia
Holla LI et al. 2011 [59]	CC	Caucasian	498	CP and H	IFN-γ +874A/T	P. gingivalis, P. intermedia, T. forsythia, Aa, T. denticola, F. nucleatum, P. micros	Not significant
TNFα							
Schulz S et al. 2008 [60]	CC	Caucasian	175	AgP, CP and H	TNFα -308G > A and -238G > A	P. gingivalis, P. intermedia, T. forsythia, Aa, T. denticola	TNFα308GG/238GG haplotype: > P. intermedia detection
Trombone APF et al. 2009 [62]	CC	Mixed	304	CP and H	TNFα -308G/A	P. gingivalis, T. forsythia, Aa, T. denticola	Not significant
Schulz S et al. 2012 [61]	CS	Caucasian	942	Cp and H (All Coronary Artery Disease patients)	TNFα 308G > A and -238G > A	P. gingivalis, P. intermedia, T. forsythia	TNFα-308 AG + AA genotype and A-allele: > P. intermedia detection

Table 2 Summary of contemporary evidence related to periodontal infectogenomics (Continued)

Authors	Study Design	Ethnicity	Number Of Patients	Clinical Groups	Analysed Gene Polymorphisms	Analysed Microbes	Associations
HLAII							
Shimomura-Kuroki J et al. 2009 [74]	CC	Japanese	64	AgP, CP and H	IL-1α −889, IL-1α + 4845, IL-1β + 3954 FcγRIIa-H/R131 HLA- DQB1	Aa, T. denticola, P. micros, F. nucleatum, C. rectus, E. nodatum, E. corrodens, C. sputigena	HLADQB1 BamHI sites in patients: > T. forsythia detection
NF-κβ							
Schulz S et al. 2010 [75]	CC	Caucasian	222	AgP, CP and H	TLR2 (Arg753Gln and Arg67Trp) NF-κβ -94ins/del ATTG	P. gingivalis, P. intermedia, T. forsythia, Aa, T. denticola	NF-κβ-94del/del: > Aa detection
VDR							
Borges et al. 2009 [64]	CC	Caucasian	60	CP and H	VDR TaqI	38 taxa	Not significant
T bet							
Cavalla et al. 2015 [63]	CC	Mixed	608	CP, CG and H	TBX21-1993 T/C	P. gingivalis, T. forsythia, T. denticola	Not significant
MMP8							
Holla LI et al. 2012 [65]	CC	Caucasian	619	CP and H	MMP8 (-799C/T and +17C/G)	P. gingivalis, P. intermedia, T. forsythia, Aa, T. denticola, P. micros, F. nucleatum	Not significant
ApoE							
Linhartova PB et al. 2015 [66]	CC	Caucasian	469	CP and H	ApoE (rs429358C/T and rs7412C/T)	P. gingivalis, P. intermedia, T. forsythia, Aa, T. denticola, P. micros, F. nucleatum	Not significant

Table 2 Summary of contemporary evidence related to periodontal infectogenomics (Continued)

Authors	Study Design	Ethnicity	Number Of Patients	Clinical Groups	Analysed Gene Polymorphisms	Analysed Microbes	Associations
PPARγ							
Hirano E et al. 2010 [67]	CS	Japanese	130	CP and H All Pregnant Females Grouped as term birth and preterm birth	PPARγPro12Ala	*P. gingivalis* *P. intermedia* *T. forsythia* *Aa*	Not significant
GWAS							
Divaris K et al. 2012 [2]	–	Caucasian and Blacks	1020 white and 123 African American participants	Healthy to severe chronic periodontitis	2,178,777 SNPs	*C. rectus* *F. nucleatum* *P. nigrescens* *P. gingivalis* *T. forsythia* *T. denticola* *P. intermedia* *Aa*	Not a significant genome wide signals. But 13 loci, including KCNK1, FBXO38, UHRF2, IL33, RUNX2, TRPS1, CAMTA1, and VAMP3, provide an evidence of association for red and orange complex microbiota, but not for *Aa*.
Rhodin K et al. 2014 [25]	–	Caucasian	1020 + 4504 from two previously conducted GWAs	Healthy to severe chronic periodontitis	18,307 genes	*C. rectus* *F. nucleatum* *P. nigrescens* *P. gingivalis* *T. forsythia* *T. denticola* *P. intermedia* *Aa*	Statistically significant association for 6 genes – 4 with severe chronic periodontitis (NIN, ABHD12B, WHAMM, AP3B2) and 2 with high periodontal pathogen colonisation (red complex – KCNK1, P. gingivalis – DAB21P).
Offenbacher S et al. 2016 [10]	–	–	975 European American For CP in the larger cohort (n = 821 severe CP, 2031 = moderate CP, 1914 = healthy/mild disease) and a German sample of 717 AgP cases and 4210 controls.	Healthy to severe chronic periodontitis and aggressive periodontitis	21,35,235 SNPs	8 periodontal pathogens divided into 6 PCTs with distinct microbial community as PCT1 with high pathogen load (Socransky trait), PCT4 with a mixed infection, PCT3, PCT5 dominated by *Aa* and *P. gingivalis*, respectively.	Genome-wide significant signals for PCT1 (CLEC19A, TRA, GGTA2P, TM9SF2, IFI16, RBMS3), PCT4 (HPVC1) and PCT5 (SLC15A4, PKP2, SNRPN). Overall, the highlighted loci included genes associated with immune response and epithelial barrier function.
Systematic review							
Nibali L et al. 2016 [80]	–	–	43 studies of candidate genes and two GWAS	Healthy to severe chronic periodontitis and aggressive periodontitis	–	Periodontal Pathogens	No evidence yet that neither IL-1 genetic polymorphisms nor any other investigated genetic polymorphisms are associated with presence and counts of subgingival microbiota.

Aa Aggregatibacter actinomycetemcomitans, AgP Aggressive Periodontitis; CS: Cross Sectional, CC Case Control, H Healthy, CG Chronic Gingivitis, HGECs Human Primary Gingival Epithelial Cultures, CP Chronic Periodontitis, L Longitudinal

The major issues concerned to the study of infectoge-nomics is the difficulty in comprehensively examining the subgingival microbiota which is further complicated by nature of microbial infection, biofilm type formed where both the symbiotic and exogenous bacteria are organised which behave as part of a complex and poly-microbial nature of periodontal infection and due to in-adequate knowledge of specific host genetic factors that are likely to affect the subgingival microbiota.

Conclusion

The functional genomics of host has crucial importance while analysing host- pathogen interactions in the patho-genesis of periodontal disease. An increased understand-ing of the genetics underpinning of interactions between the host and exogenous or symbiotic bacterial communi-ties has the potential to advance our knowledge not only of periodontitis, but also of other chronic inflammatory and microbiome-related diseases. Several risk loci identi-fied may offer promising leads for further exploration and mechanistic studies which have the potential to un-veil pathways and mechanisms that direct the host's symbiosis with healthy microflora to dysbiosis state which may predispose to the disease state. Therefore, infectogenomics may serve as a useful model to study the relationship between host genome and microbial challenge. Further exploration of the concept is essential to identify infectious states, to understand the host re-sponse, to predict disease outcomes, to monitor re-sponses to antimicrobial therapies and to indicate promising new types of treatment.

Future directions

The field of periodontal infectogenomics can determine different pathogenic pathways in different forms of peri-odontitis, and possibly assist in early prevention and management of disease. Additional multicentre studies based on large population samples in different popula-tions and with high-quality phenotypes need to be con-ducted worldwide to identify the human genetic factors that predispose to invasion by pathogens and to their proliferation. Changes in gene expression profiles can also determine the type of pathogen present. Thus, gene expression patterns in the blood could serve as a win-dow into the pathogenesis and diagnosis of infectious diseases. Advances in gene expression profiling may pos-sibly provide the chance for adjunctive pharmacological treatment. Further research is needed to validate the bio-logic basis for genetic susceptibility testing, to evaluate the ability of different genotypes to predict disease initi-ation and to evaluate the effectiveness of genotyping in making diagnostic or treatment intervention strategies, especially in dental new age tissue engineering approach. However, the consideration of specific microbiota with

distinct exposure is consistent with the paradigm of peri-odontal medicine which may provide an insight into the new alternative connection of oral-systemic diseases.

Abbreviations
Aa: Aggregatibacter actinomycetemcomitans; ABHD12B: Abhydrolase Domain Containing 12B; AgP: Aggressive Periodontitis; AP3B2: Adapter Related Protein Complex 3 Beta 2 Subunit; BMP: Bone Morphogenetic Protein; CC: Case Control; CCR5: Chemokine Receptor 5; CG: Chronic Gingivitis; CP: Chronic Periodontitis; CS: Cross Sectional; DAB2IP: Disabled Homolog 2 Interacting Protein; H: Healthy; HGECs: Human Primary Gingival Epithelial Cultures; HIV: Human Immunodeficiency Virus; HLA: Human Leukocyte Antigen; IFN-γ: Interferon Gamma; IL-4RA: Interleukin -4 Receptor α Chain 43; KCNK1: Potassium Two Pore Domain Channel Subfamily K Member 1; L: Longitudinal.; MBL: Mannose Binding Ligand; MHC II: Major Histocompatibility Complex II; MMP 8: Matrix Metalloproteinases 8; NF-κβ: Nuclear Factor Kappa β; PAMPs: Pathogen Associated Molecular Patterns; PRPs: Peptidoglycan Recognition Proteins; RUNX2: Runt Related Transcription Factor 2; SNPs: Single Nucleotide Polymorphisms; Th: T Helper Cells; TNF-α: Tumor Necrosis Factor Alpha; TRPS1: Transcription Repressor GATA Binding 1; UHRF2: Ubiquitin like PHD and Ring Finger Domain 2; VAMP3: Vesicle associated Membrane Protein 3; WHAMM: WAS Protein Homolog Associated with Actin, Golgi Membranes and Microtubules

Acknowledgements
We would like to express our sincere gratitude to all the authors for contributing to the review cited in the present manuscript.

Funding
Not applicable.

Authors' contributions
All authors contributed equally to drafting the manuscript. All authors read, revised, and approved the final manuscript.

Competing interests
The authors declare that they have no competing interests.

References
1. Laddha R, Sehdev B, Saini NK, Zubedi T, Narang AK. Periodontal Infectogenomics: a review. Int J Dent Med Res. 2015;1(6):189–92.
2. Divaris K, Monda KL, North KE, Olshan AF, Lange EM, Moss K, et al. Genome-wide association study of periodontal pathogen colonization. J Dent Res. 2012;91(Suppl 7):21S–8S.
3. Nibali L, Donos N, Henderson B. Periodontal Infectogenomics. J Med Microbiol. 2009;58:1269–74.
4. Laine ML, Loos BG, Crielaard W. Gene polymorphisms in chronic periodontitis. Int J Dent. 2010;2010:324719.
5. Hart TC, Korman KS. Genetic factors in the pathogenesis of periodontitis. Periodontol. 1997;14:202–15.
6. Kinane DF, Shiba H, Hart TC. The genetic basis of periodontitis. Periodontol 2000. 2005;39:91–117.
7. Takashiba S, Naruishi K. Gene polymorphisms in periodontal health and disease. Periodontol 2000. 2006;40:94–106.
8. Nasry B, Choong C, Flamiatos E, Chai J, Kim N, Strauss S, et al. Diversity of the oral microbiome and dental health and disease. Int J Clin Med Microbiol. 2016;1:108.
9. Nibali L, Henderson B, Sadiq ST, Donos N. Genetic dysbiosis: the role of microbial insults in chronic inflammatory diseases. J Oral Microbiol. 2014;25(6):22962.
10. Offenbacher S, Divaris K, Barros SP, Moss KL, Marchesan JT, Morelli T, Zhang S, Kim S, Sun L, Beck JD, Laudes M, Munz M, Schaefer AS, North KE.

Genome-wide association study of biologically informed periodontal complex traits offers novel insights into the genetic basis of periodontal disease. Hum Mol Genet. 2016;25(10):2113–29.

11. Kellam P, Weiss RA. Infectogenomics: insights from the host genome into infectious diseases. Cell. 2006;124(4):695–7.

12. Hill AV. The genomics and genetics of human infectious disease susceptibility. Annu Rev Genomics Hum Genet. 2001;2:373–400.

13. Weatherall DJ, Clegg JB. Genetic variability in response to infection: malaria and after. Genes Immun. 2002;3(6):331–7.

14. Blekhman R, Goodrich JK, Huang K, Sun Q, Bukowski R, Spector D, et al. Host genetic variation impacts microbiome composition across human body sites. Genome Biol. 2015;16:191–201.

15. Gasche C, Nemeth M, Grundtner P, Willheim-Polli C, Ferenci P, Schwarznbacher R. Evolution of crohn's disease- associated Nod2 mutations. Immunogenetics. 2008;60(2):115–20.

16. de Silva E, Stumpf MP. HIV and the CCR5-Δ32 resistance allele. FEMS Microbiol Lett. 2004;241(1):1–12.

17. Galvani AP, Slatkin M. Evaluating plague and smallpox as historical selective pressures for the CCR5-Δ32 HIV-resistance allele. Proc Natl Acad Sci U S A. 2003;100(25):15276–9.

18. Taborda-Vanegas N, Zapata W, Rugeles MT. Genetic and immunological factors involved in natural resistance to HIV-1 infection. Open Virol J. 2011;5:35–43.

19. Kwiatkowski D. Genetic susceptibility to malaria getting complex. Curr Opin Genet Dev. 2000;10(3):320–4.

20. Drumm ML, Ziady AG, Davis PB. Genetic variation and clinical heterogeneity in cystic fibrosis. Annu Rev Pathol. 2012;7:267–82.

21. Campodónico VL, Gadjeva M, Paradis-Bleau C, Uluer A, Pier GB. Airway epithelial control of Pseudomonas aeruginosa infection in cystic fibrosis. Trends Mol Med. 2008;14(3):120–33.

22. Fernando SL, Britton WJ. Genetic susceptibility to mycobacterial disease in humans. Immunol Cell Biol. 2006;84(2):125–37.

23. Thursz M. Genetic susceptibility in chronic viral hepatitis. Antivir Res. 2001; 52(2):113–6.

24. Knights D, Lassen KG, Xavier RJ. Advances in inflammatory bowel disease pathogenesis: linking host genetics and the microbiome. Gut. 2013;62(10): 1505–10.

25. Rhodin K, Divaris K, North KE, Barros SP, Moss K, Beck JD, Offenbacher S. Chronic periodontitis genome wide association studies: gene centric and gene set enrichment analyses. J Dent Res. 2014;93(9):882–90.

26. Hajishengallis G, Maekawa T, Abe T, Hajishengallis E, Lambris JD. Complement involvement in periodontitis: molecular mechanisms and rational therapeutic approaches. Adv Exp Med Biol. 2015;865:57–74.

27. Hajishengallis G, Abe T, Maekawa T, Hajishengallis E, Lambris JD. Role of complement in host–microbe homeostasis of the periodontium. Semin Immunol. 2013;25:65–72.

28. Marianne R, Nikolaus R, Matthias S, et al. Periodontal Ehlers-Danlos syndrome is caused by mutations in C1R and C1S, which encode subcomponents C1r and C1s of complement. Am J Hum Genet. 2016;99(5):1005–14.

29. Zhan Y, Zhang R, Lv H, Song X, Xu X, Chai L, Lv W, Shang Z, Jiang Y, Zhang R. Prioritization of candidate genes for periodontitis using multiple computational tools. J Periodontol. 2014;85:1059–69.

30. Chai L, Song Y-Q, Zee K-Y, Leung WK. Single nucleotide polymorphisms of complement component 5 and periodontitis. J Periodont Res. 2010;45:301–8.

31. Liukkonen A, He Q, Gürsoy UK, Pussinen PJ, Gröndahl-Yli-Hannuksela K, Liukkonen J, Sorsa T, Suominen AL, Huumonen S, Könönen E. Mannose-binding lectin gene polymorphism in relation to periodontal infection. J Periodont Res. 2017;52:540–5.

32. Gong Y, Bi W, Cao L, Yang Y, Chen J, Yu Y. Association of CD14-260 polymorphisms, red-complex periodontopathogens and gingival crevicular fluid cytokine levels with cyclosporine A-induced gingival overgrowth in renal transplant patients. J Periodontal Res. 2013;48(2):203–12.

33. Schulz S, Zissler N, Altermann W, Klapproth J, Zimmermann U, Gläser C, et al. Impact of genetic variants of CD14 and TLR4 on subgingival periodontopathogens. Int J Immunogenet. 2008;35(6):457–64.

34. Kinane DF, Shiba H, Stathopoulou PG, Zhao H, Lappin DF, Singh A, et al. Gingival epithelial cells heterozygous for toll-like receptor 4 polymorphisms Asp299Gly and Thr399Ile are hypo-responsive to Porphyromonas gingivalis. Genes Immun. 2006;7(3):190–200.

35. Holla LI, Vokurka J, Hrdlickova B, Augustin P, Fassmann A. Association of Toll-like receptor 9 haplotypes with chronic periodontitis in Czech population. J Clin Periodontol. 2010;37(2):152–9.

36. Wolf DL, Neiderud AM, Hinckley K, Dahlén G, van de Winkel JG, Papapanou PN. Fcγ receptor polymorphisms and periodontal status: a prospective follow-up study. J Clin Periodontol. 2006;33(10):691–8.

37. Nicu EA, Van der Velden U, Everts V, Van Winkelhoff AJ, Roos D, Loos BG. Hyperreactive PMNs in FcγRIIa 131 H/H genotype periodontitis patients. J Clin Periodontol. 2007;34(1):938–45.

38. Wang Y, Sugita N, Kikuchi A, Iwanaga R, Hirano E, Shimada Y, et al. FcγRIIB-nt645+25A/G gene polymorphism and periodontitis in Japanese women with preeclampsia. Int J Immunogenet. 2012;39(6):492–500.

39. Sugita N, Iwanaga R, Kobayashi T, Yoshie H. Association of the FcγRIIBnt645 +25A/G polymorphism with the expression level of the FcγRIIb receptor, the antibody response to Porphyromonas gingivalis and the severity of periodontitis. J Periodontal Res. 2012;47(1):105–13.

40. Yoshie H, Kobayashi T, Tai H, Galicia JC. The role of genetic polymorphisms in periodontitis. Periodontol 2000. 2007;43:102–32.

41. Kaneko S, Kobayashi T, Yamamoto K, Jansen MD, van de Winkel JG, Yoshie H. A novel polymorphism of FcαRI (CD89) associated with aggressive periodontitis. Tissue Antigens. 2004;63(6):572–7.

42. Socransky SS, Haffajee AD, Smith C, Duff GW. Microbiological parameters associated with IL-1 gene polymorphisms in periodontitis patients. J Clin Periodontol. 2000;27(11):810–8.

43. Cullinan MP, Westerman B, Hamlet SM, Palmer JE, Faddy MJ, Lang NP, Seymour GJ. A longitudinal study of interleukin-1 gene polymorphisms and periodontal disease in a general adult population. J Clin Periodontol. 2001;28(12):1137–44.

44. Cantore S, Mirgaldi R, Ballini A, Coscia MF, Scacco S, Papa F, et al. Cytokine gene polymorphisms associate with microbiological agents in periodontal disease: our experience. Int J Med Sci. 2014;11(7):674–9.

45. Papapanou PN, Neiderud AM, Sandros J, Dahlén G. Interleukin-1 gene polymorphism and periodontal status. A case-control study. J Clin Periodontol. 2001;28(5):389–96.

46. Gonçalves LS, Ferreira SM, Souza CO, Colombo AP. Influence of IL-1 gene polymorphism on the periodontal microbiota of HIV infected Brazilian individuals. Braz Oral Res. 2009;23(4):452–9.

47. Ferreira SB Jr, Trombone AP, Repeke CE, Cardoso CR, Jr MW, Santos CF, et al. An interleukin-1β single nucleotide polymorphism at position 3954 and red complex periodontopathogens independently and additively modulate the levels of IL-1β in diseased periodontal tissues. Infect Immun. 2008;76(8):3725–34.

48. Kowalski J, Górska R, Dragan M, Kozak I. Clinical state of the patients with periodontitis, IL-1 polymorphism and pathogens in periodontal pocket – is there a link? (an introductory report). Adv Med Sci. 2006;51(Suppl 1):9–12.

49. Reichert S, Machulla HK, Klapproth J, Zimmermann U, Reichert Y, Gläser C, et al. Interleukin-2 -330 and 166 gene polymorphisms in relation to aggressive or chronic periodontitis and the presence of periodontopathic bacteria. J Periodontal Res. 2009;44(5):628–35.

50. Finoti LS, Anovazzi G, Pigossi SC, Corbi SC, Teixeira SR, Braido GV, et al. Periodontopathogens levels and clinical response to periodontal therapy in individuals with the interleukin 4 haplotype of susceptibility to chronic periodontitis. Int J Microbiol. Res Rev. 2013;1(2):039–47.

51. Bartova J, Linhartova PB, Podzimek S, Janatova T, Svobodova K, Fassmann A, et al. The effect of IL-4 gene polymorphisms on cytokine production in patients with chronic periodontitis and in healthy controls. Mediat Inflamm. 2014;2014:185757.

52. Reichert S, Stein JM, Klapproth J, Zimmermann U, Reichert Y, Gläser C, et al. The genetic impact of the Q551R interleukin-4 receptor alpha polymorphism for aggressive or chronic periodontitis and the occurrence of periodontopathic bacteria. Arch Oral Biol. 2011;56(12):1485–93.

53. Finoti LS, Corbi SC, Anovazzi G, Teixeira SR, Capela MV, Tanaka MH, et al. Pathogen levels and clinical response to periodontal treatment in patients with interleukin 8 haplotypes. Pathog Dis. 2013;69:21–8.

54. Finoti LS, Corbi SC, Anovazzi G, Teixeira SR, Steffens JP, Secolin R, et al. Association between IL8 haplotypes and pathogen levels in chronic periodontitis. Eur J Clin Microbiol Infect Dis. 2013;32(10):1333–40.

55. Barilova Linhartova P, Vokurka J, Poskerova H, Fassmann A, Izakovicova Holla L. Haplotype analysis of interleukin-8 gene polymorphisms in chronic and aggressive periodontitis. Mediat Inflamm. 2013;2013:342351.

56. Reichert S, Machulla HK, Klapproth J, Zimmermann U, Reichert Y, Gläser CH, et al. The interleukin-10 promoter haplotype ATA is a putative risk factor for aggressive periodontitis. J Periodontal Res. 2008;43(1):40–7.

57. Nibali L, Donos N, Farrell S, Ready D, Pratten J, Tu YK, D'Aiuto F. Association between interleukin-6 -174 polymorphism and Aggregatibacter actinomycetemcomitans in chronic periodontitis. J Periodontol. 2010;81(12):1814–9.

58. Reichert S, Machulla HK, Klapproth J, Zimmermann U, Reichert Y, Gläser C, et al. Interferon-gamma and interleukin-12 gene polymorphisms and their relation to aggressive and chronic periodontitis and key periodontal pathogens. J Periodontol. 2008;79(8):1434–43.

59. Holla LI, Hrdlickova B, Linhartova P, Fassmann A. Interferon-γ +874A/T polymorphism in relation to generalized chronic periodontitis and the presence of periodontopathic bacteria. Arch Oral Biol. 2011;56(2):153–8.

60. Schulz S, Machulla HK, Altermann W, Klapproth J, Zimmermann U, Gläser C, et al. Genetic markers of tumour necrosis factor α in aggressive and chronic periodontitis. J Clin Periodontol. 2008;35(6):493–500.

61. Schulz S, Schlitt A, Lutze A, Lischewski S, Seifert T, Dudakliewa T, et al. The importance of genetic variants in TNFα for periodontal disease in a cohort of coronary patients. J Clin Periodontol. 2012;39(8):699–706.

62. Trombone AP, Cardoso CR, Repeke CE, Ferreira SB Jr, Martins W Jr, Campanelli AP, et al. Tumor necrosis factor-alpha -308G/a single nucleotide polymorphism and red-complex periodontopathogens are independently associated with increased levels of tumor necrosis factor-alpha in diseased periodontal tissues. J Periodontal Res. 2009;44(5):598–608.

63. Cavalla F, Biguetti CC, Colavite PM, Silveira EV, Jr MW, Letra A, et al. TBX21-1993T/C (rs4794067) polymorphism is associated with increased risk of chronic periodontitis and increased T-bet expression in periodontal lesions, but does not significantly impact the IFN-γ transcriptional level or the pattern of periodontophatic bacterial infection. Virluence. 2015;6(3):293–304.

64. Borges MA, Figueiredo LC, Brito RB Jr, Faveri M, Feres M. Microbiological composition associated with vitamin D receptor gene polymorphism in chronic periodontitis. Braz Oral Res. 2009;23(2):203–8.

65. Holla LI, Hrdlickova B, Vokurka J, Fassmann A. Matrix metalloproteinase 8 (MMP8) gene polymorphisms in chronic periodontitis. Arch Oral Biol. 2012; 57(2):188–96.

66. Borilova Linhartova P, Bartova J, Poskerova H, Machal J, Vokurka J, Fassmann A, Izakovicova Holla L. Apolipoprotein E gene polymorphisms in relation to chronic periodontitis, periodontopathic bacteria, and lipid levels. Arch Oral Biol. 2015;60(3):456–62.

67. Hirano E, Sugita N, Kikuchi A, Shimada Y, Sasahara J, Iwanaga R, et al. Peroxisome proliferator-activated receptor gamma polymorphism and periodontitis in pregnant japanese women. J Periodontol. 2010;81(6):897–906.

68. Nibali L, Ready DR, Parkar M, Brett PM, Wilson M, Tonetti MS, Griffiths GS. Gene polymorphisms and the prevalence of key periodontal pathogens. J Dent Res. 2007;86(5):416–20.

69. Nibali L, Tonetti MS, Ready D, Parkar M, Brett PM, Donos N, D'Aiuto F. Interleukin-6 polymorphisms are associated with pathogenic bacteria in subjects with periodontitis. J Periodontol. 2008;79(4):677–83.

70. Nibali L, Madden I, Franch Chillida F, Heitz-Mayfield L, Brett P, Donos N. IL6–174 genotype associated with *Aggregatibacter actinomycetemcomitans* in Indians. Oral Dis. 2011;17(2):233–7.

71. Schulz S, Stein JM, Altermann W, Klapproth J, Zimmermann U, Reichert Y, et al. Single nucleotide polymorphisms in interleukin-1gene cluster and subgingival colonization with *Aggregatibacter actinomycetemcomitans* in patients with aggressive periodontitis. Hum Immunol. 2011;72(10):940–6.

72. Krátká Z, Bártová J, Krejsa O, Otčenášková M, Janatová T, Dušková J. Interleukin-1 gene polymorphisms as assessed in a 10-year study of patients with early-onset periodontitis. Folia Microbiol. 2007;52(2):183–8.

73. Takeuchi-Hatanaka K, Ohyama H, Nishimura F, Kato-Kogoe N, Soga Y, Matsushita S, et al. Polymorphisms in the 5' flanking region of IL12RB2 are associated with susceptibility to periodontal diseases in the Japanese population. J Clin Periodontol. 2008;35(4):317–23.

74. Shimomura-Kuroki J, Yamashita K, Shimooka S. *Tannerella forsythia* and the HLA-DQB1 allele are associated with susceptibility to periodontal disease in Japanese adolescents. Odontology. 2009;97(1):32–7.

75. Schulz S, Hierse L, Altermann W, Klapproth J, Zimmermann U, Reichert Y, et al. The del/del genotype of the nuclear factor-κB -94ATTG polymorphism and its relation to aggressive periodontitis. J Periodontal Res. 2010;45(3): 396–403.

76. Agerbaek MR, Lang NP, Persson GR. Microbiological composition associated with interleukin-1 gene polymorphism in subjects undergoing supportive periodontal therapy. J Periodontol. 2006;77(8):1397–402.

77. Jansson H, Hamberg K, De Bruyn H, Bratthall G. Clinical consequences of IL-1 genotype on early implant failures in patients under periodontal maintenance. Clin Implant Dent Relat Res. 2005;7(1):51–9.

78. Luo Y, Gong Y, Yu Y. Interleukin-10 gene promoter polymorphisms are associated with cyclosporin A-induced gingival overgrowth in renal transplant patients. Arch Oral Biol. 2013;58(9):1199–207.

79. Deppe H, Mücke T, Wagenpfeil S, Kesting M, Karl J, Noe S, Sculean A. Are selected IL-1 polymorphisms and selected subgingival microorganisms significantly associated to periodontitis in type 2 diabetes patients? A clinical study. BMC Oral Health. 2015;15(1):143–50.

80. Nibali L, Di Iorio A, Onabolu O, Lin GH. Periodontal infectogenomics: systematic review of associations between host genetic variants and subgingival microbial detection. J Clin Periodontol. 2016;43(11):889–900.

81. Kobayashi T, van der Pol WL, van de Winkel JG, Hara K, Sugita N, Westerdaal NA, Yoshie H, Horigome T. Relevance of IgG receptor IIIb (CD16) polymorphism to handling of *Porphyromonas gingivalis*: implications for the pathogenesis of adult periodontitis. J Periodontal Res. 2000;35(2):65–73.

82. Nibali L, Pelekos G, D'Aiuto F, Chaudhary N, Habeeb R, Ready D, et al. Influence of IL-6 haplotypes on clinical and inflammatory response in aggressive periodontitis. Clin Oral Investig. 2013;17(4):1235–42.

21

Zoledronic acid exacerbates inflammation through M1 macrophage polarization

Junya Kaneko[1,3], Toshinori Okinaga[1], Hisako Hikiji[2*], Wataru Ariyoshi[1], Daigo Yoshiga[3], Manabu Habu[3], Kazuhiro Tominaga[3] and Tatsuji Nishihara[1]

Abstract

Background: Zoledronic acid (Zol), one of the bisphosphonates, is frequently utilized for the treatment of osteoporosis and bone metastasis. However, the onset of medication-related osteonecrosis of the jaw (MRONJ) following dental treatments has become a serious issue. We reported previously that osteonecrosis can be induced by Zol and lipopolysaccharide (LPS) in vivo, suggesting the involvement of Zol in inflammation. Macrophages are divided into M1/M2 macrophages. M1 macrophages are involved in the induction and exacerbation of inflammation and express proinflammatory mediators including interleukin (IL)-1. On the other hand, M2 macrophages are associated with anti-inflammatory reactions through the expression of anti-inflammatory cytokines, such as IL-10. In the present study, we clarified the effects of Zol on M1/M2 macrophage polarization in vitro.

Methods: Human monocytic THP-1 cells were polarized to macrophage-like cells by phorbol 12-myristate 13-acetate (PMA), and, after culturing for an additional 24 h with or without Zol, then polarized to M1 macrophages by LPS or to M2 macrophages by IL-4. Cell viability was examined by the WST-8 assay. Gene expression was confirmed by the real-time polymerase chain reaction. Protein expression was detected by western blotting and enzyme-linked immunosorbent assays.

Results: Zol treatment upregulated the expression of IL-1β mRNA and protein through NLRP3 inflammasome activation in LPS-treated THP-1 cells. Zol treatment did not affect the expression of IL-10, IL-1ra, or CD206 in IL-4-treated THP-1 cells.

Conclusions: Zol enhanced LPS-induced M1, but not M2, macrophage polarization through the NLRP3 inflammasome-dependent pathway, resulting in the production of inflammatory cytokines in THP-1 cells.

Keywords: Zoledronic acid, Macrophage polarization, Inflammation

Background

Nitrogen-containing bisphosphonates, including zoledronic acid (Zol), are widely used as anti-bone-resorptive agents, primarily for the treatment of osteoporosis, Paget's disease of the bone, multiple myeloma, hypercalcemia due to malignancy, and other bone-resorptive diseases. The onset of medication-related osteonecrosis of the jaw (MRONJ) has become a serious issue. Dental treatment such as tooth extraction triggers the MRONJ in the patients taking anti-bone-resorptive agents. The clinical symptoms often seen in MRONJ including pain, swelling, paresthesia, suppuration, and intraoral/extraoral fistula

continue for a long time [1]. Marx et al. reported the first case of osteonecrosis of the jaw (ONJ) in 2003 [2, 3]. Since then, the number of patients with ONJ has been increasing yearly. Bisphosphonates are one of the most well-known agents that cause ONJ [4]. We reported that the combined use of Zol and lipopolysaccharide (LPS) in vivo induced ONJ and osteonecrosis of the femur in rats, suggesting that Zol is involved in the inflammatory response during the progression of MRONJ [5–7].

Macrophages are derived from monocytes and move out into extravascular tissues under inflammatory or non-inflammatory conditions, playing different roles according to their surrounding environment [8]. Oral macrophages also play important roles in the inflammatory response, as well as in signaling to resolve inflammation, and promote healing and regeneration [9].

---

* Correspondence: r09hikiji@fa.kyu-dent.ac.jp
[2]School of Oral Health Sciences, Kyushu Dental University, Kitakyushu, Fukuoka 803-8580, Japan
Full list of author information is available at the end of the article

Macrophages are divided into M1 and M2 macrophage types [10]. While investigating the factors that regulate macrophage arginine metabolism, Mills et al. found that macrophages activated in mouse strains with T helper type (Th)1 and Th2 backgrounds differed qualitatively in their ability to respond to the classic stimulation of interferon (IFN)-γ or LPS or both and defined an important metabolic difference in the pathway. They proposed that these be termed M1 and M2 macrophage responses [11]. Macrophages are polarized into the M1 macrophages, when exposed to classical activators such as LPS and IFN-γ [12]. Macrophages are polarized into the M2 from when exposed to alternative activators such as interleukin (IL)-4 or IL-13 [12]. M1-polarized macrophages produce pro-inflammatory cytokines, such as IL-1β, and infiltrate into injured tissues soon after damage [13]. M2-polarized macrophages are major resident macrophages and appear at late stages of repair and remodeling in injured tissue [14]. In our previous study, we have revealed that Zol activated NF-κB by enhancing IκB-α degradation suggesting the involvement of M1-polarized macrophages [15]. Therefore, we hypothesized that Zol might be involved in M1 but not M2 macrophage polarization, resulting in the inflammatory function in MRONJ. It is interesting to know the role of Zol in M1- or M2-polarized macrophages to probe into the cause of Zol-induced MRONJ. Therefore, in the present study, we investigated the effect of Zol on M1/M2 macrophage polarization in vitro and revealed that Zol and LPS synergistically enhanced proinflammatory character of THP-1 cells via activation of inflammasome.

Methods
Cell culture conditions
The human monocytic cell line, THP-1 (JCRB0112.1; JCRB Cell Bank, Osaka, Japan), was cultured in RPMI 1640 medium (Gibco Laboratories, Grand Island, NY, USA), supplemented with 5% heat-inactivated fetal bovine serum (FBS; CORNING, NY, USA), penicillin G (100 U/ml) (Nacalai Tesque, Kyoto, Japan), and streptomycin (100 mg/ml; Wako Pure Chemical Industries, Osaka, Japan) at 37 °C with 5% CO_2. THP-1 cells were seeded at 2×10^6 cells/well in six-well plates (Iwaki, Chiba, Japan) and cultured in RPMI 1640 medium containing 5% FBS and 100 ng/ml phorbol 12-myristate 13-acetate (PMA) (Sigma-Aldrich, St. Louis, MO, USA). After culturing overnight, cells were washed with phosphate-buffered saline (PBS; pH 7.2). THP-1 cells were then treated with or without Zol (10 μM; Sigma-Aldrich). After culturing for an additional 24 h with or without Zol, LPS from *Escherichia coli* (100 ng/ml; Sigma–Aldrich) or IL-4 (50 ng/ml; R&D Systems, Minneapolis, MN, USA) were added.

Reagents
Anti-IL-1β, anti-apoptosis-associated speck-like protein containing a caspase recruitment domain (ASC), and anti-cluster of differentiation (CD) 206 polyclonal antibodies were obtained from Santa Cruz Biotechnology (Santa Cruz, CA, USA). Anti-caspase-1 p-20 and NOD-like receptor protein 3 (NLRP3) monoclonal antibodies were obtained from Adipogen Life Sciences (San Diego, CA, USA). An anti-β-actin monoclonal antibody was obtained from Sigma–Aldrich. In some experiments, 5 mM ATP (Sigma–Aldrich) was applied to LPS-treated THP-1 cells for 30 min before collecting samples.

WST-8 assay
Cell viability was determined using the tetrazolium salt, WST-8 (2-(2-methoxy-4-nitrophenyl)-3-(4-nitrophenyl)-5-(2,4-disulfophenyl)-2H-tetrazolium, monosodium salt) (Dojindo Laboratories, Kumamoto, Japan). THP-1 cells $(4 \times 10^5$/well) were seeded in 96-well plates in RPMI 1640 containing 5% FBS and 100 ng/ml PMA. After culturing overnight, cells were washed with PBS (pH 7.2) twice and then exposed to Zol for 48 h. WST-8 solution (10 μl) was then added to each well, followed by incubation for 2 h. Absorbance at 450 nm was measured using a Multiscan JX microplate reader (Thermo Electron, Kanagawa, Japan).

RNA extraction and real-time reverse transcriptase-polymerase chain reaction (RT-PCR) analysis.

THP-1 cells were harvested, centrifuged at 4 °C, and stored at − 80 °C. RNA was extracted from cell pellets using a Cica Geneus RNA Prep Kit (KANTO CHEMICAL, Tokyo, Japan) according to the manufacturer's instructions. Total RNA was used for cDNA synthesis using ReverTra Ace qPCR RT Master Mix (TOYOBO, Osaka, Japan) according to the manufacturer's instructions. Primers for real-time RT-PCR were designed using Primer Express 3.0 software (Applied Biosystems, Foster City, CA, USA). Reactions were prepared using Brilliant III Ultra-Fast SYBR Green QPCR Master Mix With Low ROX (Agilent Technologies, Santa Clara, CA, USA). Detection was performed with an AriaMx Real-Time PCR System (Agilent Technologies). Relative changes in gene expression were calculated by the comparative CT (ΔΔCT) method. Total cDNA abundance between samples was normalized using primers specific for the β-actin gene.

The primers used for real-time RT-PCR were as follows: human *IL-1β* (GenBank accession no. NM_000576), forward 5′-TCAGCCAATCTTCATTGCTCAA-3′ and reverse 5′-TGGCGAGCTCAGGTACTTCTG-3′; human *IL-1ra* (GenBank accession no. NM_173842), forward 5′-CTCCTCTTCCTGTTCCATTCAG-3′ and reverse 5′-AAGGTCTTCTGGTTAACATCCC-3′; human *IL-10* (GenBank accession no. NM_000572), forward 5′-GCTG GAGGACTTTAAGGGTTAC-3′ and reverse 5′-GATG

TCTGGGTCTTGGTTCTC-3′; human *CD206* (GenBank accession no. NM_002438), forward 5′-GGACGTGGC TGTGGATAAAT-3′ and reverse 5′-ACCCAGAAG ACGCATGTAAAG-3′; and human *β-actin* (GenBank accession no. E0 1094), forward 5′-GCGCGGCTACAGCT TCA-3′ and reverse 5′-CTTAATGTCACGCACGATT TCC-3′.

Western blotting analysis

Following treatments, cells were lysed in sodium dodecyl sulfate (SDS) lysis buffer (50 mM Tris–HCl and 2% SDS; pH 6.8) containing a protease inhibitor mixture (Nacalai Tesque). Then, the protein content of the samples was determined using a protein assay reagent (Bio-Rad, Hercules, CA, USA). Protein samples (20 µg) were subjected to electrophoresis on SDS-polyacrylamide gels and electroblotted onto polyvinylidene fluoride membranes. The membranes were blocked for 30 min with Blocking One (Nacalai Tesque) and incubated with the primary antibodies for 2 h. After washing with Tris-buffered saline containing 0.1% Tween 20 (TBS-T), the membranes were incubated with the secondary antibody for 1 h. After washing with TBS-T, immunodetection was performed using the ECL Prime Western Blotting Detection Reagent (GE Healthcare, Little Chalfont, UK) and a ChemiDoc XRS Plus imaging system (Bio-Rad). Densitometric analysis of protein bands in the western blots was performed by Image Lab software (Bio-Rad). Data were normalized to β-actin expression and are expressed as means ± standard deviation (SD) of triplicate cultures.

Enzyme-linked immunosorbent assay (ELISA) analysis

Supernatants from THP-1 cells were collected at 0–48 h following LPS treatments. Secreted cytokine levels were assessed using human IL-1β/IL-1F2 Quantikine HS and human IL-1ra/IL-1F3 Quantikine ELISA kits (R&D Systems) according to the manufacturer's instructions.

Silencing of ASC expression by specific siRNA

siRNA targeting was used to knock down ASC expression in THP-1 cells. siRNAs against human ASC and siRNA control were purchased from Nacalai Tesque. A NEPA21 Super Elec-troporator (Nepa Gene Co., Ltd., Chiba, Japan) was used to deliver siRNA into cells according to the manufacturer's instructions. In brief, 1×10^6 cells were suspended in 100 µL of RPMI 1640 and transfected with siRNA at a final concentration of 300 nM.

Statistical analysis

All data are expressed as means ± SD of three individual experiments with similar results obtained in each experiment. Statistical differences were determined using unpaired Student's *t* test. A value of $P < 0.05$ was considered as statistically significant.

Results

Zol enhanced IL-1β expression and the secretion of mature IL-1β during M1 macrophage differentiation

THP-1 cells were exposed to Zol for 48 h after PMA treatment. From the result of the WST-8 assay (Fig. 1a), 10 µM Zol was used for subsequent experiments to minimize its toxic effects on cell viability [15, 16].

LPS is known to polarize monocytes/macrophages to M1 macrophages [17]. Zol upregulated the expression of IL-1β mRNA, one of the major inflammatory cytokines, as well as M1 macrophage markers, in LPS-treated THP-1 cells. In contrast, Zol downregulated the expression of interleukin-1 receptor antagonist (IL-1ra) mRNA, which is a naturally occurring cytokine preventing the biologic response to IL-1 [18], in LPS-treated THP-1 cells (Fig. 1b; *$P < 0.05$, **$P < 0.01$).

Zol upregulated the secretion of mature IL-1β, an active form of IL-1β that is cleaved from an inactive precursor, in LPS-treated THP-1 cells. On the other hand, Zol downregulated the secretion of IL-1ra in LPS-treated THP-1 cells (Fig. 1c; **$P < 0.01$).

Zol enhanced the expression of inflammasome-associated molecules during M1 macrophage differentiation

The NLRP3 inflammasome is crucial for the formation of mature IL-1β. Therefore, we investigated the expression of NLRP3 inflammasome-associated proteins in LPS-treated THP-1 cells by western blot analysis. Among NLRP3 inflammasome-associated molecules, several proteins, including NLRP3, caspase-1 p20 precursor, cleaved caspase-1 p20, IL-1β precursor, and mature IL-1β, and ASC, were investigated. Zol upregulated the expression of NLRP3, cleaved caspase-1 p20, IL-1β precursor, and mature IL-1β in LPS-treated THP-1 cells. Caspase-1 p20 precursor and ASC were constitutively expressed throughout the experimental time (Fig. 2).

To show the role of NLRP3 inflammasome in IL-1β expression and secretion of IL-1β in LPS-treated THP-1 cells, loss of function study of a NLRP3 inflammasome-associated molecule, ASC, was performed by siRNA. Silencing of ASC downregulated the protein expression of the mature IL-1β (Fig. 3a). Furthermore, silencing of ASC reduced the amount of secreted IL-1β (Fig. 3b).

Zol had no effect on mRNA and protein expression of M2 macrophage-related molecules during M2 macrophage differentiation

IL-4 polarizes monocytes/macrophages to M2 macrophages [19]. Zol did not have any effect on the mRNA and protein expression of CD206, a well-known M2 macrophage marker [20], in IL-4-treated THP-1 cells (Fig. 4a). Furthermore, Zol had no effect on the expression of IL-10 mRNA, one of the cytokines produced by M2 macrophages, and IL-1ra mRNA, a highly expressed

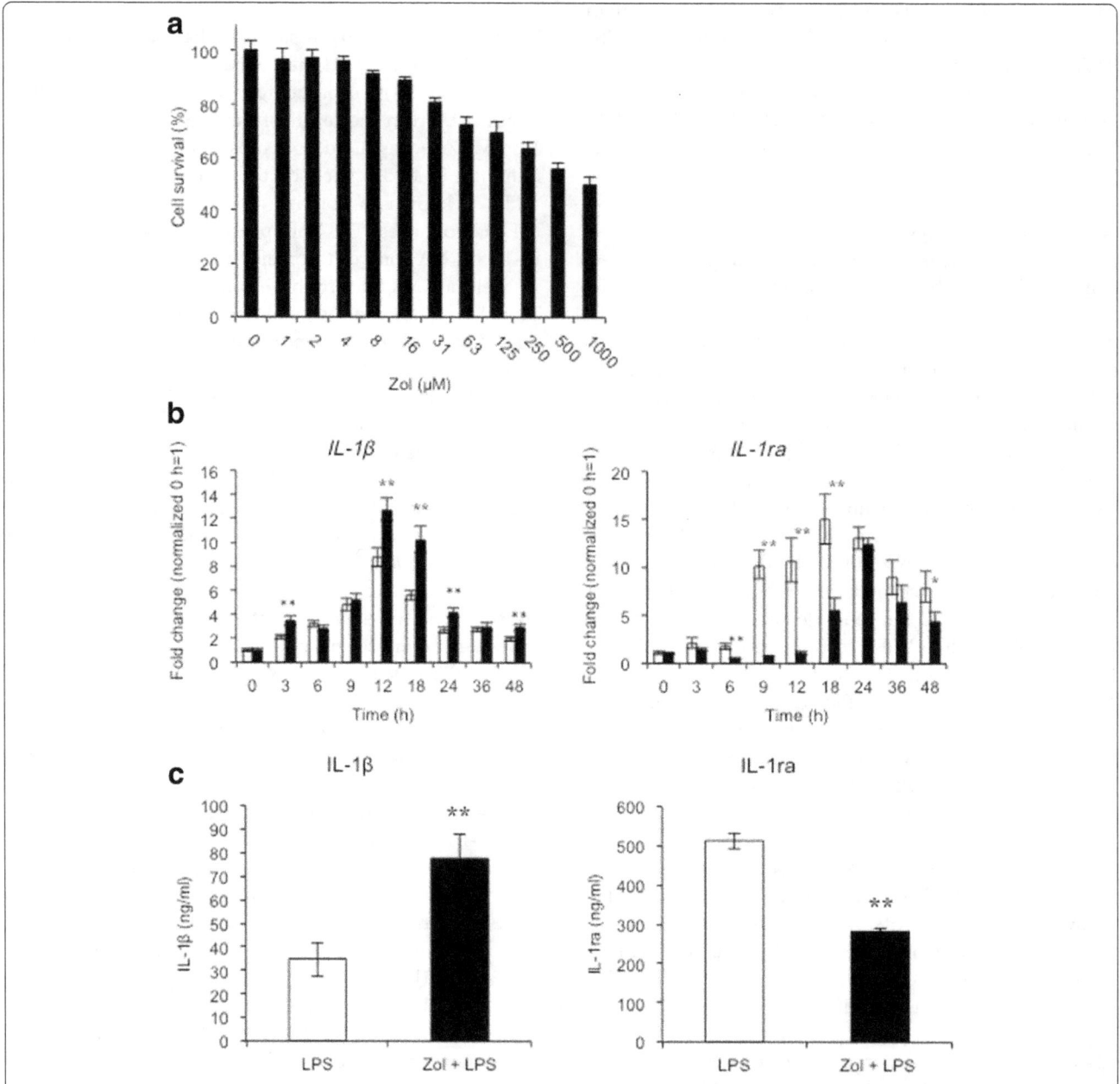

Fig. 1 Effects of zoledronic acid on the expression of M1/M2 macrophage markers in LPS-treated THP-1 cells. THP-1 cells were treated overnight with 100 ng/ml PMA, then washed and incubated for 24 h. **a** Cell viability was assessed using a WST-8 assay after treatment with Zol (1–1000 nM) for 48 h. **b** THP-1 cells were incubated with or without Zol for 24 h and then treated with 100 ng/ml LPS. Open bars represent LPS-treated THP-1 cells; filled bars represent Zol and LPS-treated THP-1 cells. Zol upregulated the expression of IL-1β mRNA and downregulated the expression of IL-1ra mRNA in LPS-treated THP-1 cells (* $P < 0.05$, ** $P < 0.01$ vs. cells treated with LPS alone). **c** ATP was applied to LPS-treated cells for 30 min before collecting samples. The secretion of IL-1β at 18 h and IL-1ra at 36 h was detected by ELISA. Zol upregulated the secretion of IL-1β and downregulated the secretion of IL-1ra in LPS-treated THP-1 cells (** $P < 0.01$ vs. cells treated with LPS alone)

molecule in M2 macrophages, in IL-4-treated THP-1 cells (Fig. 4b) [12].

Discussion

Zol enhances the production of proinflammatory cytokines [15, 21, 22] suggesting that Zol polarizes macrophages toward an M1 phenotype. In the current study, we showed

that Zol upregulated the expression of IL-1β mRNA and protein, and downregulated the expression of IL-1ra mRNA and protein, during M1 macrophage differentiation (Fig. 1). We have shown that Zol polarizes macrophages toward an M1 phenotype, but not an M2 phenotype and that Zol and LPS synergistically enhance proinflammatory character of THP-1 cells via activation of inflammasome.

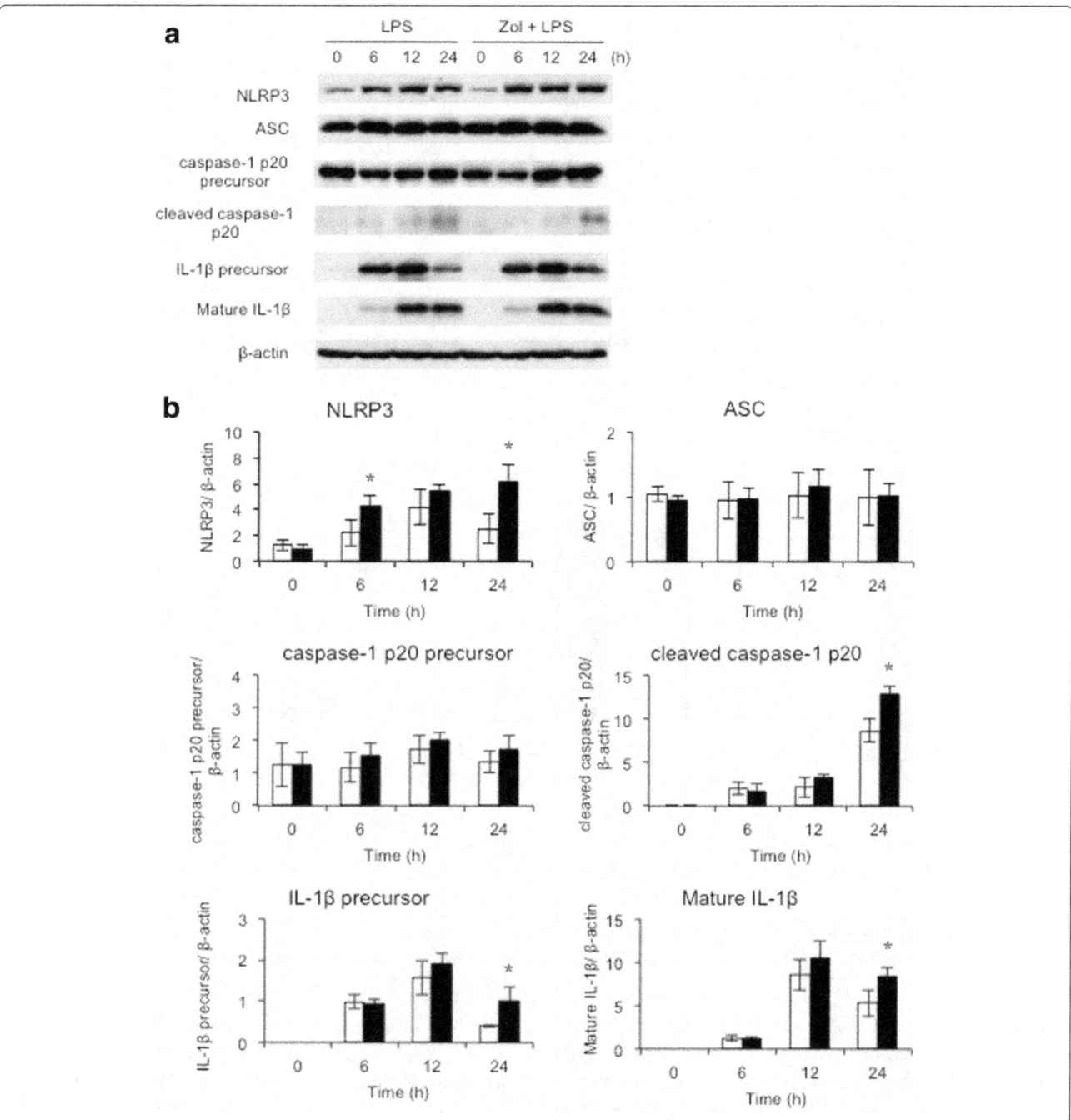

Fig. 2 Effects of zoledronic acid on the expression of inflammasome-associated proteins. THP-1 cells were treated overnight with 100 ng/ml PMA, washed with PBS, and incubated with or without Zol for 24 h. THP-1 cells were then treated with 100 ng/ml LPS. ATP was applied to LPS-treated cells for 30 min before collecting samples. **a** Protein expression was detected by western blotting. **b** Band intensities were measured by scanning densitometry. Data were normalized to β-actin expression. Open bars represent LPS-treated THP-1 cells; filled bars represent Zol and LPS-treated THP-1 cells. Zol promoted the expression of NLRP3, cleaved caspase-1 p20, IL-1β precursor, and mature IL-1β proteins in LPS-treated THP-1 cells (*$P < 0.05$ vs. cells treated with LPS alone)

In in vitro experiments, concentration of Zol at more than 10 μM is commonly used to investigate its effect on cells [15, 16, 23]. Clinically, the serum concentration of Zol is about 1.5 μM [24]. However, the serum concentration of Zol does not necessarily reflect the concentration of this compound affecting the cells in vivo. Therefore, 10 μM Zol was used for our experiments.

LPS stimulates inflammation through the production of cytokines such as IL-1β, finally resulting in the production of anti-inflammatory molecules like IL-1ra [25].

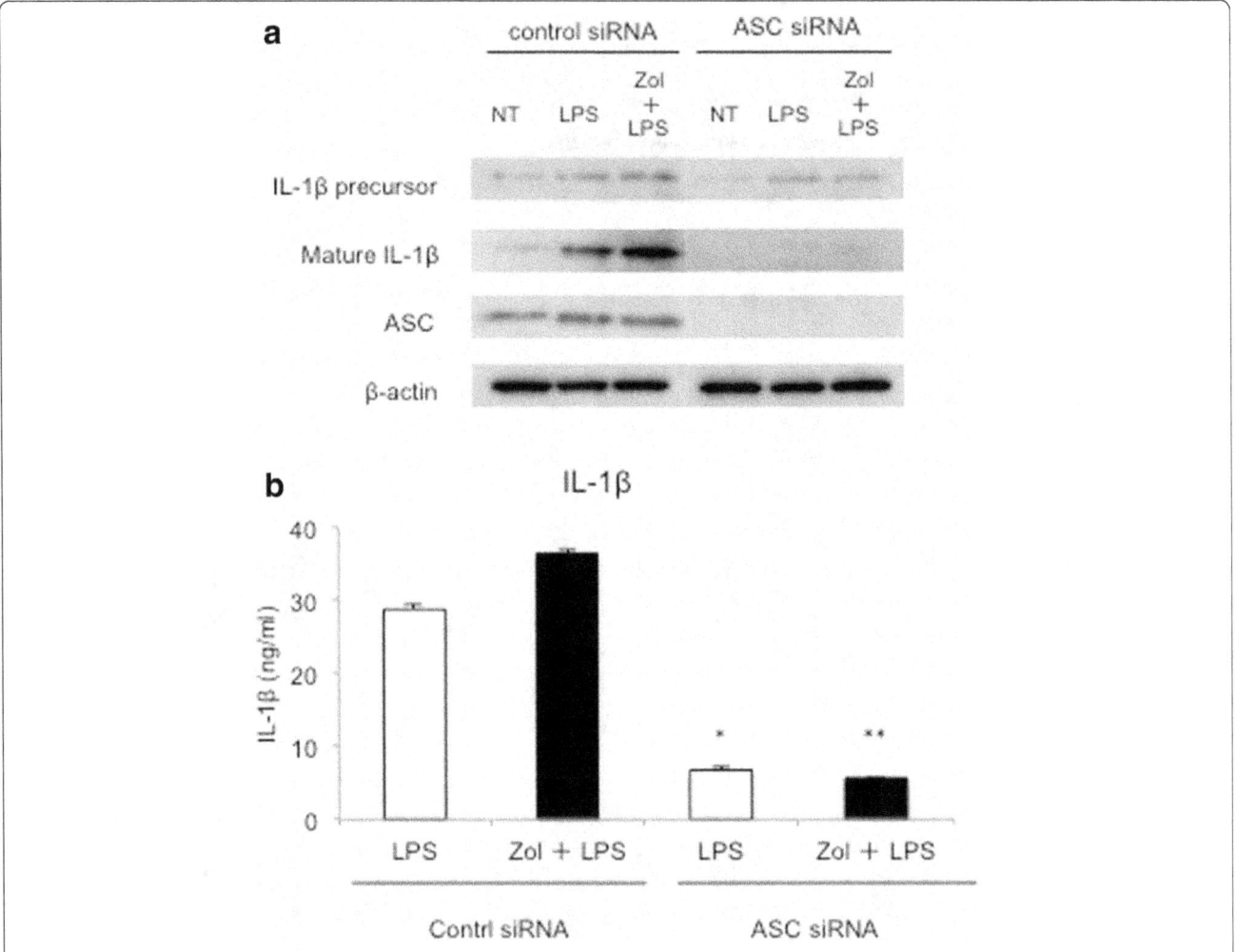

Fig. 3 Role of NLRP3 in IL-1β secretion induced in LPS-treated THP-1 cells. THP-1 cells were treated with siRNA against ASC, incubated overnight with 100 ng/ml PMA, washed with PBS, and incubated further with or without Zol for another 24 h. THP-1 cells were then treated with 100 ng/ml LPS. ATP was applied to LPS-treated cells for 30 min before collecting samples. **a** Protein expression was detected by western blotting. Silencing of ASC downregulated the expression of the mature IL-1β in LPS-treated THP-1 cells. **b** The secretion of IL-1β was detected by ELISA. Open bars represent LPS-treated THP-1 cells; filled bars represent Zol and LPS-treated THP-1 cells. Silencing of ASC reduced the secretion of IL-1β in LPS-treated THP-1 cells (*$P < 0.01$ vs. control siRNA THP-1 cells treated with LPS alone, ** $P < 0.01$ vs. control siRNA THP-1 cells treated with Zol and LPS)

Therefore, it is not surprising that LPS upregulates the expression of IL-1ra during M1 macrophage differentiation (Fig. 1). On the other hand, IL-1ra also serves as a marker of the anti-inflammatory response [26]. In the current study, Zol suppressed the expression of IL-1ra in LPS-treated THP-1 cells as compared with Zol-non-treated and LPS-treated cells. These results suggest that Zol extinguished the anti-inflammatory response in THP-1 cells. Importantly, Zol had no effect on mRNA and protein expression of M2 macrophage-related molecules such as IL-10, IL-1ra, and CD206 during M2 macrophage differentiation induced by IL-4 treatment (Fig. 4). These results clearly show that Zol prompts the differentiation of M1 but not M2 macrophages.

Various signaling pathways are reportedly involved in Zol-induced macrophage polarization [15, 21, 22]. Among these, the inflammasome is a large intracellular protein complex that recruits and activates caspase-1 which, in turn, cleaves the proform of IL-1β to its biologically active and secreted form [27]. The NLRP3 inflammasome is critical for the formation of mature IL-1β [28]. NLRP3 is the intracellular receptor of inflammasomes, and ATP activates NLRP3 [29, 30]. It is also well-known that ATP stimulates the secretion of mature IL-1β [31]. Because Zol treatment upregulated the mRNA and protein expression of IL-1β in our study, we investigated the effects of Zol on NLRP3 inflammasome activation by using ATP as a second signal to NLRP3. Zol upregulated the protein expression of NLRP3 and caspase-1 in LPS-treated THP-1 cells (Fig. 2). Silencing of ASC is reported to inhibit IL-1β release in LPS-treated THP-1 cells [32]. We have found that silencing of ASC downregulated the protein expression of

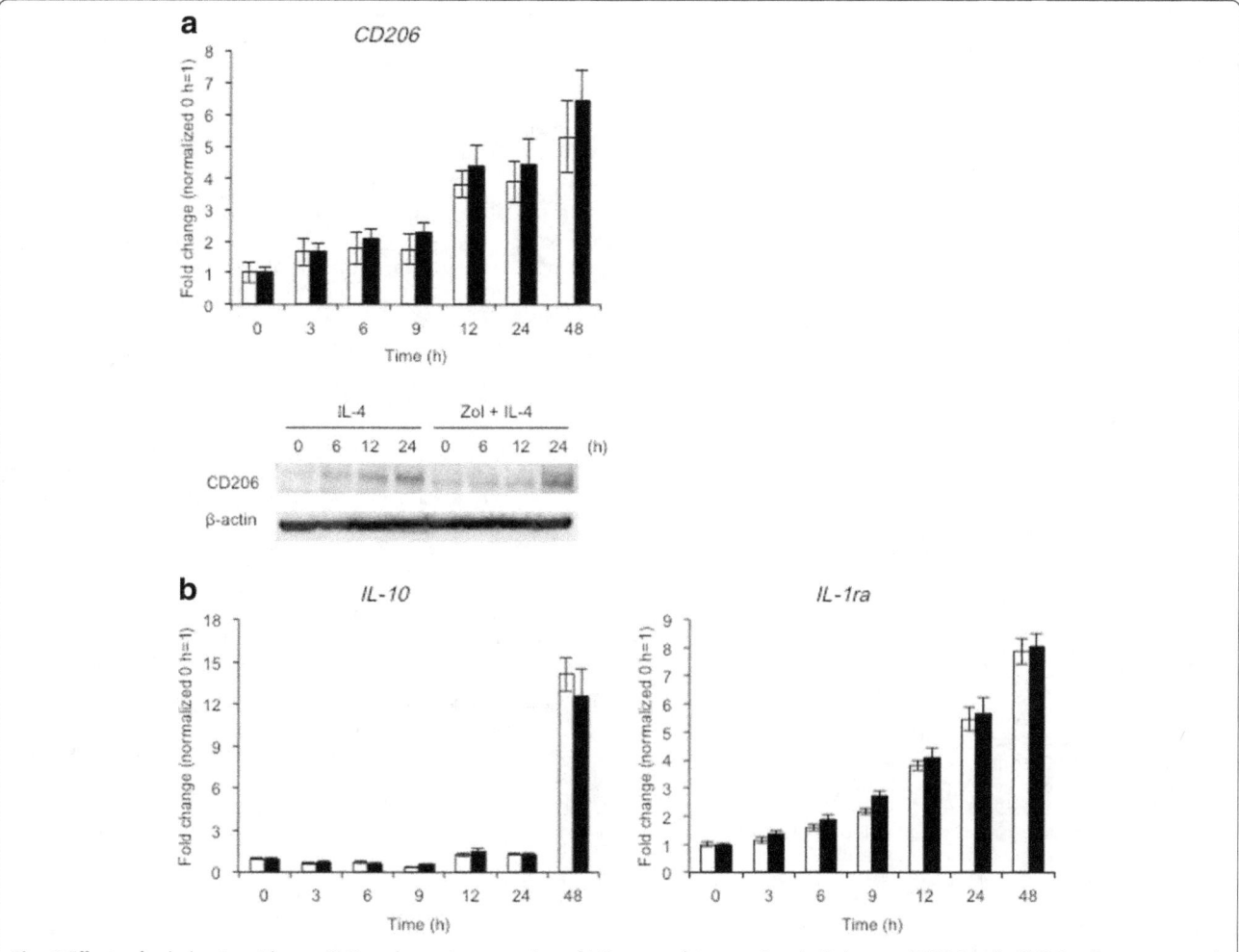

Fig. 4 Effects of zoledronic acid on mRNA and protein expression of M2 macrophage markers in IL-4-treated THP-1 cells. THP-1 cells were treated overnight with 100 ng/ml PMA, washed with PBS, and incubated with or without Zol for 24 h. THP-1 cells were then treated with 50 ng/ml IL-4. mRNA expression was detected by the real-time RT-PCR. Protein expression was detected by western blotting. Open bars represent IL-4-treated THP-1 cells; filled bars represent Zol and IL-4-treated THP-1 cells. **a** Zol did not affect the mRNA and protein expression of CD206 in IL-4-treated THP-1 cells. **b** Zol did not affect the mRNA expression of IL-10 and IL-1ra in IL-4-treated THP-1 cells

the mature IL-1β and reduced the secretion of IL-1β in LPS-treated THP-1 cells (Fig. 3). These results suggest that NLRP3 inflammasome molecules are involved in the maturation of IL-1β and the secretion of IL-1β. In total, our results demonstrate that Zol upregulates M1 macrophage differentiation through the NLRP3 inflammasome-dependent pathway. Additional research is required to investigate how inflammasome receptors other than NLRP3 may play a role in Zol-induced M1 macrophage polarization.

Conclusions

We have shown directly that Zol enhanced LPS-induced M1, but not M2, macrophage polarization through the NLRP3 inflammasome-dependent pathway, resulting in the production of inflammatory cytokines in THP-1 cells.

Abbreviations
ASC: Apoptosis-associated speck-like protein containing a caspase recruitment domain; ATP: Adenosine triphosphate; CD206: Cluster of differentiation 206; ELISA: Enzyme-linked immunosorbent assay; FBS: Fetal bovine serum; IL-10: Interleukin-10; IL-13: Interleukin-13; IL-1ra: Interleukin-1 receptor antagonist; IL-1β: Interleukin-1β; IL-4: Interleukin-4; LPS: Lipopolysaccharide; mRNA: Messenger ribonucleic acid; NLRP3: Nod-like receptor 3; PBS: Phosphate-buffered saline; PMA: Phorbol 12-myristate 13-acetate; RT-PCR: Reverse transcription-polymerase chain reaction; Zol: Zoledronic acid

Funding
This study was supported by JSPS KAKENHI Grants 16H05545 and 15K11083.

Author's contributions
The authors equally contributed to the preparation of this review. All authors read and approved the final manuscript.

Competing interests
The authors declare that they have no competing interests.

Author details
[1]Division of Infections and Molecular Biology, Department of Health Promotion, Kyushu Dental University, Kitakyushu, Fukuoka 803-8580, Japan. [2]School of Oral Health Sciences, Kyushu Dental University, Kitakyushu, Fukuoka 803-8580, Japan. [3]Division of Oral and Maxillofacial Surgery, Department of Science of Physical Functions, Kyushu Dental University, Kitakyushu, Fukuoka 803-8580, Japan.

References

1. Yoneda T, Hagino H, Sugimoto T, Ohta H, Takahashi S, Soen S, et al. Bisphosphonate-related osteonecrosis of the jaw: position paper from the Allied Task Force Committee of Japanese Society for Bone and Mineral Research, Japan Osteoporosis Society, Japanese Society of Periodontology, Japanese Society for Oral and Maxillofacial Radiology, and Japanese Society of Oral and Maxillofacial Surgeons. J Bone Miner Metab. 2010;28(4):365–83.

2. Marx RE. Pamidronate (Aredia) and zoledronate (Zometa) induced avascular necrosis of the jaws: a growing epidemic. J Oral Maxillofac Surg. 2003;61(9): 1115–7.

3. Assaf AT, Smeets R, Riecke B, Weise E, Gröbe A, Blessmann M, et al. Incidence of bisphosphonate-related osteonecrosis of the jaw in consideration of primary diseases and concomitant therapies. Anticancer Res. 2013;33(9):3917–24.

4. Rosella D, Papi P, Giardino R, Cicalini E, Piccoli L, Pompa G. Medication-related osteonecrosis of the jaw: clinical and practical guidelines. J Int Soc Prev Community Dent. 2016;6(2):97–104.

5. Tsurushima H, Kokuryo S, Sakaguchi O, Tanaka J, Tominaga K. Bacterial promotion of bisphosphonate-induced osteonecrosis in Wistar rats. Int J Oral Maxillofac Surg. 2013;42(11):1481–7.

6. Sakaguchi O, Kokuryo S, Tsurushima H, Tanaka J, Habu M, Uehara M, et al. Lipopolysaccharide aggravates bisphosphonate-induced osteonecrosis in rats. Int J Oral Maxillofac Surg. 2015;44(4):528–34.

7. Tanaka J, Kokuryo S, Yoshiga D, Tsurushima H, Sakaguchi O, Habu M, et al. An osteonecrosis model induced by oral bisphosphonate in ovariectomised rats. Oral Dis. 2015;21(8):969–76.

8. Ariel A, Maridonneau-Parini I, Rovere-Querini P, Levine JS, Mühl H. Macrophages in inflammation and its resolution. Front Immunol. 2012;3:324.

9. Hasturk H, Kantarci A, Van Dyke TE. Oral inflammatory diseases and systemic inflammation: role of the macrophage. Front Immunol. 2012;3:118.

10. Solinas G, Germano G, Mantovani A, Allavena P. Tumor-associated macrophages (TAM) as major players of the cancer-related inflammation. J Leukoc Biol. 2009;86(5):1065–73.

11. Mills CD, Kincaid K, Alt JM, Heilman MJ, Hill AM. M-1/M-2 macrophages and the Th1/Th2 paradigm. J Immunol. 2000;164(12):6166–73.

12. Martinez FO, Gordon S. The M1 and M2 paradigm of macrophage activation: time for reassessment. F1000Prime Rep. 2014;6:13.

13. Arnold L, Henry A, Poron F, Baba-Amer Y, van Rooijen N, Plonquet A, et al. Inflammatory monocytes recruited after skeletal muscle injury switch into antiinflammatory macrophages to support myogenesis. J Exp Med. 2007; 204(5):1057–69.

14. Biswas SK, Mantovani A. Orchestration of metabolism by macrophages. Cell Metab. 2012;15(4):432–7.

15. Muratsu D, Yoshiga D, Taketomi T, Onimura T, Seki Y, Matsumoto A, et al. Zoledronic acid enhances lipopolysaccharide-stimulated proinflammatory reactions through controlled expression of SOCS1 in macrophages. PLoS One. 2013;8(7):e67906.

16. Tanaka Y, Nagai Y, Dohdoh M, Oizumi T, Ohki A, Kuroishi T, et al. In vitro cytotoxicity of zoledronate (nitrogen-containing bisphosphonate: NBP) and/ or etidronate (non-NBP) in tumour cells and periodontal cells. Arch Oral Biol. 2013;58(6):628–37.

17. Mosmann TR, Coffman RL. TH1 and TH2 cells: different patterns of lymphokine secretion lead to different functional properties. Annu Rev Immunol. 1989;7:145–73.

18. Petrasek J, Bala S, Csak T, Lippai D, Kodys K, Menashy V, et al. IL-1 receptor antagonist ameliorates inflammasome-dependent alcoholic steatohepatitis in mice. J Clin Invest. 2012;122(10):3476–89.

19. Abramson SL, Gallin JI. IL-4 inhibits superoxide production by human mononuclear phagocytes. J Immunol. 1990;144(2):625–30.

20. Jablonski KA, Amici SA, Webb LM, Ruiz-Rosado JD, Popovich PG, Partida-Sanchez S, et al. Novel markers to delineate murine M1 and M2 macrophages. PLoS One. 2015;10(12):e0145342.

21. Scheller EL, Hankenson KD, Reuben JS, Krebsbach PH. Zoledronic acid inhibits macrophage SOCS3 expression and enhances cytokine production. J Cell Biochem. 2011;112(11):3364–72.

22. Coscia M, Quaglino E, Iezzi M, Curcio C, Pantaleoni F, Riganti C, et al. Zoledronic acid repolarizes tumour-associated macrophages and inhibits mammary carcinogenesis by targeting the mevalonate pathway. J Cell Mol Med. 2010;14(12):2803–15.

23. Tai TW, Su FC, Chen CY, Jou IM, Lin CF. Activation of p38 MAPK-regulated Bcl-xL signaling increases survival against zoledronic acid-induced apoptosis in osteoclast precursors. Bone. 2014;67:166–74.

24. DR's Net Pharmacist Net. Novartis Pharma. 2016. https://drs-net.novartis.co.jp/SysSiteAssets/common/pdf/zom/pi/pi_zom_r.pdf.

25. Striz I. Cytokines of the IL-1 family: recognized targets in chronic inflammation underrated in organ transplantations. Clin Sci (Lond). 2017; 131(17):2241–56.

26. Rőszer T. Understanding the mysterious M2 macrophage through activation markers and effector mechanisms. Mediat Inflamm. 2015;2015:816460.

27. Okinaga T, Ariyoshi W, Nishihara T. Aggregatibacter actinomycetemcomitans invasion induces interleukin-1β production through reactive oxygen species and Cathepsin B. J Interf Cytokine Res. 2015;35(6):431–40.

28. Cullen SP, Kearney CJ, Clancy DM, Martin SJ. Diverse activators of the NLRP3 Inflammasome promote IL-1β secretion by triggering necrosis. Cell Rep. 2015;11(10):1535–48.

29. Gombault A, Baron L. Couillin I. ATP release and purinergic signaling in NLRP3 inflammasome activation. Front Immunol. 2012;3:414.

30. Jo EK, Kim JK, Shin DM, Sasakawa C. Molecular mechanisms regulating NLRP3 inflammasome activation. Cell Mol Immunol. 2016;13(2):148–59.

31. Grahames CB, Michel AD, Chessell IP, Humphrey PP. Pharmacological characterization of ATP- and LPS-induced IL-1beta release in human monocytes. Br J Pharmacol. 1999;127(8):1915–21.

32. Netea MG, Nold-Petry CA, Nold MF, Joosten LA, Opitz B, van der Meer JH, et al. Differential requirement for the activation of the inflammasome for processing and release of IL-1beta in monocytes and macrophages. Blood. 2009;113(10):2324–35.

22

The etiopathogenesis of atopic dermatitis: barrier disruption, immunological derangement, and pruritus

Pawinee Rerknimitr[1,2], Atsushi Otsuka[1*], Chisa Nakashima[1] and Kenji Kabashima[1,3*]

Abstract

Atopic dermatitis (AD) is a common chronic skin inflammatory disorder characterized by recurrent eczema accompanied by an intractable itch that leads to an impaired quality of life. Extensive recent studies have shed light on the multifaceted pathogenesis of the disease. The complex interplay among skin barrier deficiency, immunological derangement, and pruritus contributes to the development, progression, and chronicity of the disease. Abnormalities in filaggrin, other stratum corneum constituents, and tight junctions induce and/or promote skin inflammation. This inflammation, in turn, can further deteriorate the barrier function by downregulating a myriad of essential barrier-maintaining molecules. Pruritus in AD, which may be due to hyperinnervation of the epidermis, increases pruritogens, and central sensitization compromises the skin integrity and promotes inflammation. There are unmet needs in the treatment of AD. Based on the detailed evidence available to date, certain disease mechanisms can be chosen as treatment targets. Numerous clinical trials of biological agents are currently being conducted and are expected to provide treatments for patients suffering from AD in the future. This review summarizes the etiopathogenesis of the disease and provides a rationale for choosing the novel targeted therapy that will be available in the future.

Keywords: Atopic dermatitis, Immunology, Pathogenesis, Innate, Adaptive, Filaggrin

Background

Atopic dermatitis (AD) is a chronic inflammatory skin disorder that affects one fifth of the population in developed countries [1]. The disease is characterized by recurrent eczema accompanied by a chronic intractable itch that leads to an impaired quality of life [2–4]. The onset of AD occurs primarily in childhood and is thought to precede allergic disorders mediated by an immunoglobulin E (IgE) sensitization to environmental antigens, namely, asthma and allergic rhinoconjunctivitis, the so-called atopic march [5–8]. Moreover, there are increasing evidence that AD is associated with systemic diseases and may be considered as a systemic disorder [9, 10]. The prevalence of AD in children is 15 to 25% [11]. Seventy percent of patients outgrow during late childhood

[12]. However, many remain affected [13, 14], and some may experience a new disease onset in adulthood [1].

Though extensive recent studies have shed light on the understanding of AD, the exact pathogenesis of the disease remains obscure. The complex interplay among genetics, environmental factors, microbiota, skin barrier deficiency, immunological derangement, and possibly autoimmunity contributes to the development of the disease [15–17]. This review aims to summarize the current understanding of the pathogenesis of AD with a focus on the major etiopathogenesis: barrier disruption, immunological derangement, and pruritus.

Skin barrier disruption
Stratum corneum and tight junction
The skin serves as a barrier to protect the body from outside dangers, such as microbes and toxic substances. The epidermis includes four main layers: the stratum corneum (SC), stratum granulosum (SG), stratum spinosum, and stratum basale. SC is the outermost part of the

* Correspondence: otsukamn@kuhp.kyoto-u.ac.jp; kaba@kuhp.kyoto-u.ac.jp
[1]Department of Dermatology, Kyoto University Graduate School of Medicine, 54 Shogoin-Kawara, Sakyo, Kyoto 606-8507, Japan
Full list of author information is available at the end of the article

epidermis and is composed of denucleated corneocytes embedded in intercellular lipids (often called "bricks and mortar") [18], whereas tight junctions (TJs) are intercellular junctions that regulate the paracellular transport of water and solutes [19]. Skin barrier disruption in AD occurs as a result of an aberration of both components.

SC homeostasis relies greatly on filaggrin (FLG) and its metabolic process. The term filaggrin is short for "filament-aggregating protein," indicating that it is a protein that binds with keratin intermediate filaments and is responsible for the integral structural component [20]. FLG is formed and stored as profilaggrin polymers in keratohyalin granules in SG. At the interface between SG and SC, profilaggrin polymers are cleaved into FLG monomers by certain proteases, such as CAP1 [21] and SASPase [22, 23]. These monomers then assemble with keratin intermediate filaments to strengthen SC. Finally, at the upper SC, FLG is degraded into amino acids, urocanic acid (UCA), and pyrrolidine carboxylic acid (PCA). UCA is responsible for the acid mantle of the skin, and PCA provides natural moisturizing factors in the skin. This degradation process is mediated by proteases, namely, caspase 14 [24], calpain 1 [25], and bleomycin hydrolase [25].

Networks of TJs are found in the intercellular spaces of SG and regulate the paracellular transport of water, ions, and solutes [19, 26]. Strands of TJs are composed of the transmembrane portion in which claudins and occludins represent the most abundant constituents. Zonula occludens (ZO) is the major cytosolic scaffolding proteins responsible for the TJ assembly [27].

The importance of TJs in barrier function has been clearly demonstrated: mice with claudin-1 deficiency die within a day after birth with wrinkling skin [28]. Importantly, TJ aberration is associated with AD since human AD epidermis has a reduced expression of claudin-1, claudin-23 [29], and ZO-1 [30] and shows evidence of impaired barrier function. In addition, polymorphisms of *CLDN1*-encoding claudin-1 are found in AD patients [29].

Filaggrin and its role in the pathogenesis of AD

FLG is essential for controlling transepidermal water loss and maintaining SC hydration [31, 32] and for the cornification and organization of the epidermis [31, 33]. FLG is known to be decreased in the epidermis of AD patients [34], and null mutation in FLG is the strongest risk factor for AD [35]. FLG haploid insufficiency further confers the risk of developing of several atopic diseases, including asthma, food allergy, and allergic rhinitis [36].

FLG deficiency also leads to an increase in skin pH, which, in turn, enhances the function of serine proteases kallikrein (KLK)5, KLK7, and KLK14, which are responsible for corneocyte shedding [37]. These activated KLKs can increase the production of interleukin (IL)-1α and IL-1β from corneocytes [38]. Moreover, by binding to the protease-activated receptor type 2 (PAR2) on keratinocytes, KLKs can induce thymic stromal lymphopoietin (TSLP) production that further promotes inflammation [39, 40].

The analysis with Flg mutant mice

The importance of FLG in the pathogenesis of AD is supported by the evidence that mice with Flg deficiency, e.g., flaky tail ($Matt^{ma/ma}Flg^{ft/ft}$) mice and Flg mutant ($Flg^{ft/ft}$) mice on a proallergic BALB/c background, exhibit a spontaneous AD phonotype [7, 41–43]. Of note, the flaky tail mice harbor double gene mutations, *Flg* and matted (*ma*), both of which affect the skin barrier in a different fashion. Abnormality in *Flg* leads to an aberrant profilaggrin polypeptide expression while *ma* mutation gives rise to the matted hair and spontaneous dermatitis phenotype [41, 44]. In addition, the derangement in proteases required for profilaggrin and Flg processing also gives rise to impairment of the skin barrier and SC dehydration, as observed in mice deficient in CAP1 [21], SASPase [22], and caspase 14 [24].

Furthermore, increased allergen penetration is observed in Flg-deficient mice, e.g., Flg-null mice [45] and flaky tail mice [46], and augmented responses in contact hypersensitivity are detected [45]. Allergen penetration results in inflammasome and protease activation [47]. Additionally, a reduction in FLG predisposes microbial colonization in the skin [32], partly due to the loss of the acid mantle resulting from the decrease in FLG breakdown products [48] combined with the indirect neutralizing effects of FLG to α-toxin of *Staphylococcus aureus* [49]. This effect is known to be mediated by the secretion of sphingomyelinase, an enzyme stored in the lamellar bodies of keratinocytes in which FLG is required for proper secretion [49–51]. Intriguingly, by promoting Flg expression in NC/Nga mice, development of the AD phenotype in the mice is attenuated, and upregulating FLG may be one of the approaches to improve AD [52].

Sweating is known to be attenuated in AD, which may be a result of acrosyringium obstruction caused by abnormalities in the sweat duct structures and/or derangement in the common sudomotor nerves that control sweating [53, 54]. Recently, it has been demonstrated that a sweat duct obstruction is observed in Flg mutant mice and that sweating is consequently reduced. These findings suggest that FLG may also contribute to the integrity of the acrosyringeal wall [55]. The immunologic modulation of FLG in the development of AD is summarized in Fig. 1.

Other SC components and their relationship with AD

Intercellular lipids are a fundamental part of SC and are regarded as the mortar in the brick and mortar model of the epidermis. These lipids are composed of ceramides,

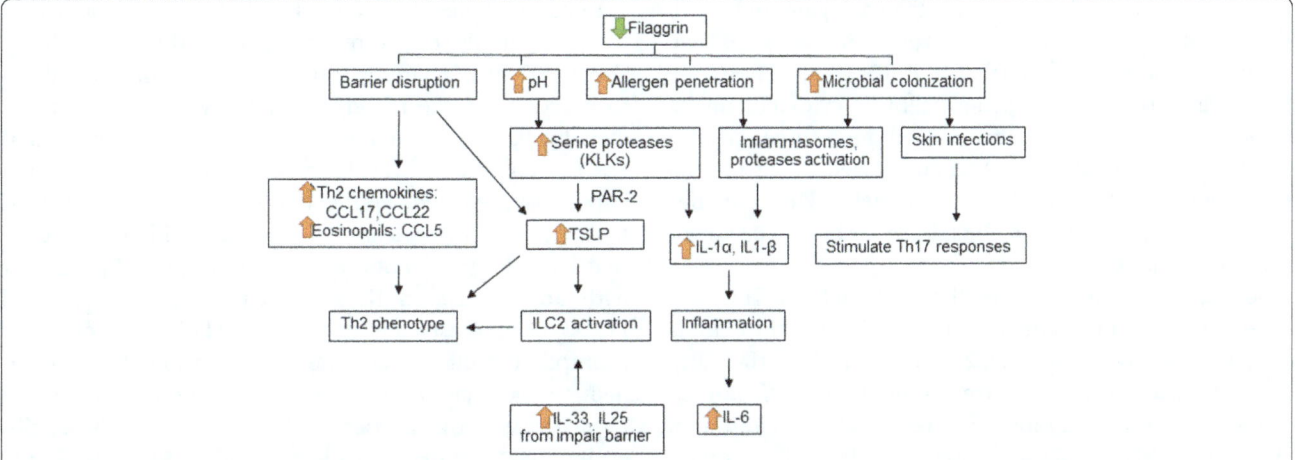

Fig. 1 Immunologic modulation of filaggrin (FLG) in the development of atopic dermatitis. Decreased FLG exacerbates skin inflammation in many ways. Th2 phenotype skewing occurs because of barrier disruption and keratinocyte injuries that stimulate thymic stromal lymphopoietin (TSLP), Th2, and eosinophil-recruiting chemokines together with IL-33 and IL-25 released from keratinocytes. Moreover, the loss of the acid mantle in the epidermis also promotes TSLP secretion via protease-activated receptor type 2 (PAR-2) activation by increased serine proteases. Enhanced allergen penetration and microbial colonization activate inflammasomes and the Th17 pathway that complicate the pathogenesis of AD in a later state

free fatty acids, and cholesterol in a ratio of 1:1:1 M [18]. The lipid precursors are formed and stored in the lamellar bodies of SG and are released into the extracellular space when the keratinocytes differentiate into SC [18]. Abnormalities in the enzymes responsible for lipid processing and the transportation of lamellar bodies across the cells give rise to a myriad of barrier-insufficient skin diseases. For example, mutations of the genes that encode the enzymes 12R-lipoxygenase and epidermal lipoxygenase 3 are associated with autosomal recessive congenital ichthyosis (ARCI) [56]. It is of note that transmembrane protein 79/mattrin (Tmem79/Matt), a five-transmembrane protein of lamellar bodies, is essential in the lamellar body secretory system and that flaky tail ($Matt^{ma/ma}Flg^{ft/ft}$) mice and Tmem79 (ma/ma) mice with ma mutation exhibit spontaneous AD-like dermatitis [44, 57]. Moreover, in the human counterpart, a meta-analysis revealed that a missense mutation in the human $MATT$ gene is associated with AD [57].

Corneocyte shedding is tightly regulated by serine proteases and serine protease inhibitors as mentioned above. Serine protease inhibitors include lymphoepithelial Kazal-type 5 serine protease inhibitor (LEKTI), which is encoded by the serine protease inhibitor Kazal-type 5 ($SPINK5$) [58]. Disorders involving mutation and genetic polymorphisms of the genes that encode KLKs and LEKTI exhibit AD-like phenotypes [59–61]. For instance, Netherton syndrome is caused by $SPINK5$ mutations. Patients with this disease exhibit severe dermatitis, allergic rhinoconjunctivitis, asthma, and a high serum IgE level [60]. Moreover, recent studies show that polymorphisms in $SPINK5$ are related to AD [61, 62]. Skin barrier dysfunction and cutaneous inflammation due to aberrant immunologic

responses are critical for AD development [1, 63]. The initial trigger, however, remains a subject of debate. Although null mutation of the FLG gene poses the strongest risk for AD, 60% of individuals who carry the gene do not have AD symptoms [36]. On the contrary, a significant portion of AD patients do not have FLG mutation [36]. It is thus evident that additional factors are needed to develop the disease. In fact, recent genome-wide association studies reported ten new loci that are associated with AD and show a relationship with autoimmune regulation, especially in innate signaling and T cell activation [35, 64]. In the following section, immunological derangement in AD will be discussed.

The immunopathogenesis of AD
Keratinocytes

Acute skin barrier disruption promotes T helper (Th)2 skewing. Keratinocyte-derived cytokines such as TSLP [65], which is known to promote the AD-like phenotype [66], IL-25, IL-33, and granulocyte-macrophage colony-stimulating factor (GM-CSF) influence innate lymphoid cells (ILCs) and increase the production of Th2 chemokines: CCL17 (thymus- and activation-regulated chemokine (TARC)), CCL22, and an eosinophil chemoattractant: CCL5 (regulated upon activation, normal T cell expressed and secreted (RANTES)) [67]. In addition to promoting Th2 cell recruitment, CCL17 has been reported to enhance keratinocyte proliferation and implicate in AD development [68].

ILCs, basophils, eosinophils, and mast cells

ILCs are a novel group of innate immune cells developed from a common lymphoid progenitor [69]. Although the morphology of ILCs resembles that of lymphoid cells, ILCs do not carry an antigen receptor. Instead, they have similar transcription factors as T cell subsets. Therefore, ILCs are capable of producing hallmark cytokines in the same fashion. ILCs can be divided into three groups: ILC1, ILC2, and ILC3. ILC2, characterized by having the transcription factor GATA3 and producing Th2 cytokines (IL-4, IL-5, and IL-13), is considered to be important in the pathogenesis of AD.

Several studies have shown that, although few ILCs are observed in normal human skin, in AD, the skin is infiltrated markedly by the ILC2 subset [70, 71]. IL-5 and IL-13 released from ILC2 are essential and sufficient to induce AD lesions in mouse models [71, 72]. In addition, ILC2 can drive Th2 responses in vivo [71]. Certain epithelial-derived cytokines and eicosanoids, namely, TSLP [71], IL-25 [73], IL-33 [73, 74], and prostaglandin D2 (PGD2) [75, 76], can activate ILC2 whereas E-cadherin [73] is known to have an inhibitory effect. In addition, ILC2 can also respond to hematopoietic cell-derived cytokines, IL-2 and IL-7 [72]. Importantly, IL-4 from basophils can directly activate ILC2 and bring about AD-like inflammation [77]. The immunomodulatory actions of the aforementioned cytokines are mediated by ligation with the corresponding receptors that are present on the ILC2. In AD, where the epidermal barrier is breached, epithelial-derived cytokines (TSLP, IL-25, IL-33) are released. In addition, FLG deficiency that leads to a reduction in E-cadherin [73, 78] together with an increase in IL-4 derived from basophils and PGD2 from mast cells is present. These environments promptly recruit and activate ILC2 and initiate the cutaneous inflammation observed in AD. The complex interplay between the barrier dysfunction, ILC2, basophils, eosinophils, and mast cells is involved in AD [69, 79–82], as shown in Fig. 2.

In addition to cytokines and chemokines, the neurotransmitter dopamine is involved in mast cell activation and Th2 skewing in AD. Mast cells and Th2 cells bear dopamine receptors, the D1-like receptor group. Upon

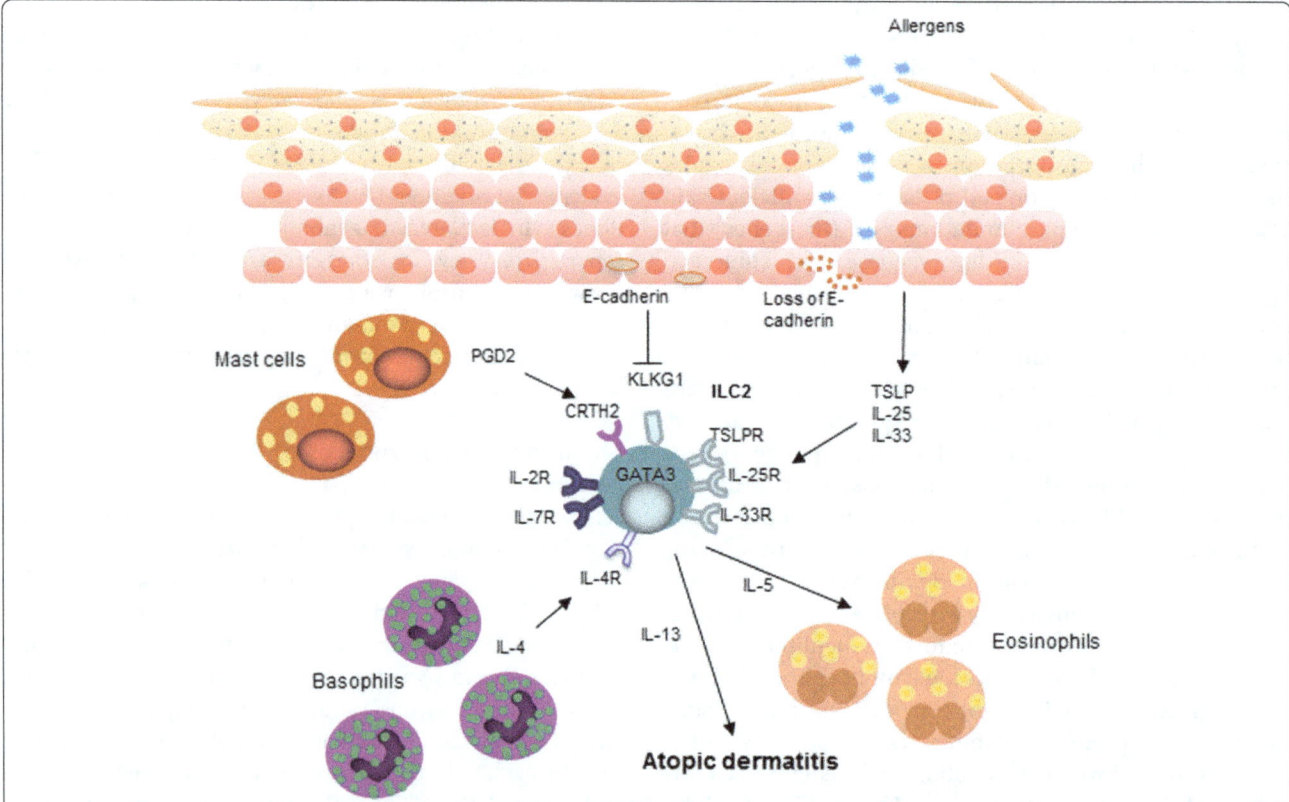

Fig. 2 Interplay among the barrier dysfunction, innate lymphoid cell (ILC)2, basophils, eosinophils, and mast cells. Barrier disruption leads to the production and release of epithelial-derived cytokines, namely, thymic stromal lymphopoietin (TSLP), IL-25, and IL-33. Upon ligation with the corresponding receptors on ILC2, TSLP receptor (TSLPR), IL-25 receptor (IL-25R, also known as IL17RB), and IL-33 receptor (IL-33R or ST2), ILC2 is activated to release Th2 cytokines, e.g., IL-5 and IL-13. In addition, IL-4 from basophils which are found in proximity to ILC2 in AD skin lesions can directly activate ILC2. PGD2, presumably from mast cell degranulation, also contributes to the recruitment of ILC2 into the skin as well as the induction of ILC2 Th2 cytokine production. In contrast, cell adhesion molecules, E-cadherin, on keratinocytes, are known to have an inhibitory effect on ILC2. Nevertheless, loss of E-cadherin is observed in FLG-deficient individuals. Therefore, skin inflammation is enhanced as there is an increase in stimulatory but a decrease in inhibitory stimuli

ligand binding, mast cells are degranulated and Th2 cells are activated, observed by an increase in the ratio of IL-4 to IFN-γ mRNA expression [83]. As psychoneuro-immunology plays a role in many skin diseases, results from the study might explain the worsening of AD symptoms after a psychological strain.

Dendritic cells (DCs)

DCs are professional antigen-presenting cells that capture antigens, allergens, and microbes, to prime naïve T cells into immunogenic or tolerogenic subsets, and act as a bridge between innate and adaptive immunity [84]. In the steady state of the skin, Langerhans cells (LCs) reside in the epidermis, and groups of dermal DCs (DDCs) are found in the dermis. It has been suggested that DCs initiate AD in humans, although it remains unclear which cutaneous DC subsets initiate epicutaneous sensitization.

LCs perform surface antigen surveillance and recognition by extending their dendrites through the TJs to take up the antigens [85]. LCs' function in this regard has been reported to induce Th2 responses as LCs efficiently drive naïve CD4$^+$ T cells into Th2 cells [86]. It is speculated that a breach in TJs may enhance penetration of foreign antigens, which are then taken up by LCs, amplifying Th2 cutaneous inflammation.

LCs are also responsible for the initiation of AD under the influence of TSLP [63, 87, 88]. Nakajima et al. demonstrated that LCs are essential to the induction of clinical manifestations and IgE elevation in a mouse model upon epicutaneous sensitization with the protein antigen ovalbumin (OVA) via the action of TSLP and its receptors presented on LCs [87]. TSLP is abundantly expressed in keratinocytes of lesional and non-lesional skin in AD patients as a result of both skin barrier dysfunction and proinflammatory cytokines, such as IL-1β, tumor necrosis factor (TNF)-α, IL-4, and IL-13 in AD [65, 89]. Importantly, TSLP can trigger DC migration to the draining lymph nodes [90], and LCs treated with TSLP drive naïve T cells to Th2 phenotypes [91]. All of these events lead to a Th2 bias in the acute stage of AD.

During the inflammatory state of AD, myeloid inflammatory DCs, namely, inflammatory dendritic epidermal cells (IDECs), are recruited [92]. DCs in the skin of AD patients are well characterized by the presence of a high-affinity receptor for IgE (FcεRI) that renders these DCs to induce T cell responses effectively [92]. A wide spectrum and amount of foreign surface and penetrating antigens, microbes, and allergens are encountered in AD skin due to the breach in the epidermis and the barrier dysfunction [92].

The cross-linking of FcεRI with IgE on the LC surface in an in vitro study leads to a release of chemokines, for example, IL-6, CCL22, CCL17, and CCL2, which can recruit Th2 cells and other immune cells, importantly, IDECs [93]. A patch test study showed that IDECs rapidly migrate into the epidermis of patch-tested lesions [94]. IDECs are key DCs in amplifying skin inflammation as they can migrate to the draining lymph nodes and prime naïve T cell into interferon (IFN)-γ- and IL-18-producing T cells [93]. Therefore, IDECs are considered to be important in the switching of Th2 to Th1 in chronic AD [94].

Another interesting feature of AD is a decreased plasmacytoid DC (pDC) number in AD skin compared to that expected to be observed in skin inflammatory conditions [95]. This can be explained by a lack of chemoattractant for pDCs, i.e., chemerin, in AD skin [96] and a paucity of skin-homing molecules in the blood pDCs of AD patients [97] in combination with the Th2 milieu in the skin [84]. pDCs are crucial in immune responses against viral infections. The reduced number and improper function of pDCs observed in AD skin can thus contribute to a susceptibility to viral infections [97].

Th2/Th1 paradigm shift

AD is traditionally viewed as a Th2-mediated allergic disease with increased IgE production, eosinophilia, mast cell activation, and overexpression of Th2 cytokines IL-4, IL-5, and IL-13 [63, 98]. Th2 polarization and barrier defects are closely related. TSLP, IL-25, and IL-33 are upregulated in the epithelium after environmental signals [11]. Keratinocytes are the main source of TSLP, which is crucial in the induction of Th2 skewing in AD skin by the activation of LCs and DCs [99]. In turn, Th2 cytokines IL-4 and IL-13 can induce keratinocytes to express TSLP [100]. In addition, Th2 cytokines can inhibit the expression of Toll-like receptors (TLRs), which dampens host defense against infections [100]. Moreover, IL-4 and IL-13 have negative impacts on skin barrier function. FLG, loricrin, and involucrin, the integral components of SC, are downregulated with Th2 cytokines, regardless of FLG genotypes [101, 102]. Keratinocyte differentiation is perturbed by Th2 cytokines via STAT3 and STAT6 activation, and topical Janus kinase (JAK) inhibitors can restore epithelial function by suppressing STAT3 signaling [103]. B cell class switching and increased IgE synthesis are also induced by IL-4. Based on this supporting evidence, suppression of Th2 cytokines appeared to be useful in alleviating AD symptoms [104–106]. Recently, a novel biological agent, the anti-IL-4 receptor antibody dupilumab, has been studied in clinical trials and found to be promising for the treatment of AD [107].

Th17

Th17 cells have the capacity to produce IL-17A, IL-17F, IL-22, and IL-26 upon stimulation [108]. Indeed, IL-17 can induce S100 protein and proinflammatory cytokine expression, which are responsible for eosinophil- and neutrophil-mediated inflammation [109, 110]. Many studies have suggested the involvement of Th17 in the pathogenesis of AD. For instance, it is reported that epicutaneous sensitization in mice with OVA typically leads to AD-like dermatitis and the cutaneous expression of IL-17 and IL-17-producing T cells in the draining lymph nodes and spleen, as well as increased serum IL-17 levels [111]. In addition, a study that used a repeated hapten application to induce AD in mice showed that IL-17A is necessary for the development of skin inflammation, IL-4 production, and IgG1 and IgE induction [112]. Interestingly, IL-17A is detected in the AD-like dermatitis of flaky tail mice [42, 46, 113]. Consistently, analysis of the peripheral blood of severe AD patients reveals an increased number of IL-17-producing cells [114, 115].

AD can be divided into two types: extrinsic and intrinsic AD. Patients with extrinsic AD typically have an elevated IgE level, harbor *FLG* mutation with a disruptive barrier, exhibit an early onset, and traditionally have a Th2-dominant response. On the other hand, intrinsic AD patients exhibit different features [116–118]. Patients with intrinsic AD usually do not show an elevated IgE level, do not harbor *FLG* mutation, exhibit with an adult onset, and are associated with more Th17 and Th22 immune activation than extrinsic AD patients [119]. Essentially, a study that compared phenotypes between European/American versus Asian AD showed that Asian AD skin exhibits more epidermal hyperplasia and parakeratosis that skewed toward psoriasis features. It is of note that higher Th17 activation is observed in Asian AD; this needs to be considered in the selection of treatments for different populations [120].

Antimicrobial peptides
Atopic skin is characterized by increased *S. aureus* colonization and/or infections with a loss of microbial diversity during flares [121]. This may be explained partly by the reduction in antimicrobial peptides (AMPs) of the skin. In homeostasis, AMPs, such as S100 protein psoriasin, ribonuclease (RNase) 7, dermcidin, and lactoferrin, are constitutively present in the epidermis and serve as one of the first-line protections against microbes. Upon challenges with danger signals/organisms, additional AMPs, namely, human beta-defensins (hBD)-2, hBD-3 and cathelicidin (LL-37), are upregulated [122]. In the past, it was thought that the reduction in hBD-2, hBD-3, and LL-37 levels in AD epidermis was one of the causes of *S. aureus* overgrowth [123]. This can be explained by the fact that skin inflammation in AD is predominantly mediated by Th2 cytokines (IL-4, IL-13) in the acute phase of the disease [63] and that the Th2 cytokine milieu is known to suppress the production of the AMPs [124]. Recent findings, however, have shown that

the induction of the AMPs hBD-2, hBD-3, and LL-37 was not impaired in AD [125]. These productions may not be sufficient to tackle the infections or the AMP functions may be disturbed [126]. Interestingly, *Escherichia coli* infection is rarely encountered in AD, and the major AMP family that combats this microbe is the S100 proteins, which consist of S100A7 (psoriasin), S100A8, and S100A9 [124]. An increase in S100 proteins in patients with AD has been reported [124, 125]. In addition, S100 proteins have proinflammatory properties that can further promote skin inflammation and inhibit keratinocyte differentiation, complicating the barrier dysfunction [126, 127].

Recent interesting studies have shown that TSLP exists in two different isoforms, i.e., short and long forms, both of which exhibit different functions. In the skin and gut, the short form is constitutively expressed, which is responsible for maintaining tissue homeostasis and acts as antimicrobial peptides [128, 129]. In contrast, the long form predominates and possesses proinflammatory activity under inflammatory states, such as in the lesional skin of AD [128, 130].

Pattern recognition receptors (PRRs) recognize vital and highly conserved molecular structures of microorganisms, so-called pathogen-associated molecular patterns (PAMPs), and danger signals, damage-associated molecular patterns (DAMPs). Upon receptor ligation, signaling pathways are stimulated and result in the production of cytokines with biological effects. In the skin, PRRs are found in keratinocytes and other innate immune cells [131] and are known to be involved in the pathogenesis of AD. TLRs are the most well-characterized PRRs. Other PPRs include NOD-like receptors (NLRs), RIG-I-like receptors (RLRs), and C-type lectin receptors (CLRs).

TLR2 is a major ligand for *S. aureus* [132] that has a unique ability to form either a homodimer or a heterodimer with TLR1 or TLR6 to expand their binding spectrum capability [133]. Bacterial lipoteichoic acid (LTA) found in *S. aureus*-infected AD lesions can bind to TLR2, which then exerts immunologic responses. Interestingly, a single nucleotide polymorphism (SNP) of TLR2 has been reported to be associated with severe AD and implicated in an increase in *S. aureus* infections [134, 135]. Moreover, intracellular muramyl dipeptide (MDP) derived from *S. aureus* peptidoglycan is recognized by NOD2, NLR family, within keratinocytes [136]. It is of note that NOD2-deficient mice exhibit an increased susceptibility to subcutaneous *S. aureus* infection [137], and polymorphisms in the NOD2 gene are associated with human AD [138].

Interestingly, peptidoglycan from *S. aureus* induces signaling through NOD-2 coupled with TLR stimulation which efficiently induces DCs to produce IL-12p70 and IL-23, which drive Th1 and Th17 responses, respectively [139]. This may in part explain the shift of Th2-

dominated to Th1/Th17-co-dominated inflammation in the chronic stage of AD where multiple PRRs are engaged [133].

S. aureus and AD

The cutaneous microbiome plays an important role in the skin during homeostasis and in the disease state. This is especially evident in AD in which skin colonization with S. aureus is found in almost 90% of lesional skin and 55 to 75% of non-lesional skin [5]. Skin infections and the toxin from S. aureus further exacerbate the cutaneous proinflammatory state [140]. Importantly, skin colonization with S. aureus produces superantigens that also stimulate Th17 responses by increasing IL-17 production [140, 141]. Indeed, in AD patients with skin infections, a rise in the percentage of Th17 cells in peripheral blood has been found [142]. S. aureus can worsen barrier impairment [143]; releases proteases, enzymes, and cytolytic toxins that induce cell injuries [143, 144]; and engages PRRs and exerts inflammation [145]. Its toxic shock syndrome toxin 1 (TSST-1) and enterotoxins (SEs) act as superantigens to activate a large number of T cells [146], promote T cell recruitment to the skin [147], and exert superantigen-specific IgE [148]. Additionally, S. aureus δ-toxin can stimulate mast cell degranulation [149]. These summarized events eventually deteriorate the disease state of AD [150].

Pruritus

Itch or pruritus is one of the most disturbing symptoms that characterize AD and can in fact significantly impair the quality of life of affected individuals [151]. Pruritus in AD is a result of the complex interplay among many factors. Although the exact pathogenesis remains unknown, recent studies have shown that hyperinnervation of the epidermis, an increase in several itch mediators/pruritogens, and central sensitization of itch are evident in AD.

Hyperinnervation of AD skin

The sprouting of nerve fibers is under a balanced homeostasis between nerve sprouting factors, e.g., nerve growth factor (NGF), amphiregulin, and gelatinase versus nerve retraction factors, e.g., semaphorin 3A (Sema3A) and anosmin-1 [152]. An increase in nerve fiber density in the epidermis is reported in AD [153, 154]. This is partly explained by the elevation of NGF that is observed in the plasma of AD patients [155] and a decrease in Sema3A that is detected in the lesional AD epidermis [156].

In addition to the hyperinnervation of the skin, a lower threshold for activation of the sensory nerve fibers is also observed in AD, and these events mutually function to increase the excitability of the sensory nerves [157].

This hypersensitivity of the primary itch-sensing neurons may contribute to alloknesis, pruritus resulting from non-pruritogenic stimuli [158], which is a well-observed phenomenon in AD patients [159]. Interestingly, artemin, a glial cell-derived neurotrophic factor (GDNF)-related family, is reported to be important in warm inducing itch because artemin is upregulated in fibroblasts from AD lesions, and an intradermal injection of artemin in mice leads to an increased number and sprouting of peripheral nerves together with thermal hyperalgesia [160, 161].

Itch mediators/pruritogens

Several itch mediators and their corresponding receptors are reported to be responsible for itch in AD: histamine (H), especially the role of H1 and H4 receptors (H1R and H4R) [157, 162], certain proteases (including tryptase, dust mites, and S. aureus [151]), substance P [63, 151], IL-31 [163, 164], TSLP [165], and endothelin-1 [166].

Recently, much interest has been focused on the role of IL-31-induced pruritus. IL-31 is predominantly produced by Th2 cells, and its receptor, which comprises IL-31 receptor α (IL-31RA) and oncostatin M receptor β (OSMRβ), is expressed in peripheral nerve fibers, dorsal root ganglions (DRGs), and keratinocytes [167, 168]. Upon its ligand binding, IL-31 signaling is mediated by activation of the JAK-signal transducer and activator of transcription (STAT) (STAT-1/5 and ERK-1/2), mitogen-activated protein kinase, and phosphoinositide-3-kinase (PI3K) signaling pathways [169, 170]. The IL-31 level is elevated in AD skin as well as in the serum [163, 171]. The IL-31 serum level correlates with the disease severity [172]. Clinical trials related to anti-IL-31 receptor (nemolizumab) and anti-IL-31 (BMS-981164) as treatments for AD are currently being conducted [173].

Central sensitization of pruritus in AD

The role played by the central nervous system in terms of the itch associated with AD has been investigated to a lesser extent compared to that of peripheral innervation. A study that used functional magnetic resonance imaging with arterial spin labelling, however, showed an increase in the activation of the anterior cingulate cortex and dorsolateral prefrontal cortex in human AD subjects compared with that of healthy controls [174]. These results suggest a central sensitization in AD individuals. Importantly, cognitive and affective processes play a pivotal role in the interpretation and perception of pruritus [151]. This is evident in AD, as several psychotropic drugs, including antidepressants, can attenuate the itch severity in some patients [175].

In addition to the brain itself, the activation of STAT3 in the astrocytes of the spinal dorsal horn has been shown to be involved in chronic pruritus. This activation results in the production of lipocalin-2 that enhances pruritus and may lead to a vicious itch-scratch cycle [176]. It is of note that astrocytes are a subtype of glial cells of the central nervous system [151].

The complex interplay among itch, barrier disruption, and immunologic aberration is illustrated in Fig. 3. Pruritus is known to induce scratching behavior that introduces or worsens breaches in the skin. On the other hand, in dry skin model mice, epidermal barrier dysfunction is observed together with an increase in the number of epidermal nerve fibers [177]. With regard to the relationship between pruritus and the immune responses, once the barrier is disrupted from scratching, e.g., in an experimental tape stripping procedure, Th2 chemokines (CCL17 and CCL22) and eosinophil-recruiting chemokines (CCL5) are increasingly produced by keratinocytes [67]. Moreover, tape stripping also results in TSLP production in the skin [65]. Consequently, Th2 skewing ensues. Conversely, immune responses can induce itch via the secretion of a myriad of cytokines that can act as pruritogens, namely, TSLP, IL-2, IL-31, IL-4, and IL-13 [157].

Novel AD treatments
Based on the growing knowledge of the complex pathophysiology of AD, many novel targeted therapies are currently in clinical trials. Table 1 summarizes these novel treatments [11, 173, 178–180].

Anti-IL-4 receptor, dupilumab
Based on the importance of IL-4 in inducing AD inflammation and barrier impairment, studies have examined

how to attenuate its function. The central focus with a growing number of evidence is dupilumab, a fully humanized monoclonal antibody against the IL-4 receptor α subunit (IL-4Rα). This subunit is shared by IL-4 and IL-13; therefore, by blocking IL-4Ra, both IL-4 and IL-13 are inhibited [181].

Several phase II studies have shown the efficacy of dupilumab in improving clinical outcomes, biomarkers, and the transcriptome level in AD patients [181–183]. Moreover, a recent phase III study has confirmed the findings in a larger number of patients [184]. Although further studies with long-term follow-up periods are needed, dupilumab appears to be a promising treatment modality for AD.

IL-13 antagonist
IL-13 belongs to the Th2 cytokine lineage that can bind to both IL-4 and IL-13 receptors; therefore, the functions of IL-4 and IL-13 are considered to be similar [11]. IL-13 is important in B cell activation and differentiation and in promoting IgE production by B cells [178]. Lebrikizumab and tralokinumab are monoclonal antibodies against IL-13. Their roles in AD treatment are currently being explored in current phase II studies (ClinicalTrials.gov identifier: NCT02340234 and NCT02347176).

IL-23p40 antagonist
The fact that Th1 and Th17 cells are involved in the pathogenesis of AD has led to a trial of ustekinumab in AD. Ustekinumab is a fully human monoclonal antibody against the receptor p40 subunit, shared by IL-12 and

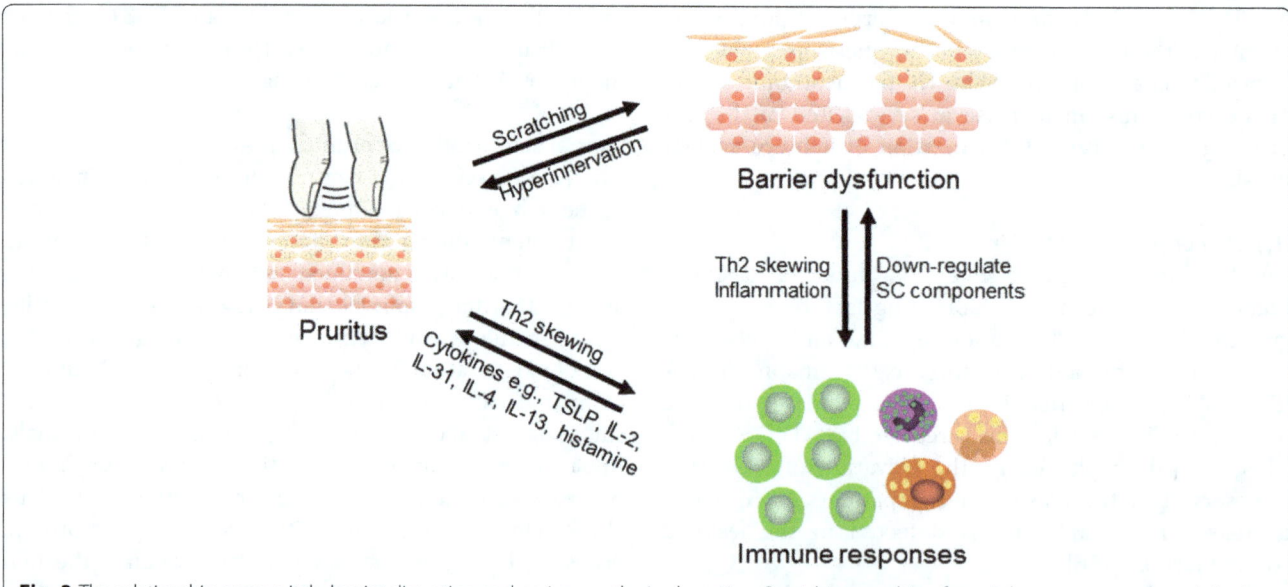

Fig. 3 The relationship among itch, barrier disruption and an immunologic aberration. Scratching resulting from itch can worsen a breach in the skin. Dry skin promotes itch by increasing the density of epidermal nerve fibers. Scratching also promotes Th2 chemokines, eosinophil-recruiting chemokines, and thymic stromal lymphopoietin (TSLP). Conversely, immune responses can induce itch via the secretion of a myriad of cytokines that can act as pruritogens

Table 1 Novel AD treatments. The table is modified from Heratizadeh and Werfel [178], Lauffer and Ring [179], Noda et al. [180], Nomura and Kabashima [173], and Werfel et al. [11]

Mechanism of action	Route	Compound	Company	Type of clinical trial	Result
Targeting pathogenic cytokines and their cognate receptors					
IL-4/IL-13 receptor α-chain antagonist	SC	Dupilumab	Regeneron	Phase III	Improvement in clinical outcomes, pruritus, and quality of life
IL-13 antagonist	SC	Lebrikizumab	Roche	Phase II	Not yet available
	SC	Tralokinumab	AstraZeneca	Phase II	Not yet available
IL-23p40 antagonist	SC	Ustekinumab	Janssen	Phase II	Not yet available
IL-22 antagonist	IV	Fezakinumab	Pfizer	Phase II	Not yet available
IL-31 receptor antagonist	SC	Nemolizumab	Roche	Phase II	Improvement in pruritus and EASI score
IL-31 antagonist	SC, IV	BMS-981164	Bristol-Myers Squibb	Phase I	Not yet available
IL-1R1 antagonist	SC	Anakinra	Sobi	Phase I	Unpublished
IL-6	SC, IV	Tocilizumab	Genentech	Case series	Improvement in EASI score
Targeting pathogenic molecules					
PDE-4 inhibitors	Topical	Crisaborole	Anacor	Phase III	ISGA score success
	Topical	E6005	Eisai	Phase II	EASI score and SCORAD improvement
	Topical	DRM02	QLT	Phase II	Not yet available
	Oral	Apremilast	Celgene	Phase II	EASI score improvement
CRTh2 antagonist	Oral	ODC-9101	Oxagen	Phase II	Not yet available
	Oral	Fevipiprant	Novartis	Phase II	Not yet available
JAK inhibitor	Topical	Tofacitinib	Pfizer	Phase II	Decrease in EASI score
	Oral	Pf-04965842	Pfizer	Phase II	Not yet available
TSLP antagonist	SC	Tezepelumab	Amgen	Phase II	Not yet available
Targeting IgE					
IgE antagonist	SC	Omalizumab	Novartis	Stopped after proof-of-concept study	Heterogeneous results
	SC	Ligelizumab	Novartis	Phase II	Not yet available

Abbreviations: PDE phosphodiesterase, *CRTh2* chemoattractant receptor-homologous molecule expressed on Th2 lymphocytes, *JAK*, Janus kinase, *TSLP* thymic stromal lymphopoietin, *SC* subcutaneous injection, *IV* intravenous, *ISGA* Investigator's Static Global Assessment, *SCORAD* SCORing Atopic Dermatitis, *EASI* Eczema Area and Severity Index

IL-23, which are required for the development and maintenance of Th17 and Th1 cells [179]. Notably, a recent phase II study showed no significant differences in clinical efficacy (SCORAD50) between ustekinumab and placebo in adult AD patients, which may be explained by an inappropriate dosing regimen [185]. Another phase II study is being evaluated (NCT01806662).

IL-31 receptor antagonist and IL-31 antagonist

IL-31 is an important mediator of both itch and inflammation [186, 187]. Nemolizumab, an IL-31 receptor antagonist, has been shown to significantly reduce itch and improve the Eczema Area and Severity Index (EASI) score in AD patients [188]. Additionally, a result from a phase I/Ib study suggests that nemolizumab is well tolerated and seems to be beneficial, especially in alleviating troublesome pruritus [189].

Phosphodiesterase (PDE)-4 inhibitors

PDE is a crucial regulator of cytokine production, and PDE-4 is the most abundant isoenzyme found in human leukocytes [190]. In addition, T and B cells, macrophages, monocytes, neutrophils, and eosinophils also express PDE-4 [191]. Inhibition of PDE-4 resulted in an accumulation of intracellular cyclic adenosine monophosphate (cAMP), which in turn inhibits proinflammatory cytokine transcription and production [192]. It is also known that AD mononuclear leukocytes exhibit increased cAMP-PDE activity that leads to inflammation [193].

PDE-4 inhibitors have been developed in both topical and orally administered forms. Clinical trials evaluating the efficacy of these drugs are detailed in Table 1. Topical PDE-4 inhibitors, e.g., crisaborole [194] and E6005 [195], demonstrate clinical efficacy for AD in phase II and III clinical trials, respectively. Moreover, apremilast, an oral PDE-4 inhibitor that has been used in various inflammatory diseases, including psoriasis, has shown promising results for AD in a recent phase II study [196].

Chemoattractant receptor-homologous molecule expressed on Th2 lymphocytes (CRTh2)

CRTh2 is a prostaglandin D2 receptor that is expressed in Th2 cells, ILC2, eosinophils, and basophils [197, 198]. Activation of CRTh2 induces Th2 cell, ILC2, and eosinophil chemotaxis and promotes their cytokine production [197, 199]. CRTh2 inhibitors are currently in clinical trials for allergic diseases such as asthma and AD. For AD, the results are not yet available (NCT01785602 and NCT02002208).

JAK inhibitor

The JAK-STAT signaling pathway involves a family of cytoplasmic protein tyrosine kinases that is essential for the induction of the cellular responses of many pivotal pathogenic cytokines in AD, namely, IL-4/IL-13 [103]. Furthermore, the activation of eosinophils, the maturation of B cells, and the suppression of regulatory T cells (Tregs) are mediated through the JAK-STAT signaling pathway [200]. Indeed, JTE052, a JAK inhibitor, has been shown to decrease STAT3 activation and leads to an improvement in the skin barrier and an upregulation of filaggrin in a murine AD model [103]. Moreover, the JAK inhibitor can inhibit IFN-γ, IL-13, and IL-17A production from antigen-specific T cells and decrease differentiation and proliferation of effector memory T cells in the draining lymph nodes in the sensitization phase of a murine contact hypersensitivity (CHS) model [201]. Therefore, it appears to be promising as a treatment of various inflammatory dermatoses. JAK inhibitors have been investigated as a treatment for psoriasis and alopecia totalis [202]. In addition, a greater percentage change from baseline (a reduction) in the EASI score was observed in a phase II clinical trial involving topical tofacitinib [203]. Additional studies are currently underway (Table 1).

TSLP antagonist

As mentioned earlier, TSLP is crucial for Th2 skewing and is of great importance in inflammation and itching in AD. This makes TSLP as a promising target molecule to improve AD. Tezepelumab, its antagonist, is currently being studied (NCT02525094).

Other possible biologics for AD that have been studied include drugs that target IgE and B cells, as an increase in B cells and IgE is commonly observed in AD patients [204]. But the outcomes of the treatment with omalizumab, a humanized, monoclonal anti-IgE antibody, in multiple case reports and few control trials have appeared inconclusive [205–207].

In addition, rituximab, a chimeric monoclonal antibody against CD20 that depletes immature and mature B cells, also shows conflicting results [208–210]. Further investigation of omalizumab and rituximab for this indication has therefore been discontinued. Ligelizumab, a new anti-IgE antibody that exhibits a stronger IgE inhibitory effect compared to that of omalizumab [211] may, however, be beneficial for AD and is currently in a phase II trial (NCT01552629).

In summary, there are several promising therapies in the pipeline to satisfy the unmet needs of AD treatment [212]. Further insights into the disease mechanisms will tremendously improve the treatment outcomes and improve the quality of life for individuals with AD.

Conclusions

The skin barrier, innate and adaptive immunity, and pruritus mutually orchestrate skin inflammation in AD. The pathogenesis of the disease is complex and many aspects require further clarification. Based on the detailed evidence available to date, certain disease mechanisms can be chosen as treatment targets. Many clinical trials of biological agents are currently being conducted. These new drugs in the pipeline may satisfy the unmet needs in the treatment of AD.

Abbreviations

AD: Atopic dermatitis; CRTh2: Chemoattractant receptor-homologous molecule expressed on Th2 lymphocytes; DCs: Dendritic cells; EASI: Eczema Area and Severity Index; FLG: Filaggrin; ILCs: Innate lymphoid cells; ISGA: Investigator's Static Global Assessment; JAK: Janus kinase; LCs: Langerhans cells; pDC: Plasmacytoid DC; PDE: Phosphodiesterase; SC: Stratum corneum; SCORAD: SCORing Atopic Dermatitis; SG: Stratum granulosum; STAT: Signal transducer and activator of transcription; TARC: Thymus- and activation-regulated chemokine (also known as CCL17); TJs: Tight junctions; TLR: Toll-like receptor; TSLP: Thymic stromal lymphopoietin

Acknowledgements

PR thanks the Skin and Allergy Research Unit, Chulalongkorn University, for their support. This work was supported in part by Grants-in-Aid for Scientific Research from the Ministry of Education, Culture, Sports, Science and Technology, the Japan Agency for Medical Research and Development (AMED), and the Ministry of Health, Labour and Welfare Sciences (MHLW) and by Precursory Research for Embryonic Science and Technology.

Funding

This work was supported in part by Grants-in-Aid for Scientific Research from the Ministries of Education, Culture, Sports, Science and Technology, Japan Agency for Medical Research and Development (AMED) and by the Ministry of Health, Labour and Welfare Sciences (MHLW) research grants, and Precursory Research for Embryonic Science and Technology.

Authors' contributions

PR, AO, CN, and KK conceived and designed the work. PR collected the data. PR, CN, AO, and KK analyzed and interpreted the data. PR, CN, and AO drafted the article. PR, AO, CN, KK critically revised the article. PR, AO, CN, and KK gave final approval of the version to be published.

Competing interests

The authors declare that they have no competing interests.

Author details
[1]Department of Dermatology, Kyoto University Graduate School of Medicine, 54 Shogoin-Kawara, Sakyo, Kyoto 606-8507, Japan. [2]Division of Dermatology, Department of Medicine, Faculty of Medicine, Skin and Allergy Research Unit, Chulalongkorn University, Bangkok, Thailand. [3]Singapore Immunology Network (SIgN) and Institute of Medical Biology, Agency for Science, Technology and Research (A*STAR), Biopolis, Singapore.

References
1. Weidinger S, Novak N. Atopic dermatitis. Lancet. 2016;387:1109–22.
2. Wallach D, Taieb A. Atopic dermatitis/atopic eczema. Chem Immunol Allergy. 2014;100:81–96.
3. Beattie PE, Lewis-Jones MS. A comparative study of impairment of quality of life in children with skin disease and children with other chronic childhood diseases. Br J Dermatol. 2006;155:145–51.
4. Holm JG, Agner T, Clausen ML, Thomsen SF. Quality of life and disease severity in patients with atopic dermatitis. J Eur Acad Dermatol Venereol. 2016;30:1760–7.
5. Bieber T. Atopic dermatitis. N Engl J Med. 2008;358:1483–94.
6. Alduraywish SA, Lodge CJ, Campbell B, Allen KJ, Erbas B, Lowe AJ, et al. The march from early life food sensitization to allergic disease: a systematic review and meta-analyses of birth cohort studies. Allergy. 2016;71:77–89.
7. Saunders SP, Moran T, Floudas A, Wurlod F, Kaszlikowska A, Salimi M, et al. Spontaneous atopic dermatitis is mediated by innate immunity, with the secondary lung inflammation of the atopic march requiring adaptive immunity. J Allergy Clin Immunol. 2016;137:482–91.
8. Lee HJ, Lee NR, Kim BK, Jung M, Kim DH, Moniaga CS, et al. Acidification of stratum corneum prevents the progression from atopic dermatitis to respiratory allergy. Exp Dermatol. 2017;26:66–72.
9. Brunner PM, Silverberg JI, Guttman-Yassky E, Paller AS, Kabashima K, Amagai M, et al. Increasing comorbidities suggest that atopic dermatitis is a systemic disorder. J Invest Dermatol. 2017;137:18–25.
10. Nomura T, Kayama T, Okamura E, Ogino K, Uji A, Yoshimura N, et al. Severe atopic dermatitis accompanied by autoimmune retinopathy. Eur J Dermatol. 2013;23:263–4.
11. Werfel T, Allam JP, Biedermann T, Eyerich K, Gilles S, Guttman-Yassky E, et al. Cellular and molecular immunologic mechanisms in patients with atopic dermatitis. J Allergy Clin Immunol. 2016;138:336–49.
12. Illi S, von Mutius E, Lau S, Nickel R, Gruber C, Niggemann B, et al. The natural course of atopic dermatitis from birth to age 7 years and the association with asthma. J Allergy Clin Immunol. 2004;113:925–31.
13. Margolis JS, Abuabara K, Bilker W, Hoffstad O, Margolis DJ. Persistence of mild to moderate atopic dermatitis. JAMA Dermatol. 2014;150:593–600.
14. Mortz CG, Andersen KE, Dellgren C, Barington T, Bindslev-Jensen C. Atopic dermatitis from adolescence to adulthood in the TOACS cohort: prevalence, persistence and comorbidities. Allergy. 2015;70:836–45.
15. Kabashima K, Otsuka A, Nomura T. Linking air pollution to atopic dermatitis. Nat Immunol. 2016;18:5–6.
16. Dainichi T, Hanakawa S, Kabashima K. Classification of inflammatory skin diseases: a proposal based on the disorders of the three-layered defense systems, barrier, innate immunity and acquired immunity. J Dermatol Sci. 2014;76:81–9.
17. Kashiwakura J, Okayama Y, Furue M, Kabashima K, Shimada S, Ra C, et al. Most highly cytokinergic IgEs have polyreactivity to autoantigens. Allergy Asthma Immunol Res. 2012;4:332–40.
18. Egawa G, Kabashima K. Multifactorial skin barrier deficiency and atopic dermatitis: essential topics to prevent the atopic march. J Allergy Clin Immunol. 2016;138:350–358.e1.
19. Kirschner N, Houdek P, Fromm M, Moll I, Brandner JM. Tight junctions form a barrier in human epidermis. Eur J Cell Biol. 2010;89:839–42.
20. Steinert PM, Cantieri JS, Teller DC, Lonsdale-Eccles JD, Dale BA. Characterization of a class of cationic proteins that specifically interact with intermediate filaments. Proc Natl Acad Sci U S A. 1981;78:4097–101.
21. Leyvraz C, Charles RP, Rubera I, Guitard M, Rotman S, Breiden B, et al. The epidermal barrier function is dependent on the serine protease CAP1/Prss8. J Cell Biol. 2005;170:487–96.
22. Matsui T, Miyamoto K, Kubo A, Kawasaki H, Ebihara T, Hata K, et al. SASPase regulates stratum corneum hydration through profilaggrin-to-filaggrin processing. EMBO Mol Med. 2011;3:320–33.
23. Egawa G, Doi H, Miyachi Y, Kabashima K. Skin tape stripping and cheek swab method for a detection of filaggrin. J Dermatol Sci. 2013;69:263–5.
24. Hoste E, Kemperman P, Devos M, Denecker G, Kezic S, Yau N, et al. Caspase-14 is required for filaggrin degradation to natural moisturizing factors in the skin. J Invest Dermatol. 2011;131:2233–41.
25. Kamata Y, Taniguchi A, Yamamoto M, Nomura J, Ishihara K, Takahara H, et al. Neutral cysteine protease bleomycin hydrolase is essential for the breakdown of deiminated filaggrin into amino acids. J Biol Chem. 2009;284:12829–36.
26. Brandner JM, Kief S, Grund C, Rendl M, Houdek P, Kuhn C, et al. Organization and formation of the tight junction system in human epidermis and cultured keratinocytes. Eur J Cell Biol. 2002;81:253–63.
27. Niessen CM. Tight junctions/adherens junctions: basic structure and function. J Invest Dermatol. 2007;127:2525–32.
28. Furuse M, Hata M, Furuse K, Yoshida Y, Haratake A, Sugitani Y, et al. Claudin-based tight junctions are crucial for the mammalian epidermal barrier: a lesson from claudin-1-deficient mice. J Cell Biol. 2002;156:1099–111.
29. De Benedetto A, Rafaels NM, McGirt LY, Ivanov AI, Georas SN, Cheadle C, et al. Tight junction defects in patients with atopic dermatitis. J Allergy Clin Immunol. 2011;127:773–786.e1-7.
30. Yuki T, Tobiishi M, Kusaka-Kikushima A, Ota Y, Tokura Y. Impaired tight junctions in atopic dermatitis skin and in a skin-equivalent model treated with interleukin-17. PLoS One. 2016;11:e0161759.
31. Brown SJ, McLean WH. One remarkable molecule: filaggrin. J Invest Dermatol. 2012;132:751–62.
32. Thyssen JP, Kezic S. Causes of epidermal filaggrin reduction and their role in the pathogenesis of atopic dermatitis. J Allergy Clin Immunol. 2014;134:792–9.
33. Pendaries V, Malaisse J, Pellerin L, Le Lamer M, Nachat R, Kezic S, et al. Knockdown of filaggrin in a three-dimensional reconstructed human epidermis impairs keratinocyte differentiation. J Invest Dermatol. 2014;134:2938–46.
34. Palmer CN, Irvine AD, Terron-Kwiatkowski A, Zhao Y, Liao H, Lee SP, et al. Common loss-of-function variants of the epidermal barrier protein filaggrin are a major predisposing factor for atopic dermatitis. Nat Genet. 2006;38:441–6.
35. Paternoster L, Standl M, Waage J, Baurecht H, Hotze M, Strachan DP, et al. Multi-ancestry genome-wide association study of 21,000 cases and 95,000 controls identifies new risk loci for atopic dermatitis. Nat Genet. 2015;47:1449–56.
36. Irvine AD, McLean WH, Leung DY. Filaggrin mutations associated with skin and allergic diseases. N Engl J Med. 2011;365:1315–27.
37. Brattsand M, Stefansson K, Lundh C, Haasum Y, Egelrud T. A proteolytic cascade of kallikreins in the stratum corneum. J Invest Dermatol. 2005;124:198–203.
38. Kezic S, O'Regan GM, Lutter R, Jakasa I, Koster ES, Saunders S, et al. Filaggrin loss-of-function mutations are associated with enhanced expression of IL-1 cytokines in the stratum corneum of patients with atopic dermatitis and in a murine model of filaggrin deficiency. J Allergy Clin Immunol. 2012;129:1031–1039.e1031.
39. Briot A, Deraison C, Lacroix M, Bonnart C, Robin A, Besson C, et al. Kallikrein 5 induces atopic dermatitis-like lesions through PAR2-mediated thymic stromal lymphopoietin expression in Netherton syndrome. J Exp Med. 2009;206:1135–47.
40. Moniaga CS, Jeong SK, Egawa G, Nakajima S, Hara-Chikuma M, Jeon JE, et al. Protease activity enhances production of thymic stromal lymphopoietin and basophil accumulation in flaky tail mice. Am J Pathol. 2013;182:841–51.
41. Moniaga CS, Egawa G, Kawasaki H, Hara-Chikuma M, Honda T, Tanizaki H, et al. Flaky tail mouse denotes human atopic dermatitis in the steady state and by topical application with Dermatophagoides pteronyssinus extract. Am J Pathol. 2010;176:2385–93.
42. Moniaga CS, Kabashima K. Filaggrin in atopic dermatitis: flaky tail mice as a novel model for developing drug targets in atopic dermatitis. Inflamm Allergy Drug Targets. 2011;10:477–85.
43. Ewald DA, Noda S, Oliva M, Litman T, Nakajima S, Li X, et al. Major differences between human atopic dermatitis and murine models, as determined by using global transcriptomic profiling. J Allergy Clin Immunol. 2017;139(2):562–71.
44. Sasaki T, Shiohama A, Kubo A, Kawasaki H, Ishida-Yamamoto A, Yamada T, et al. A homozygous nonsense mutation in the gene for Tmem79, a

component for the lamellar granule secretory system, produces spontaneous eczema in an experimental model of atopic dermatitis. J Allergy Clin Immunol. 2013;132:1111–1120.e1114.

45. Kawasaki H, Nagao K, Kubo A, Hata T, Shimizu A, Mizuno H, et al. Altered stratum corneum barrier and enhanced percutaneous immune responses in filaggrin-null mice. J Allergy Clin Immunol. 2012;129:1538–1546.e1536.

46. Fallon PG, Sasaki T, Sandilands A, Campbell LE, Saunders SP, Mangan NE, et al. A homozygous frameshift mutation in the mouse Flg gene facilitates enhanced percutaneous allergen priming. Nat Genet. 2009;41:602–8.

47. Jeong SK, Kim HJ, Youm JK, Ahn SK, Choi EH, Sohn MH, et al. Mite and cockroach allergens activate protease-activated receptor 2 and delay epidermal permeability barrier recovery. J Invest Dermatol. 2008;128:1930–9.

48. Miajlovic H, Fallon PG, Irvine AD, Foster TJ. Effect of filaggrin breakdown products on growth of and protein expression by Staphylococcus aureus. J Allergy Clin Immunol. 2010;126:1184–1190.e1183.

49. Brauweiler AM, Bin L, Kim BE, Oyoshi MK, Geha RS, Goleva E, et al. Filaggrin-dependent secretion of sphingomyelinase protects against staphylococcal alpha-toxin-induced keratinocyte death. J Allergy Clin Immunol. 2013;131:421–427.e421-422.

50. Mildner M, Jin J, Eckhart L, Kezic S, Gruber F, Barresi C, et al. Knockdown of filaggrin impairs diffusion barrier function and increases UV sensitivity in a human skin model. J Invest Dermatol. 2010;130:2286–94.

51. Scharschmidt TC, Man MQ, Hatano Y, Crumrine D, Gunathilake R, Sundberg JP, et al. Filaggrin deficiency confers a paracellular barrier abnormality that reduces inflammatory thresholds to irritants and hapten. J Allergy Clin Immunol. 2009;124:496–506.e491-496.

52. Otsuka A, Doi H, Egawa G, Maekawa A, Fujita T, Nakamizo S, et al. Possible new therapeutic strategy to regulate atopic dermatitis through upregulating filaggrin expression. J Allergy Clin Immunol. 2014;133:139–146.e131-110.

53. Matsui S, Murota H, Takahashi A, Yang L, Lee JB, Omiya K, et al. Dynamic analysis of histamine-mediated attenuation of acetylcholine-induced sweating via GSK3beta activation. J Invest Dermatol. 2014;134:326–34.

54. Murota H, Matsui S, Ono E, Kijima A, Kikuta J, Ishii M, et al. Sweat, the driving force behind normal skin: an emerging perspective on functional biology and regulatory mechanisms. J Dermatol Sci. 2015;77:3–10.

55. Rerknimitr P, Tanizaki H, Yamamoto Y, Amano W, Nakajima S, Nakashima C, et al. Decreased Filaggrin Level May Lead to Sweat Duct Obstruction in Filaggrin Mutant Mice. J Invest Dermatol. 2017;137(1):248–51.

56. Eckl KM, de Juanes S, Kurtenbach J, Natebus M, Lugassy J, Oji V, et al. Molecular analysis of 250 patients with autosomal recessive congenital ichthyosis: evidence for mutation hotspots in ALOXE3 and allelic heterogeneity in ALOX12B. J Invest Dermatol. 2009;129:1421–8.

57. Saunders SP, Goh CS, Brown SJ, Palmer CN, Porter RM, Cole C, et al. Tmem79/Matt is the matted mouse gene and is a predisposing gene for atopic dermatitis in human subjects. J Allergy Clin Immunol. 2013;132:1121–9.

58. Deraison C, Bonnart C, Lopez F, Besson C, Robinson R, Jayakumar A, et al. LEKTI fragments specifically inhibit KLK5, KLK7, and KLK14 and control desquamation through a pH-dependent interaction. Mol Biol Cell. 2007;18:3607–19.

59. Vasilopoulos Y, Sharaf N, di Giovine F, Simon M, Cork MJ, Duff GW, et al. The 3′-UTR AACCins5874 in the stratum corneum chymotryptic enzyme gene (SCCE/KLK7), associated with atopic dermatitis; causes an increased mRNA expression without altering its stability. J Dermatol Sci. 2011;61:131–3.

60. Chavanas S, Bodemer C, Rochat A, Hamel-Teillac D, Ali M, Irvine AD, et al. Mutations in SPINK5, encoding a serine protease inhibitor, cause Netherton syndrome. Nat Genet. 2000;25:141–2.

61. Walley AJ, Chavanas S, Moffatt MF, Esnouf RM, Ubhi B, Lawrence R, et al. Gene polymorphism in Netherton and common atopic disease. Nat Genet. 2001;29:175–8.

62. Zhao LP, Di Z, Zhang L, Wang L, Ma L, Lv Y, et al. Association of SPINK5 gene polymorphisms with atopic dermatitis in Northeast China. J Eur Acad Dermatol Venereol. 2012;26:572–7.

63. Kabashima K. New concept of the pathogenesis of atopic dermatitis: interplay among the barrier, allergy, and pruritus as a trinity. J Dermatol Sci. 2013;70:3–11.

64. Hirota T, Takahashi A, Kubo M, Tsunoda T, Tomita K, Sakashita M, et al. Genome-wide association study identifies eight new susceptibility loci for atopic dermatitis in the Japanese population. Nat Genet. 2012;44:1222–6.

65. Oyoshi MK, Larson RP, Ziegler SF, Geha RS. Mechanical injury polarizes skin dendritic cells to elicit a T(H)2 response by inducing cutaneous thymic stromal lymphopoietin expression. J Allergy Clin Immunol. 2010;126:976–84.

66. Yoo J, Omori M, Gyarmati D, Zhou B, Aye T, Brewer A, et al. Spontaneous atopic dermatitis in mice expressing an inducible thymic stromal lymphopoietin transgene specifically in the skin. J Exp Med. 2005;202:541–9.

67. Onoue A, Kabashima K, Kobayashi M, Mori T, Tokura Y. Induction of eosinophil- and Th2-attracting epidermal chemokines and cutaneous late-phase reaction in tape-stripped skin. Exp Dermatol. 2009;18:1036–43.

68. Nakahigashi K, Kabashima K, Ikoma A, Verkman AS, Miyachi Y, Hara-Chikuma M. Upregulation of aquaporin-3 is involved in keratinocyte proliferation and epidermal hyperplasia. J Invest Dermatol. 2011;131:865–73.

69. Kim BS. Innate lymphoid cells in the skin. J Invest Dermatol. 2015;135:673–8.

70. Bruggen MC, Bauer WM, Reininger B, Clim E, Captarencu C, Steiner GE, et al. In Situ Mapping of Innate Lymphoid Cells in Human Skin: Evidence for Remarkable Differences between Normal and Inflamed Skin. J Invest Dermatol. 2016;136(12):2396–405.

71. Kim BS, Siracusa MC, Saenz SA, Noti M, Monticelli LA, Sonnenberg GF, et al. TSLP elicits IL-33-independent innate lymphoid cell responses to promote skin inflammation. Sci Transl Med. 2013;5:170ra116.

72. Roediger B, Kyle R, Yip KH, Sumaria N, Guy TV, Kim BS, et al. Cutaneous immunosurveillance and regulation of inflammation by group 2 innate lymphoid cells. Nat Immunol. 2013;14:564–73.

73. Salimi M, Barlow JL, Saunders SP, Xue L, Gutowska-Owsiak D, Wang X, et al. A role for IL-25 and IL-33-driven type-2 innate lymphoid cells in atopic dermatitis. J Exp Med. 2013;210:2939–50.

74. Imai Y, Yasuda K, Sakaguchi Y, Haneda T, Mizutani H, Yoshimoto T, et al. Skin-specific expression of IL-33 activates group 2 innate lymphoid cells and elicits atopic dermatitis-like inflammation in mice. Proc Natl Acad Sci U S A. 2013;110:13921–6.

75. Xue L, Salimi M, Panse I, Mjosberg JM, McKenzie AN, Spits H, et al. Prostaglandin D2 activates group 2 innate lymphoid cells through chemoattractant receptor-homologous molecule expressed on TH2 cells. J Allergy Clin Immunol. 2014;133:1184–94.

76. Honda T, Kabashima K. Prostanoids in allergy. Allergol Int. 2015;64:11–6.

77. Kim BS, Wang K, Siracusa MC, Saenz SA, Brestoff JR, Monticelli LA, et al. Basophils promote innate lymphoid cell responses in inflamed skin. J Immunol. 2014;193:3717–25.

78. Nakai K, Yoneda K, Hosokawa Y, Moriue T, Presland RB, Fallon PG, et al. Reduced expression of epidermal growth factor receptor, E-cadherin, and occludin in the skin of flaky tail mice is due to filaggrin and loricrin deficiencies. Am J Pathol. 2012;181:969–77.

79. Morita H, Moro K, Koyasu S. Innate lymphoid cells in allergic and nonallergic inflammation. J Allergy Clin Immunol. 2016;138:1253–64.

80. Otsuka A, Nonomura Y, Kabashima K. Roles of basophils and mast cells in cutaneous inflammation. Semin Immunopathol. 2016;38:563–70.

81. Otsuka A, Kabashima K. Mast cells and basophils in cutaneous immune responses. Allergy. 2015;70:131–40.

82. Nakashima C, Otsuka A, Kitoh A, Honda T, Egawa G, Nakajima S, et al. Basophils regulate the recruitment of eosinophils in a murine model of irritant contact dermatitis. J Allergy Clin Immunol. 2014;134:100–7.

83. Mori T, Kabashima K, Fukamachi S, Kuroda E, Sakabe J, Kobayashi M, et al. D1-like dopamine receptors antagonist inhibits cutaneous immune reactions mediated by Th2 and mast cells. J Dermatol Sci. 2013;71:37–44.

84. Gros E, Novak N. Cutaneous dendritic cells in allergic inflammation. Clin Exp Allergy. 2012;42:1161–75.

85. Kubo A, Nagao K, Yokouchi M, Sasaki H, Amagai M. External antigen uptake by Langerhans cells with reorganization of epidermal tight junction barriers. J Exp Med. 2009;206:2937–46.

86. Klechevsky E, Morita R, Liu M, Cao Y, Coquery S, Thompson-Snipes L, et al. Functional specializations of human epidermal Langerhans cells and CD14+ dermal dendritic cells. Immunity. 2008;29:497–510.

87. Nakajima S, Igyarto BZ, Honda T, Egawa G, Otsuka A, Hara-Chikuma M, et al. Langerhans cells are critical in epicutaneous sensitization with protein antigen via thymic stromal lymphopoietin receptor signaling. J Allergy Clin Immunol. 2012;129:1048–1055.e1046.

88. Elentner A, Finke D, Schmuth M, Chappaz S, Ebner S, Malissen B, et al. Langerhans cells are critical in the development of atopic dermatitis-like inflammation and symptoms in mice. J Cell Mol Med. 2009;13:2658–72.

89. Ziegler SF. The role of thymic stromal lymphopoietin (TSLP) in allergic disorders. Curr Opin Immunol. 2010;22:795–9.

90. Fernandez MI, Heuze ML, Martinez-Cingolani C, Volpe E, Donnadieu MH, Piel M, et al. The human cytokine TSLP triggers a cell-autonomous dendritic cell migration in confined environments. Blood. 2011;118:3862–9.

91. Ebner S, Nguyen VA, Forstner M, Wang YH, Wolfram D, Liu YJ, et al. Thymic stromal lymphopoietin converts human epidermal Langerhans cells into antigen-presenting cells that induce proallergic T cells. J Allergy Clin Immunol. 2007;119:982–90.

92. Novak N. An update on the role of human dendritic cells in patients with atopic dermatitis. J Allergy Clin Immunol. 2012;129:879–86.

93. Novak N, Valenta R, Bohle B, Laffer S, Haberstok J, Kraft S, et al. FcepsilonRI engagement of Langerhans cell-like dendritic cells and inflammatory dendritic epidermal cell-like dendritic cells induces chemotactic signals and different T-cell phenotypes in vitro. J Allergy Clin Immunol. 2004;113:949–57.

94. Kerschenlohr K, Decard S, Przybilla B, Wollenberg A. Atopy patch test reactions show a rapid influx of inflammatory dendritic epidermal cells in patients with extrinsic atopic dermatitis and patients with intrinsic atopic dermatitis. J Allergy Clin Immunol. 2003;111:869–74.

95. Wollenberg A, Wagner M, Gunther S, Towarowski A, Tuma E, Moderer M, et al. Plasmacytoid dendritic cells: a new cutaneous dendritic cell subset with distinct role in inflammatory skin diseases. J Invest Dermatol. 2002;119:1096–102.

96. Albanesi C, Scarponi C, Pallotta S, Daniele R, Bosisio D, Madonna S, et al. Chemerin expression marks early psoriatic skin lesions and correlates with plasmacytoid dendritic cell recruitment. J Exp Med. 2009;206:249–58.

97. Novak N, Allam JP, Hagemann T, Jenneck C, Laffer S, Valenta R, et al. Characterization of FcepsilonRI-bearing CD123 blood dendritic cell antigen-2 plasmacytoid dendritic cells in atopic dermatitis. J Allergy Clin Immunol. 2004;114:364–70.

98. Moy AP, Murali M, Kroshinsky D, Duncan LM, Nazarian RM. Immunologic overlap of helper T-cell subtypes 17 and 22 in erythrodermic psoriasis and atopic dermatitis. JAMA Dermatol. 2015;151:753–60.

99. Nygaard U, Hvid M, Johansen C, Buchner M, Folster-Holst R, Deleuran M, et al. TSLP, IL-31, IL-33 and sST2 are new biomarkers in endophenotypic profiling of adult and childhood atopic dermatitis. J Eur Acad Dermatol Venereol. 2016;30:1930–8.

100. Kim JE, Kim JS, Cho DH, Park HJ. Molecular mechanisms of cutaneous inflammatory disorder: atopic dermatitis. Int J Mol Sci. 2016;17.

101. Howell MD, Kim BE, Gao P, Grant AV, Boguniewicz M, Debenedetto A, et al. Cytokine modulation of atopic dermatitis filaggrin skin expression. J Allergy Clin Immunol. 2007;120:150–5.

102. Kim BE, Leung DY, Boguniewicz M, Howell MD. Loricrin and involucrin expression is down-regulated by Th2 cytokines through STAT-6. Clin Immunol. 2008;126:332–7.

103. Amano W, Nakajima S, Kunugi H, Numata Y, Kitoh A, Egawa G, et al. The Janus kinase inhibitor JTE-052 improves skin barrier function through suppressing signal transducer and activator of transcription 3 signaling. J Allergy Clin Immunol. 2015;136:667–677.e667.

104. Mitsuishi T, Kabashima K, Tanizaki H, Ohsawa I, Oda F, Yamada Y, et al. Specific substance of Maruyama (SSM) suppresses immune responses in atopic dermatitis-like skin lesions in DS-Nh mice by modulating dendritic cell functions. J Dermatol Sci. 2011;63:184–90.

105. Watcharanurak K, Nishikawa M, Takahashi Y, Kabashima K, Takahashi R, Takakura Y. Regulation of immunological balance by sustained interferon-gamma gene transfer for acute phase of atopic dermatitis in mice. Gene Ther. 2013;20:538–44.

106. Hattori K, Nishikawa M, Watcharanurak K, Ikoma A, Kabashima K, Toyota H, et al. Sustained exogenous expression of therapeutic levels of IFN-gamma ameliorates atopic dermatitis in NC/Nga mice via Th1 polarization. J Immunol. 2010;184:2729–35.

107. Thaçi D, Simpson EL, Beck LA, Bieber T, Blauvelt A, Papp K, et al. Efficacy and safety of dupilumab in adults with moderate-to-severe atopic dermatitis inadequately controlled by topical treatments: a randomised, placebo-controlled, dose-ranging phase 2b trial. Lancet. 2016;387(10013):40–52.

108. Nomura T, Kabashima K, Miyachi Y. The panoply of alphabetaT cells in the skin. J Dermatol Sci. 2014;76:3–9.

109. Jin S, Park CO, Shin JU, Noh JY, Lee YS, Lee NR, et al. DAMP molecules S100A9 and S100A8 activated by IL-17A and house-dust mites are increased in atopic dermatitis. Exp Dermatol. 2014;23:938–41.

110. Park H, Li Z, Yang XO, Chang SH, Nurieva R, Wang YH, et al. A distinct lineage of CD4 T cells regulates tissue inflammation by producing interleukin 17. Nat Immunol. 2005;6:1133–41.

111. He R, Oyoshi MK, Jin H, Geha RS. Epicutaneous antigen exposure induces a Th17 response that drives airway inflammation after inhalation challenge. Proc Natl Acad Sci U S A. 2007;104:15817–22.

112. Nakajima S, Kitoh A, Egawa G, Natsuaki Y, Nakamizo S, Moniaga CS, et al. IL-17A as an inducer for Th2 immune responses in murine atopic dermatitis models. J Invest Dermatol. 2014;134:2122–30.

113. Oyoshi MK, Murphy GF, Geha RS. Filaggrin-deficient mice exhibit TH17-dominated skin inflammation and permissiveness to epicutaneous sensitization with protein antigen. J Allergy Clin Immunol. 2009;124:485–493.e481.

114. Toda M, Leung DY, Molet S, Boguniewicz M, Taha R, Christodoulopoulos P, et al. Polarized in vivo expression of IL-11 and IL-17 between acute and chronic skin lesions. J Allergy Clin Immunol. 2003;111:875–81.

115. Koga C, Kabashima K, Shiraishi N, Kobayashi M, Tokura Y. Possible pathogenic role of Th17 cells for atopic dermatitis. J Invest Dermatol. 2008;128:2625–30.

116. Tokura Y. Extrinsic and intrinsic types of atopic dermatitis. J Dermatol Sci. 2010;58:1–7.

117. Kabashima-Kubo R, Nakamura M, Sakabe J, Sugita K, Hino R, Mori T, et al. A group of atopic dermatitis without IgE elevation or barrier impairment shows a high Th1 frequency: possible immunological state of the intrinsic type. J Dermatol Sci. 2012;67:37–43.

118. Mori T, Ishida K, Mukumoto S, Yamada Y, Imokawa G, Kabashima K, et al. Comparison of skin barrier function and sensory nerve electric current perception threshold between IgE-high extrinsic and IgE-normal intrinsic types of atopic dermatitis. Br J Dermatol. 2010;162:83–90.

119. Suarez-Farinas M, Dhingra N, Gittler J, Shemer A, Cardinale I, de Guzman SC, et al. Intrinsic atopic dermatitis shows similar TH2 and higher TH17 immune activation compared with extrinsic atopic dermatitis. J Allergy Clin Immunol. 2013;132:361–70.

120. Noda S, Suarez-Farinas M, Ungar B, Kim SJ, de Guzman SC, Xu H, et al. The Asian atopic dermatitis phenotype combines features of atopic dermatitis and psoriasis with increased TH17 polarization. J Allergy Clin Immunol. 2015;136:1254–64.

121. Kong HH, Oh J, Deming C, Conlan S, Grice EA, Beatson MA, et al. Temporal shifts in the skin microbiome associated with disease flares and treatment in children with atopic dermatitis. Genome Res. 2012;22:850–9.

122. Harder J, Schroder JM, Glaser R. The skin surface as antimicrobial barrier: present concepts and future outlooks. Exp Dermatol. 2013;22:1–5.

123. Ong PY, Ohtake T, Brandt C, Strickland I, Boguniewicz M, Ganz T, et al. Endogenous antimicrobial peptides and skin infections in atopic dermatitis. N Engl J Med. 2002;347:1151–60.

124. Glaser R, Meyer-Hoffert U, Harder J, Cordes J, Wittersheim M, Kobliakova J, et al. The antimicrobial protein psoriasin (S100A7) is upregulated in atopic dermatitis and after experimental skin barrier disruption. J Invest Dermatol. 2009;129:641–9.

125. Harder J, Dressel S, Wittersheim M, Cordes J, Meyer-Hoffert U, Mrowietz U, et al. Enhanced expression and secretion of antimicrobial peptides in atopic dermatitis and after superficial skin injury. J Invest Dermatol. 2010;130:1355–64.

126. Schittek B. The antimicrobial skin barrier in patients with atopic dermatitis. Curr Probl Dermatol. 2011;41:54–67.

127. Son ED, Kim HJ, Kim KH, Bin BH, Bae IH, Lim KM, et al. S100A7 (psoriasin) inhibits human epidermal differentiation by enhanced IL-6 secretion through IkappaB/NF-kappaB signalling. Exp Dermatol. 2016;25:636–41.

128. Fornasa G, Tsilingiri K, Caprioli F, Botti F, Mapelli M, Meller S, et al. Dichotomy of short and long thymic stromal lymphopoietin isoforms in inflammatory disorders of the bowel and skin. J Allergy Clin Immunol. 2015;136:413–22.

129. Bjerkan L, Schreurs O, Engen SA, Jahnsen FL, Baekkevold ES, Blix IJ, et al. The short form of TSLP is constitutively translated in human keratinocytes and has characteristics of an antimicrobial peptide. Mucosal Immunol. 2015;8:49–56.

130. Bjerkan L, Sonesson A, Schenck K. Multiple functions of the new cytokine-based antimicrobial peptide thymic stromal lymphopoietin (TSLP). Pharmaceuticals (Basel). 2016;9.

131. Kupper TS, Fuhlbrigge RC. Immune surveillance in the skin: mechanisms and clinical consequences. Nat Rev Immunol. 2004;4:211–22.

132. Stoll H, Dengjel J, Nerz C, Gotz F. Staphylococcus aureus deficient in lipidation of prelipoproteins is attenuated in growth and immune activation. Infect Immun. 2005;73:2411–23.

133. Skabytska Y, Kaesler S, Volz T, Biedermann T. The role of innate immune

signaling in the pathogenesis of atopic dermatitis and consequences for treatments. Semin Immunopathol. 2016;38:29–43.

134. Ahmad-Nejad P, Mrabet-Dahbi S, Breuer K, Klotz M, Werfel T, Herz U, et al. The toll-like receptor 2 R753Q polymorphism defines a subgroup of patients with atopic dermatitis having severe phenotype. J Allergy Clin Immunol. 2004;113:565–7.

135. Mrabet-Dahbi S, Dalpke AH, Niebuhr M, Frey M, Draing C, Brand S, et al. The Toll-like receptor 2 R753Q mutation modifies cytokine production and Toll-like receptor expression in atopic dermatitis. J Allergy Clin Immunol. 2008;121:1013–9.

136. Voss E, Wehkamp J, Wehkamp K, Stange EF, Schroder JM, Harder J. NOD2/CARD15 mediates induction of the antimicrobial peptide human beta-defensin-2. J Biol Chem. 2006;281:2005–11.

137. Hruz P, Zinkernagel AS, Jenikova G, Botwin GJ, Hugot JP, Karin M, et al. NOD2 contributes to cutaneous defense against Staphylococcus aureus through alpha-toxin-dependent innate immune activation. Proc Natl Acad Sci U S A. 2009;106:12873–8.

138. Macaluso F, Nothnagel M, Parwez Q, Petrasch-Parwez E, Bechara FG, Epplen JT, et al. Polymorphisms in NACHT-LRR (NLR) genes in atopic dermatitis. Exp Dermatol. 2007;16:692–8.

139. Volz T, Nega M, Buschmann J, Kaesler S, Guenova E, Peschel A, et al. Natural Staphylococcus aureus-derived peptidoglycan fragments activate NOD2 and act as potent costimulators of the innate immune system exclusively in the presence of TLR signals. Faseb J. 2010;24:4089–102.

140. Miller LS, Cho JS. Immunity against Staphylococcus aureus cutaneous infections. Nat Rev Immunol. 2011;11:505–18.

141. Islander U, Andersson A, Lindberg E, Adlerberth I, Wold AE, Rudin A. Superantigenic Staphylococcus aureus stimulates production of interleukin-17 from memory but not naive T cells. Infect Immun. 2010;78:381–6.

142. Czarnowicki T, Gonzalez J, Shemer A, Malajian D, Xu H, Zheng X, et al. Severe atopic dermatitis is characterized by selective expansion of circulating TH2/TC2 and TH22/TC22, but not TH17/TC17, cells within the skin-homing T-cell population. J Allergy Clin Immunol. 2015;136:104–115.e107.

143. Hepburn L, Hijnen DJ, Sellman BR, Mustelin T, Sleeman MA, May RD, et al. The complex biology and contribution of Staphylococcus aureus in atopic dermatitis, current and future therapies. Br J Dermatol. 2016. doi:10.1111/bjd.15139. [Epub ahead of print].

144. Hirasawa Y, Takai T, Nakamura T, Mitsuishi K, Gunawan H, Suto H, et al. Staphylococcus aureus extracellular protease causes epidermal barrier dysfunction. J Invest Dermatol. 2010;130:614–7.

145. Takeuchi O, Akira S. Pattern recognition receptors and inflammation. Cell. 2010;140:805–20.

146. Spaulding AR, Satterwhite EA, Lin YC, Chuang-Smith ON, Frank KL, Merriman JA, et al. Comparison of Staphylococcus aureus strains for ability to cause infective endocarditis and lethal sepsis in rabbits. Front Cell Infect Microbiol. 2012;2:18.

147. Leung DY, Travers JB, Giorno R, Norris DA, Skinner R, Aelion J, et al. Evidence for a streptococcal superantigen-driven process in acute guttate psoriasis. J Clin Invest. 1995;96:2106–12.

148. Leung DY, Harbeck R, Bina P, Reiser RF, Yang E, Norris DA, et al. Presence of IgE antibodies to staphylococcal exotoxins on the skin of patients with atopic dermatitis. Evidence for a new group of allergens. J Clin Invest. 1993;92:1374–80.

149. Nakamura Y, Oscherwitz J, Cease KB, Chan SM, Munoz-Planillo R, Hasegawa M, et al. Staphylococcus delta-toxin induces allergic skin disease by activating mast cells. Nature. 2013;503:397–401.

150. Nakamizo S, Egawa G, Honda T, Nakajima S, Belkaid Y, Kabashima K. Commensal bacteria and cutaneous immunity. Semin Immunopathol. 2015;37:73–80.

151. Kido-Nakahara M, Furue M, Ulzii D, Nakahara T. Itch in atopic dermatitis. Immunol Allergy Clin North Am. 2017;37:113–22.

152. Kamo A, Tominaga M, Tengara S, Ogawa H, Takamori K. Inhibitory effects of UV-based therapy on dry skin-inducible nerve growth in acetone-treated mice. J Dermatol Sci. 2011;62:91–7.

153. Urashima R, Mihara M. Cutaneous nerves in atopic dermatitis. A histological, immunohistochemical and electron microscopic study. Virchows Arch. 1998;432:363–70.

154. Tominaga M, Tengara S, Kamo A, Ogawa H, Takamori K. Psoralen-ultraviolet A therapy alters epidermal Sema3A and NGF levels and modulates epidermal innervation in atopic dermatitis. J Dermatol Sci. 2009;55:40–6.

155. Toyoda M, Nakamura M, Makino T, Hino T, Kagoura M, Morohashi M. Nerve growth factor and substance P are useful plasma markers of disease activity in atopic dermatitis. Br J Dermatol. 2002;147:71–9.

156. Tominaga M, Ogawa H, Takamori K. Decreased production of semaphorin 3A in the lesional skin of atopic dermatitis. Br J Dermatol. 2008;158:842–4.

157. Mollanazar NK, Smith PK, Yosipovitch G. Mediators of chronic pruritus in atopic dermatitis: getting the itch out? Clin Rev Allergy Immunol. 2016;51:263–92.

158. Han L, Dong X. Itch mechanisms and circuits. Annu Rev Biophys. 2014;43:331–55.

159. Ikoma A, Steinhoff M, Stander S, Yosipovitch G, Schmelz M. The neurobiology of itch. Nat Rev Neurosci. 2006;7:535–47.

160. Murota H, Katayama I. Evolving understanding on the aetiology of thermally provoked itch. Eur J Pain. 2016;20:47–50.

161. Murota H, Izumi M, Abd El-Latif MIA, Nishioka M, Terao M, Tani M, et al. Artemin causes hypersensitivity to warm sensation, mimicking warmth-provoked pruritus in atopic dermatitis. J Allergy Clin Immunol. 2012;130:671–682.e674.

162. Cowden JM, Zhang M, Dunford PJ, Thurmond RL. The histamine H4 receptor mediates inflammation and pruritus in Th2-dependent dermal inflammation. J Invest Dermatol. 2010;130:1023–33.

163. Sonkoly E, Muller A, Lauerma AI, Pivarcsi A, Soto H, Kemeny L, et al. IL-31: a new link between T cells and pruritus in atopic skin inflammation. J Allergy Clin Immunol. 2006;117:411–7.

164. Dillon SR, Sprecher C, Hammond A, Bilsborough J, Rosenfeld-Franklin M, Presnell SR, et al. Interleukin 31, a cytokine produced by activated T cells, induces dermatitis in mice. Nat Immunol. 2004;5:752–60.

165. Wilson SR, Thé L, Batia LM, Beattie K, Katibah GE, McClain SP, et al. The epithelial cell-derived atopic dermatitis cytokine TSLP activates neurons to induce itch. Cell. 2013;155:285–95.

166. Kido-Nakahara M, Buddenkotte J, Kempkes C, Ikoma A, Cevikbas F, Akiyama T, et al. Neural peptidase endothelin-converting enzyme 1 regulates endothelin 1-induced pruritus. J Clin Invest. 2014;124:2683–95.

167. Heise R, Neis MM, Marquardt Y, Joussen S, Heinrich PC, Merk HF, et al. IL-31 receptor alpha expression in epidermal keratinocytes is modulated by cell differentiation and interferon gamma. J Invest Dermatol. 2009;129:240–3.

168. Kato A, Fujii E, Watanabe T, Takashima Y, Matsushita H, Furuhashi T, et al. Distribution of IL-31 and its receptor expressing cells in skin of atopic dermatitis. J Dermatol Sci. 2014;74(3):229–35.

169. Cornelissen C, Marquardt Y, Czaja K, Wenzel J, Frank J, Lüscher-Firzlaff J, et al. IL-31 regulates differentiation and filaggrin expression in human organotypic skin models. J Allergy Clin Immunol. 2012;129:426–433.e428.

170. Kasraie S, Niebuhr M, Werfel T. Interleukin (IL)-31 activates signal transducer and activator of transcription (STAT)-1, STAT-5 and extracellular signal-regulated kinase 1/2 and down-regulates IL-12p40 production in activated human macrophages. Allergy. 2013;68:739–47.

171. Raap U, Wieczorek D, Gehring M, Pauls I, Ständer S, Kapp A, et al. Increased levels of serum IL-31 in chronic spontaneous urticaria. Exp Dermatol. 2010;19:464–6.

172. Raap U, Wichmann K, Bruder M, Ständer S, Wedi B, Kapp A, et al. Correlation of IL-31 serum levels with severity of atopic dermatitis. J Allergy Clin Immunol. 2008;122:421–3.

173. Nomura T, Kabashima K. Advances in atopic dermatitis in 2015. J Allergy Clin Immunol. 2016;138:1548–55.

174. Ishiuji Y, Coghill RC, Patel TS, Oshiro Y, Kraft RA, Yosipovitch G. Distinct patterns of brain activity evoked by histamine-induced itch reveal an association with itch intensity and disease severity in atopic dermatitis. Brit J Dermatol. 2009;161:1072–80.

175. Leslie TA, Greaves MW, Yosipovitch G. Current topical and systemic therapies for itch. Handb Exp Pharmacol. 2015;226:337–56.

176. Shiratori-Hayashi M, Koga K, Tozaki-Saitoh H, Kohro Y, Toyonaga H, Yamaguchi C, et al. STAT3-dependent reactive astrogliosis in the spinal dorsal horn underlies chronic itch. Nat Med. 2015;21:927–31.

177. Tominaga M, Ozawa S, Tengara S, Ogawa H, Takamori K. Intraepidermal nerve fibers increase in dry skin of acetone-treated mice. J Dermatol Sci. 2007;48:103–11.

178. Heratizadeh A, Werfel T. Anti-inflammatory therapies in atopic dermatitis. Allergy. 2016;71:1666–75.

179. Lauffer F, Ring J. Target-oriented therapy: emerging drugs for atopic dermatitis. Expert Opin Emerg Drugs. 2016;21:81–9.

180. Noda S, Krueger JG, Guttman-Yassky E. The translational revolution and use of biologics in patients with inflammatory skin diseases. J Allergy Clin Immunol. 2015;135:324–36.

181. Beck LA, Thaci D, Hamilton JD, Graham NM, Bieber T, Rocklin R, et al. Dupilumab treatment in adults with moderate-to-severe atopic dermatitis. N Engl J Med. 2014;371:130–9.

182. Simpson EL, Gadkari A, Worm M, Soong W, Blauvelt A, Eckert L, et al. Dupilumab therapy provides clinically meaningful improvement in patient-reported outcomes (PROs): a phase IIb, randomized, placebo-controlled, clinical trial in adult patients with moderate to severe atopic dermatitis (AD). J Am Acad Dermatol. 2016;75:506–15.

183. Hamilton JD, Suarez-Farinas M, Dhingra N, Cardinale I, Li X, Kostic A, et al. Dupilumab improves the molecular signature in skin of patients with moderate-to-severe atopic dermatitis. J Allergy Clin Immunol. 2014;134:1293–300.

184. Simpson EL, Bieber T, Guttman-Yassky E, Beck LA, Blauvelt A, Cork MJ, et al. Two phase 3 trials of dupilumab versus placebo in atopic dermatitis. N Engl J Med. 2016;375:2335–48.

185. Khattri S, Brunner PM, Garcet S, Finney R, Cohen SR, Oliva M, et al. Efficacy and safety of ustekinumab treatment in adults with moderate-to-severe atopic dermatitis. Exp Dermatol. 2017;26(1):28–35.

186. Otsuka A, Tanioka M, Nakagawa Y, Honda T, Ikoma A, Miyachi Y, et al. Effects of cyclosporine on pruritus and serum IL-31 levels in patients with atopic dermatitis. Eur J Dermatol. 2011;21:816–7.

187. Otsuka A, Honda T, Doi H, Miyachi Y, Kabashima K. An H1-histamine receptor antagonist decreases serum interleukin-31 levels in patients with atopic dermatitis. Br J Dermatol. 2011;164:455–6.

188. Kabashima K, Furue M, Hanifin J, Pulka G, Mlynarczyk I, Wollenberg A. Humanized anti-interleukin-31 receptor A antibody nemolizumab (CIM331) suppresses pruritus and improves eczema in patients with moderate-to-severe atopic dermatitis. J Invest Dermatol. 2016;136:S161.

189. Nemoto O, Furue M, Nakagawa H, Shiramoto M, Hanada R, Matsuki S, et al. The first trial of CIM331, a humanized antihuman interleukin-31 receptor A antibody, in healthy volunteers and patients with atopic dermatitis to evaluate safety, tolerability and pharmacokinetics of a single dose in a randomized, double-blind, placebo-controlled study. Br J Dermatol. 2016;174:296–304.

190. Chan SC, Reifsnyder D, Beavo JA, Hanifin JM. Immunochemical characterization of the distinct monocyte cyclic AMP-phosphodiesterase from patients with atopic dermatitis. J Allergy Clin Immunol. 1993;91:1179–88.

191. Felding J, Sorensen MD, Poulsen TD, Larsen J, Andersson C, Refer P, et al. Discovery and early clinical development of 2-{6-[2-(3,5-dichloro-4-pyridyl)acetyl]-2,3-dimethoxyphenoxy}-N-propylacetamide (LEO 29102), a soft-drug inhibitor of phosphodiesterase 4 for topical treatment of atopic dermatitis. J Med Chem. 2014;57:5893–903.

192. Souness JE, Aldous D, Sargent C. Immunosuppressive and anti-inflammatory effects of cyclic AMP phosphodiesterase (PDE) type 4 inhibitors. Immunopharmacology. 2000;47:127–62.

193. Grewe SR, Chan SC, Hanifin JM. Elevated leukocyte cyclic AMP-phosphodiesterase in atopic disease: a possible mechanism for cyclic AMP-agonist hyporesponsiveness. J Allergy Clin Immunol. 1982;70:452–7.

194. Paller AS, Tom WL, Lebwohl MG, Blumenthal RL, Boguniewicz M, Call RS, et al. Efficacy and safety of crisaborole ointment, a novel, nonsteroidal phosphodiesterase 4 (PDE4) inhibitor for the topical treatment of atopic dermatitis (AD) in children and adults. J Am Acad Dermatol. 2016;75:494–503.e494.

195. Ohba F, Matsuki S, Imayama S, Matsuguma K, Hojo S, Nomoto M, et al. Efficacy of a novel phosphodiesterase inhibitor, E6005, in patients with atopic dermatitis: an investigator-blinded, vehicle-controlled study. J Dermatolog Treat. 2016;27:467–72.

196. Volf EM, Au SC, Dumont N, Scheinman P, Gottlieb AB. A phase 2, open-label, investigator-initiated study to evaluate the safety and efficacy of apremilast in subjects with recalcitrant allergic contact or atopic dermatitis. J Drugs Dermatol. 2012;11:341–6.

197. Wojno ED, Monticelli LA, Tran SV, Alenghat T, Osborne LC, Thome JJ, et al. The prostaglandin D(2) receptor CRTH2 regulates accumulation of group 2 innate lymphoid cells in the inflamed lung. Mucosal Immunol. 2015;8:1313–23.

198. Iwasaki M, Nagata K, Takano S, Takahashi K, Ishii N, Ikezawa Z. Association of a new-type prostaglandin D2 receptor CRTH2 with circulating T helper 2 cells in patients with atopic dermatitis. J Invest Dermatol. 2002;119:609–16.

199. Pettipher R, Hansel TT. Antagonists of the prostaglandin D2 receptor CRTH2. Drug News Perspect. 2008;21:317–22.

200. Bao L, Zhang H, Chan LS. The involvement of the JAK-STAT signaling pathway in chronic inflammatory skin disease atopic dermatitis. Jakstat. 2013;2:e24137.

201. Amano W, Nakajima S, Yamamoto Y, Tanimoto A, Matsushita M, Miyachi Y, et al. JAK inhibitor JTE-052 regulates contact hypersensitivity by downmodulating T cell activation and differentiation. J Dermatol Sci. 2016;84:258–65.

202. Samadi A, Ahmad Nasrollahi S, Hashemi A, Nassiri-Kashani M, Firooz A. Janus kinase (JAK) inhibitors for the treatment of skin and hair disorders: a review of literature. J Dermatol Treat. 2017;22:1–11.

203. Bissonnette R, Papp KA, Poulin Y, Gooderham M, Raman M, Mallbris L, et al. Topical tofacitinib for atopic dermatitis: a phase IIa randomized trial. Brit J Dermatol. 2016;175:902–11.

204. Czarnowicki T, Gonzalez J, Bonifacio KM, Shemer A, Xiangyu P, Kunjravia N, et al. Diverse activation and differentiation of multiple B-cell subsets in patients with atopic dermatitis but not in patients with psoriasis. J Allergy Clin Immunol. 2016;137:118–129.e115.

205. Krathen RA, Hsu S. Failure of omalizumab for treatment of severe adult atopic dermatitis. J Am Acad Dermatol. 2005;53:338–40.

206. Vigo PG, Girgis KR, Pfuetze BL, Critchlow ME, Fisher J, Hussain I. Efficacy of anti-IgE therapy in patients with atopic dermatitis. J Am Acad Dermatol. 2006;55:168–70.

207. Belloni B, Ziai M, Lim A, Lemercier B, Sbornik M, Weidinger S, et al. Low-dose anti-IgE therapy in patients with atopic eczema with high serum IgE levels. J Allergy Clin Immunol. 2007;120:1223–5.

208. Simon D, Hosli S, Kostylina G, Yawalkar N, Simon HU. Anti-CD20 (rituximab) treatment improves atopic eczema. J Allergy Clin Immunol. 2008;121:122–8.

209. Ponte P, Lopes MJ. Apparent safe use of single dose rituximab for recalcitrant atopic dermatitis in the first trimester of a twin pregnancy. J Am Acad Dermatol. 2010;63:355–6.

210. Sediva A, Kayserova J, Vernerova E, Polouckova A, Capkova S, Spisek R, et al. Anti-CD20 (rituximab) treatment for atopic eczema. J Allergy Clin Immunol. 2008;121:1515–6. author reply 1516-1517.

211. Arm JP, Bottoli I, Skerjanec A, Floch D, Groenewegen A, Maahs S, et al. Pharmacokinetics, pharmacodynamics and safety of QGE031 (ligelizumab), a novel high-affinity anti-IgE antibody, in atopic subjects. Clin Exp Allergy. 2014;44:1371–85.

212. Saeki H, Nakahara T, Tanaka A, Kabashima K, Sugaya M, Murota H, et al. Clinical practice guidelines for the management of atopic dermatitis 2016. J Dermatol. 2016;43:1117–45.

23

Morphology regulation in vascular endothelial cells

Kiyomi Tsuji-Tamura[1,2]* and Minetaro Ogawa[1]

Abstract

Morphological change in endothelial cells is an initial and crucial step in the process of establishing a functional vascular network. Following or associated with differentiation and proliferation, endothelial cells elongate and assemble into linear cord-like vessels, subsequently forming a perfusable vascular tube. In vivo and in vitro studies have begun to outline the underlying genetic and signaling mechanisms behind endothelial cell morphology regulation. This review focuses on the transcription factors and signaling pathways regulating endothelial cell behavior, involved in morphology, during vascular development.

Keywords: Vasculature, Endothelial cells, Angiogenesis, Morphology, Elongation

Background
Vascular system development
During the earliest stages of embryonic development, vascular formation occurs in connection with blood cell formation (hematopoiesis) [1, 2]. There are various theories about the origin of endothelial cells, but the mesoderm has been reported to generate an endothelial cell progenitor (angioblast) and a common progenitor of hematopoietic cells and endothelial cells (hemangioblast) [3] (Fig. 1). De novo vascularization, or vasculogenesis, is accomplished by endothelial cells derived from these mesodermal progenitors. During this process, cells form a primitive vessel network that serves as the basis for the mature vascular system [4]. New blood vessels are then formed from pre-existing ones and spread into avascular areas. This process, in which the network of early primitive vessels is expanded, is defined as angiogenesis [5]. Subsequently, vasculature undergoes remodeling in an ordered manner. Initiation of endothelial cell specification into arteries and veins appears to occur before forming structural arteries and veins [6]. Vasculature maturation results when new blood vessels recruit and are linked to vascular smooth muscle cells and pericytes. In addition, a population of endothelial cells

known as the hemogenic endothelium reportedly generates hematopoietic stem cells directly [3, 7–10].

Specification of angioblasts to either arterial or venous endothelial cells is established prior to forming blood vessel structures [11–13]. The receptor tyrosine kinase EphB4 and its transmembrane ligand ephrinB2 are demonstrated to be significant factors for arteriovenous definition [14]. The binding of vascular endothelial growth factor (VEGF) to its receptor VEGFR2, also known as KDR/Flk1, induces the expression of ephrinB2 through Notch signaling in arterial-fated precursor cells [15]. The specification of venous endothelial cells appears to set as the default in the absence of Notch signaling. Moreover, it has been reported that chicken ovalbumin upstream promoter-transcription factor II (COUP-TFII), which specifically expressed in venous endothelial cells, suppresses Notch signaling, leading in maintain vein identity [16]. After that, a subpopulation of venous endothelial cells acquires the expression of prospero homeobox 1 (Prox1) transcription factors, leading to specification of lymphatic endothelial cells [13, 17, 18]. COUP-TFII directly interacts with Prox1 and also controls lymphatic cell fate [19].

The process of vascular development requires various and complicated endothelial cell angiogenic behaviors. As endothelial cells proliferate, migrate, and undergo morphological changes such as elongating and sprouting, they assemble into a solid linear mass called a vascular cord. Following this, tubulogenesis occurs through

---

* Correspondence: ktamuratsuji@den.hokudai.ac.jp
[1]Department of Cell Differentiation, Institute of Molecular Embryology and Genetics, Kumamoto University, Kumamoto 860-0811, Japan
[2]Present Address: Oral Biochemistry and Molecular Biology, Department of Oral Health Science, Faculty of Dental Medicine and Graduate School of Dental Medicine, Hokkaido University, Sapporo 060-8586, Japan

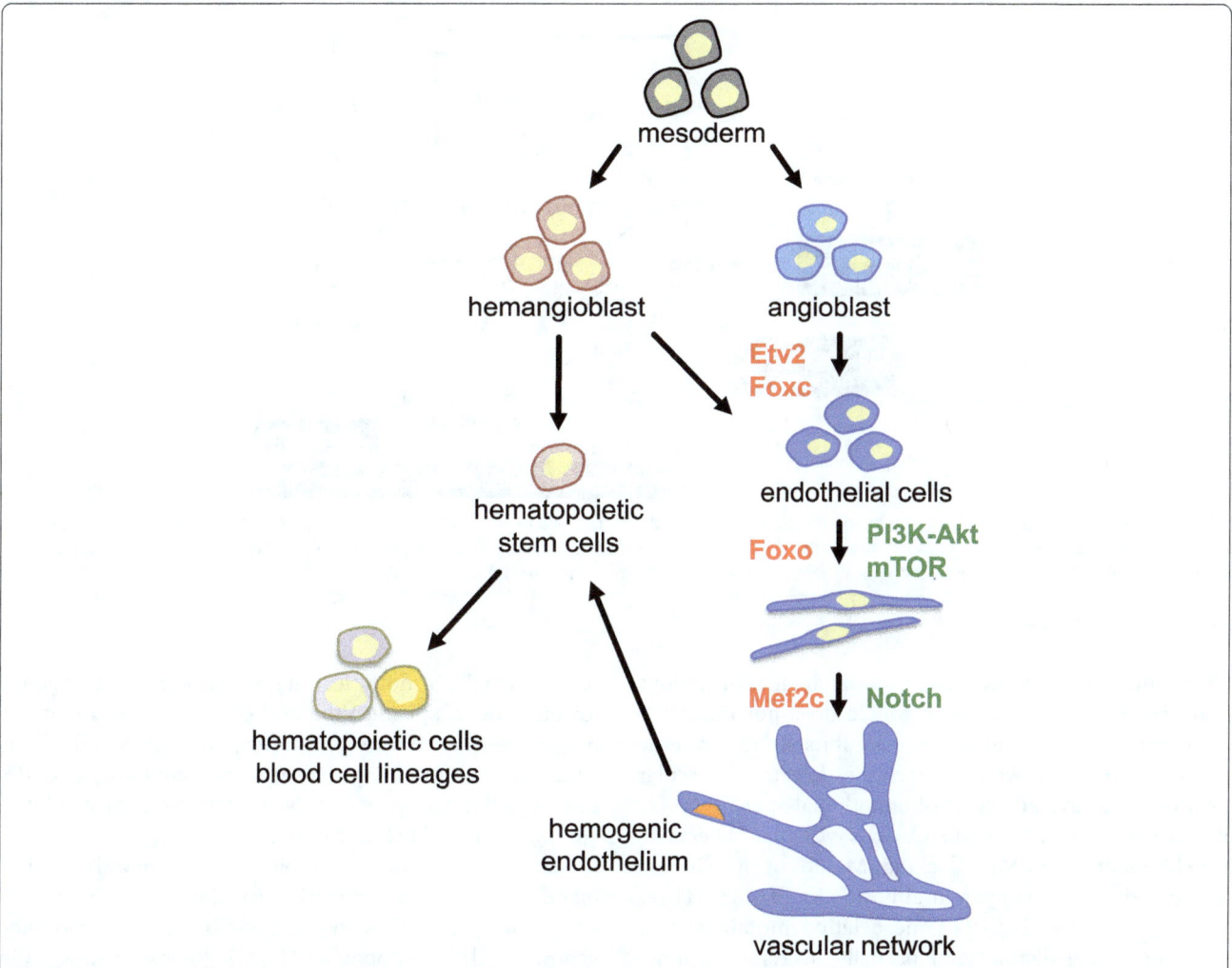

Fig. 1 Schematic model of early vascular development. Endothelial cells are derived from mesodermal precursors: angioblasts and hemangioblasts. They form vascular networks by undergoing morphological changes. Possible transcription factors (red) and signaling molecules (green) controlling each process are shown. During early vascular development, hematopoietic lineages arise from hemangioblasts or hemogenic endothelium

lumen formation at the center of the cord [20]. These processes are orchestrated at the genetic and signaling levels [21, 22]. In this review, we concentrate on transcriptional regulators and signaling pathways required for endothelial cell regulation, especially on morphology, during vascular formation (Fig. 2).

Transcriptional regulation of endothelial cell morphology
During vascularization, endothelial cells acquire specific morphological features to form vascular structures.

Although vasculature morphology has been studied widely both in vivo and in vitro, no key transcriptional signal initiating these morphological changes has yet been identified. Endothelial specification and vascular morphological change are closely related processes that occur in a partially simultaneous or sequential manner. Thus, it is unclear whether common transcriptional factors are involved in these processes or whether vascular

morphology is regulated by specific factors. We discuss several transcriptional factors, including Mef2, Ets, and Forkhead, that may play important roles in early vascular development [4, 21, 22].

Mef2 transcription factors
Myocyte enhancer factor 2 (Mef2) is a member of MADS box transcription enhancer factor family. Mef2 is an important cellular development regulator in multiple cell types in muscle, vascular, neural, and immune tissues [23–25]. In vertebrates, there are four MEF2 genes: Mef2a, Mef2b, Mef2c, and Mef2d. The expression of Mef2a, Mef2c, and Mef2d can be detected in the cardiovasculature network during early embryonic development [26, 27] and endothelial cells in vivo and in vitro [28, 29], pointing to a potential role for Mef2 in vascular development. Mef2a-null mice exhibit mitochondrial deficiency in cardiac muscle and perinatal lethality [30].

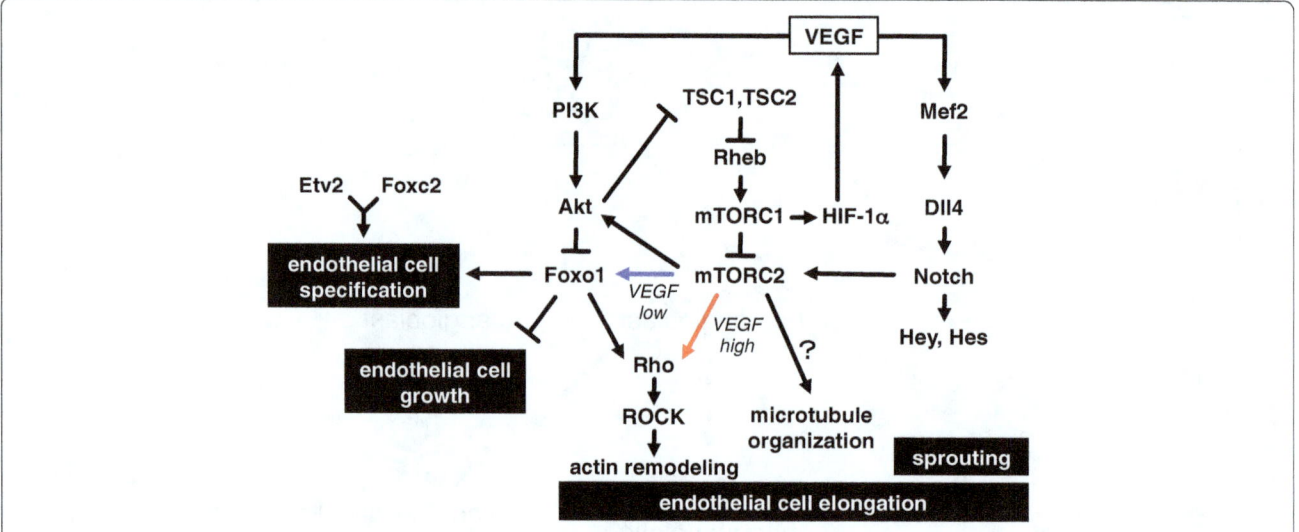

Fig. 2 Schematic model of transcription factor and signaling molecule interactions in endothelial cell functions. VEGF regulates endothelial cell functions through interaction and association with PI3K-Akt, mTOR, and Notch signaling. Foxo1-dependent (blue) and Foxo1-independent (red) pathways for endothelial cell elongation are shown. Pathway depends on environmental levels of VEGF

Mef2c-null mice show severe vascular malformations and die by E9.5 [28]. Loss of Mef2c does not affect the endothelial cell specification but inhibits smooth muscle cell differentiation, which causes the defects of vascular network. However, deletion of endothelial-specific Mef2c in mice does not result in obvious vascular defects in development [31]. Mice lacking Mef2b or Mef2d are viable and show no apparent abnormality [32, 33]. These phenotypes for each Mef2 gene deletion mutant appear to demonstrate distinct and partially overlapping functions among Mef2 members.

Mef2 factors have been demonstrated to regulate sprouting angiogenesis. In the presence of VEGF, these factors regulate the transcriptional activation of a Notch ligand Delta-like ligand 4 (Dll4) in endothelial cells [29]. Induced endothelial deletion of both Mef2a and Mef2c suppresses sprouting angiogenesis in mouse retina. In contrast, Mef2c has been shown to negatively regulate angiogenesis [34]. Mef2c overexpression inhibits VEGF-induced tube formation in HUVEC on collagen gel cultures, while Mef2 inhibition in a dominant-negative mutant enhances basal tube formation.

Ets and Foxc transcription factors

De Val et al. described a conserved endothelial cell-specific enhancer identified from the Mef2c gene [35, 36]. The enhancer contains a composite DNA binding site, referred to as the FOX:ETS motif. Etv2, also known as ER71 or Etsrp71, which is an ETS family transcription factor. Forkhead box C2 (Foxc2), also known as Mfh-1, is a member of the forkhead box (Fox) family of transcription factors. Etv2 in combination with Foxc2 binds

to the FOX:ETS motif, leading to the activation of genes for endothelial specification and establishment. Endothelial gene enhancers or promoters, such as Mef2c, Flk1, Tie2, Tal1, Notch4, and VE-cadherin, contain FOX:ETS motifs and thus appear to be under the control of the combination of Etv2 and Foxc2.

Loss of Etv2 causes a complete lack of endothelial and blood cells whereby mutant mice die by E10.5 [2, 37], suggesting that Etv2 is an indispensable factor in vasculogenesis and hematopoiesis. Foxc2 knockout mice die prenatally and perinatally, with cardiovascular system, skeletal structure, and lymphatic vascular system malformations; however, major vessels remain [38, 39]. Foxc1 expression has been reported to overlap with that of Foxc2. Foxc1 knockout mice also die prenatally and perinatally, with similar abnormalities as mutants lacking Foxc2 [40–42]. Foxc1 and Foxc2 compound null mice die by E9.5 and display more severe cardiovascular system abnormalities compared with mice lacking either Foxc1 or Foxc2 [42–44]. Moreover, Foxc1 is also able to bind to the FOX:ETS motif [36]. These findings indicate redundant roles of Foxc1 and Foxc2 during vasculature development [45].

We previously demonstrated that the Mef2c enhancer with the FOX:ETS motif is activated in endothelial cell precursors derived from murine embryonic stem (ES) cells [46, 47]. Activation is induced continuously in differentiated endothelial cells with a flat polygonal shape, and cells with an elongated shape stimulated by a high concentration of VEGF. Therefore, activation of the FOX:ETS motif may participate in endothelial cell lineage specification, but it is not necessarily connected to changes in endothelial cell morphology.

Foxo transcription factors

The forkhead box O (Foxo) transcription factor family contains four members: Foxo1, Foxo3, Foxo4, and Foxo6. This family is generally associated with promoting cell cycle arrest as well as inducing apoptosis and oxidative stress resistance [48, 49]. High Foxo1 expression can be observed in developing embryonic vasculature. Foxo1-deficient mice can provide insight into the role Foxo1 plays in vascular morphology during embryonic development [50, 51]. While Foxo1-null embryos have differentiated endothelial cells, they exhibit severe vascular defects including underdevelopment of branchial arches and malformation of dorsal aorta, thus resulting in death near embryonic days 10.5–11. This phenotype is mimicked by endothelial cell-specific deletion of Foxo1 in mice [52], suggesting that Foxo1 expression in endothelial cells is required for vascular structure formation in vivo.

ES cell-derived Foxo1-deficient endothelial cells do not exhibit cell elongation in response to VEGF [50]. They show actin-microtubule cytoskeleton disorganization and fail to interact with smooth muscle cells [53], suggesting a potential role of Foxo1 in cytoskeletal remodeling and smooth muscle cell recruitment. Conversely, Foxo1 may be required for endothelial growth control during postnatal vascular development or in mature endothelial cells. Inducible endothelial cell-specific disruption of Foxo1 enhances endothelial proliferation and leads to hyperplastic vasculature during retinal angiogenesis in mice [54]. Foxo1 appears to confer quiescence in endothelial cells by reducing metabolic activity via suppressed Myc signaling. Combined deletion of Foxo1, Foxo3, and Foxo4 in mice causes hemangiomas, which is increasing along with aging process [55]. Foxo1 overexpression suppresses migration and matrigel tube formation in human umbilical vein endothelial cells (HUVEC) [56]. Moreover, Foxo1 may bind less strongly to the FOX:ETS motif than FoxC1 or FoxC2 [36]. These findings suggest that Foxo1 may regulate multiple discrete endothelial cell functions during vascularization. Although multiple factors have been demonstrated that appear to be regulated by Foxo1, including Ang2, CXCR4, PDGF-B, and Flk1 [56], the transcriptional targets involved with changes in endothelial morphology remain unclear.

Foxo1, Foxo3, and Foxo4 have highly conserved amino acids [57]. However, Foxo3- and Foxo4-null mice are viable and outwardly normal, with no detectable vascular formation abnormalities comparable to those observed in Foxo1-null mice [50, 51]. Foxo6-null mice also develop normally and do not show any vascular malformation [58]. The redundant functions of Foxo subtypes have been demonstrated with in vitro experiments. Foxo3 induction in Foxo1-deficient endothelial cells derived from ES cells alleviates morphological abnormalities during the late, but not early, differentiation stage [59]. Foxo3 as well as Foxo1 overexpression inhibits migration and tube formation in HUVEC [56]. Foxo3 may partially overlap with Foxo1 in regulating endothelial cell functions.

Signaling regulation of endothelial cell morphology

VEGF is a well-known angiogenic factor that regulates various endothelial functions including survival, proliferation, migration, differentiation, and vascular permeability [60, 61]. The VEGF pathway interacts and associates with multiple pathways, such as PI3K-Akt, mTOR, and Notch signaling [62, 63], and transmits signals to cells during angiogenesis.

VEGF signaling

The signaling of VEGF and VEGFR2 plays an indispensable role in vascular development as well as regulates multiple angiogenic processes, including vascular growth and homeostasis [60, 64]. Heterozygous disruption of VEGF in mice causes abnormal blood vessel formation, resulting in embryonic death by E12 [65, 66]. VEGFR2-deficient mice die by E9.5 due to underdeveloped hematopoietic and endothelial cells [67]. These experiments identify the critical function of VEGF-VEGFR2 in vascular development. VEGF binds to and activates VEGFR2, leading to activation of intracellular signals such as protein kinase C (PKC), mitogen-activated protein kinase (MAPK), phosphatidyl inositol 3-kinase (PI3K)/Akt, also known as protein kinase B (PKB), and focal adhesion kinase (FAK). These signals regulate endothelial cell proliferation, migration, survival, and permeability [60]. VEGF has been reported to induce Mef2c expression and regulate endothelial cell functions such as migration or tube formation [68, 69].

Many studies demonstrate the important role VEGF plays in both physiological angiogenesis and pathological or therapeutic angiogenesis. Aberrant VEGF production in a tumor environment is induced through activation of hypoxia-inducible factor 1α (HIF-1α) mostly under hypoxia and results in the formation of disorganized and leaky tumor vessels [60, 70]. These abnormal vascular networks prevent the delivery of anti-cancer drugs to the tumor. Therefore, normalization of tumor vasculature has been proposed as a potential therapeutic strategy in cancer treatment [71–73]. VEGF has also been applied in tissue engineering to gain neovascularization due to its strong induction of angiogenesis [74, 75]. However, over-secretion of VEGF in myoblasts reportedly leads to hemangioma when transplanted into mouse muscle [76]. Although VEGF is required for vascular formation and maintenance, an appropriate level of VEGF in each environment is crucial.

We recently demonstrated that pharmacological inhibition of PI3K-Akt and mammalian target of rapamycin complex 1 (mTORC1) signaling can induce endothelial cell elongation without excess VEGF stimulation [47]. ES-derived endothelial cells require a low level of VEGF for growth. When stimulated by high levels of VEGF, these cells show over-growth and a shift from a flat, polygonal shape to a long, elongated shape (Fig. 3) [46, 47, 59]. However, PI3K-Akt or mTORC1 signaling inhibition also induces endothelial cell elongation in the presence of low levels of VEGF. These results indicate that PI3K-Akt and mTORC1 negatively regulate endothelial cell elongation.

PI3K-Akt signaling

PI3K-Akt signaling is activated by growth factors and angiogenic factors such as insulin, VEGF, and angiopoietin [77–79]. The serine/threonine protein kinase Akt is phosphorylated and activated by phosphoinositide-dependent kinase 1 (PDK1) when it binds to phosphatidylinositol-3,4,5-trisphosphate (PIP3) produced by PI3K. Phosphatase and tensin homolog deleted on chromosome 10 (PTEN) suppresses PI3K signaling through dephosphorylation of PIP3. Activated Akt negatively or positively regulates downstream targets to control various cellular functions including cell survival, proliferation, and metabolism. PI3K-Akt signaling has been shown to increase VEGF expression by producing the HIF-1α protein, thereby inducing angiogenesis [80, 81]. The binding of VEGF and VEGFR2 appears to increase mTORC1 activation through PI3K-Akt signaling, leading to endothelial cell survival and growth [77, 82, 83].

PI3K isoforms are divided into three classes: class I, class II, and class III [78, 84]. Blocking class IA PI3K signaling through general or endothelial cell-specific inactivation of p110α subunits in mice results in embryonic lethality by E12.5 due to severe vascular defects including an underdeveloped vascular plexus and poorly remodeled, enlarged vessels [85]. Endothelial cell-specific loss of class IA PI3K signaling through ablation of p85α and p85β subunits also causes embryonic lethality at E11.5 due to hemorrhaging [86]. These mice show normal phenotypes during early

vasculogenesis but later show severe microvessel dilation and red blood cell congestion. General or endothelial cell-specific class II PI3K-C2α-deleted mice die between E10.5 and E12.5 due to vascular abnormalities, including microvessel dilation, hemorrhaging, and reduced branching [87]. These findings suggest that these signaling pathways are not involved in the initial stages of vascular development but are required for subsequent vascular remodeling and integrity.

Akt has three isoforms (Akt1, Akt2, and Akt3) that have partially overlapping and specific functions. Akt1 has been demonstrated to play a central role in angiogenesis [77] Akt1-deficient mice are viable but show reduced body weight [88, 89]. In vascular structure, loss of Akt1 causes decreased vascularization and reduced phosphorylation of endothelial nitric-oxide synthase (eNOS) in the placenta [89]. Postnatal deletion of endothelial-specific Akt1 in mice leads to delayed angiogenesis in mouse retina [90]. Endothelial coverage and radial outgrowth are also reduced in mouse retina. These findings indicate that PI3K and Akt are essential signaling molecules in vascular development.

Foxo1 is reportedly phosphorylated by PI3K-Akt signaling then translocalized from the nucleus to the cytoplasm, which results in suppression of its transcriptional activity [91, 92]. Inhibition of PI3K-Akt signaling by LY294002 or Akt inhibitor VIII induces endothelial cell elongation in the presence of low levels of VEGF [47]. In contrast, Foxo1-deficient endothelial cells fail to respond to PI3K-Akt inhibition even in the presence of excess VEGF. These findings imply that PI3K-Akt inhibition induces endothelial cell elongation by activating Foxo1. Thus, PI3K-Akt signaling appears to negatively regulate the elongation of endothelial cells. Ola et al. reported that PI3K signaling inhibition improves vascular defects in a mouse vascular malformation caused by blocking of bone morphogenetic protein (BMP) 9/10 or Activin receptor-like kinase 1 (Alk1) [92]. Loss of BMP9/10 or Alk1 increases Akt and Foxo1 phosphorylation in endothelial

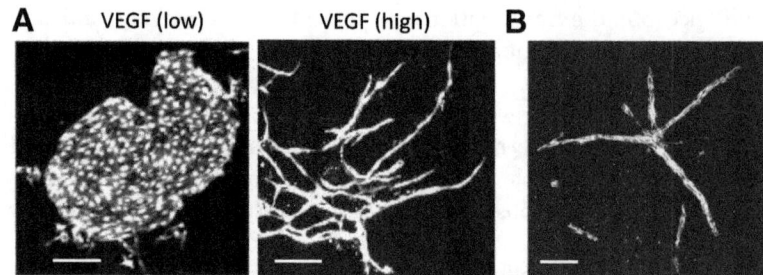

Fig. 3 Elongation of endothelial cells derived from ES cells. **a** In the co-culture system with OP9 stromal feeder cells, ES-derived endothelial cells form a round colony in the presence of a low level of VEGF, which produced by OP9 cells (left panel). These cells form long elongated structures, when stimulated by a high level of VEGF (right panel). Scale bar 200 μm. **b** ES-derived endothelial cells form vessel-like structures in the 3D collagen gel culture. Scale bar 100 μm

cells. These findings suggest PI3K-Akt signaling plays a key role in regulating endothelial cell morphology.

mTOR signaling

mTOR signaling is a crucial mediator in cell survival, proliferation, metabolism, and tumorigenesis [93]. mTOR is a serine/threonine protein kinase that forms two functionally distinct complexes, mTORC1 and mTORC2. The role of mTORC1 signaling in tumor angiogenesis is well understood. The GTP-bound active form of Ras homolog enriched in brain (Rheb) interacts and activates mTORC1, which drives VEGF secretion in tumor cells by inducing HIF-1α, promoting fragile tumor vessels [62, 77, 94]. Rheb is inactivated by tuberous sclerosis 1 (TSC1) and TSC2, which enhance conversion to the GDP-bound inactive form of Rheb due to its GAP activity. TSC2 is phosphorylated and inactivated by Akt [95, 96]. Thus, PI3K-Akt signaling is involved in mTORC1 activation.

Phenotypic analysis highlights critical players of mTOR signaling in embryonic development using general or endothelial cell-specific knockout mice. Regulatory-associated proteins of MTOR, complex 1 (Raptor) is an essential component of mTORC1. RPTOR independent companion of MTOR, complex 2 (Rictor) is an essential component of mTORC2. Raptor-deficient mice die early in development [97]; embryos appear to show proliferation defects during the blastocyst stage. Loss of endothelial cell-specific Raptor also results in embryonic death [98]. Conversely, mice lacking Rictor display a normal phenotype until E9.5, after which they die mid-gestation, around E11.5 [97, 99]. Endothelial cell specific-loss of Rictor also leads to embryonic death around E11.5–12.5 [98, 100]. The loss of Rictor has been shown to cause reduced or delayed peripheral vascularization in mice [100]. These findings suggest that mTORC1 and mTORC2 signaling is required for fetal development and embryonic angiogenesis.

We have previously demonstrated that mTORC1 inhibition by rapamycin or everolimus induces ES cell-derived endothelial cell elongation in the presence of low levels of VEGF [47]. This elongation requires mTORC2 and depends upon Foxo1. mTORC1 has been reported to inhibit mTORC2 signaling by activating p70 ribosomal protein S6 kinase 1 (S6K1), which phosphorylates Rictor [101, 102]. Therefore, the inhibition of mTORC1 may lead to endothelial cell elongation by compensating for mTORC2 signal activation. It is well known that mTORC2 signaling results in phosphorylation and deactivation of Foxo by activating Akt during regulation of cell proliferation and survival [97, 103–106]. However, Foxo1 is required to induce endothelial cell elongation during low VEGF conditions [47]. Although Foxo1 is a prevalent factor in endothelial morphology, mTORC1 inhibition in combination with high VEGF levels can induce endothelial cell elongation in a Foxo1-independent manner. Disruption

of mTORC2 signaling by the genetic loss or decline of Rictor can inhibit the vascular assembly or angiogenic sprouting stimulated by VEGF in endothelial cells on matrix cultures [98, 107]. Thus, mTORC2 signaling in association with high VEGF levels appears to drive endothelial cell elongation independently of Foxo1.

mTORC2 can control actin cytoskeleton organization, which is linked to cell morphology. Knockdown of Rictor prevents actin fiber assembly and fibroblast cell spreading [108]. mTORC2 regulates the actin cytoskeleton through Rho GTPase Rac. On the other hand, downregulation of Rictor reduces phosphorylation of protein Kinase Cα (PKCα) and causes prominent organization of cytoplasmic actin fiber and reduced cortical actin in Hela cells [109]. Although the function of mTORC2 in actin organization may depend on cell type, these findings suggest that mTORC2 is a major factor in regulating the actin cytoskeleton. Downregulation of Rictor inhibits the actin stress fiber formation stimulated by VEGF in endothelial cells [107]. Endothelial cell elongation induced by PI3K-Akt or mTORC1 inhibition requires actin remodeling by activating Rho-ROCK signaling [46, 47]. Moreover, our recent study shows that dual inhibition of mTORC1/mTORC2 by KU0063794, but not mTORC1-specific inhibition by everolimus, remarkably impairs both actin and microtubule organization, inhibiting endothelial cell elongation [110]. The defects appear to result from disorderly microtubule distribution or stability. These findings suggest the mTOR signaling pathway is an important signaling node that modulates endothelial cell elongation by shaping the actin and microtubule cytoskeleton. Further studies are necessary to elucidate the mechanisms of mTOR signaling in endothelial cell morphological change.

Notch signaling

Four Notch receptors (Notch1, Notch2, Notch3, and Notch4), as well as five Notch transmembrane ligands of the Delta-Serrate-Lag (DSL) type, Jagged1 and 2 (Jag1 and Jag2), and Delta-like 1, 3, and 4 (Dll1, Dll3, and Dll4), are found in mammals [63, 111]. Notch signaling is involved in multiple stages of vascular development, including proliferation, migration, and arterial-venous endothelial cell fate determination [112]. Notch signaling is initiated by interactions between the Notch receptor and its ligand, which leads to the cleavage and release of the Notch intracellular domain (NICD). The NICD translocates to the nucleus and binds to a recombination signal binding protein for immunoglobulin kappa J region (RBP-j), also known as CBF1/Igkjrb/PBPjk. They then upregulate the expression of their target genes, hairy and enhancer of split (Hes) or Hes-related with YRPW motif (Hey). Hes1 suppresses PTEN expression, resulting in PI3K-Akt signal activation [113]. Further, non-canonical Notch signaling has been reported to interact with mTORC2 [114, 115]. NICD regulates cell survival through the activation of Akt, depending on mTORC2.

Notch signaling, together with VEGF, controls sprouting angiogenesis through endothelial cell specification. Endothelial cells are specialized to tip cells and stalk cells in sprouting angiogenesis [5, 116, 117]. Tip cells lead and guide blood vessel sprouts, and stalk cells follow tip cells and form sprout elongation. In tip cells, VEGF signaling induces the expression of Dll4, which binds to and activates Notch signaling in neighboring stalk cells and suppresses stalk cell VEGFR expression. As tip cells expressing Dll4 receive stronger VEGF stimulation, they acquire the higher motility and sprouting activity, resulting in further angiogenesis. This Dll4-Notch signaling is antagonized in stalk cells by Jagged1, which modulates the base of emerging vessel sprouts. Notch signaling attenuation or heterozygous Dll4 deletion in mice increases the number of tip cells and enhances cell proliferation, causing excessive vessel sprouting and branching defect [118, 119]. Thus, Notch signaling is essential in controlling angiogenic sprouting.

Loss of Notch1 in mice leads to embryonic lethality by E11.5 [120, 121], whereas Notch4-deficient mice are viable and exhibit no phenotypic defects [122]. However, deleting both Notch1 and Notch4 genes in mice causes embryonic lethality due to more severe vascular defects than Notch1 knockout mice [122]. Double-deletion mutants have normal vasculogenesis, but fail to perform vascular remodeling. This suggests a partially redundant function of Notch1 and Notch4 during vascular development. Similar findings were reported in RBP-j-deleted mice [122, 123]. Heterozygous deletion of Dll4 in mice also causes similar vascular defects to those in Notch1 and Notch4 double-deletion mutants, although vascular remodeling defects are less severe [123]. Hey1 and Hey2 as well as Hes1 and Hes5 show subtype redundancy in vascular development. Hey1-deficient mice develop normally [124], and Hey2-deficient mice do not show apparent embryonic vessel development defects but have postnatal cardiac hypertrophy [125]. Loss of both Hey1 and Hey2 leads to embryonic death by E11.5 due to defects of vascular development [124, 126]. In these mutants, early vasculogenesis is normal but large vessels do not form in the yolk sac and poor development of large vessels frequently occurs in the embryo, highlighting defects in vascular remodeling. Mice lacking either Hes1 or Hes5 exhibit no obvious abnormalities during vascular development, whereas general or endothelial-specific Hes1 deletion mutants on a Hes5-null background show defects in brain vascular remodeling [127].

In human arterial endothelial cells, VEGF induces Notch1 and Dll4 expression through the PI3K-Akt pathway [128]. Activation of Notch signaling using NICD or

Hes1 expression enhances network and cord formation in a three-dimensional model, whereas blocking Notch signaling using a dominant-negative form of RBP-j partially inhibits the network formation stimulated by VEGF. Moreover, Notch1 signaling is activated by fluid shear stress in human aortic endothelial cells [129]. Fluid shear stress is a biophysical trigger of morphological change in endothelial cells, although flow-induced shape is not identical to the vessel-like elongation of ES cell-derived endothelial cells in response to VEGF (Fig. 3). It has been established that fluid flow induces each endothelial cells to elongate in parallel to the direction of flow and causes actin filament alignment [129, 130]. Reduced expression of Notch1 in vivo and in vitro has been shown to prevent endothelial cell elongation in response to flow as well as promote endothelial cell proliferation [129]. These findings suggest that Notch signaling plays an important role in modifying endothelial cell morphology.

Vascular regeneration
Transcription factors and signaling molecules required for vascular regeneration in adulthood have been reported. The expression of Etv2 is very low or absent in adult, however, its expression is upregulated in endothelial cells following ischemic injury [131]. Deletion of endothelial-specific Etv2 impairs neovascularization in mouse hindlimb ischemia model. The overexpression of Etv2 improves vessel formation after ischemia. Moreover, ischemic injury upregulates Dll4 expression in microvascular endothelial cells of normoperfused muscles [132]. Dll4 inhibition in a soluble mutant impairs blood flow recovery and neovascularization after ischemia in muscle. On the other hand, Foxo transcription factor is reported to negatively regulate postnatal neovascularization. Deleting Foxo3 gene in mice causes the enhanced reperfusion and the increased capillary density in hind limb ischemia [56]. These factors are critical for vascular formation during embryonic development, moreover, involved in positively or negatively regulate vascular regeneration following injury.

Conclusion
Comprehending the mechanisms regulating vascular structure formation is crucial to gain insight into both the physiological angiogenic process as well as diseases surrounding pathological angiogenesis. Abnormal or excessive angiogenesis is linked to increased tumor development [60, 70]. In diabetic patients, uncontrolled formation or deficiency of vessels, known as disordered angiogenesis, contributes to mortality and disability [133]. Furthermore, establishing functional vascular networks is key for tissue and organ regeneration in tissue engineering [74, 75].

Transgenic lines (Table 1) or cultured models (Fig. 3) help to visualize vascular structure or cell shape, facilitating

Table 1 Mouse phenotypes

Disrupted gene		Phenotype	References
Mef2 transcription factors			
Mef2a		Perinatal death (cardiac sudden death), mitochondrial defects	[30]
Mef2b		Normal cardiac development	[32]
Mef2c		Embryonic death by day 9.5, cardiovascular defects, defects of smooth muscle cell differentiation	[28]
Mef2c (endothelial-specific deletion)		Promotion of vascular growth in oxygen-induced retinopathy	[31]
Mef2d		Resistance to cardiac hypertrophy induced by pressure overload	[33]
Ets and Foxc transcription factors			
Etv2		Embryonic death by day 10.5, defects of blood and vessel development	[2, 37]
Etv2 (endothelial-specific deletion)		No obvious phenotype in steady state condition	[131]
Foxc1		Prenatal and perinatal death, cardiovascular abnormalities, skeletal defects	[40–42]
Foxc2		Prenatal and perinatal death, cardiovascular and lymphatic abnormalities, skeletal defects	[38, 39]
Foxc1 and Foxc2		Embryonic death by day 9.5, more severe defects of cardiovascular and lymphatic development than Foxc1 or Foxc2-null mice	[41, 43, 44]
Foxo transcription factors			
Foxo1		Embryonic death by day 10.5–11, vasculature defects	[50, 51]
Foxo1 (endothelial-specific deletion)		Embryonic death by day 11, vasculature defects	[52]
Foxo3		Age-dependent infertility, abnormality of ovarian follicular development	[50, 51]
Foxo4		Normal	[50, 51]
Foxo6		Defects of memory consolidation	[58]
VEGF signaling			
VEGF (heterozygous deletion)		Embryonic death by day 12, abnormality of vascular development	[65, 66]
VEGFR2	VEGF receptor	Embryonic death by day 9.5, defects of hematopoietic and endothelial cell development	[67]
PI3K-Akt signaling			
p110α (general or endothelial-specific inactivation)	Class IA PI3K subunit	Embryonic death by day 12.5, vascular defects	[85]
p85α and p85β	Class IA PI3K subunit	Embryonic death by day 11.5, vascular defects, hemorrhage	[86]
PI3K-C2α (general or endothelial-specific deletion)	Class II PI3K subunit	Embryonic death by days 11.5–12.5, vascular defects, hemorrhage	[87]
Akt1		Growth retardation, reduction of vascularization in placenta	[88, 89]
Akt1 (endothelial-specific postnatal deletion)		Reduction of vascular development in retina	[90]
mTOR signaling			
Raptor	mTORC1 subunit	Embryonic death at early stages of development	[97]
Raptor (endothelial cell-specific deletion)		Embryonic death	[98]
Rictor	mTORC2 subunit	Embryonic death by day 11.5, growth arrest, placental abnormalities	[97, 99]
Rictor (endothelial cell-specific deletion)		Embryonic death by days 11.5–12.5, growth retardation, reduction of peripheral vascularization	[98, 100]

Table 1 Mouse phenotypes *(Continued)*

Disrupted gene		Phenotype	References
Notch signaling			
Notch1	Notch receptor	Embryonic death by day 11.5, delayed and disorganized somitogenesis	[120, 121]
Notch4	Notch receptor	Normal	[122]
Notch1 and Notch4		More severe phenotype than Notch1-null mice, defects of vascular remodeling	[122]
Dll4 (heterozygous deletion)	Notch ligand	Similar to phenotype of Notch1 and Notch4-null mice, defects of vascular remodeling	[123]
RBP-j	Notch transcriptional effector	Defects of vascular remodeling and somite formation	[123]
Hey1	Notch target gene	Normal	[124]
Hey2	Notch target gene	Cardiac hypertrophy after birth	[125]
Hey1 and Hey2		Embryonic death by days 9.5–11.5, defects of vascular remodeling, hemorrhage	[124, 126]
Hes1	Notch target gene	No obvious phenotype in vascular development	[127]
Hes5	Notch target gene	Normal	[127]
Hes1 and Hes5 (general or endothelial-specific deletion of Hes1 on Hes5-null background)		Defects of vascular remodeling in the brain	[127]

evaluation of vascular morphology. However, the mechanisms modulating endothelial cell morphological change are not well understood compared with endothelial cell differentiation or proliferation. This may be due to the intricate behaviors of endothelial cells and the diverse roles played by angiogenic factors. Accurately classifying endothelial cell events during vascular development is difficult, as events occur in spatially and temporally similar or related contexts. Furthermore, as described in the literature, relevant factors and signaling molecules frequently have overlapping functions or associated interactions. Consequently, it may be even more important to investigate and reveal specific molecules or mechanisms associated with endothelial cell morphological change. A deeper understanding of vascular development holds promise for developing new therapeutics regulating vascular function.

Abbreviations

Alk1: Activin receptor-like kinase 1; BMP: Bone morphogenetic protein; COUP-TFII: Chicken ovalbumin upstream promoter-transcription factor II; Dll1, Dll3, and Dll4: Delta-like 1, 3, and 4; DSL: Delta-Serrate-Lag; eNOS: Endothelial nitric-oxide synthase; ES cells: Embryonic stem cells; FAK: Focal adhesion kinase; Fox: Forkhead box; Hes: Hairy and enhancer of split; Hey: Hairy/enhancer-of-split related with YRPW motif; HIF-1α: Hypoxia-inducible factor 1α; HUVEC: Human umbilical vein endothelial cells; Jag1 and Jag2: Jagged1 and 2; MADS: MCM1, Agamous, Deficiens, Serum-response factor; MAPK: Mitogen-activated protein kinase; Mef2: Myocyte enhancer factor 2; mTORC1: Mammalian target of rapamycin complex 1 or mechanistic target of rapamycin complex 1; NICD: Notch intracellular domain; PDK1: Phosphoinositide-dependent kinase 1; PI3K: Phosphatidyl inositol 3-kinase; PIP3: Phosphatidylinositol-3,4,5-trisphosphate; PKB: Protein kinase B; PKCα: Protein Kinase Cα; Prox1: Prospero homeobox 1; PTEN: Phosphatase and tensin homolog deleted on chromosome 10; Raptor: Regulatory associated protein of MTOR, complex 1; RBP-j: Recombination signal binding protein for immunoglobulin kappa J region; Rheb: Ras homolog enriched in brain; Rictor: RPTOR independent companion of MTOR, complex 2; S6K1: p70 ribosomal protein S6 kinase 1; TSC1: Tuberous sclerosis 1; VEGF: Vascular endothelial growth factor

Acknowledgements

We gratefully thank the members of the Department of Cell Differentiation and the Liaison Laboratory Research Promotion Center, Institute of Molecular Embryology and Genetics, Kumamoto University, and Oral Biochemistry and Molecular Biology, Department of Oral Health Science, Faculty of Dental Medicine and Graduate School of Dental Medicine, Hokkaido University.

Funding

This work was supported by Japan Society for the Promotion of Science (grant numbers KAKENHI 24792237 and 15K11259), and the program of the Joint Usage/Research Center for Developmental Medicine, Institute of Molecular Embryology and Genetics, Kumamoto University.

Authors' contributions

KTT designed the review topic. KTT and MO contributed to the drafting of the manuscript. Both authors read and approved the final manuscript.

Competing interests

The authors declare that they have no competing interests.

References

1. Stainier DY, Weinstein BM, Detrich HW 3rd, Zon LI, Fishman MC. Cloche, an early acting zebrafish gene, is required by both the endothelial and hematopoietic lineages. Development. 1995;121(10):3141–50.

2. Lee D, Park C, Lee H, Lugus JJ, Kim SH, Arentson E, Chung YS, Gomez G, Kyba M, Lin S, Janknecht R, Lim DS, Choi K. ER71 acts downstream of BMP, Notch, and Wnt signaling in blood and vessel progenitor specification. Cell Stem Cell. 2008;2(5):497–507.

3. Bautch VL. Stem cells and the vasculature. Nat Med. 2011;17(11):1437–43.

4. Conway EM, Collen D, Carmeliet P. Molecular mechanisms of blood vessel growth. Cardiovasc Res. 2001;49(3):507–21.

5. Ribatti D, Crivellato E. "Sprouting angiogenesis", a reappraisal. Dev Biol. 2012;372(2):157–65.

6. Herbert SP, Huisken J, Kim TN, Feldman ME, Houseman BT, Wang RA, Shokat KM, Stainier DY. Arterial-venous segregation by selective cell sprouting: an alternative mode of blood vessel formation. Science. 2009;326(5950):294–8.

7. Boisset JC, van Cappellen W, Andrieu-Soler C, Galjart N, Dzierzak E, Robin C. In vivo imaging of haematopoietic cells emerging from the mouse aortic endothelium. Nature. 2010;464(7285):116–20.

8. Yokomizo T, Dzierzak E. Three-dimensional cartography of hematopoietic clusters in the vasculature of whole mouse embryos. Development. 2010; 137(21):3651–61.

9. Zovein AC, Hofmann JJ, Lynch M, French WJ, Turlo KA, Yang Y, Becker MS, Zanetta L, Dejana E, Gasson JC, Tallquist MD, Iruela-Arispe ML. Fate tracing reveals the endothelial origin of hematopoietic stem cells. Cell Stem Cell. 2008;3(6):625–36.

10. Tanzir A, Tsuji-Tamura K, Ogawa M. CXCR4 signaling negatively modulates the bipotential state of hemogenic endothelial cells derived from embryonic stem cells by attenuating the endothelial potential. Stem Cells. 2016;34(12):2814–24.

11. Zhong TP, Childs S, Leu JP, Fishman MC. Gridlock signalling pathway fashions the first embryonic artery. Nature. 2001;414(6860):216–20.

12. dela Paz NG, D'Amore PA. Arterial versus venous endothelial cells. Cell Tissue Res. 2009;335(1):5–16.

13. Kume T. Specification of arterial, venous, and lymphatic endothelial cells during embryonic development. Histol Histopathol. 2010;25(5):637–46.

14. Wang HU, Chen ZF, Anderson DJ. Molecular distinction and angiogenic interaction between embryonic arteries and veins revealed by ephrin-B2 and its receptor Eph-B4. Cell. 1998;93(5):741–53.

15. Lawson ND, Vogel AM, Weinstein BM. Sonic hedgehog and vascular endothelial growth factor act upstream of the Notch pathway during arterial endothelial differentiation. Dev Cell. 2002;3(1):127–36.

16. You LR, Lin FJ, Lee CT, DeMayo FJ, Tsai MJ, Tsai SY. Suppression of Notch signalling by the COUP-TFII transcription factor regulates vein identity. Nature. 2005;435(7038):98–104.

17. Srinivasan RS, Dillard ME, Lagutin OV, Lin FJ, Tsai S, Tsai MJ, Samokhvalov IM, Oliver G. Lineage tracing demonstrates the venous origin of the mammalian lymphatic vasculature. Genes Dev. 2007;21(19):2422–32.

18. Oliver G, Srinivasan RS. Endothelial cell plasticity: how to become and remain a lymphatic endothelial cell. Development. 2010;137(3):363–72.

19. Yamazaki T, Yoshimatsu Y, Morishita Y, Miyazono K, Watabe T. COUP-TFII regulates the functions of Prox1 in lymphatic endothelial cells through direct interaction. Genes Cells. 2009;14(3):425–34.

20. Charpentier MS, Conlon FL. Cellular and molecular mechanisms underlying blood vessel lumen formation. BioEssays. 2014;36(3):251–9.

21. De Val S. Key transcriptional regulators of early vascular development. Arterioscler Thromb Vasc Biol. 2011;31(7):1469–75.

22. Park C, Kim TM, Malik AB. Transcriptional regulation of endothelial cell and vascular development. Circ Res. 2013;112(10):1380–400.

23. Pon JR, Marra MA. MEF2 transcription factors: developmental regulators and emerging cancer genes. Oncotarget. 2016;7(3):2297–312.

24. Potthoff MJ, Olson EN. MEF2: a central regulator of diverse developmental programs. Development. 2007;134(23):4131–40.

25. Tirziu D, Simons M. Endothelium as master regulator of organ development and growth. Vasc Pharmacol. 2009;50(1–2):1–7.

26. Edmondson DG, Lyons GE, Martin JF, Olson EN. Mef2 gene expression marks the cardiac and skeletal muscle lineages during mouse embryogenesis. Development. 1994;120(5):1251–63.

27. Subramanian SV, Nadal-Ginard B. Early expression of the different isoforms of the myocyte enhancer factor-2 (MEF2) protein in myogenic as well as non-myogenic cell lineages during mouse embryogenesis. Mech Dev. 1996;57(1):103–12.

28. Lin Q, Lu J, Yanagisawa H, Webb R, Lyons GE, Richardson JA, Olson EN. Requirement of the MADS-box transcription factor MEF2C for vascular development. Development. 1998;125(22):4565–74.

29. Sacilotto N, Chouliaras KM, Nikitenko LL, Lu YW, Fritzsche M, Wallace MD, Nornes S, Garcia-Moreno F, Payne S, Bridges E, Liu K, Biggs D, Ratnayaka I, Herbert SP, Molnar Z, Harris AL, Davies B, Bond GL, Bou-Gharios G, Schwarz JJ, De Val S. MEF2 transcription factors are key regulators of sprouting angiogenesis. Genes Dev. 2016;30(20):2297–309.

30. Naya FJ, Black BL, Wu H, Bassel-Duby R, Richardson JA, Hill JA, Olson EN. Mitochondrial deficiency and cardiac sudden death in mice lacking the MEF2A transcription factor. Nat Med. 2002;8(11):1303–9.

31. Xu Z, Gong J, Maiti D, Vong L, Wu L, Schwarz JJ, Duh EJ. MEF2C ablation in endothelial cells reduces retinal vessel loss and suppresses pathologic retinal neovascularization in oxygen-induced retinopathy. Am J Pathol. 2012;180(6):2548–60.

32. Lin Q, Schwarz J, Bucana C, Olson EN. Control of mouse cardiac morphogenesis and myogenesis by transcription factor MEF2C. Science. 1997;276(5317):1404–7.

33. Kim Y, Phan D, van Rooij E, Wang DZ, McAnally J, Qi X, Richardson JA, Hill JA, Bassel-Duby R, Olson EN. The MEF2D transcription factor mediates stress-dependent cardiac remodeling in mice. J Clin Invest. 2008;118(1):124–32.

34. Sturtzel C, Testori J, Schweighofer B, Bilban M, Hofer E. The transcription factor MEF2C negatively controls angiogenic sprouting of endothelial cells depending on oxygen. PLoS One. 2014;9(7):e101521.

35. De Val S, Anderson JP, Heidt AB, Khiem D, Xu SM, Black BL. Mef2c is activated directly by Ets transcription factors through an evolutionarily conserved endothelial cell-specific enhancer. Dev Biol. 2004;275(2):424–34.

36. De Val S, Chi NC, Meadows SM, Minovitsky S, Anderson JP, Harris IS, Ehlers ML, Agarwal P, Visel A, Xu SM, Pennacchio LA, Dubchak I, Krieg PA, Stainier DY, Black BL. Combinatorial regulation of endothelial gene expression by ets and forkhead transcription factors. Cell. 2008;135(6):1053–64.

37. Ferdous A, Caprioli A, Iacovino M, Martin CM, Morris J, Richardson JA, Latif S, Hammer RE, Harvey RP, Olson EN, Kyba M, Garry DJ. Nkx2-5 transactivates the Ets-related protein 71 gene and specifies an endothelial/endocardial fate in the developing embryo. Proc Natl Acad Sci U S A. 2009;106(3):814–9.

38. Iida K, Koseki H, Kakinuma H, Kato N, Mizutani-Koseki Y, Ohuchi H, Yoshioka H, Noji S, Kawamura K, Kataoka Y, Ueno F, Taniguchi M, Yoshida N, Sugiyama T, Miura N. Essential roles of the winged helix transcription factor MFH-1 in aortic arch patterning and skeletogenesis. Development. 1997;124(22):4627–38.

39. Petrova TV, Karpanen T, Norrmen C, Mellor R, Tamakoshi T, Finegold D, Ferrell R, Kerjaschki D, Mortimer P, Yla-Herttuala S, Miura N, Alitalo K. Defective valves and abnormal mural cell recruitment underlie lymphatic vascular failure in lymphedema distichiasis. Nat Med. 2004;10(9):974–81.

40. Kume T, Deng KY, Winfrey V, Gould DB, Walter MA, Hogan BL. The forkhead/winged helix gene Mf1 is disrupted in the pleiotropic mouse mutation congenital hydrocephalus. Cell. 1998;93(6):985–96.

41. Winnier GE, Kume T, Deng K, Rogers R, Bundy J, Raines C, Walter MA, Hogan BL, Conway SJ. Roles for the winged helix transcription factors MF1 and MFH1 in cardiovascular development revealed by nonallelic noncomplementation of null alleles. Dev Biol. 1999;213(2):418–31.

42. Kume T, Jiang H, Topczewska JM, Hogan BL. The murine winged helix transcription factors, Foxc1 and Foxc2, are both required for cardiovascular development and somitogenesis. Genes Dev. 2001;15(18):2470–82.

43. Seo S, Fujita H, Nakano A, Kang M, Duarte A, Kume T. The forkhead transcription factors, Foxc1 and Foxc2, are required for arterial specification and lymphatic sprouting during vascular development. Dev Biol. 2006;294(2):458–70.

44. Seo S, Kume T. Forkhead transcription factors, Foxc1 and Foxc2, are required for the morphogenesis of the cardiac outflow tract. Dev Biol. 2006;296(2):421–36.

45. Papanicolaou KN, Izumiya Y, Walsh K. Forkhead transcription factors and cardiovascular biology. Circ Res. 2008;102(1):16–31.

46. Tsuji-Tamura K, Sakamoto H, Ogawa M. ES cell differentiation as a model to study cell biological regulation of vascular development. In: Atwood CS, ed. Embryonic stem cells: the hormonal regulation of pluripotency and embryogenesis: InTech, 2011:581–606.

47. Tsuji-Tamura K, Ogawa M. Inhibition of the PI3K/Akt and mTORC1 signaling pathways promotes the elongation of vascular endothelial cells. J Cell Sci. 2016;129:1165–78.

48. Carlsson P, Mahlapuu M. Forkhead transcription factors: key players in development and metabolism. Dev Biol. 2002;250(1):1–23.

49. Eijkelenboom A, Burgering BM. FOXOs: signalling integrators for homeostasis maintenance. Nat Rev Mol Cell Biol. 2013;14(2):83–97.

50. Furuyama T, Kitayama K, Shimoda Y, Ogawa M, Sone K, Yoshida-Araki K, Hisatsune H, Nishikawa S, Nakayama K, Nakayama K, Ikeda K, Motoyama N, Mori N. Abnormal angiogenesis in Foxo1 (Fkhr)-deficient mice. J Biol Chem. 2004;279(33):34741–9.

51. Hosaka T, Biggs WH 3rd, Tieu D, Boyer AD, Varki NM, Cavenee WK, Arden KC. Disruption of forkhead transcription factor (FOXO) family members in mice reveals their functional diversification. Proc Natl Acad Sci U S A. 2004;101(9):2975–80.

52. Dharaneeswaran H, Abid MR, Yuan L, Dupuis D, Beeler D, Spokes KC, Janes L, Sciuto T, Kang PM, Jaminet SS, Dvorak A, Grant MA, Regan ER, Aird WC. FOXO1-mediated activation of Akt plays a critical role in vascular homeostasis. Circ Res. 2014;115(2):238–51.

53. Park SH, Sakamoto H, Tsuji-Tamura K, Furuyama T, Ogawa M. Foxo1 is essential for in vitro vascular formation from embryonic stem cells. Biochem Biophys Res Commun. 2009;390(3):861–6.

54. Wilhelm K, Happel K, Eelen G, Schoors S, Oellerich MF, Lim R, Zimmermann B, Aspalter IM, Franco CA, Boettger T, Braun T, Fruttiger M, Rajewsky K, Keller C, Bruning JC, Gerhardt H, Carmeliet P, Potente M. FOXO1 couples metabolic activity and growth state in the vascular endothelium. Nature. 2016;529(7585):216–20.

55. Paik JH, Kollipara R, Chu G, Ji H, Xiao Y, Ding Z, Miao L, Tothova Z, Horner JW, Carrasco DR, Jiang S, Gilliland DG, Chin L, Wong WH, Castrillon DH, DePinho RA. FoxOs are lineage-restricted redundant tumor suppressors and regulate endothelial cell homeostasis. Cell. 2007;128(2):309–23.

56. Potente M, Urbich C, Sasaki K, Hofmann WK, Heeschen C, Aicher A, Kollipara R, DePinho RA, Zeiher AM, Dimmeler S. Involvement of Foxo transcription factors in angiogenesis and postnatal neovascularization. J Clin Invest. 2005;115(9):2382–92.

57. Obsil T, Obsilova V. Structural basis for DNA recognition by FOXO proteins. Biochim Biophys Acta. 2011;1813(11):1946–53.

58. Salih DA, Rashid AJ, Colas D, de la Torre-Ubieta L, Zhu RP, Morgan AA, Santo EE, Ucar D, Devarajan K, Cole CJ, Madison DV, Shamloo M, Butte AJ, Bonni A, Josselyn SA, Brunet A. FoxO6 regulates memory consolidation and synaptic function. Genes Dev. 2012;26(24):2780–801.

59. Matsukawa M, Sakamoto H, Kawasuji M, Furuyama T, Ogawa M. Different roles of Foxo1 and Foxo3 in the control of endothelial cell morphology. Genes Cells. 2009;14(10):1167–81.

60. Cross MJ, Claesson-Welsh L. FGF and VEGF function in angiogenesis: signalling pathways, biological responses and therapeutic inhibition. Trends Pharmacol Sci. 2001;22(4):201–7.

61. Hoeben A, Landuyt B, Highley MS, Wildiers H, Van Oosterom AT, De Bruijn EA. Vascular endothelial growth factor and angiogenesis. Pharmacol Rev. 2004;56(4):549–80.

62. Karar J, Maity A. PI3K/AKT/mTOR pathway in angiogenesis. Front Mol Neurosci. 2011;4:51.

63. Thomas JL, Baker K, Han J, Calvo C, Nurmi H, Eichmann AC, Alitalo K. Interactions between VEGFR and Notch signaling pathways in endothelial and neural cells. Cell Mol Life Sci. 2013;70(10):1779–92.

64. Cebe-Suarez S, Zehnder-Fjallman A, Ballmer-Hofer K. The role of VEGF receptors in angiogenesis; complex partnerships. Cell Mol Life Sci. 2006; 63(5):601–15.

65. Carmeliet P, Ferreira V, Breier G, Pollefeyt S, Kieckens L, Gertsenstein M, Fahrig M, Vandenhoeck A, Harpal K, Eberhardt C, Declercq C, Pawling J, Moons L, Collen D, Risau W, Nagy A. Abnormal blood vessel development and lethality in embryos lacking a single VEGF allele. Nature. 1996;380(6573):435–9.

66. Ferrara N, Carver-Moore K, Chen H, Dowd M, Lu L, O'Shea KS, Powell-Braxton L, Hillan KJ, Moore MW. Heterozygous embryonic lethality induced by targeted inactivation of the VEGF gene. Nature. 1996;380(6573):439–42.

67. Shalaby F, Rossant J, Yamaguchi TP, Gertsenstein M, Wu XF, Breitman ML, Schuh AC. Failure of blood-island formation and vasculogenesis in Flk-1-deficient mice. Nature. 1995;376(6535):62–6.

68. Maiti D, Xu Z, Duh EJ. Vascular endothelial growth factor induces MEF2C and MEF2-dependent activity in endothelial cells. Invest Ophthalmol Vis Sci. 2008;49(8):3640–8.

69. Xu J, Cao S, Wang L, Xu R, Chen G, Xu Q. VEGF promotes the transcription of the human PRL-3 gene in HUVEC through transcription factor MEF2C. PLoS One. 2011;6(11):e27165.

70. Azzi S, Hebda JK, Gavard J. Vascular permeability and drug delivery in cancers. Front Oncol. 2013;3:211.

71. Tong YJ, Zhang M, Zou P, Guo R. Inhibiting effect of vascular endothelial growth factor (VEGF) antisense oligodeoxynucleotides on VEGF expression in U937 cell. Zhongguo Shi Yan Xue Ye Xue Za Zhi. 2004;12(2):151–3.

72. Falcon BL, Hashizume H, Koumoutsakos P, Chou J, Bready JV, Coxon A, Oliner JD, McDonald DM. Contrasting actions of selective inhibitors of angiopoietin-1 and angiopoietin-2 on the normalization of tumor blood vessels. Am J Pathol. 2009;175(5):2159–70.

73. Carmeliet P, Jain RK. Principles and mechanisms of vessel normalization for cancer and other angiogenic diseases. Nat Rev Drug Discov. 2011;10(6):417–27.

74. Jabbarzadeh E, Starnes T, Khan YM, Jiang T, Wirtel AJ, Deng M, Lv Q, Nair LS, Doty SB, Laurencin CT. Induction of angiogenesis in tissue-engineered scaffolds designed for bone repair: a combined gene therapy-cell transplantation approach. Proc Natl Acad Sci U S A. 2008;105(32):11099–104.

75. Chung JC, Shum-Tim D. Neovascularization in tissue engineering. Cell. 2012;1(4):1246–60.

76. Ozawa CR, Banfi A, Glazer NL, Thurston G, Springer ML, Kraft PE, McDonald DM, Blau HM. Microenvironmental VEGF concentration, not total dose, determines a threshold between normal and aberrant angiogenesis. J Clin Invest. 2004;113(4):516–27.

77. Jiang BH, Liu LZ. PI3K/PTEN signaling in angiogenesis and tumorigenesis. Adv Cancer Res. 2009;102:19–65.

78. Chalhoub N, Baker SJ. PTEN and the PI3-kinase pathway in cancer. Annu Rev Pathol. 2009;4:127–50.

79. Gonzalez E, McGraw TE. The Akt kinases: isoform specificity in metabolism and cancer. Cell Cycle. 2009;8(16):2502–8.

80. Jiang BH, Zheng JZ, Aoki M, Vogt PK. Phosphatidylinositol 3-kinase signaling mediates angiogenesis and expression of vascular endothelial growth factor in endothelial cells. Proc Natl Acad Sci U S A. 2000;97(4):1749–53.

81. Jiang BH, Jiang G, Zheng JZ, Lu Z, Hunter T, Vogt PK. Phosphatidylinositol 3-kinase signaling controls levels of hypoxia-inducible factor 1. Cell Growth Differ. 2001;12(7):363–9.

82. Gerber HP, McMurtrey A, Kowalski J, Yan M, Keyt BA, Dixit V, Ferrara N. Vascular endothelial growth factor regulates endothelial cell survival through the phosphatidylinositol 3'-kinase/Akt signal transduction pathway. Requirement for Flk-1/KDR activation. J Biol Chem. 1998;273(46):30336–43.

83. Dayanir V, Meyer RD, Lashkari K, Rahimi N. Identification of tyrosine residues in vascular endothelial growth factor receptor-2/FLK-1 involved in activation of phosphatidylinositol 3-kinase and cell proliferation. J Biol Chem. 2001;276(21):17686–92.

84. Hawkins PT, Stephens LR. PI3K signalling in inflammation. Biochim Biophys Acta. 2015;1851(6):882–97.

85. Graupera M, Guillermet-Guibert J, Foukas LC, Phng LK, Cain RJ, Salpekar A, Pearce W, Meek S, Millan J, Cutillas PR, Smith AJ, Ridley AJ, Ruhrberg C, Gerhardt H, Vanhaesebroeck B. Angiogenesis selectively requires the p110alpha isoform of PI3K to control endothelial cell migration. Nature. 2008;453(7195):662–6.

86. Yuan TL, Choi HS, Matsui A, Benes C, Lifshits E, Luo J, Frangioni JV, Cantley LC. Class 1A PI3K regulates vessel integrity during development and tumorigenesis. Proc Natl Acad Sci U S A. 2008;105(28):9739–44.

87. Yoshioka K, Yoshida K, Cui H, Wakayama T, Takuwa N, Okamoto Y, Du W, Qi X, Asanuma K, Sugihara S, Aki S, Miyazawa H, Biswas K, Nagakura C, Ueno M, Iseki S, Schwartz RJ, Okamoto H, Sasaki T, Matsui O, Asano M, Adams RH, Takakura N, Takuwa Y. Endothelial PI3K-C2alpha, a class II PI3K, has an essential role in angiogenesis and vascular barrier function. Nat Med. 2012;18(10):1560–9.

88. Chen WS, Xu PZ, Gottlob K, Chen ML, Sokol K, Shiyanova T, Roninson I, Weng W, Suzuki R, Tobe K, Kadowaki T, Hay N. Growth retardation and

increased apoptosis in mice with homozygous disruption of the Akt1 gene. Genes Dev. 2001;15(17):2203–8.

89. Yang ZZ, Tschopp O, Hemmings-Mieszczak M, Feng J, Brodbeck D, Perentes E, Hemmings BA. Protein kinase B alpha/Akt1 regulates placental development and fetal growth. J Biol Chem. 2003;278(34):32124–31.

90. Lee MY, Luciano AK, Ackah E, Rodriguez-Vita J, Bancroft TA, Eichmann A, Simons M, Kyriakides TR, Morales-Ruiz M, Sessa WC. Endothelial Akt1 mediates angiogenesis by phosphorylating multiple angiogenic substrates. Proc Natl Acad Sci U S A. 2014;111(35):12865–70.

91. Tang ED, Nunez G, Barr FG, Guan KL. Negative regulation of the forkhead transcription factor FKHR by Akt. J Biol Chem. 1999;274(24):16741–6.

92. Ola R, Dubrac A, Han J, Zhang F, Fang JS, Larrivee B, Lee M, Urarte AA, Kraehling JR, Genet G, Hirschi KK, Sessa WC, Canals FV, Graupera M, Yan M, Young LH, Oh PS, Eichmann A. PI3 kinase inhibition improves vascular malformations in mouse models of hereditary haemorrhagic telangiectasia. Nat Commun. 2016;7:13650.

93. Kim LC, Cook RS, Chen J. mTORC1 and mTORC2 in cancer and the tumor microenvironment. Oncogene. 2017;36(16):2191–201.

94. Dodd KM, Yang J, Shen MH, Sampson JR, Tee AR. mTORC1 drives HIF-1alpha and VEGF-A signalling via multiple mechanisms involving 4E-BP1, S6K1 and STAT3. Oncogene. 2015;34(17):2239–50.

95. Kwiatkowski DJ, Manning BD. Tuberous sclerosis: a GAP at the crossroads of multiple signaling pathways. Hum Mol Genet. 2005;14 Spec No. 2:R251–8.

96. Okumura N, Yoshida H, Kitagishi Y, Murakami M, Nishimura Y, Matsuda S. PI3K/AKT/PTEN signaling as a molecular target in leukemia angiogenesis. Adv Hematol. 2012;2012:843085.

97. Guertin DA, Stevens DM, Thoreen CC, Burds AA, Kalaany NY, Moffat J, Brown M, Fitzgerald KJ, Sabatini DM. Ablation in mice of the mTORC components raptor, rictor, or mLST8 reveals that mTORC2 is required for signaling to Akt-FOXO and PKCalpha, but not S6K1. Dev Cell. 2006;11(6):859–71.

98. Wang S, Amato KR, Song W, Youngblood V, Lee K, Boothby M, Brantley-Sieders DM, Chen J. Regulation of endothelial cell proliferation and vascular assembly through distinct mTORC2 signaling pathways. Mol Cell Biol. 2015;35(7):1299–313.

99. Shiota C, Woo JT, Lindner J, Shelton KD, Magnuson MA. Multiallelic disruption of the rictor gene in mice reveals that mTOR complex 2 is essential for fetal growth and viability. Dev Cell. 2006;11(4):583–9.

100. Aimi F, Georgiopoulou S, Kalus I, Lehner F, Hegglin A, Limani P, Gomes de Lima V, Ruegg MA, Hall MN, Lindenblatt N, Haas E, Battegay EJ, Humar R. Endothelial Rictor is crucial for midgestational development and sustained and extensive FGF2-induced neovascularization in the adult. Sci Rep. 2015;5:17705.

101. Julien LA, Carriere A, Moreau J, Roux PP. mTORC1-activated S6K1 phosphorylates Rictor on threonine 1135 and regulates mTORC2 signaling. Mol Cell Biol. 2010;30(4):908–21.

102. Sun J, Liu Y, Moreno S, Baudry M, Bi X. Imbalanced mechanistic target of rapamycin C1 and C2 activity in the cerebellum of Angelman syndrome mice impairs motor function. J Neurosci. 2015;35(11):4706–18.

103. Sarbassov DD, Guertin DA, Ali SM, Sabatini DM. Phosphorylation and regulation of Akt/PKB by the rictor-mTOR complex. Science. 2005;307(5712):1098–101.

104. Rini BI, Atkins MB. Resistance to targeted therapy in renal-cell carcinoma. Lancet Oncol. 2009;10(10):992–1000.

105. Zoncu R, Efeyan A, Sabatini DM. mTOR: from growth signal integration to cancer, diabetes and ageing. Nat Rev Mol Cell Biol. 2011;12(1):21–35.

106. Song MS, Salmena L, Pandolfi PP. The functions and regulation of the PTEN tumour suppressor. Nat Rev Mol Cell Biol. 2012;13(5):283–96.

107. Farhan MA, Carmine-Simmen K, Lewis JD, Moore RB, Murray AG. Endothelial cell mTOR complex-2 regulates sprouting angiogenesis. PLoS One. 2015;10(8):e0135245.

108. Jacinto E, Loewith R, Schmidt A, Lin S, Ruegg MA, Hall A, Hall MN. Mammalian TOR complex 2 controls the actin cytoskeleton and is rapamycin insensitive. Nat Cell Biol. 2004;6(11):1122–8.

109. Sarbassov DD, Ali SM, Kim DH, Guertin DA, Latek RR, Erdjument-Bromage H, Tempst P, Sabatini DM. Rictor, a novel binding partner of mTOR, defines a rapamycin-insensitive and raptor-independent pathway that regulates the cytoskeleton. Curr Biol. 2004;14(14):1296–302.

110. Tsuji-Tamura K, Ogawa M. Dual inhibition of mTORC1 and mTORC2 perturbs cytoskeletal organization and impairs endothelial cell elongation. Biochem Biophys Res Commun. 2018;497(1):326–31.

111. Yavropoulou MP, Maladaki A, Yovos JG. The role of Notch and Hedgehog signaling pathways in pituitary development and pathogenesis of pituitary adenomas. Hormones (Athens). 2015;14(1):5–18.

112. Iso T, Hamamori Y, Kedes L. Notch signaling in vascular development. Arterioscler Thromb Vasc Biol. 2003;23(4):543–53.

113. Palomero T, Sulis ML, Cortina M, Real PJ, Barnes K, Ciofani M, Caparros E, Buteau J, Brown K, Perkins SL, Bhagat G, Agarwal AM, Basso G, Castillo M, Nagase S, Cordon-Cardo C, Parsons R, Zuniga-Pflucker JC, Dominguez M, Ferrando AA. Mutational loss of PTEN induces resistance to NOTCH1 inhibition in T-cell leukemia. Nat Med. 2007;13(10):1203–10.

114. Perumalsamy LR, Nagala M, Banerjee P, Sarin A. A hierarchical cascade activated by non-canonical Notch signaling and the mTOR-Rictor complex regulates neglect-induced death in mammalian cells. Cell Death Differ. 2009;16(6):879–89.

115. Crabtree JS, Singleton CS, Miele L. Notch signaling in neuroendocrine tumors. Front Oncol. 2016;6:94.

116. Eilken HM, Adams RH. Dynamics of endothelial cell behavior in sprouting angiogenesis. Curr Opin Cell Biol. 2010;22(5):617–25.

117. Siekmann AF, Affolter M, Belting HG. The tip cell concept 10 years after: new players tune in for a common theme. Exp Cell Res. 2013;319(9):1255–63.

118. Hellstrom M, Phng LK, Hofmann JJ, Wallgard E, Coultas L, Lindblom P, Alva J, Nilsson AK, Karlsson L, Gaiano N, Yoon K, Rossant J, Iruela-Arispe ML, Kalen M, Gerhardt H, Betsholtz C. Dll4 signalling through Notch1 regulates formation of tip cells during angiogenesis. Nature. 2007;445(7129):776–80.

119. Suchting S, Freitas C, le Noble F, Benedito R, Breant C, Duarte A, Eichmann A. The Notch ligand Delta-like 4 negatively regulates endothelial tip cell formation and vessel branching. Proc Natl Acad Sci U S A. 2007;104(9):3225–30.

120. Swiatek PJ, Lindsell CE, del Amo FF, Weinmaster G, Gridley T. Notch1 is essential for postimplantation development in mice. Genes Dev. 1994;8(6):707–19.

121. Conlon RA, Reaume AG, Rossant J. Notch1 is required for the coordinate segmentation of somites. Development. 1995;121(5):1533–45.

122. Krebs LT, Xue Y, Norton CR, Shutter JR, Maguire M, Sundberg JP, Gallahan D, Closson V, Kitajewski J, Callahan R, Smith GH, Stark KL, Gridley T. Notch signaling is essential for vascular morphogenesis in mice. Genes Dev. 2000;14(11):1343–52.

123. Krebs LT, Shutter JR, Tanigaki K, Honjo T, Stark KL, Gridley T. Haploinsufficient lethality and formation of arteriovenous malformations in Notch pathway mutants. Genes Dev. 2004;18(20):2469–73.

124. Fischer A, Schumacher N, Maier M, Sendtner M, Gessler M. The Notch target genes Hey1 and Hey2 are required for embryonic vascular development. Genes Dev. 2004;18(8):901–11.

125. Gessler M, Knobeloch KP, Helisch A, Amann K, Schumacher N, Rohde E, Fischer A, Leimeister C. Mouse gridlock: no aortic coarctation or deficiency, but fatal cardiac defects in Hey2 −/− mice. Curr Biol. 2002;12(18):1601–4.

126. Kokubo H, Miyagawa-Tomita S, Nakazawa M, Saga Y, Johnson RL. Mouse hesr1 and hesr2 genes are redundantly required to mediate Notch signaling in the developing cardiovascular system. Dev Biol. 2005;278(2):301–9.

127. Kitagawa M, Hojo M, Imayoshi I, Goto M, Ando M, Ohtsuka T, Kageyama R, Miyamoto S. Hes1 and Hes5 regulate vascular remodeling and arterial specification of endothelial cells in brain vascular development. Mech Dev. 2013;130(9–10):458–66.

128. Liu ZJ, Shirakawa T, Li Y, Soma A, Oka M, Dotto GP, Fairman RM, Velazquez OC, Herlyn M. Regulation of Notch1 and Dll4 by vascular endothelial growth factor in arterial endothelial cells: implications for modulating arteriogenesis and angiogenesis. Mol Cell Biol. 2003;23(1):14–25.

132. Caporali A, Meloni M, Vollenkle C, Bonci D, Sala-Newby GB, Addis R,

129. Mack JJ, Mosqueiro TS, Archer BJ, Jones WM, Sunshine H, Faas GC, Briot A, Aragon RL, Su T, Romay MC, McDonald AI, Kuo CH, Lizama CO, Lane TF, Zovein AC, Fang Y, Tarling EJ, de Aguiar Vallim TQ, Navab M, Fogelman AM, Bouchard LS, Iruela-Arispe ML. NOTCH1 is a mechanosensor in adult arteries. Nat Commun. 2017;8(1):1620.

130. Katoh K, Kano Y, Ookawara S. Role of stress fibers and focal adhesions as a mediator for mechano-signal transduction in endothelial cells in situ. Vasc Health Risk Manag. 2008;4(6):1273–82.

131. Park C, Lee TJ, Bhang SH, Liu F, Nakamura R, Oladipupo SS, Pitha-Rowe I, Capoccia B, Choi HS, Kim TM, Urao N, Ushio-Fukai M, Lee DJ, Miyoshi H, Kim BS, Lim DS, Apte RS, Ornitz DM, Choi K. Injury-mediated vascular regeneration requires endothelial ER71/ETV2. Arterioscler Thromb Vasc Biol. 2016;36(1):86–96.

Spinetti G, Losa S, Masson R, Baker AH, Agami R, le Sage C, Condorelli G, Madeddu P, Martelli F, Emanueli C. Deregulation of microRNA-503 contributes to diabetes mellitus-induced impairment of endothelial function and reparative angiogenesis after limb ischemia. Circulation. 2011;123(3):282–91.

133. Cheng R, Ma JX. Angiogenesis in diabetes and obesity. Rev Endocr Metab Disord. 2015;16(1):67–75.

24

Functional similarities of microRNAs across different types of tissue stem cells in aging

Koichiro Watanabe, Yasuaki Ikuno, Yumi Kakeya, Hirotaka Kito, Aoi Matsubara, Mizuki Kaneda, Yu Katsuyama and Hayato Naka-Kaneda[*]

Abstract

Restoration of tissue homeostasis by controlling stem cell aging is a promising therapeutic approach for geriatric disorders. The molecular mechanisms underlying age-related dysfunctions of specific types of adult tissue stem cells (TSCs) have been studied, and various microRNAs were recently reported to be involved. However, the central roles of microRNAs in stem cell aging remain unclear. Interest in this area was sparked by murine heterochronic parabiosis experiments, which demonstrated that systemic factors can restore the functions of TSCs. Age-related changes in secretion profiles, termed the senescence-associated secretory phenotype, have attracted attention, and several pro- and anti-aging factors have been identified. On the other hand, many microRNAs are linked with the age-dependent dysregulations of various physiological processes, including "stem cell aging." This review summarizes microRNAs that appear to play common roles in stem cell aging.

Keywords: Stem cell aging, microRNA, miR-17, miR-125b, miR-181a, SASP

Background

Overcoming age-related diseases and elongating the healthy lifespan are emerging issues for aging societies. Dysfunctions of aged tissue stem cells (TSCs) contribute to loss of tissue homeostasis, including reductions in lymphopoiesis and the long-term repopulating abilities of hematopoietic stem/progenitor cells (HSCs) [1, 2], the muscle repair capacity of skeletal muscle satellite cells [3], and the multipotency of mesenchymal stem/stromal cells (MSCs) [4]. The restoration of TSC functions in murine heterochronic parabiosis experiments triggered interest in the rejuvenation of aged TSCs [5]. Thereafter, several pro-aging [6–12] and anti-aging [13–16] systemic factors were identified, although some of the findings are conflicting [17]. Senescent cells secrete a myriad of inflammatory factors, referred to as the senescence-associated secretory phenotype (SASP) [18]. Clearance of senescent cells delays the induction of various geriatric pathologies, supporting the concept that the

SASP promotes aging in a non-cell-autonomous fashion [19, 20]. Several lines of evidence indicated that age-related TSC dysfunctions and tissue-level pathologies can be improved by manipulating (reversing) cell-extrinsic/systemic conditions, at least in part.

We previously identified growth differentiation factor 6 (Gdf6; also known as Bmp13 and CDMP-2) as a regenerative factor secreted by young MSCs [21, 22]. Upregulation of human GDF6 restores the differentiation potential of old MSCs in vitro and reverses multiple age-related pathologies in vivo. miR-17 and its paralogues miR-106a and 106b (miR-17/106) regulate not only differentiation potential but also expression of some secretory factors, including Gdf6, and are implicated in the decline of these functions with age. Many microRNAs are associated with age-related dysfunctions of several types of TSCs. Here, we review microRNAs, which are commonly downregulated with age and induced dysregulation of cytogenesis, proliferation, and inflammation in multiple TSCs, and discuss functional similarities of microRNAs across different types of TSCs in aging.

---

* Correspondence: hayato@belle.shiga-med.ac.jp
Department of Anatomy, Shiga University of Medical Science, Seta Tsukinowa-cho, Otsu, Shiga 520-2192, Japan

miR-17 family (miR-17-92a, 106b-25, and 106a-363 clusters)

miR-17 family members play essential and pleiotropic roles in development, metabolism, diseases, tumorigenesis, and aging [23, 24]. We first identified miR-17/106 family members as key regulators of the neurogenic-to-gliogenic switch in developing neural stem/progenitor cells (NSCs) by controlling the "competence" necessary for NSCs to respond to gliogenic cell-extrinsic signals [25, 26]. Next, we found that downregulation of miR-17/106 induces a decline in differentiation potential and dysregulated expression of secretory factors in old MSCs [22]. Another group also reported a relationship between miR-17/106 and an age-dependent decrease in the osteogenic potential of MSCs [27]. miR-17/106 also regulate the proliferation and development of HSCs [28–30]. Other reports studied the impact of miR-17 overexpression in vivo. Transgenic mice expressing miR-17 exhibit delayed tissue growth and have an elongated lifespan [31, 32]. Epidemiologic studies reported that miR-17 family members are upregulated in centenarians, which supports the hypothesis that these microRNAs are important for the young healthy conditions and involved in human aging [33, 34].

miR-125b

A myeloid skewing phenotype and a decline in engraftment capability have long been recognized as age-related dysfunctions of old HSCs [1]. miR-125b is expressed in HSCs, and overexpression of miR-125b predominantly expands lymphoid-biased HSCs [35]. In addition, miR-125b can increase the level of myeloid progenitors [36]. Both reports showed that miR-125b overexpression increases the engraftment capabilities of HSCs and progenitors in transplantation assays into irradiated mice. Moreover, reduction of miR-125b increases expression levels of the chemokine CCL4 with age [37]. miR-125b

activates and is activated by the NF-κB pathway [38, 39] is sometimes regarded as an "inflamma-miR," which is implicated in the regulation of immune and inflammatory responses [40]. miR-125b directly suppresses p53 expression in developing NSCs. miR-125b is expressed throughout zebrafish embryos and is enriched in the brain, while loss of miR-125b elevates p53 expression and triggers p53-dependent apoptosis in these embryos [41]. miR-125b is also expressed in MSCs [42], epidermal stem cells [43], and some types of tumor cells [44–48]. Interestingly, lin-4, a Caenorhabditis elegans homolog of miR-125b, is a heterochronic gene and generates the temporal pattern of many cell lineages during development [49], and is related to lifespan and tissue aging via its control of the insulin/insulin-like growth factor–1 pathway [50]. Overexpression of lin-4 elongates lifespan, whereas loss-of mutation accelerates tissue aging and shortens it.

miR-181 family (miR-181a/b/c/d)

Chronic inflammation accelerates systemic aging [10]. miR-181 family members have anti-inflammatory functions and are categorized as inflamma-miRs, together with miR-125b [40]. miR-181 regulates the differentiation of multiple types of TSCs, such as HSCs [51], myoblasts (activated progenitor cells) [52], MSCs [53], and some types of cancer stem cells [54–56]. We confirmed that miR-181 family members are downregulated with age in multiple TSCs (HSCs, MSCs, and intestinal stem cells). However, they continue to be expressed in differentiated cells and function pleiotropically. The age-dependent decline in miR-181a expression induces functional defects in CD4+ T cells [57]. miR-181a is downregulated in old pancreatic beta cells and necessary for their proliferation [58]. Extracellular vesicles derived from brain metastatic cancer cells contain miR-181c and can destroy and pass through the blood-brain barrier

Table 1 Functional similarities of microRNAs in different types of TSCs

microRNA family	Differentiation (specification)	Proliferation, survival, and apoptosis	Secretion and inflammation	Tumorigenesis	Others
miR-17/106	MSCs (↑Ad, ↑Os) [22, 27] NSCs (↑N, ↓G) [25] HSCs (↑B, ↑Ly, ↑My) [28–30]	↑HSCs [28–30]	MSCs (↑Gdf6 and etc.) [22]	Lymphoma [28–30]	
miR-125b	HSCs (↑Ly, ↑My) [35, 36] MSCs (↑Ad, ↑Os) [42] Skin stem cells (↓Epi, ↓Oil, ↓HF) [43]	↑HSCs [35, 36] ↑NSCs [41] ↑Skin stem cells [43]	HSCs (↓CCL4, ↑NF-κB, ↓TNFAIP3) [37, 39, 40]	Breast cancer [44] Hepatocellular carcinoma [45] Leukemia [46] Skin tumor [47] Stomach adenocarcinoma [48]	↑HSC engraftment [35, 36]
miR-181	HSCs (↑Ly) [51] Myoblasts (↑Muscle) [52]	↑Beta cells [58]	HSCs (↓IL-1α, ↓c-fos, ↓NF-κB) [40] MSCs (↑IL-6) [53]	Hepatic cancer stem cells [54] Breast cancer [55] Leukemia [56]	↑T cell receptor sensitivity [57] ↑Blood-brain barrier destruction [59]

↑: promotion/positive regulation, ↓: inhibition/negative regulation, Ad: adipocytes, Os: Osteoblasts, N: neurons, G: glial cells, B: B cells, Ly: lymphocytes, My: myeloid cells, Epi: epidermal cells, Oil: oil-gland cells, HF: hair follicle cells

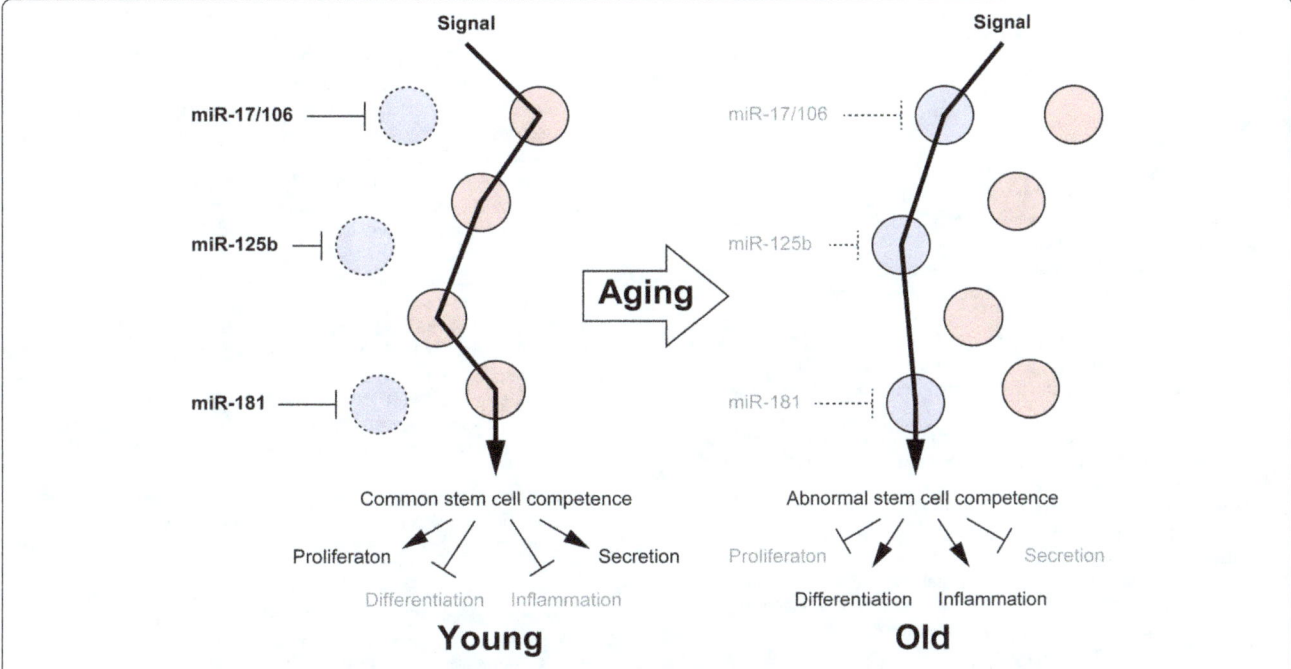

Fig. 1 Schematic diagram of the disruption of microRNA-mediated stem cell competence. Decline in microRNAs for regulation of stem cell functions induces disruption of proper stem cell competence and dysfunctions

[59]. The critical roles of miR-181 in age-related cell-intrinsic dysfunctions of TSCs are unclear. The old TSCs with downregulated miR-181 family members would generate abnormal somatic cells, which have something dysfunctions, and these cells may contribute to the disturbance of tissue homeostasis.

Commonality of microRNA functions among various types of TSCs

Recent studies have revealed that a part of microRNAs appear to play common roles in stem cell aging (Table 1). In fact, many microRNAs, including miR-17 family, miR-125b, and miR-181 family members, show similar expression pattern, namely they are expressed at higher levels during proliferating phase and downregulated with age. This is supported by a report concerning the classification of tumor cells derived from various tissues based on their microRNA, not their mRNA, expression profiles, suggesting that the existence of functionally common microRNAs, at least, for proliferation and undifferentiated states [60]. We have focused on microRNA-mediated "competence regulation," which is responsible for the responsiveness to the various cell-extrinsic signals, as the fundamental machinery controlling the properties of TSCs, and miR-17 family members are key regulators in this context [22, 25, 61]. In our previous study, we revealed that miR-17/106 switches the usages of JAK-STAT and BMP pathways from neurogenic to gliogenic signals [25]. In young states, microRNAs regulate signal transduction correctly. Downregulation of microRNAs with age should induce deregulation of

signal transduction and reflect abnormal phenotypes to signals (Fig. 1). All miR-17, miR-125b, miR-181 family members are downregulated various old TSCs and downregulation of them suppresses cytogenesis, proliferation, and secretion of homeostatic factors and promotes inflammation and tumorigenesis (Table 1).

Conclusions

Some microRNAs have similar functions in different types of TSCs. Downregulation of these specific-microRNAs induces similar age-related dysfunctions of TSCs. These microRNAs may define the "young competence" by specifying the signal pathways with suppression of their regulon, including signal mediators and transcription factors. Further investigation of the roles of the other microRNAs in stem cell aging will help to elucidate the central molecular machinery of the aging and develop the next-generation therapeutic methods for geriatric diseases.

Abbreviations
Gdf6: Growth differentiation factor 6; HSCs: Hematopoietic stem/progenitor cells; miR-17/106: miR-17, miR-106a, and 106b; MSCs: Mesenchymal stem/stromal cells; NSCs: Neural stem/progenitor cells; SASP: Senescence-associated secretory phenotype; TSCs: Tissue stem cells

Funding
This work was supported by the Uehara Memorial Foundation and JSPS KAKENHI Grant Number JP16K08602.

Authors' contributions
HNK drafted and completed the manuscript. All authors read and approved the final manuscript.

Competing interests
The authors declare that they have no competing interests.

References
1. Sudo K, Ema H, Morita Y, Nakauchi H. Age-associated characteristics of murine hematopoietic stem cells. J Exp Med. 2000;192(9):1273–80.
2. Rossi DJ, Bryder D, Zahn JM, Ahlenius H, Sonu R, Wagers AJ, Weissman IL. Cell intrinsic alterations underlie hematopoietic stem cell aging. Proc Natl Acad Sci U S A. 2005;102(26):9194–9.
3. Renault V, Thornell LE, Eriksson PO, Butler-Browne G, Mouly V. Regenerative potential of human skeletal muscle during aging. Aging Cell. 2002; 1(2):132–9.
4. Zhou S, Greenberger JS, Epperly MW, Goff JP, Adler C, Leboff MS, Glowacki J. Age-related intrinsic changes in human bone-marrow-derived mesenchymal stem cells and their differentiation to osteoblasts. Aging Cell. 2008;7(3):335–43.
5. Conboy IM, Conboy MJ, Wagers AJ, Girma ER, Weissman IL, Rando TA. Rejuvenation of aged progenitor cells by exposure to a young systemic environment. Nature. 2005;433(7027):760–4.
6. Acosta JC, O'Loghlen A, Banito A, Guijarro MV, Augert A, Raguz S, Fumagalli M, Da Costa M, Brown C, Popov N, et al. Chemokine signaling via the CXCR2 receptor reinforces senescence. Cell. 2008;133(6):1006–18.
7. Salminen A, Ojala J, Kaarniranta K, Haapasalo A, Hiltunen M, Soininen H. Astrocytes in the aging brain express characteristics of senescence-associated secretory phenotype. Eur J Neurosci. 2011;34(1):3–11.
8. Villeda SA, Luo J, Mosher KI, Zou B, Britschgi M, Bieri G, Stan TM, Fainberg N, Ding Z, Eggel A, et al. The ageing systemic milieu negatively regulates neurogenesis and cognitive function. Nature. 2011;477(7362):90–4.
9. Naito AT, Sumida T, Nomura S, Liu ML, Higo T, Nakagawa A, Okada K, Sakai T, Hashimoto A, Hara Y, et al. Complement C1q activates canonical Wnt signaling and promotes aging-related phenotypes. Cell. 2012;149(6): 1298–313.
10. Jurk D, Wilson C, Passos JF, Oakley F, Correia-Melo C, Greaves L, Saretzki G, Fox C, Lawless C, Anderson R, et al. Chronic inflammation induces telomere dysfunction and accelerates ageing in mice. Nat Commun. 2014;2:4172.
11. Smith LK, He Y, Park JS, Bieri G, Snethlage CE, Lin K, Gontier G, Wabl R, Plambeck KE. Udeochu J *et al*: beta2-microglobulin is a systemic pro-aging factor that impairs cognitive function and neurogenesis. Nat Med. 2015;
12. Fry CS, Kirby TJ, Kosmac K, McCarthy JJ, Peterson CA. Myogenic progenitor cells control extracellular matrix production by fibroblasts during skeletal muscle hypertrophy. Cell Stem Cell. 2017;20(1):56–69.
13. Loffredo FS, Steinhauser ML, Jay SM, Gannon J, Pancoast JR, Yalamanchi P, Sinha M, Dall'Osso C, Khong D, Shadrach JL, et al. Growth differentiation factor 11 is a circulating factor that reverses age-related cardiac hypertrophy. Cell. 2013;153(4):828–39.
14. Elabd C, Cousin W, Upadhyayula P, Chen RY, Chooljian MS, Li J, Kung S, Jiang KP, Conboy IM. Oxytocin is an age-specific circulating hormone that is necessary for muscle maintenance and regeneration. Nat Commun. 2014; 5:4082.
15. Katsimpardi L, Litterman NK, Schein PA, Miller CM, Loffredo FS, Wojtkiewicz GR, Chen JW, Lee RT, Wagers AJ, Rubin LL. Vascular and neurogenic rejuvenation of the aging mouse brain by young systemic factors. Science. 2014;344(6184):630–4.
16. Sinha M, Jang YC, Oh J, Khong D, Wu EY, Manohar R, Miller C, Regalado SG, Loffredo FS, Pancoast JR, et al. Restoring systemic GDF11 levels reverses age-related dysfunction in mouse skeletal muscle. Science. 2014;344(6184): 649–52.
17. Egerman MA, Cadena SM, Gilbert JA, Meyer A, Nelson HN, Swalley SE, Mallozzi C, Jacobi C, Jennings LL, Clay I, et al. GDF11 increases with age and inhibits skeletal muscle regeneration. Cell Metab. 2015;22(1):164–74.
18. Coppe JP, Patil CK, Rodier F, Sun Y, Munoz DP, Goldstein J, Nelson PS, Desprez PY, Campisi J. Senescence-associated secretory phenotypes reveal cell-nonautonomous functions of oncogenic RAS and the p53 tumor suppressor. PLoS Biol. 2008;6(12):2853–68.
19. Baker DJ, Wijshake T, Tchkonia T, LeBrasseur NK, Childs BG, van de Sluis B, Kirkland JL, van Deursen JM. Clearance of p16Ink4a-positive senescent cells delays ageing-associated disorders. Nature. 2011;479(7372):232–6.
20. Baker DJ, Childs BG, Durik M, Wijers ME, Sieben CJ, Zhong J, Saltness RA, Jeganathan KB, Verzosa GC, Pezeshki A, et al. Naturally occurring p16-positive cells shorten healthy lifespan. Nature. 2016;

21. Hisamatsu D, Naka-Kaneda H. Reversing multiple age-related pathologies by controlling the senescence-associated secretory phenotype of stem cells. Neural Regen Res. 2016;11(11):1746–7.
22. Hisamatsu D, Ohno-Oishi M, Nakamura S, Mabuchi Y, Naka-Kaneda H. Growth differentiation factor 6 derived from mesenchymal stem/stromal cells reduces age-related functional deterioration in multiple tissues. Aging (Albany NY). 2016;8(6):1259–75.
23. Mogilyansky E, Rigoutsos I. The miR-17/92 cluster: a comprehensive update on its genomics, genetics, functions and increasingly important and numerous roles in health and disease. Cell Death Differ. 2013;20(12): 1603–14.
24. Dellago H, Bobbili MR, Grillari J. MicroRNA-17-5p: at the crossroads of Cancer and aging - a mini-review. Gerontology. 2017;63(1):20–8.
25. Naka-Kaneda H, Nakamura S, Igarashi M, Aoi H, Kanki H, Tsuyama J, Tsutsumi S, Aburatani H, Shimazaki T, Okano H. The miR-17/106-p38 axis is a key regulator of the neurogenic-to-gliogenic transition in developing neural stem/progenitor cells. Proc Natl Acad Sci U S A. 2014;111(4):1604–9.
26. Shimazaki T, Okano H. Heterochronic microRNAs in temporal specification of neural stem cells: application toward rejuvenation. NPJ Aging Mech Dis. 2016;2:15014.
27. Liu W, Qi M, Konermann A, Zhang L, Jin F, Jin Y. The p53/miR-17/Smurf1 pathway mediates skeletal deformities in an age-related model via inhibiting the function of mesenchymal stem cells. Aging (Albany NY). 2015; 7(3):205–18.
28. Ventura A, Young AG, Winslow MM, Lintault L, Meissner A, Erkeland SJ, Newman J, Bronson RT, Crowley D, Stone JR, et al. Targeted deletion reveals essential and overlapping functions of the miR-17 through 92 family of miRNA clusters. Cell. 2008;132(5):875–86.
29. Meenhuis A, van Veelen PA, de Looper H, van Boxtel N, van den Berge IJ, Sun SM, Taskesen E, Stern P, de Ru AH, van Adrichem AJ, et al. MiR-17/20/ 93/106 promote hematopoietic cell expansion by targeting sequestosome 1-regulated pathways in mice. Blood. 2011;118(4):916–25.
30. Li Y, Vecchiarelli-Federico LM, Li YJ, Egan SE, Spaner D, Hough MR, Ben-David Y. The miR-17-92 cluster expands multipotent hematopoietic progenitors whereas imbalanced expression of its individual oncogenic miRNAs promotes leukemia in mice. Blood. 2012;119(19):4486–98.
31. Shan SW, Lee DY, Deng Z, Shatseva T, Jeyapalan Z, Du WW, Zhang Y, Xuan JW, Yee SP, Siragam V, et al. MicroRNA MiR-17 retards tissue growth and represses fibronectin expression. Nat Cell Biol. 2009;11(8):1031–8.
32. Du WW, Yang W, Fang L, Xuan J, Li H, Khorshidi A, Gupta S, Li X, Yang BB. miR-17 extends mouse lifespan by inhibiting senescence signaling mediated by MKP7. Cell Death Dis. 2014;5:e1355.
33. Serna E, Gambini J, Borras C, Abdelaziz KM, Belenguer A, Sanchis P, Avellana JA, Rodriguez-Manas L, Vina J. Centenarians, but not octogenarians, up-regulate the expression of microRNAs. Sci Rep. 2012;2:961.
34. Gombar S, Jung HJ, Dong F, Calder B, Atzmon G, Barzilai N, Tian XL, Pothof J, Hoeijmakers JH, Campisi J, et al. Comprehensive microRNA profiling in B-cells of human centenarians by massively parallel sequencing. BMC Genomics. 2012;13:353.
35. Ooi AG, Sahoo D, Adorno M, Wang Y, Weissman IL, Park CY. MicroRNA-125b expands hematopoietic stem cells and enriches for the lymphoid-balanced and lymphoid-biased subsets. Proc Natl Acad Sci U S A. 2010;107(50): 21505–10.
36. O'Connell RM, Chaudhuri AA, Rao DS, Gibson WS, Balazs AB, Baltimore D. MicroRNAs enriched in hematopoietic stem cells differentially regulate long-term hematopoietic output. Proc Natl Acad Sci U S A. 2010;107(32): 14235–40.
37. Cheng NL, Chen X, Kim J, Shi AH, Nguyen C, Wersto R, Weng NP. MicroRNA-125b modulates inflammatory chemokine CCL4 expression in immune cells and its reduction causes CCL4 increase with age. Aging Cell. 2015;14(2):200–8.
38. Tan G, Niu J, Shi Y, Ouyang H, Wu ZH. NF-kappaB-dependent microRNA-125b up-regulation promotes cell survival by targeting p38alpha upon ultraviolet radiation. J Biol Chem. 2012;287(39):33036–47.
39. Kim SW, Ramasamy K, Bouamar H, Lin AP, Jiang D, Aguiar RC. MicroRNAs miR-125a and miR-125b constitutively activate the NF-kappaB pathway by targeting the tumor necrosis factor alpha-induced protein 3 (TNFAIP3, A20). Proc Natl Acad Sci U S A. 2012;109(20):7865–70.
40. Rippo MR, Olivieri F, Monsurro V, Prattichizzo F, Albertini MC, Procopio AD. MitomiRs in human inflamm-aging: a hypothesis involving miR-181a, miR-34a and miR-146a. Exp Gerontol. 2014;56:154–63.

41. Le MT, Teh C, Shyh-Chang N, Xie H, Zhou B, Korzh V, Lodish HF, Lim B. MicroRNA-125b is a novel negative regulator of p53. Genes Dev. 2009;23(7):862–76.

42. Yu JM, Wu X, Gimble JM, Guan X, Freitas MA, Bunnell BA. Age-related changes in mesenchymal stem cells derived from rhesus macaque bone marrow. Aging Cell. 2011;10(1):66–79.

43. Zhang L, Stokes N, Polak L, Fuchs E. Specific microRNAs are preferentially expressed by skin stem cells to balance self-renewal and early lineage commitment. Cell Stem Cell. 2011;8(3):294–308.

44. Saetrom P, Biesinger J, Li SM, Smith D, Thomas LF, Majzoub K, Rivas GE, Alluin J, Rossi JJ, Krontiris TG, et al. A risk variant in an miR-125b binding site in BMPR1B is associated with breast cancer pathogenesis. Cancer Res. 2009; 69(18):7459–65.

45. Kim JK, Noh JH, Jung KH, Eun JW, Bae HJ, Kim MG, Chang YG, Shen Q, Park WS, Lee JY, et al. Sirtuin7 oncogenic potential in human hepatocellular carcinoma and its regulation by the tumor suppressors MiR-125a-5p and MiR-125b. Hepatology. 2013;57(3):1055–67.

46. So AY, Sookram R, Chaudhuri AA, Minisandram A, Cheng D, Xie C, Lim EL, Flores YG, Jiang S, Kim JT, et al. Dual mechanisms by which miR-125b represses IRF4 to induce myeloid and B-cell leukemias. Blood. 2014;124(9): 1502–12.

47. Zhang L, Ge Y, Fuchs E. miR-125b can enhance skin tumor initiation and promote malignant progression by repressing differentiation and prolonging cell survival. Genes Dev. 2014;28(22):2532–46.

48. Kim BC, Jeong HO, Park D, Kim CH, Lee EK, Kim DH, Im E, Kim ND, Lee S, Yu BP, et al. Profiling age-related epigenetic markers of stomach adenocarcinoma in young and old subjects. Cancer Inform. 2015;14:47–54.

49. Lee RC, Feinbaum RL, Ambros V. The C. Elegans heterochronic gene lin-4 encodes small RNAs with antisense complementarity to lin-14. Cell. 1993; 75(5):843–54.

50. Boehm M, Slack F. A developmental timing microRNA and its target regulate life span in C. Elegans. Science. 2005;310(5756):1954–7.

51. Chen CZ, Li L, Lodish HF, Bartel DP. MicroRNAs modulate hematopoietic lineage differentiation. Science. 2004;303(5654):83–6.

52. Naguibneva I, Ameyar-Zazoua M, Polesskaya A, Ait-Si-Ali S, Groisman R, Souidi M, Cuvellier S, Harel-Bellan A. The microRNA miR-181 targets the homeobox protein Hox-A11 during mammalian myoblast differentiation. Nat Cell Biol. 2006;8(3):278–84.

53. Liu L, Wang Y, Fan H, Zhao X, Liu D, Hu Y, Kidd AR 3rd, Bao J, Hou Y. MicroRNA-181a regulates local immune balance by inhibiting proliferation and immunosuppressive properties of mesenchymal stem cells. Stem Cells. 2012;30(8):1756–70.

54. Ji J, Yamashita T, Budhu A, Forgues M, Jia HL, Li C, Deng C, Wauthier E, Reid LM, Ye QH, et al. Identification of microRNA-181 by genome-wide screening as a critical player in EpCAM-positive hepatic cancer stem cells. Hepatology. 2009;50(2):472–80.

55. Wang Y, Yu Y, Tsuyada A, Ren X, Wu X, Stubblefield K, Rankin-Gee EK, Wang SE. Transforming growth factor-beta regulates the sphere-initiating stem cell-like feature in breast cancer through miRNA-181 and ATM. Oncogene. 2011;30(12):1470–80.

56. Su R, Lin HS, Zhang XH, Yin XL, Ning HM, Liu B, Zhai PF, Gong JN, Shen C, Song L, et al. MiR-181 family: regulators of myeloid differentiation and acute myeloid leukemia as well as potential therapeutic targets. Oncogene. 2015; 34(25):3226–39.

57. Li G, Yu M, Lee WW, Tsang M, Krishnan E, Weyand CM, Goronzy JJ. Decline in miR-181a expression with age impairs T cell receptor sensitivity by increasing DUSP6 activity. Nat Med. 2012;

58. Tugay K, Guay C, Marques AC, Allagnat F, Locke JM, Harries LW, Rutter GA, Regazzi R. Role of microRNAs in the age-associated decline of pancreatic beta cell function in rat islets. Diabetologia. 2016;59(1):161–9.

59. Tominaga N, Kosaka N, Ono M, Katsuda T, Yoshioka Y, Tamura K, Lotvall J, Nakagama H, Ochiya T. Brain metastatic cancer cells release microRNA-181c-containing extracellular vesicles capable of destructing blood-brain barrier. Nat Commun. 2015;6:6716.

60. Lu J, Getz G, Miska EA, Alvarez-Saavedra E, Lamb J, Peck D, Sweet-Cordero A, Ebert BL, Mak RH, Ferrando AA, et al. MicroRNA expression profiles classify human cancers. Nature. 2005;435(7043):834–8.

61. Naka H, Nakamura S, Shimazaki T, Okano H. Requirement for COUP-TFI and II in the temporal specification of neural stem cells in CNS development. Nat Neurosci. 2008;11(9):1014–23.

25

Human iPS cell-engineered three-dimensional cardiac tissues perfused by capillary networks between host and graft

Hidetoshi Masumoto[1,2,3,4]* and Jun K. Yamashita[3]*

Abstract

Stem cell-based cardiac regenerative therapy is expected to be a promising strategy for the treatment of severe heart diseases. Pluripotent stem cells enabled us to reconstruct regenerated myocardium in injured hearts as an engineered tissue aiming for cardiac regeneration. To establish a long-term survival of transplanted three-dimensional (3D) engineered heart tissues in vivo, it is indispensable to induce microcapillaries into the engineered tissues after transplantation. Using temperature-responsive culture surface, we have developed pluripotent stem cell-derived cardiac tissue sheets including multiple cardiac cell lineages. The application of gelatin hydrogel microsphere between the cell sheet stacks enabled us to generate thick stacked cell sheets with functional vascular network in vivo. Another technology to generate 3D engineered cardiac tissues using cardiac cells and biomaterials also validated successful induction of vascular network originated from both host and graft-derived vascular cells.

Keywords: Capillary network, 3D cardiac tissues, Human iPS cells, Cardiac regeneration

Background

Stem cell-based cardiac regeneration is a rapidly expanding paradigm to deliver therapeutic approaches for severe cardiac disorders resistant to current therapies [1, 2]. The discovery of human induced pluripotent stem cells (iPSCs) [3] opened the door toward in vitro formulation of human myocardium aiming for cardiac regeneration. Engineered three-dimensional (3D) myocardial tissue constructs generated from human iPSCs including multiple cardiovascular lineage constructs are more likely to replicate the dynamic organization and function of native myocardium and have emerged as a robust methodology to accomplish myocardial regeneration in animal heart disease models [4–7]. In the context of cell

transplantation to the heart, the 3D construct is reported to be advantageous over single cell injection into the myocardium because of the avoidance of mechanical loss related to the cell injection [8] and/or the higher survival efficiency *in vivo* [9].

In addition with the biophysical advantages of 3D structure in cell retainment after transplantation as described above, the introduction of microcapillaries is an important factor for long-term survival of the transplanted tissue. It is assumed that the transplanted tissue survives only through the direct diffusion of oxygen and nutrition at the initial stage of the transplantation, and vascular formation perfusing the whole engineered tissue would be indispensable for the long-term survival. It means that the successful cardiac regenerative strategy requires re-vascularization mechanisms to validate long-term myocardial regeneration.

Cell sheet-based thick cardiac tissues
Cell sheet formulation is one of the principal methods to generate 3D tissues from single cells [10]. Okano et al.

* Correspondence: hidetoshi.masumoto@riken.jp; juny@cira.kyoto-u.ac.jp
[1]Clinical Translational Research Program, RIKEN Center for Biosystems Dynamics Research, 2-2-3 Minatojima-minamimachi, Chuo-ku, Kobe, Hyogo 650-0047, Japan
[3]Department of Cell Growth and Differentiation, Center for iPS Cell Research and Application (CiRA), Kyoto University, 53 Shogoin Kawahara-cho, Sakyo-ku, Kyoto 606-8507, Japan
Full list of author information is available at the end of the article

reported a novel method to generate cell sheets using poly (N-isopropylacrylamide) (PIPAAm), a temperature-responsive polymer which changes the property of culture surface from hydrophobic to hydrophilic along with the lowering of the temperature which enables us to collect the confluent cell culture as a cell-sheet shape preserving attachment molecule and extracellular proteins without enzymatical digestion or physical damage [11]. Using this method, we have reported a formulation of human iPS cell-derived "cardiac tissue sheet (CTS)" including multiple cardiac cell lineages including cardiomyocytes and vascular cells (vascular endothelial cells, and mural cells), and a successful human myocardial regeneration and functional recovery mainly mediated by paracrine mechanisms such as angiogenesis in a rat myocardial infarction model [6]. However, the extent of the engraftment was not fully satisfactory requiring additional strategies to enhance the regenerative capacity.

It is also reported that the tissue thickening by the simple layering of cell sheets is limited for less than four layers because of the central necrosis due to the shortage of oxygen and nutrition supply [12]. To overcome this problem, we developed a cell-sheet stacking method to insert gelatin hydrogel microsphere (GHM), which is a biomaterial to work as a spacer between the cell sheets securing oxygen and nutrition supply among the whole cell sheet stacks. Using this method, we have reported a successful myocardial regeneration using mouse embryonic stem cell-derived CTSs in a rat MI model [13]. The engraftment efficiency of the stacked cell sheets with GHM was > 10 times higher than those without GHM. We also revealed that the transplantation of GHM-supported CTS stacks was secured by microcapillary network between host

and graft which was verified by the injection of fluorescent dye-conjugated lectin via venous system of the host which stained the capillaries inside the graft at 4 weeks after transplantation (Fig. 1a). We stained the nuclei of cells consisting CTSs with Hoechst 33342 before transplantation and confirmed that the vasculature perfusing the engrafted tissues were composed of graft-originated vascular cells. At 3 months after CTS-stack transplantation, the graft seems to be similar with bona fide myocardium perfused with vasculature allocated in every 50 μm which is supposed to be sufficient for the perfusion of the whole regenerated myocardium (Fig. 1b).

Another method to induce vascular networks into the cell sheet-based 3D structures is to generate "vascularized cardiac cell sheets" using bioreactors [14, 15]. In the study, the authors developed a bioreactor system using a femoral muscle-based and a synthetic collagen gel-based vascular beds which can provide fair perfusion throughout the 12-layered cell sheets. This novel system may also serve as a technology to induce vascular networks inside the engineered tissues.

Biomaterial-supported engineered cardiac tissue
Another format of 3D cardia tissue is biomaterials-supported engineered tissues which strongly support the structural stiffness of the artificial tissue structure [4, 16–18]. Taking advantages of a 3D cardiac tissue formation technology using rat [19] or chick [20] embryonic cardiac cells and a combination of biomaterials (collagen I, Matrigel), we have developed self-pulsating human iPS-derived engineered cardiac tissues (hiPS-C-ECTs) with cylindrical [5] and mesh-like [7] shapes.

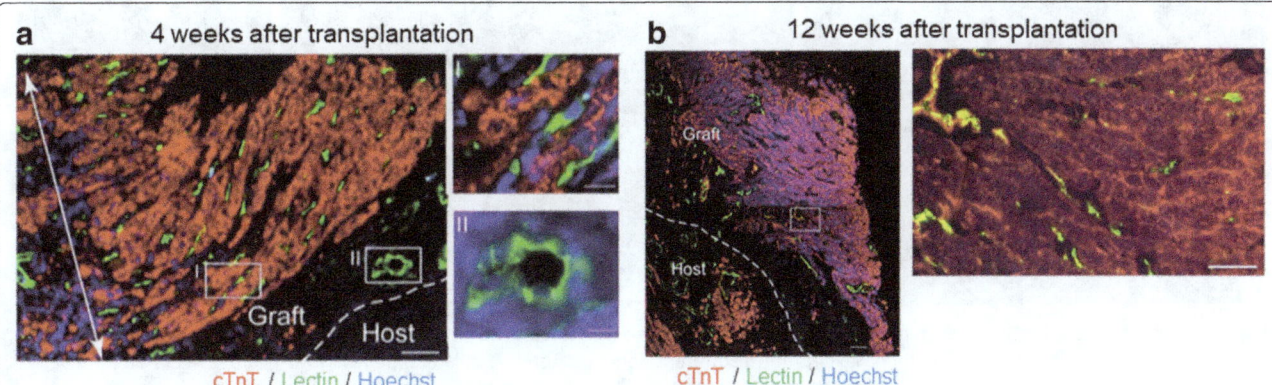

Fig. 1 Vascular network formation after mouse embryonic stem cell-derived thick cardiac tissue sheets with gelatin hydrogel microsphere. cTnT immunostaining for lectin (represents perfused vasculature)-perfused rat heart. Cardiomyocytes (cTnT, red), perfused vessels (lectin-stained, green), and pre-stained graft nuclei (Hoechst, blue). **a** Four weeks after transplantation. Note that thick regenerated myocardium (double-headed arrow) supported by dense perfused capillary networks (green) were formed. Capillaries (I) and larger vessels (II) in the graft (green) were largely Hoechst-positive. **b** Twelve weeks after transplantation. High magnification image of white box in the right panel. A compact myocardial tissue with capillary vessels was formed. cTnT, cardiac troponin T. Scale bars 100 μm in (**b**) (left), 50 μm in (**a**) and (**b**) (right), 10 μm in (**a**) (I-II). Referred from reference no. 13 with modifications

The incorporation of multiple cardiac cell lineages into the hiPSC-ECTs enhanced the tissue function including tissue stiffness evaluated by the measurement of Young's modulus, cardiomyocyte alignment, and sarcomeric ultrastructural maturation shown by transmission electron microscopy. The formulation of multiple lineages also validated a better force-frequency relationship which is known to be a parameter for tissue maturation [21].

The transplantation of hiPSC-ECTs onto a rat MI model revealed an increase of capillaries around the grafted tissue and a fair vascular network formation throughout the regenerated myocardium at 4 weeks after transplantation [5]. The injection of fluorescent dye-conjugated lectin via venous system of the host rat validated that the vascular network was functional to perfuse the regenerated myocardium (Fig. 2a). The immunohistochemical analyses for human nucleic antigen, specific for human cells, and von Willebrand factor, a specific marker for endothelial cells, showed that the vasculature inside the regenerated myocardium was composed of both host human and recipient rat cells (Fig. 2b). These results indicate that the transplanted hiPSC-ECTs can survive through the mechanism of vascular network formation between host and graft.

Mechanisms and significance of perfusion among engineered 3D constructs in vivo

In 3D cardiac tissue formats introduced above, the microcapillary network formation throughout the tissue contributed to the long-term survival of the tissues. It is possible that the mechanism of vascular network formation in vivo includes two different biological processes: (1) Angiogenesis mediated by paracrine factors from transplanted engineered tissues, and (2) physical contribution of transplanted vascular cells which can be incorporated into newly formed vasculatures inside the regenerated myocardium. The sufficient vascular formation by the collaboration of these processes might be advantageous for long-term 3D graft survival and a successful cardiac regenerative therapy. On the other hand, the required extent of in vitro vascular formulation prior to in vivo transplantation is still controversial. It may depend on the balance of the in vitro conditions such as cellular composition/maturation or culture microenvironment, and in vivo conditions of transplanted site such as oxygen concentration or vascular supply which depends on disease conditions of the recipient heart (Fig. 3). It requires further investigations to optimize the suitable formulation for an efficient vascular network formation in vivo and functional integration between host and graft.

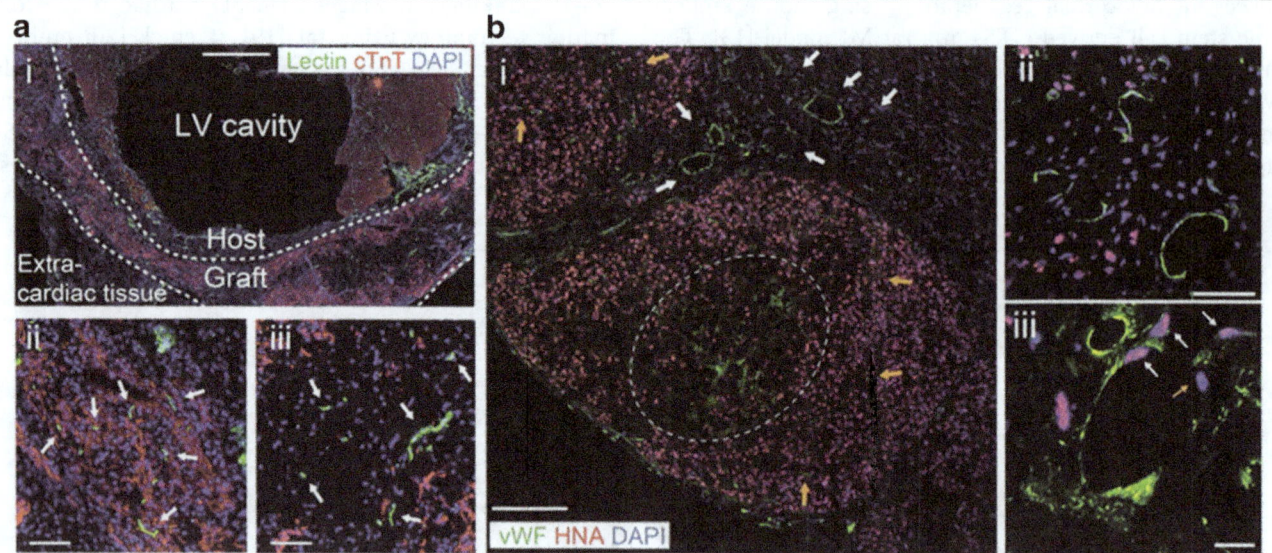

Fig. 2 Vascular network formation after human iPS cell-derived engineered cardiac tissues (hiPSC-ECTs) transplantation onto a rat myocardial infarction model. **a** cTnT immunostaining for lectin (represents perfused vasculature)-perfused rat heart 4 weeks after implantation of hiPSC-ECTs. (i) Lower magnification image. (ii) and (iii) Higher magnification images. Perfused vasculature among (ii) and at central area (iii) of regenerated myocardium (arrows). **b** vWF (endothelial cell marker) and HNA double immunostaining. (i) Lower magnification image. White arrows indicate promoted capillary formation around grafted tissue. Orange arrows indicate penetrating vasculature. White dotted line indicates vasculature in the center of grafted tissue. (ii) and (iii) Higher magnification images. (ii) Prominent host-derived (HNA⁻) vascular formation around regenerated myocardium. (iii) chimeric vasculature composed of both host (HNA⁻; orange arrow) and graft (HNA⁺; white arrows) vascular cells. cTnT, cardiac troponin-T; DAPI, 4, 6 diamidino-2-phenylindole; LV, left ventricle; vWF, von Willebrand factor; HNA, human nucleic antigen. Scale bars 1 mm in (**a**) (i), 200 μm in (**b**) (i), 100 μm in (**a**) (ii, iii), 50 μm in (**b**) (ii), 20 μm in (**b**) (iii). Referred from reference no. 5 with modifications

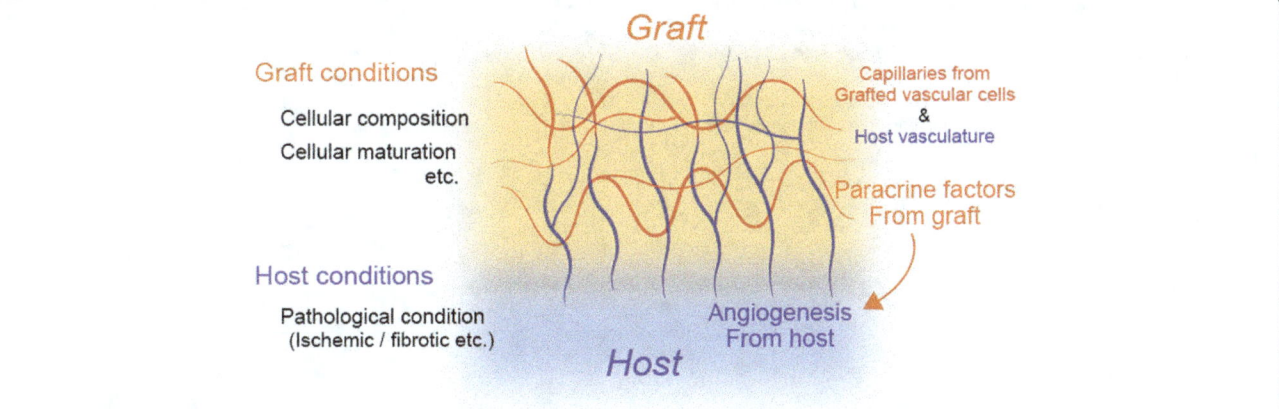

Fig. 3 Schematic summary of the mechanism of capillary formation in 3D cardiac tissue. Biological interaction between host and graft results in capillary formation throughout the graft securing long-term graft survival

Conclusion

In the present review, we introduced various strategies to induce microcapillaries for 3D engineered cardiac tissues aiming to promote the effectiveness of stem cell-based cardiac regenerative therapy. Further investigations for the post-transplantation vascularization are anticipated.

Authors' contributions
HM and JKY wrote the manuscript. Both authors read and approved the final manuscript.

Competing interests
The authors declare that they have no competing interests.

Author details
[1]Clinical Translational Research Program, RIKEN Center for Biosystems Dynamics Research, 2-2-3 Minatojima-minamimachi, Chuo-ku, Kobe, Hyogo 650-0047, Japan. [2]Clinical Translational Research Program, RIKEN Center for Developmental Biology, Kobe, Japan. [3]Department of Cell Growth and Differentiation, Center for iPS Cell Research and Application (CiRA), Kyoto University, 53 Shogoin Kawahara-cho, Sakyo-ku, Kyoto 606-8507, Japan. [4]Department of Cardiovascular Surgery, Kyoto University Graduate School of Medicine, Kyoto, Japan.

References

1. Menasche P. Cell therapy trials for heart regeneration - lessons learned and future directions. Nat Rev Cardiol. 2018; In press
2. Wu R, Hu X, Wang J. Concise review: optimized strategies for stem cell-based therapy in myocardial repair: clinical translatability and potential limitation. Stem Cells. 2018;36:482–500.
3. Takahashi K, Tanabe K, Ohnuki M, et al. Induction of pluripotent stem cells from adult human fibroblasts by defined factors. Cell. 2007;131:861–72.
4. Zimmermann WH, Melnychenko I, Wasmeier G, et al. Engineered heart tissue grafts improve systolic and diastolic function in infarcted rat hearts. Nat Med. 2006;12:452–8.
5. Masumoto H, Nakane T, Tinney JP, et al. The myocardial regenerative potential of three-dimensional engineered cardiac tissues composed of multiple human iPS cell-derived cardiovascular cell lineages. Sci Rep. 2016;6:29933.
6. Masumoto H, Ikuno T, Takeda M, et al. Human iPS cell-engineered cardiac tissue sheets with cardiomyocytes and vascular cells for cardiac regeneration. Sci Rep. 2014;4:6716.
7. Nakane T, Masumoto H, Tinney JP, et al. Impact of cell composition and geometry on human induced pluripotent stem cells-derived engineered cardiac tissue. Sci Rep. 2017;7:45641.
8. Teng CJ, Luo J, Chiu RCJ, et al. Massive mechanical loss of microspheres with direct intramyocardial injection in the beating heart: implications for cellular cardiomyoplasty. J Thorac Cardiovasc Surg. 2006;132:628–32.
9. Sekine H, Shimizu T, Dobashi I, et al. Cardiac cell sheet transplantation improves damaged heart function via superior cell survival in comparison with dissociated cell injection. Tissue Eng Part A. 2011;17:2973–80.
10. Masumoto H, Yamashita JK. Strategies in cell therapy for cardiac regeneration. Inflamm Regen. 2013;33:114–20.
11. Okano T, Yamada N, Sakai H, et al. A novel recovery-system for cultured-cells using plasma-treated polystyrene dishes grafted with poly (N-Isopropylacrylamide). J Biomed Mater Res. 1993;27:1243–51.
12. Shimizu T, Sekine H, Yang J, et al. Polysurgery of cell sheet grafts overcomes diffusion limits to produce thick, vascularized myocardial tissues. FASEB J. 2006;20:708–10.
13. Matsuo T, Masumoto H, Tajima S, et al. Efficient long-term survival of cell grafts after myocardial infarction with thick viable cardiac tissue entirely from pluripotent stem cells. Sci Rep. 2015;5:16842.
14. Sakaguchi K, Shimizu T, Okano T. Construction of three-dimensional vascularized cardiac tissue with cell sheet engineering. J Control Release. 2015;205:83–8.
15. Sekine H, Shimizu T, Okano T. Cell sheet tissue engineering for heart failure. In: Nakanishi T, Markwald RR, Baldwin HS, et al., editors. Etiology and Morphogenesis of Congenital Heart Disease: From Gene Function and Cellular Interaction to Morphology. Tokyo: Springer; 2016. p. 19–24. https://www.springer.com/la/book/9784431546276.
16. Eschenhagen T, Zimmermann WH. Engineering myocardial tissue. Circ Res. 2005;97:1220–31.
17. Tulloch NL, Muskheli V, Razumova MV, et al. Growth of engineered human myocardium with mechanical loading and vascular coculture. Circ Res. 2011;109:47–59.
18. Ruan JL, Tulloch NL, Razumova MV, et al. Mechanical stress conditioning and electrical stimulation promote contractility and force maturation of induced pluripotent stem cell-derived human cardiac tissue. Circulation. 2016;134:1557–67.
19. Fujimoto KL, Clause KC, Liu LJ, et al. Engineered fetal cardiac graft preserves its cardiomyocyte proliferation within postinfarcted myocardium and sustains cardiac function. Tissue Eng A. 2011;17:585–96.

20. Tobita K, Liu LJ, Janczewski AM, et al. Engineered early embryonic cardiac tissue retains proliferative and contractile properties of developing embryonic myocardium. Am J Physiol Heart Circ Physiol. 2006;291:H1829–37.

21. Ronaldson-Bouchard K, Ma SP, Yeager K, et al. Advanced maturation of human cardiac tissue grown from pluripotent stem cells. Nature. 2018;556:239–43.

26

Piezoelectric smart biomaterials for bone and cartilage tissue engineering

Jaicy Jacob, Namdev More, Kiran Kalia and Govinda Kapusetti[*]

Abstract

Tissues like bone and cartilage are remodeled dynamically for their functional requirements by signaling pathways. The signals are controlled by the cells and extracellular matrix and transmitted through an electrical and chemical synapse. Scaffold-based tissue engineering therapies largely disturb the natural signaling pathways, due to their rigidity towards signal conduction, despite their therapeutic advantages. Thus, there is a high need of smart biomaterials, which can conveniently generate and transfer the bioelectric signals analogous to native tissues for appropriate physiological functions. Piezoelectric materials can generate electrical signals in response to the applied stress. Furthermore, they can stimulate the signaling pathways and thereby enhance the tissue regeneration at the impaired site. The piezoelectric scaffolds can act as sensitive mechanoelectrical transduction systems. Hence, it is applicable to the regions, where mechanical loads are predominant. The present review is mainly concentrated on the mechanism related to the electrical stimulation in a biological system and the different piezoelectric materials suitable for bone and cartilage tissue engineering.

Keywords: Piezoelectricity, Piezoelectric materials, Bone, Cartilage, Tissue regeneration, Electroactive scaffolds, Mechanical stimulation

Background

Smart materials are in general discussed to the materials, which can reversibly modify one or more of its functional or structural properties, according to the imposed external stimulus or to the modifications in their surrounding conditions [1]. The external stimulus includes physical (temperature, light, electric or magnetic fields), chemical (pH) and mechanical stimuli (stress and strain). Piezoelectric materials are considered as smart materials owing to the fact that these materials can transduce the mechanical pressure acting on it to the electrical signals (called direct piezoelectric effect) and electrical signals to mechanical signals (called converse piezoelectric effect) [2]. The basic requirement of material to exhibit piezoelectricity depends on its crystal lattice structure and the lack of a center of symmetry [3]. Pierre Curie and Jacques Curie in 1880 have discovered the phenomenon. The word *"piezo"* originates from the Greek word *"piezein"* meaning pressure [4].

Piezoelectric materials have a wide variety of electronic applications such as transducers, actuators and sensors. Moreover, piezoelectric materials have significant applications in tissue engineering as an electroactive scaffold for tissue repair and regeneration. They can deliver variable electrical stimulus without an external power source [5]. The electrical stimulation resulting from piezoelectric scaffold can regenerate and repair the tissues by definite pathways [6]. The piezoelectric scaffolds with optimized properties can produce suitable bioelectrical signals, similar to the natural extracellular matrix (ECM), which has observed during remodeling phenomenon in bone and cartilage [7].

The electro-active scaffolds are most significant in tissue engineering where the electrical stimulation is relevant for the tissue repair or regeneration, such as, neuronal tissue repair, bone and cartilage repair and regeneration etc. [8]. Tissues like bone, cartilage, dentin, tendon and keratin can demonstrate direct piezoelectricity [9]. Collagen is a fiber-like structure and it is major constituent in bone and cartilage, responsible for the piezoelectric property [10]. Due to the piezoelectric property of collagen, it can generate electric signals in response to internal forces. These

* Correspondence: govindphysics@gmail.com
Department of Medical Devices, National Institute of Pharmaceutical Education and Research, Ahmedabad 380054, India

signals transmitted through ECM to the voltage-gated channels in the cell membrane. Mainly, the osteocyte cells are involved in mechanotransduction and they communicate with other cells such as osteoblasts and osteoclasts. The activation of these channels transmits the intracellular signals to the nucleus, leads to the activation of signaling cascades, responsible for the cellular events such as matrix production, cell growth and tissue repair [11]. Hence, the electro-active scaffolds, which mimics the piezoelectric coefficients of natural tissues may be a suitable approach for the repair and regeneration of skeletal tissues like bone and cartilage.

Bone and cartilage are dense connective tissues, which consist mainly cells and extracellular matrix (ECM) (Fig. 1). In general, ECM consists two main cell types immature and mature, the immature cell in cartilage and bone are chondroblast and osteoblast, respectively. Vitally, the blast cells have the capacity to cell division and further it secretes the ECM. Subsequently the blast cells differentiate into mature cells like chondrocytes and osteocytes, in cartilage and bone respectively. Matured cells are mostly encompassing in conserving the matrix and it has limited capacity for cell division and matrix production [12].

Other cells present in the matrix are fibroblasts, macrophages, adipocytes and mast cells.

ECM is well distributed among the cells, and provides a microenvironment to perform their regular activities and functions. Besides, via ECM, the signals are transmitted to the cell membrane receptors, which activates intracellular signaling cascades and this provides stimuli to the nucleus [13]. The stimuli will further regulate the transcription of several proteins, which have a significant role to regulate cell functionality. Beyond these, ECM can regulate their size and shape according to the changes in the external loads [14]. The characteristic of ECM differs based on the embedded cell type. The bone has rigid/inflexible ECM, while; cartilage has flexible ECM due to the presence of different cells. Further, structurally cartilage is avascular, but all connective tissues including bone are highly vascular.

Generally, ECM structure comprises a hydrated network of glycosaminoglycan chains, with various interwoven protein fibrils and fibers. The bone has abundant ECM, composed of 25% water, 25% organic collagen fibers and 50% crystallized mineral salts [15]. The inorganic mineral salts in the form of microcrystalline, such as hydroxyapatite $[Ca_{10} (PO4)_6 (OH)_2]$ confer the hardness and mostly rigidity of the bone [16]. The mineral salts like calcium hydroxide and calcium phosphate combined to form centrosymmetric hydroxyapatite nanocrystals, which further combines with other mineral salts and ions such as magnesium, fluoride and manganese. These crystals were deposited in the network of collagen fibers, which further undergoing a process called calcination. The entire process is initiated by bone formation cells (osteoblasts) [15]. Compact bone has mostly type I collagen and has the piezoelectric coefficient approximately 0.7pC/N [17].

The ECM of cartilage comprises of collagen (type II, VI, IX, X and XI), proteoglycan, non-collagenous proteins and tissue fluid. Collagen is strong and flexible structure and can resist the pulling forces [18]. Among all, cartilage is compose of 90–95% type II collagen and the primary function is to resist tension [19]. The piezoelectric collagen can influence the cell membrane receptors and ultimately the nucleus owing to electrical charge alterations in response to functional loads [20].

The deformities and injuries in hard tissues like, bone and cartilage can occur, primarily, due to mechanical trauma and various disease conditions. The osteoporosis, paget disease, ricket, osteomalacia, osteoarthritis, osteomyelitis, and osteosarcoma mainly contribute bone degeneration [21]. Cartilage degeneration is primarily, due to gaut, osteoarthritis, acromegaly and alkeptonuric ochronosis [22].

Conventional therapies include pharmacological treatments such as, estrogens and selective estrogen receptor modulator (e.g. tamoixifen, ralaoxifen and nafoxidine) [23], biphosphonates (e.g. alendronate, zoledronate and pomidronate) [24], anti-inflammatory molcules (e.g. NSAID, indomethacine and aspirin) [25]. However, major limitation

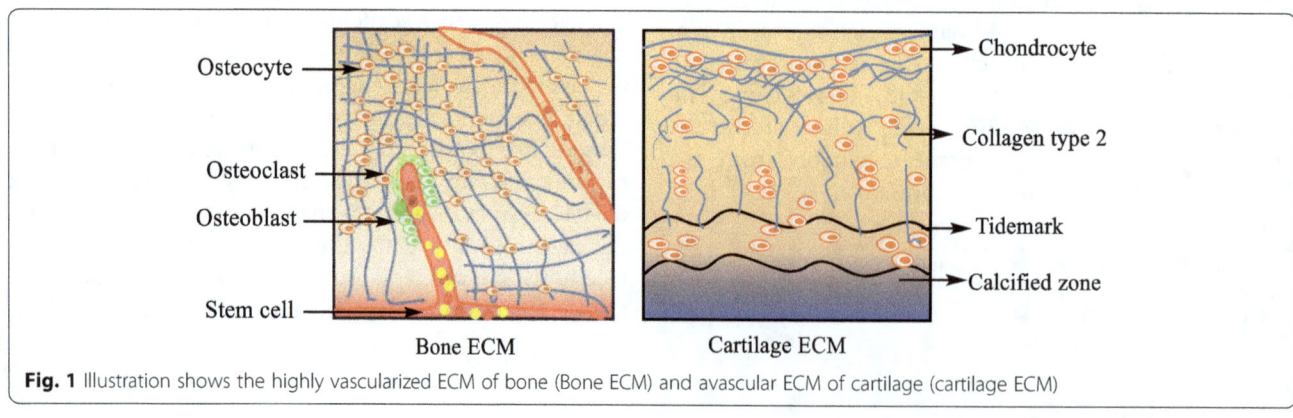

Fig. 1 Illustration shows the highly vascularized ECM of bone (Bone ECM) and avascular ECM of cartilage (cartilage ECM)

of the pharmacological therapies are disease dependent, less effective in case of critical degeneration, lack of site specificity and drug associated toxicity [26]. Surgical intervention is an important treatment choice; the major practices are autograft, allograft, xenograft, bone marrow stimulation, mosacoplsty and autologous chondrocyte implantation. The surgical practices have success rate up to some extent, the major limitations come from; donor site morbidity, due to secondary surgery associated with autograft and allograft. Furthermore, immunogenic rejection and disease transmission as consequence of allograft and xenograft practices [27–29]. Bone marrow stimulation has poor regenerative capacity and the regenerated cartilage has low biomechanical integrity [30], the donor site morbidity also associated with mosiacplasty [31]. The autologous chondrocyte implantation is a costly practice and complicated process, it is not recommended for osteoarthritis [32].

In recent years, researchers are seen tissue engineering approach as an effective alternative for hard tissue regeneration and repair. The advanced tissue engineering methodology is a mutli-displinary technique. It is an amalgamation of engineering and the life science principle for the repair, replace, maintain, or enhance the function of a tissue and related organ. The tissue engineering aspects broadly covers the cell seeded, growth factor implanted, drug loaded and other bioactive molecule loaded scaffolds [33]. Basically, the cell based therapy utilizes various cell types like, mesenchymal stem cells (MSCs), embryonic stem cells (ESCs) and induced pluripotent stem cells (iPSC) [34, 35]. The growth factor such as transforming growth factor-β, bone morphogenic protein – 2, bone morphogenic protein-4 etc. are frequently used in bone and cartilage tissue engineering [36]. Various causes restrict the use of cell-based and growth factor based therapies for cartilage and bone regeneration exercises. In cell-based therapies; chondrogenic and osteogenic potentials differ from their source, cell senescence, unpredictable differentiation because of improper microenvironment, the initial insufficient nutrient and hypoxic condition at implanted site lead to irregular outcomes. The growth factor based therapies are highly expensive, involves complicate experimental process, high instability, hazy selection (no standard criteria for the selection of growth factor), dose related complications, short half-life and scalability [37–43]. Hence, there is a high need of safe and effective alternatives to regeneration and repair of complex tissue like bone and cartilage.

The advancement in material science and engineering to develop specialized materials to crack the baffling problems by introducing so-called smart materials in various applications [44–46]. The smart material is described as, variation of at least one property of material is stable, reproducible and significant, when material is subjected to external stimuli. It is well reported that, the classification of smart materials typically depend on its output response, which includes piezoelectric materials, materials develop stable and reproducible electric signals, when mechanical stresses applied and vice-versa; large deformations can be induced and recovered in presence of temperature or stress variations in shape memory smart materials; temperature responsive materials, pH sensitive materials, self-healing materials and thermoelectric materials etc. [47–49].

Piezoelectricity has shown its strong effectiveness in natural pathways, specifically at the site where the collagen implicated activities. The compressive force on collagen triggers the re-organization of dipole moment and generates negative charges on the surface [50]. The generated charge prompts the electrical stimulation to the cells, leads to the opening of voltage-gated calcium channels. The increased activity of intracellular calcium concentration activates the calmodulin, which subsequently stimulates the activation of calcineurin. The calcineurin dephosphorylates NF-AT (Nuclear Factor of Activated Cells), which further translocate into the nucleus, where it binds co-operatively with other transcription factors to regulatory regions of the inducible genes. These genes further induce the translation of several growth factors like Transforming Growth Factorβ (TGF β), Bone Morphogenetic Protein (BMP) etc. which are responsible for the regulation of ECM production as well as up/ down regulation of several proteins and cellular metabolism [38, 51]. Various studies were reported that the electrical stimulation can produce TGF β through calcium/ calmodulin pathway and the TGF β is the potential key factor to promote the cellular processes including cell growth and differentiation, extracellular matrix synthesis, inflammation and tissue repair (Fig. 2). These pleiotropic actions of TGFβ are due to its involvement in either inhibition or stimulation of some common regulatory pathways responsible for the cellular events [52]. It is an important growth factor for the formation of bone and cartilage [53].

In general, tensile/compression forces acting on the piezoelectric scaffolds generates the electrical stimulation and transfers it to the surrounding cells, promotes the cell signaling pathways, responsible for the growth factor synthesis (Scheme 1). The mechanism behind the conversion of mechanical stimuli into biochemical signals remains elusive [54]. It is well evident that the piezoelectric collagen stimulates the cell proliferation (tissue regeneration) by electrical stimuli via mechanotrasduction. The collagen possesses polar hexagonal crystalline unit and it is primarily responsible for piezoelectricity [55]. The literature strongly suggests that the collagen rich bone converts the functional stresses into electrical stimulations for regeneration and remodeling. The electrical stimulation is largely contributes in cell phynotypic change [56]. Mechanical stimulation has

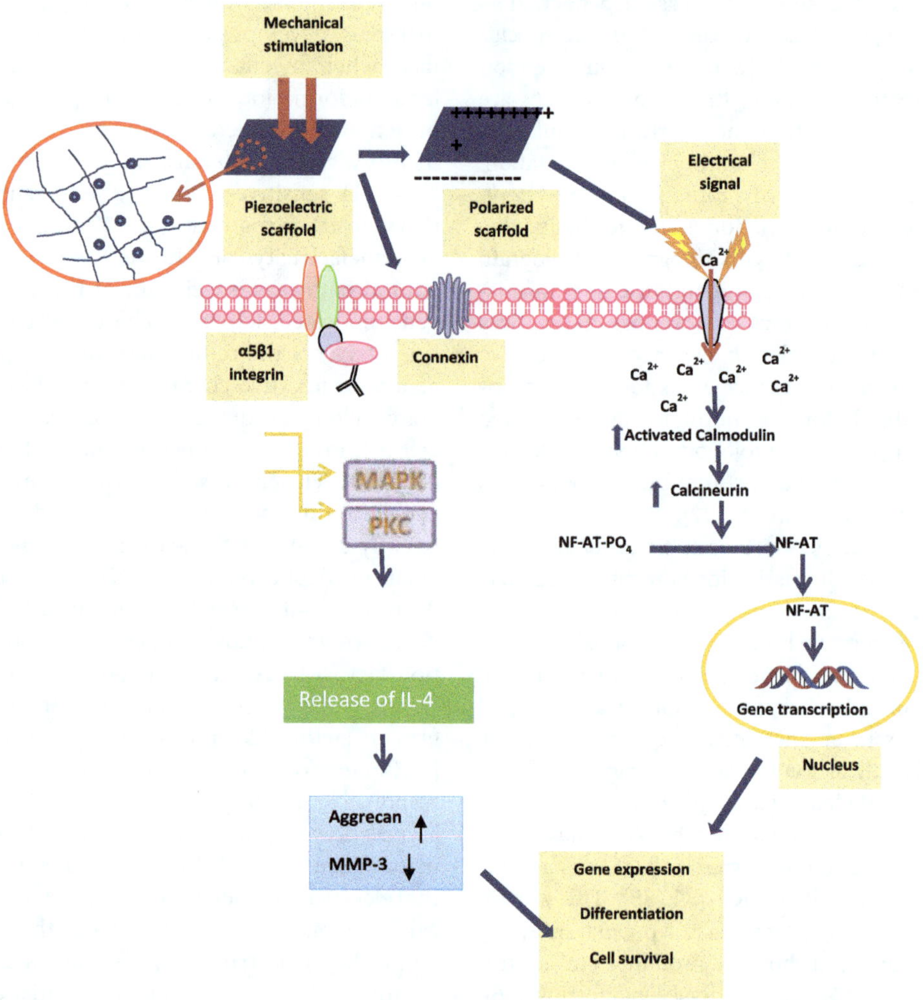

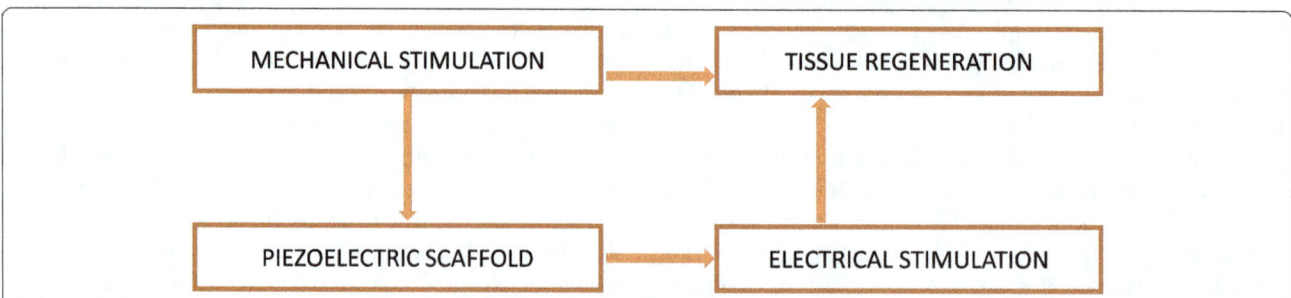

Fig. 2 Schematic diagram of ca^{2+} signal transduction pathway and other miscellaneous pathways activate in response to the electrical and mechanical stimulations. The mechanical stimulation on piezoelectric scaffold will result in the electrical signal generation and which will stimulate the voltage-gated ca^{2+} channel. Further increase in the intracellular Ca^{2+} concentration activates the calmodulin (an abbreviation of the calcium-modulated protein) and which will further activate the calcineurin (calcium and calmodulin-dependent serine/threonine protein phosphatase). The activated calcineurin dephosphorylates the NF-AT and it will translocate to the nucleus, where it acts in conjunction with other associated proteins as transcription factors. Also the mechanical stimulation itself can activate the mechanoreceptors present in the membrane and which will lead to the activation of PKC and MAPK signaling cascades. These cascades will result in the synthesis of proteoglycan and inhibition of IL-1, responsible for the breakdown of proteoglycan

Scheme 1 Representing the tissue regeneration in response to the mechanical stimulation on the piezoelectric scaffold. The mechanical force on the piezoelectric scaffold generates the electrical stimulus for enhanced tissue regeneration. At the same time, applied mechanical stress can simultaneously augments the tissue regeneration in predefined signaling pathways

some major constrains like, sensitization of bone cell, age related issue like higher the age poor the regenerative capacity [57]. The mechanotransduction pathway involves the stretch-activated ion channels, $\alpha 5\beta 1$ and an autocrine/paracrine interleukin-4 (IL-4) loop (Fig. 2) [58]. The $\alpha 5\beta 1$ integrin is a major mechanoreceptor present in the chondrocyte and bone cells [59]. The activation of $\alpha 5\beta 1$ integrin as a result of the mechanical stresses, followed by translocation of the protein kinase C (PKC) to the cell membrane. Hence, the integrin-dependent PKC associated signaling cascades including Ras/Rac dependent MAP Kinase pathway has been activated [60]. The activation of PKC increases the activation of proteoglycan synthesis, inhibits the interleukin-1 (IL-1) induced proteoglycan breakdown and inhibition of proteoglycan synthesis [58].

Piezoelectric materials

To induce piezoelectric property in the scaffold, the best possible way is to select appropriate piezoelectric material; either, piezoelectric polymer or ceramic or polymer-ceramic composite for fabrication of bio-scaffold. Hence, piezoelectric materials are best suits for biomedical applications, where the electromechanical transduction involves. The property possesses to the material due to lack of center of symmetry [61]. The deformation of such materials results in the development of charges of opposite polarity on opposite faces of crystals. Fundamentally this is due to the separation of the center of neutrality of charges on the crystal lattice as the material is deformed along certain axes. The term applies to some polycrystalline, inorganic materials and some inorganic substances [9]. Piezoelectric materials can also be classifies as piezoelectric polymers and piezoelectric ceramics. The piezoelectric ceramics are included in the polycrystalline class [62]. Piezoelectric materials are using either alone or as a composite in tissue engineering.

Piezoelectric polymers

The properties of piezoelectric polymers are different from inorganic crystals, since these possess the advantage of processing flexibility. Mechanically, polymers have high strength and high impact resistance as compared to inorganic materials. Structural requirements of piezoelectric polymers are (1) the presence of permanent molecular dipoles (2) the ability to align or orient the molecular dipoles (3) the ability to sustain the alignment once it is achieve and (4) the ability of the material to undergo large strains when mechanically stressed [63]. The piezoelectric polymers, which are used in tissue engineering for cartilage and bone as follows:

PVDF (poly(vinylidene fluoride))

PVDF is a best known piezoelectric copolymer with the piezoelectric coefficient of 20 pC/N [64]. Due to its high flexibility and non-toxicity, PVDF have been used for a variety of biomedical applications, from tissue engineering scaffolds to implantable self-powered devices [65]. PVDF-TrFE and barium titanate piezoelectric composite membrane has been reported as charge generator to promote the bone regeneration [66]. Martins et al. were well demonstrated the potential application of PVDF scaffolds in skeletal muscle regeneration. After corona poling of the PVDF scaffolds the formed negatively charged surfaces promote better cell adhesion and proliferation of myoblast cells [67]. The piezoelectric PVDF scaffold has been largely promoting the osteogenic differentiation of human adipose-derived stem cells [68]. A novel piezoelectric actuator device based on PVDF has been demonstrated to effectively stimulate the bone growth at the bone-implant interface by the use of converse piezoelectric effect [69]. Furthermore, PVDF and PVDF-TrFE has been reported for neural tissue regeneration [70]. The PVDF is well known biocompatible thermoplastic polymer. It has high chemical and physical resistance. Still when it expose to the extreme alkaline condition it tends to degrade but not suitable for biological environment [71]. However, the PVDF is a non-biodegradable polymer which limits its applicability in tissue engineering [72].

P(VDF-TrFE)

It is a copolymer of vinylidene fluoride (VDF) and trifluoroethylene (TrFE). The copolymer has been demonstrated highest piezoelectric coefficient (30 pC/N) among the polymers [73]. It was reported that the copolymer is cytocompatible and shown positive influence on cell adhesion and cell proliferation [74]. The polymer has an ability to regenerate the different type of tissues like, bone, skin, cartilage and tendon [75].The electrospun nanofibrous based scaffold of PVDF-TrFE copolymer have been regenerated neural and articular cartilage very efficiently [5]. The piezoelectric fibers can be stimulated the differentiable cells into mature phenotype and have an ability to promote stem cell-induced tissue repair [7]. Currently, the blends of polymers for bone and cartilage tissue engineering are gaining more importance. Furthermore, the PVDF and PVDF-TrFE have been blended with starch or cellulose-like natural polymer to develop suitable scaffold structures for tissue repair and regeneration, particularly for bone tissue engineering. The starch or cellulose is blended to produce a porous structure to support tissue growth [76].

PHBV (poly- 3- hydroxybutyrate-3-hydroxy valerate)

PHBV is a member of PHAs and it is gaining importance in biomedical field because of its biocompatibility, biodegradability and its thermoplasticity [77]. Moreover, it has longer degradation time than other biocompatible polymer and remarkably it has piezoelectric coefficient (1.3 pC/N) similar to human bone [78, 79]. The studies had been reported the collagen-PHBV matrices for cartilage tissue engineering because of its biocompatibility and more extended biodegradation rate [80]. PHBV has been degraded by enzymatic degradation mechanism, subsequent hydrolysis and release the carbon dioxide [81]. Biodegradable PHBV-HA composite had been demonstrated for bone tissue engineering [77]. Similarly various studies had been reported the use of PHBV as matrices for cartilage and bone regeneration while, the utilization of piezoelectric property of PHBV for bone and cartilage regeneration is not till reported.

Polyamides

Polyamides and polypeptides possess piezoelectricity by odd numbered Nylons and peptide (CONH) bonds, respectively [64]. Odd nylons (nylons-5, nylons-7) contains even numbered methylene groups and one amide group on each monomer unit. Due to the presence of one amide group, odd numbered nylon results net dipole moment (3.7 D) [82]. The piezoelectric polarization proceeds as a consequence of the stress-induced internal rotation of the peptide bonds [83]. The piezoelectric coefficient (d_{31}) for nylon is 3 pC/N at 25 °C and 14 pC/N at 107 °C [82]. Wang et al., have been reported that polyamide-hydroxyapatite composite promotes the osteogenesis by 12 weeks of implantation [84]. Also studies had been reported that the polyamides are applicable for cartilage repair or regeneration as a polymeric matrix. But proper modifications are required to promote the cell attachment and proliferation of chondrocytes [85]. Lack of degradation pattern of the polyamides has limited applications in tissue engineering.

Poly-l-lactic acid (PLLA)

Poly-L-lactic acid is a biodegradable and biocompatible polymer, along with it has a large shear piezoelectric coefficient. The piezoelectric shear coefficient of PLLA (d_{14}) is – 10 pC/N [73]. Due to its helical structure, it doesn't require poling for generation of piezoelectricity. Moreover, the mechanical orientation of molecules in the crystals and the quasi-crystalline region is enough to generate piezoelectricity. Fukada, et al. has demonstrated that implantation of PLLA can promote the bone growth in the response of its piezoelectric polarization [86]. PLLA has huge clinical application in orthopedics such as screws and pins, due to its strong mechanical properties. The PLLA is degraded by hydrolytic degradation and the byproduct is PLA, which is nontoxic and water-soluble. The degradable PLLA has been well documented for rapid bone regeneration by consuming its piezoelectric property [73].

Biopolymers

Natural polymers are gaining more importance in tissue engineering because of their degradability and low toxicity. More than that, the polymers have offer biological signaling, cell adhesion, cell responsive degradation and remodeling [17]. Meanwhile, their use as a unique scaffold material has often compromise owing to their inadequate physical properties, together with the possible loss of biological properties during formulations. Moreover, appropriate screening and processing are required to avoid the disease transmission and immune rejection. While suitable chemical or physical processing will help to overcome these issues [87].

Cellulose

Cellulose is the most abundant natural polymer on earth and it has a piezoelectric property with a shear piezoelectric coefficient (d_{14}) 0.2 pC/N [88]. It has large number biomedical applications, due to excellent biocompatibility, high tensile strength and impersonates with biological environment, despite its water content and nanofibrous structure. While, it has a small pore size or the dense mesh formation of fibers limits the cell infiltration. However this can be overcome by the incorporation of proper porogens. Moreover, studies have been demonstrated that the ability of cellulose to promote cellular adhesion particularly chondrocytes, osteocytes, endothelial cells and smooth muscle cells [89]. Hence, it is appropriate piezoelectric material for both bone and cartilage tissue engineering.

Collagen

Collagen is a biological protein and vital component of the ECM like bone, cartilage, tendon, teeth and blood vessels, where it responsible for the structural and mechanical support [90]. It is a natural piezoelectric material with piezoelectric coefficient ranges from 0.2 to 2.0 pC/N [79]. Additionally, it is suitable as a biomaterial in tissue engineering due to its biocompatibility, good cell binding properties, hydrophilicity, low antigenicity, absorbability in the body etc. [17]. The researchers had been reported the application of collagen scaffold in bone healing [91]. Similarly the collagen-hydroxyapatite piezoelectric composite scaffold has been proved as a suitable structure for cellular growth and bone healing [92]. Also the collagen-calcium phosphate composite scaffolds are reported for cartilage tissue engineering. Studies with collagen-calcium phosphate composite scaffolds are demonstrated the average filling ratio of the defect area with the newly formed cartilage tissue at week eight and twenty is about 81% and 96%, respectively [80]. However, it has certain limitations like low mechanical stiffness, rapid degradation and toxicity by addition of crosslinking agents.

Chitin

Chitin is a natural polysaccharide and is the structural component of the cuticles of crustaceans, insects and mollusks. It has a piezoelectric structure with piezoelectric coefficient ranges from 0.2–1.5 pC/N depending upon its source [79]. Chitosan is a polymer which is obtained by the deacetylation of chitin, has a number of biomedical applications such as wound healing and carriers for controlled drug delivery etc. [93]. By making it composite with other suitable filler components it is suitable for bone and cartilage regeneration. Chitin largely favors for biomedical applications, since it is a hydrophilic material, which promotes cell adhesion, cell proliferation, differentiation and it offers well biocompatibility [17]. But, low mechanical properties and inability to maintain predefined shape, limits its use in tissue engineering particularly for hard tissue applications.

Piezoceramics

A large number of piezoceramics are available with a very high piezoelectric coefficient, such as lead zirconate titanate (PZT), barium titanate (BT), zinc oxide (ZnO), potassium sodium niobate (KNN), lithium sodium potassium niobate (LNPN) and boron nitride nanotubes (BNNT). The common concern related piezoceramics in tissue engineering is its cytotoxicity. In general, lead contained ceramics have limited application in tissue engineering due to their toxic nature. The PZT possess the very high piezoelectric constant ranges from 200 to 350 pC/N is a highly cytotoxicity [94]. Hence, PZT would not be preferred in tissue engineering application and the lead-free piezo ceramics could be an alternative choice. Other ceramic also have dose dependent toxicity so they are applicable for tissue engineering up to some extent.

Barium Titanate

Barium titanate (BT) is highly biocompatible with d_{33} coefficient of 191pC/N [3]. It has been reported that the BT nanoparticles have demonstrated cytocompatibility, even at higher concentrations like 100 μg/ml [95]. The studies have been demonstrated that the PLGA matrix reinforced with BT nanoparticles supports the cell attachment and proliferation of osteoblast and osteocytes [96]. Also, TiO_2 powders have the ability to improve the osteoconductivity hence have improved efficacy to promote osteoblast adhesion [97]. Significantly, it has been reported that the piezoelectric property of BT has a positive influence on the cellular proliferation [98]. Furthermore, the incorporation of barium titanate nanoparticles into the polymeric matrix would improve the mechanical properties of the composite scaffold structure [99]. Hence, it is quite evident that the piezoelectric

BT has an ability to promote the cellular activities in tissue engineering applications.

Zinc oxide

Zinc has a critical role in cell proliferation and differentiation in the biological system by modulating the activity of different enzymes including transcription factors, metalloproteinase and polymerases [100]. Piezoelectric zinc oxide has not shown any toxic effects in micrometer and larger size ranges [101], but it has been demonstrated toxicity in nano size due to the production of reactive oxygen species [102]. Significant results has reported on zinc oxide nanoparticles dispersed in the polymeric scaffold along with hypoxia have shown ability to synthesis cartilage [103]. According to Material Safe Data Sheet (MSDS) databases LD50 of acute oral ZnO is 7950 mg/kg for mice shows no significant toxicity [104]. Moreover, the cytotoxicity of the nanoparticles can be reduced by chemical and physical modification for medical application [102].

Potassium sodium Niobate (KNN) and lithium sodium potassium Niobate (LKNN)

KNN and LKNN are lead free piezoelectric ceramic materials with piezoelectric coefficient 63 pC/N and 98 pC/N, respectively [105]. Addition of lithium (Li) has largely enhanced piezoelectric properties, while it would increase the cytotoxicity due to the release of Li ions when it is exposed to the bioenvironment [65]. The electric charge of the ferroelectric lithium niobate crystals enhances the proliferation and osteoblastic activity to rapid bone regeneration [106]. It has been reported that the utilization of piezoelectric property of KNN in drug delivery devices and also it is applicable for bone, cartilage, skin and nerve repair and regeneration [107].

Boron nitride

Boron nitride nanotube has superior piezoelectric property than that of piezoelectric polymers [108]. Researchers are exploited BNNTs as nano vectors to carry electrical /mechanical stimuli on demand within a cellular system. After BNNT internalization, the electrical stimulation has conveyed to tissue or/ cell culture using a wireless mechanical source (i.e., ultrasound) (Fig. 3). Its cytocompatibility can be improved by improving its dispersibility in the solvents. It is reported that its dispersibility can be improved by non-covalent polymeric wrapping or by using non-toxic surfactants, which has been increased its potential for biomedical application [109]. The proper functionalization of BNNT with glycol-chitosan or the addition of surfactant poly-L-lysine (PLL) or polyethyleneimine (PEI) results in the formation of BNNT dispersion and improves the cytocompatibility of BNNT [110]. The studies have been

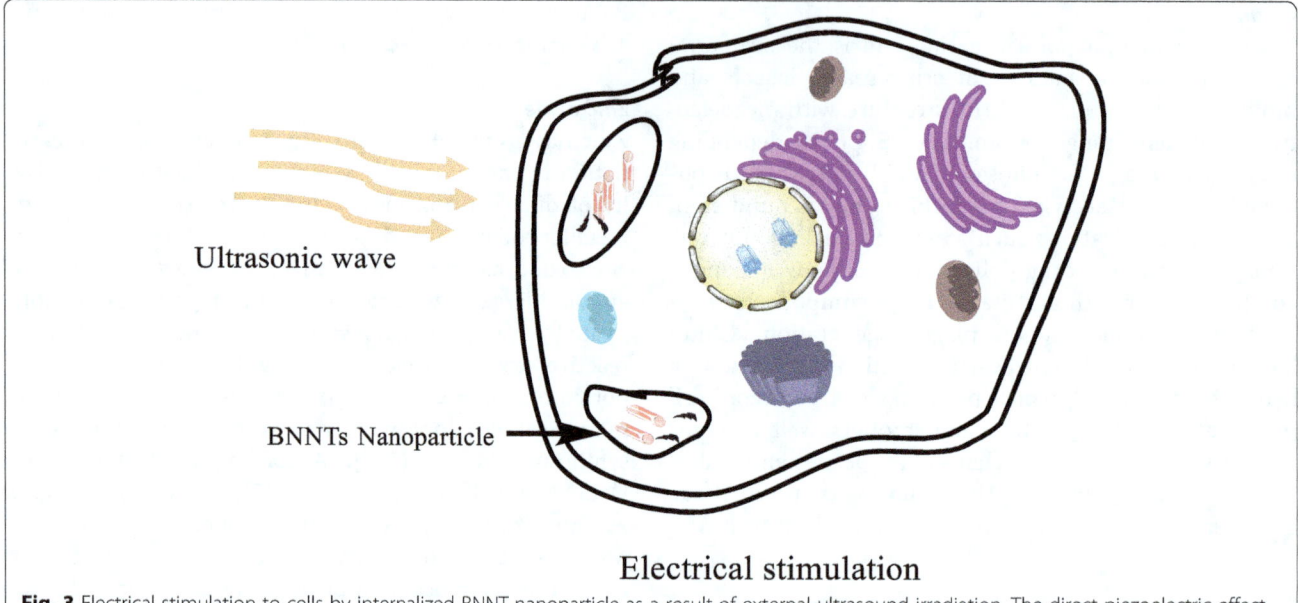

Fig. 3 Electrical stimulation to cells by internalized BNNT nanoparticle as a result of external ultrasound irradiation. The direct piezoelectric effect applied on BNNTs and ultrasonic wave as mechanical stress to convert into electrical stimuli for enhanced cell differentiation

demonstrated that biodegradable polymeric scaffold reinforced with BNNT has a positive influence on osteoblast proliferation and differentiation [111, 112]. The studies report that the BNNT has a negative influence on the chondrocytes, fibroblast and smooth muscle cells. It decreases the adhesion of chondrocytes, fibroblasts and smooth muscle cells while it can increase the adhesion of osteoblast cells [110]. Moreover, it has excellent mechanical properties and highly crucial for orthopedic applications [113]. Hence BNNT is an excellent material for bone tissue engineering.

Future prospective

Piezoelectric collagen fibers are present in cartilage and bone, but the function of piezoelectricity is not yet fully investigated. The piezoelectric material can act as a mechanoelectrical transducer. The electroactive scaffolds can generate the electric field in response to minute mechanical vibrations. Also the scaffold of piezoelectric material can be tuned the effective electric field characteristics of the natural ECM observed during development, regeneration or repair of the tissues. The scaffold can directly influence the osteoblast or chondroblast cells and can promote its adhesion and proliferation, further the production of ECM and thereby repair of damaged sites. Moreover it can stimulate the mesenchymal stem cells directly and further its differentiation into chondroblasts or osteoblasts. Therefore, the smart piezoelectric biomaterials require strong attention towards tissue engineering, particularly bone, cartilage and nerve regeneration. These materials will offer natural physiological conditions like ECM to regulate the signaling pathways to stimulate the

regeneration mechanism. Significantly, the piezoelectric scaffolds can enhance the cell functionality without the addition of growth factors and drug molecules. The stimulating factors implanted treatments are highly expensive, highly instable (extra and random growth of tissue), complicated selection criteria (lack of dose optimization criteria) and dose related complications. Even more, the stimulating factors implanted scaffolds, further compacted the treatment procedure. Therefore, the smart piezoelectric material based scaffolds can be better alternative to aforementioned conventional therapies. The smart scaffold utilizes the functional loads as stimulating factor to regenerate the tissue by effect. The tissue regeneration can be regulated by natural feedback system to maintain the integration of the system. Hence, the class of piezoelectric materials has huge research and market scope for advanced tissue engineering therapies.

Conclusion

The present review provides the brief insight about the importance of the alternative technologies like smart materials in regenerative medicine. The detailed information about various piezoelectric materials for bone and cartilage tissue engineering has been presented in the report. Numerous piezoelectric materials are available and proved its effectiveness in the field of sensors; actuators etc. while the exploration of their biomedical applications are exponentially increased in last decade. Piezoelectric polymers/ biopolymers like, PHBV, PLLA, PVDF, collagen and cellulose etc. have been discussed in detail in terms of applications and their physical properties. Piezoceramics have been debated for their applications for hard tissue regeneration with various forms. Hence, the piezoelectric smart materials are best possible futuristic materials for regenerative medicine.

Abbreviations

BMP: Bone Morphogenetic Protein; BNNT: Boron nitride nanotubes; BT: Barium titanate; ECM: Extracellular matrix; IL-1: Interleukin-1; IL-4: Interleukin-4; KNN: potassium sodium niobate; Li: Lithium; LKNN: Lithium sodium potassium niobate; LNPN: Lithium sodium potassium niobate; NF-AT: Nuclear Factor of Activated Cells; PEI: Polyethylene imine; PHBV: Poly(3-hydroxybutyrate-co-3-hydroxyvalerate); PKC: Protein kinase; PLL: Poly-L-lysine; PLLA: Poly-L-Lactic acid; PVDF: Poly(vinylidene fluoride); PZT: Lead zirconate titanate; TGF β: Transforming Growth Factorβ; TrFE: Trifluoroethylene; ZnO: Zinc oxide

Acknowledgements

The authors would like to thank all our laboratory members for their helpful and constructive comments the manuscript.

Funding

Not applicable (no funding for the study).

Authors' contributions

Ms. Jaicy Jacob and Mr. Namdev More have collected the entire literature and make the draft of the review. The topic has been suggested by Govinda Kapusetti and Kiran Kalia, further all corrections have been carried out for the final manuscript for the publication. All authors read and approved the final manuscript.

Competing interests

The authors declare that they have no competing interests.

References

1. Lee SJ, Yoo JJ, Atala A. Biomaterials and tissue engineering. In: Clinical Regenerative Medicine in Urology. Singapore: Springer; 2018. p. 17–51.
2. Mason WP. Piezoelectricity, its history and applications. The Journal of the Acoustical Society of America. 1981;70(6):1561–6.
3. Mindlin R. Elasticity, piezoelectricity and crystal lattice dynamics. J Elast. 1972;2(4):217–82.
4. Mould R. Pierre Curie, 1859–1906. Curr Oncol. 2007;14(2):74.
5. Arinzeh T, Collins G, Lee Y-S. System and method for a piezoelectric scaffold for nerve growth and repair. In: Google Patents; 2016.
6. Minary-Jolandan M. Yu M-F: nanoscale characterization of isolated individual type I collagen fibrils: polarization and piezoelectricity. Nanotechnology. 2009;20(8):085706.
7. Arinzeh TL, Weber N, Jaffe M. Electrospun electroactive polymers for regenerative medicine applications. In: Google Patents; 2016.
8. Shastri VR, Schmidt CE, Langer RS, Vacanti JP. Neuronal stimulation using electrically conducting polymers. In: Google patents; 2000.
9. Bassett CAL. Biologic significance of piezoelectricity. Calcif Tissue Int. 1967; 1(1):252–72.
10. Halperin C, Mutchnik S, Agronin A, Molotskii M, Urenski P, Salai M, Rosenman G. Piezoelectric effect in human bones studied in nanometer scale. Nano Lett. 2004;4(7):1253–6.
11. Miara B, Rohan E, Zidi M, Labat B. Piezomaterials for bone regeneration design—homogenization approach. Journal of the Mechanics and Physics of Solids. 2005;53(11):2529–56.
12. Huey DJ. Hu JC, Athanasiou KA: unlike bone, cartilage regeneration remains elusive. Science. 2012;338(6109):917–21.
13. Tuzlakoglu K, Bolgen N, Salgado A, Gomes ME, Piskin E, Reis R. Nano-and micro-fiber combined scaffolds: a new architecture for bone tissue engineering. J Mater Sci Mater Med. 2005;16(12):1099–104.
14. Grodzinsky AJ, Levenston ME, Jin M, Frank EH. Cartilage tissue remodeling in response to mechanical forces. Annu Rev Biomed Eng. 2000;2(1):691–713.
15. Poole AR, Kojima T, Yasuda T, Mwale F, Kobayashi M, Laverty S. Composition and structure of articular cartilage: a template for tissue repair. Clin Orthop Relat Res. 2001;391:S26–33.
16. Huber M, Trattnig S, Lintner F. Anatomy, biochemistry, and physiology of articular cartilage. Investig Radiol. 2000;35(10):573–80.
17. Puppi D, Chiellini F, Piras A, Chiellini E. Polymeric materials for bone and cartilage repair. Prog Polym Sci. 2010;35(4):403–40.
18. Eyre D. Articular cartilage and changes in arthritis: collagen of articular cartilage. Arthritis Research & Therapy. 2001;4(1):30.
19. Muir H, Bullough P, Maroudas A. The distribution of collagen in human articular cartilage with some of its physiological implications. Bone & Joint Journal. 1970;52(3):554–63.
20. Reddi AH. Morphogenesis and tissue engineering of bone and cartilage: inductive signals, stem cells, and biomimetic biomaterials. Tissue Eng. 2000; 6(4):351–9.
21. Lane NE. Metabolic bone disease. Curr Opin Rheumatol. 2007;19(4):363.
22. Mankin HJ. The reaction of articular cartilage to injury and osteoarthritis. N Engl J Med. 1974;291(24):1285–92.
23. Riggs BL, Hartmann LC. Selective estrogen-receptor modulators—mechanisms of action and application to clinical practice. N Engl J Med. 2003;348(7):618–29.
24. Giusti A, Hamdy NA, Papapoulos SE. Atypical fractures of the femur and bisphosphonate therapy: a systematic review of case/case series studies. Bone. 2010;47(2):169–80.
25. Allen HL, Wase A, Bear W. Indomethacin and aspirin: effect of nonsteroidal anti-inflammatory agents on the rate of fracture repair in the rat. Acta Orthop Scand. 1980;51(1–6):595–600.
26. Rodan GA, Martin TJ. Therapeutic approaches to bone diseases. Science. 2000;289(5484):1508–14.
27. Fishman JA, Greenwald MA, Grossi PA. Transmission of infection with human allografts: essential considerations in donor screening. Clin Infect Dis. 2012;55(5):720–7.
28. Cypher TJ, Grossman JP. Biological principles of bone graft healing. The Journal of foot and ankle surgery. 1996;35(5):413–7.
29. Jackson DW, Windler GE, Simon TM. Intraarticular reaction associated with the use of freeze-dried, ethylene oxide-sterilized bone-patella tendon-bone allografts in the reconstruction of the anterior cruciate ligament. Am J Sports Med. 1990;18(1):1–11.
30. Steadman JR, Briggs KK, Rodrigo JJ, Kocher MS, Gill TJ, Rodkey WG. Outcomes of microfracture for traumatic chondral defects of the knee: average 11-year follow-up. Arthroscopy: The Journal of Arthroscopic & Related Surgery. 2003;19(5):477–84.
31. Nehrer S, Minas T. Treatment of articular cartilage defects. Investig Radiol. 2000;35(10):639–46.
32. Grande DA, Pitman MI, Peterson L, Menche D, Klein M. The repair of experimentally produced defects in rabbit articular cartilage by autologous chondrocyte transplantation. J Orthop Res. 1989;7(2):208–18.
33. Nerem RM, Sambanis A. Tissue engineering: from biology to biological substitutes. Tissue Eng. 1995;1(1):3–13.
34. Wu Q, Yang B, Hu K, Cao C, Man Y, Wang P. Deriving osteogenic cells from induced pluripotent stem cells for bone tissue engineering. Tissue Eng B Rev. 2017;23(1):1–8.
35. Wan C, He Q, Li G. Allogenic peripheral blood derived mesenchymal stem cells (MSCs) enhance bone regeneration in rabbit ulna critical-sized bone defect model. J Orthop Res. 2006;24(4):610–8.
36. Nakashima M, Nagasawa H, Yamada Y, Reddi AH. Regulatory role of transforming growth factor-β, bone morphogenetic protein-2, and protein-4

on gene expression of extracellular matrix proteins and differentiation of dental pulp cells. Dev Biol. 1994;162(1):18–28.

37. Sakaguchi Y, Sekiya I, Yagishita K, Muneta T. Comparison of human stem cells derived from various mesenchymal tissues: superiority of synovium as a cell source. Arthritis & Rheumatology. 2005;52(8):2521–9.

38. More N, Kapusetti G. Piezoelectric material–a promising approach for bone and cartilage regeneration. Med Hypotheses. 2017;108:10–6.

39. van Beuningen HM, Glansbeek HL, van der Kraan PM, van den Berg WB. Differential effects of local application of BMP-2 or TGF-β1 on both articular cartilage composition and osteophyte formation. Osteoarthr Cartil. 1998;6(5):306–17.

40. Koga H, Engebretsen L, Brinchmann JE, Muneta T, Sekiya I. Mesenchymal stem cell-based therapy for cartilage repair: a review. Knee Surg Sports Traumatol Arthrosc. 2009;17(11):1289–97.

41. Cancedda R, Dozin B, Giannoni P, Quarto R. Tissue engineering and cell therapy of cartilage and bone. Matrix Biol. 2003;22(1):81–91.

42. Amini AR, Laurencin CT, Nukavarapu SP. Bone tissue engineering: recent advances and challenges. Crit Rev™ Biomed Eng. 2012;40(5):363–408.

43. Ziegler J, Mayr-Wohlfart U, Kessler S, Breitig D, Günther KP. Adsorption and release properties of growth factors from biodegradable implants. J Biomed Mater Res A. 2002;59(3):422–8.

44. Mano JF. Smart polymers: applications in biotechnology and biomedicine. In: USA: Wiley Online library; 2009. p. 622.

45. Reis R, Mano J, Del Campo A. Smart instructive polymer substrates for tissue engineering. In: Smart polymers and their applications. Cambridge: Elsevier; 2014. p. 301–26.

46. Li S, Tiwari A, Prabaharan M, Aryal S. Smart polymer materials for biomedical applications. New York: Nova Science Publishers, Inc; 2011.

47. Roy D, Cambre JN, Sumerlin BS. Future perspectives and recent advances in stimuli-responsive materials. Prog Polym Sci. 2010;35(1–2):278–301.

48. Del as Heras Alarcón C, Pennadam S, Alexander C. Stimuli responsive polymers for biomedical applications. Chem Soc Rev. 2005;34(3):276–85.

49. Jeong B, Gutowska A. Lessons from nature: stimuli-responsive polymers and their biomedical applications. Trends Biotechnol. 2002;20(7):305–11.

50. Ahn AC, Grodzinsky AJ. Relevance of collagen piezoelectricity to "Wolff's law": a critical review. Med Eng Phys. 2009;31(7):733–41.

51. Xu J, Wang W, Clark C, Brighton C. Signal transduction in electrically stimulated articular chondrocytes involves translocation of extracellular calcium through voltage-gated channels. Osteoarthr Cartil. 2009;17(3):397–405.

52. Ballock RT, Heydemann A, Wakefield LM, Flanders KC, Roberts AB, Sporn MB. TGF-β1 prevents hypertrophy of epiphyseal chondrocytes: regulation of gene expression for cartilage matrix proteins and metalloproteases. Dev Biol. 1993;158(2):414–29.

53. Zhuang H, Wang W, Seldes RM, Tahernia AD, Fan H, Brighton CT. Electrical stimulation induces the level of TGF-β1 mRNA in osteoblastic cells by a mechanism involving calcium/calmodulin pathway. Biochem Biophys Res Commun. 1997;237(2):225–9.

54. Riddle RC, Donahue HJ. From streaming-potentials to shear stress: 25 years of bone cell mechanotransduction. J Orthop Res. 2009;27(2):143–9.

55. Fukada E, Yasuda I. Piezoelectric effects in collagen. Jpn J Appl Phys. 1964;3(2):117.

56. Spadaro JA. Mechanical and electrical interactions in bone remodeling. Bioelectromagnetics. 1997;18(3):193–202.

57. Huang C, Ogawa R. Mechanotransduction in bone repair and regeneration. FASEB J. 2010;24(10):3625–32.

58. Lee H-S, Millward-Sadler S, Wright M, Nuki G, Al-Jamal R, Salter D. Activation of integrin—RACK1/PKCα signalling in human articular chondrocyte mechanotransduction. Osteoarthr Cartil. 2002;10(11):890–7.

59. Litzenberger JB, Kim J-B, Tummala P, Jacobs CR. β1 integrins mediate mechanosensitive signaling pathways in osteocytes. Calcif Tissue Int. 2010; 86(4):325–32.

60. Kanno T, Takahashi T, Tsujisawa T, Ariyoshi W, Nishihara T. Mechanical stress-mediated Runx2 activation is dependent on Ras/ERK1/2 MAPK signaling in osteoblasts. J Cell Biochem. 2007;101(5):1266–77.

61. Li C, Weng G. Antiplane crack problem in functionally graded piezoelectric materials. TRANSACTIONS-AMERICAN SOCIETY OF MECHANICAL ENGINEERS. J Appl Mech. 2002;69(4):481–8.

62. Berlincourt D, Cmolik C, Jaffe H. Piezoelectric properties of polycrystalline lead titanate zirconate compositions. Proc IRE. 1960;48(2):220–9.

63. Fousek J, Cross L, Litvin D. Possible piezoelectric composites based on the flexoelectric effect. Mater Lett. 1999;39(5):287–91.

64. Setter N, Damjanovic D, Eng L, Fox G, Gevorgian S, Hong S, Kingon A, Kohlstedt H, Park N, Stephenson G. Ferroelectric thin films: review of materials, properties, and applications. J Appl Phys. 2006;100(5):051606.

65. Rajabi AH, Jaffe M, Arinzeh TL. Piezoelectric materials for tissue regeneration: a review. Acta Biomater. 2015;24:12–23.

66. Gimenes R, Zaghete MA, Bertolini M, Varela JA, Coelho LO, Silva NF Jr. Composites PVDF-TrFE/BT used as bioactive membranes for enhancing bone regeneration. In: Smart structures and materials. California: International Society for Optics and Photonics; 2004. p. 539–47.

67. Martins P, Ribeiro S, Ribeiro C, Sencadas V, Gomes A, Gama F, Lanceros-Méndez S. Effect of poling state and morphology of piezoelectric poly (vinylidene fluoride) membranes for skeletal muscle tissue engineering. RSC Adv. 2013;3(39):17938–44.

68. Ribeiro C, Pärssinen J, Sencadas V, Correia V, Miettinen S, Hytönen VP, Lanceros-Méndez S. Dynamic piezoelectric stimulation enhances osteogenic differentiation of human adipose stem cells. J Biomed Mater Res A. 2015;103(6):2172–5.

69. Reis J, Frias C, Canto e Castro C, Botelho ML, Marques AT, JAO S, Capela e Silva F, Potes J. A new piezoelectric actuator induces bone formation in vivo: a preliminary study. Biomed Res Int. 2012;2012:613403.

70. Lee Y-S, Livingston Arinzeh T. Electrospun nanofibrous materials for neural tissue engineering. Polymers. 2011;3(1):413–26.

71. Ross G, Watts J, Hill M, Morrissey P. Surface modification of poly (vinylidene fluoride) by alkaline treatment1. The degradation mechanism. Polymer. 2000;41(5):1685–96.

72. Neuss S, Apel C, Buttler P, Denecke B, Dhanasingh A, Ding X, Grafahrend D, Groger A, Hemmrich K, Herr A. Assessment of stem cell/biomaterial combinations for stem cell-based tissue engineering. Biomaterials. 2008;29(3):302–13.

73. Fukada E. New piezoelectric polymers. Jpn J Appl Phys. 1998;37(5S):2775.

74. Weber N, Lee Y-S, Shanmugasundaram S, Jaffe M, Arinzeh TL. Characterization and in vitro cytocompatibility of piezoelectric electrospun scaffolds. Acta Biomater. 2010;6(9):3550–6.

75. Valentini RF. Negatively charged polymeric electret implant. In: Google patents; 1998.

76. Pereira JD, Camargo RC, José Filho C, Alves N, Rodriguez-Perez MA, Constantino CJ. Biomaterials from blends of fluoropolymers and corn starch—implant and structural aspects. Mater Sci Eng C. 2014;36:226–36.

77. Esmaeili M, Baei MS: Fabrication of biodegradable polymer nanocomposite from copolymer synthesized by C. necator for bone tissue engineering. 2011.

78. Ke S, Huang H, Ren L, Wang Y. Nearly constant dielectric loss behavior in poly (3-hydroxybutyrate-co-3-hydroxyvalerate) biodegradable polyester. In: AIP; 2009.

79. Fukada E. History and recent progress in piezoelectric polymers. IEEE Trans Ultrason Ferroelectr Freq Control. 2000;47(6):1277–90.

80. Köse GT, Korkusuz F, Özkul A, Soysal Y, Özdemir T, Yildiz C, Hasirci V. Tissue engineered cartilage on collagen and PHBV matrices. Biomaterials. 2005; 26(25):5187–97.

81. Numata K, Abe H, Doi Y. Enzymatic processes for biodegradation of poly (hydroxyalkanoate) s crystals. Can J Chem. 2008;86(6):471–83.

82. Newman B, Chen P, Pae K, Scheinbeim J. Piezoelectricity in nylon 11. J Appl Phys. 1980;51(10):5161–4.

83. Takahashi Y, Iijima M, Fukada E. Pyroelectricity in poled thin films of aromatic polyurea prepared by vapor deposition polymerization. Jpn J Appl Phys. 1989;28(12A):L2245.

84. Wang H, Li Y, Zuo Y, Li J, Ma S, Cheng L. Biocompatibility and osteogenesis of biomimetic nano-hydroxyapatite/polyamide composite scaffolds for bone tissue engineering. Biomaterials. 2007;28(22):3338–48.

85. Naughton GK, Willoughby J. Method for repairing cartilage. In: Google Patents; 1998.

86. Fukada E. Piezoelectricity of biopolymers. Biorheology. 1995;32(6):593–609.

87. Di Martino A, Sittinger M, Risbud MV. Chitosan: a versatile biopolymer for orthopaedic tissue-engineering. Biomaterials. 2005;26(30):5983–90.

88. Kim J, Yun S, Ounaies Z. Discovery of cellulose as a smart material. Macromolecules. 2006;39(12):4202–6.

89. Zaborowska M, Bodin A, Bäckdahl H, Popp J, Goldstein A, Gatenholm P. Microporous bacterial cellulose as a potential scaffold for bone regeneration. Acta Biomater. 2010;6(7):2540–7.

90. Ferreira AM, Gentile P, Chiono V, Ciardelli G. Collagen for bone tissue regeneration. Acta Biomater. 2012;8(9):3191–200.

91. Rocha LB, Goissis G, Rossi MA. Biocompatibility of anionic collagen matrix as scaffold for bone healing. Biomaterials. 2002;23(2):449–56.

92. Silva C, Thomazini D, Pinheiro A, Aranha N, Figueiro S, Goes J, Sombra A. Collagen–hydroxyapatite films: piezoelectric properties. Mater Sci Eng B. 2001;86(3):210–8.

93. Silva C, Lima C, Pinheiro A, Góes J, Figueiro S, Sombra A. On the piezoelectricity of collagen–chitosan films. Phys Chem Chem Phys. 2001; 3(18):4154–7.

94. Savakus H, Klicker K, Newnham R. PZT-epoxy piezoelectric transducers: a simplified fabrication procedure. Mater Res Bull. 1981;16(6):677–80.

95. Ciofani G, Ricotti L, Canale C, D'Alessandro D, Berrettini S, Mazzolai B, Mattoli V. Effects of barium titanate nanoparticles on proliferation and differentiation of rat mesenchymal stem cells. Colloids Surf B: Biointerfaces. 2013;102:312–20.

96. Ciofani G, Ricotti L, Mattoli V. Preparation, characterization and in vitro testing of poly (lactic-co-glycolic) acid/barium titanate nanoparticle composites for enhanced cellular proliferation. Biomed Microdevices. 2011;13(2):255–66.

97. Liu H, Slamovich EB, Webster TJ. Increased osteoblast functions among nanophase titania/poly (lactide-co-glycolide) composites of the highest nanometer surface roughness. J Biomed Mater Res A. 2006;78(4):798–807.

98. Baxter FR, Bowen CR, Turner IG, Dent AC. Electrically active bioceramics: a review of interfacial responses. Ann Biomed Eng. 2010;38(6):2079–92.

99. Ivanova O, Williams C, Campbell T. Additive manufacturing (AM) and nanotechnology: promises and challenges. Rapid Prototyp J. 2013;19(5):353–64.

100. Shankar AH, Prasad AS. Zinc and immune function: the biological basis of altered resistance to infection. Am J Clin Nutr. 1998;68(2):447S–63S.

101. Fan Z. Lu JG: zinc oxide nanostructures: synthesis and properties. J Nanosci Nanotechnol. 2005;5(10):1561–73.

102. Rasmussen JW, Martinez E, Louka P, Wingett DG. Zinc oxide nanoparticles for selective destruction of tumor cells and potential for drug delivery applications. Expert opinion on drug delivery. 2010;7(9):1063–77.

103. Mirza EH, Pan-Pan C, Ibrahim W, Bin WMA, Djordjevic I, Pingguan-Murphy B. Chondroprotective effect of zinc oxide nanoparticles in conjunction with hypoxia on bovine cartilage-matrix synthesis. J Biomed Mater Res A. 2015; 103(11):3554–63.

104. Wang B, Feng W, Wang M, Wang T, Gu Y, Zhu M, Ouyang H, Shi J, Zhang F, Zhao Y. Acute toxicological impact of nano-and submicro-scaled zinc oxide powder on healthy adult mice. J Nanopart Res. 2008;10(2):263–76.

105. Yu S-W, Kuo S-T, Tuan W-H, Tsai Y-Y, Wang S-F. Cytotoxicity and degradation behavior of potassium sodium niobate piezoelectric ceramics. Ceram Int. 2012;38(4):2845–50.

106. Carville NC, Collins L, Manzo M, Gallo K, Lukasz BI, McKayed KK, Simpson JC, Rodriguez BJ. Biocompatibility of ferroelectric lithium niobate and the influence of polarization charge on osteoblast proliferation and function. J Biomed Mater Res A. 2015;103(8):2540–8.

107. Atanasoska L, Radhakrishnan R, Schewe S. Medical devices employing piezoelectric materials for delivery of therapeutic agents. In: Google patents; 2014.

108. Ciofani G, Raffa V, Menciassi A, Cuschieri A. Boron nitride nanotubes: an innovative tool for nanomedicine. Nano Today. 2009;4(1):8–10.

109. Ciofani G, Raffa V, Menciassi A, Dario P. Preparation of boron nitride nanotubes aqueous dispersions for biological applications. J Nanosci Nanotechnol. 2008;8(12):6223–31.

110. Ciofani G, Danti S, Genchi GG, Mazzolai B, Mattoli V. Boron nitride nanotubes: biocompatibility and potential spill-over in nanomedicine. Small. 2013;9(9–10): 1672–85.

111. Ciofani G, Danti S, D'Alessandro D, Ricotti L, Moscato S, Bertoni G, Falqui A, Berrettini S, Petrini M, Mattoli V. Enhancement of neurite outgrowth in neuronal-like cells following boron nitride nanotube-mediated stimulation. ACS Nano. 2010;4(10):6267–77.

112. Lahiri D, Rouzaud F, Richard T, Keshri AK, Bakshi SR, Kos L, Agarwal A. Boron nitride nanotube reinforced polylactide–polycaprolactone copolymer composite: mechanical properties and cytocompatibility with osteoblasts and macrophages in vitro. Acta Biomater. 2010;6(9):3524–33.

113. Nakhmanson SM, Calzolari A, Meunier V, Bernholc J, Nardelli MB. Spontaneous polarization and piezoelectricity in boron nitride nanotubes. Phys Rev B. 2003; 67(23):235406.

27

Cancer cell reprogramming to identify the genes competent for generating liver cancer stem cells

Kenly Wuputra[1†], Chang-Shen Lin[1,2†], Ming-Ho Tsai[1], Chia-Chen Ku[1], Wen-Hsin Lin[1], Ya-Han Yang[3,4], Kung-Kai Kuo[3,4] and Kazunari K. Yokoyama[1,3,5,6,7,8*]

Abstract

The cancer stem cell (CSC) hypothesis postulates that cancer originates from the malignant transformation of stem/progenitor cells and is considered to apply to many cancers, including liver cancer. Identification that CSCs are responsible for drug resistance, metastasis, and secondary tumor appearance suggests that these populations are novel obligatory targets for the treatment of cancer. Here, we describe our new method for identifying potential CSC candidates. The reprogramming of cancer cells via induced pluripotent stem cell (iPSC) technology is a novel therapy for the treatment and for the study of CSC-related genes. This technology has advantages for studying the interactions between CSC-related genes and the cancer niche microenvironment. This technology may also provide a useful platform for studying the genes involved in the generation of CSCs before and after reprogramming, and for elucidating the mechanisms underlying cancer initiation and progression. The present review summarizes the current understanding of transcription factors involved in the generation of liver CSCs from liver cancer cell-derived iPSCs and how these contribute to oncogenesis, and discusses the modeling of liver cancer development.

Keywords: c-JUN oncogene, Induced pluripotent stem cells, Liver cancer, OCT4, Reprogramming

Background

The cancer stem cell (CSC) hypothesis initially proposed for leukemia by J. Dick is now accepted [1–3]. CSCs represent a small subset of cells within a tumor that are endowed with stem-like properties such as the ability for (i) self-renewal, (ii) pluripotency, (iii) tumor formation, and (iv) drug resistance [4, 5]. Importantly, CSCs are thought to be responsible for tumor initiation, recurrence, and metastasis through the reduced sensitivity of cancer cells to chemotherapy compared with that of the original tumor cells [6]. Growing evidence about liver CSCs confirmed their resistance to therapeutic drugs such as cisplatin, 5-fuluorouracil, and so on [7].

The primary strategy for inducing liver CSCs is to first enrich the cells using classical stem cell markers of stem

cells such as CD13, CD24, CD44, CD47, CD90, CD133, epithelial cell adhesion molecule, and OV6, and then to apply functional methodologies such as side-population analysis, the ALDEFLUOR^{TM} assay, the sphere formation, and so on [8–11]. This cell population is then transplanted into immuno-deficient mice to examine its in vivo tumorigenic potential [7–9], and the cells are studied further according to their expression of various genes or signals such as Wnt, Notch, Hedgehog, Transforming growth factor β, epithelial mesenchymal transition (EMT)/mesenchymal epithelial transition (MET) signaling, epigenetic regulators, and microRNAs. The putative CSC subpopulation capable to initiating tumor development at lower cell numbers are tested further for self-renewal capacity using serial dilution of cells to identify the CSCs. Cancers are also generated as a consequence of transformation of the "driver" mutation at initiation [12–15], and then positive selection and clonal progression lead to the accumulation of "passenger" mutations required for additional growth advantages. It is generally accepted that a novel strategy

* Correspondence: kazu@kmu.edu.tw

†Equal contributors

[1]Graduate Institute of Medicine, Kaohsiung Medical University, Kaohsiung 807, Taiwan

[3]Center of Stem Cell Research, Kaohsiung Medical University, Kaohsiung 807, Taiwan

Full list of author information is available at the end of the article

is needed for the functional evaluation of both putative driver and passenger mutations, and for studying their molecular dynamics underlying cancer development.

Current cancer cell-reprogramming techniques such as somatic cell nuclear transfer [16] and the generation of induced pluripotent stem cells (iPSCs) [17–19] are used to identify oncogenic genes. In 2006, Yamanaka et al. [17] reported on the reprogramming of somatic cell into induced pluripotent stem cell-like cells (iPSLCs). The success in reprogramming a somatic cell into a stem cell-like state has led to the idea of reprogramming malignant cells back to their original state, which is well before the oncogenic transformation occurs. The generation of iPSCs from cancer cells may provide tools for exploring the mechanisms of tumor initiation and progression in vitro, for studying the heterogeneity and origin of CSCs, and for producing cancer type-specific drug discovery. However, these reprogramming methods remain a challenge because of the cancer-specific epigenetic state and chromosomal aberrations of cancer cells.

The epigenetic memory of the original cell type is important to reprogramming and is closely related to the inefficient reprogramming caused by failure of reset the epigenome to an embryonic stem cell (ESC)-like state [20]. The epigenetic state is reversible, but attempts to reprogram cancer cells have produced incomplete resetting of the cancer-associated epigenome because of tumor heterogeneity and further accumulation of oncogenic mutations. Therefore, cancer cell reprogramming is currently limited to certain cancer types and cancer-specific marks in the epigenome, which impede successful reprogramming, and the underlying mechanism has not been fully elucidated. The technique of cancer cell reprograming is one possible approach for identifying the committed genes of CSCs and for studying the mechanisms underlying the transcriptional, translational,

and epigenetic inheritance of cancer development. The characterization of epigenome and tumor suppressor gene complexes, such as p53, $p21^{Cip1}$, $p27^{Kip1}$, the Ink4 family, and the polycomb repressive complex (PRC) might identify the possible candidates for genes for reprogramming of cancer cells to CSCs.

Obstacles to cancer cell reprogramming

The reprogramming of cancer cells is less successful than the reprogramming of somatic cells [21–23]. Despite the presence of genetic alterations, melanoma cells can be reversed to the pluripotent state, such as that of the ESC, by nuclear transfer [24] (Table 1). However, the cells involved in other malignant cancer types, including breast cancer, leukemia, and lymphoma, cannot be reprogrammed, which suggests the presence of unknown barriers to reprogramming [23, 25, 26]. Similarly, embryonic carcinoma (EC) cell lines can be reprogrammed by nuclear transfer and exhibit normal preimplantation development. However, abnormal phenotypes of the clones occur, which suggests that EC cell lines possess a unique set of modifications in the epigenetic state that cannot be reprogrammed by altering the developmental potential [27]. The limited number of studies that have reported successful derivation of iPSCs from cancer cells supports the notion that the existence of cancer-specific genetic and epigenetic states hinders successful reprogramming independently of the complexity of the techniques used for reprogramming. Reprograming studies using patient-derived cancer cells have produced solid evidence of the capacity for reversal of the malignant phenotype, and this method holds great promise for breaking the seemingly irreversible state associated with cancer.

Table 1 Summary of studies of reprogramming of cancer cells from induce pluripotent stem cell technology. We have modified the summary of the table reported by Camare et al. [25, 26]

CSCs examples	Original cells	Methods of reprogramming	Karyotype	Chimeras	Teratoma/ tumor formation	Drug sensitivity
Utikal et al. (2009) [65]	Mice melanoma R454 (rasinduce cells)	Lentivirus OKM	Trisomy chromosomes 8 and 11	Yes	Yes	No tumor in the absence of Dox
Carette et al. (2010) [42]	Human leukemia KBM7 (CML)	Retrovirus OSKM Retrovirus OSK (incomplete reprogramming)	Tetraploid, chromosomes 9 and 22 Ph(+)	Not applied	Yes	Cell type specific drug sensitivity
Miyoshi et al. (2010) [43]	Human gastrointestinal cancer cells	Retrovirus and lentivirus + lipofectamine OSKM	Abnormal	Not applied	Yes	Post iPSC cells—more sensitive to 5-Fu and differentiation inducing drug
Kuo et al. (2016) [59]	Human HepG2 liver cancer cells and mouse hepatocytes-iPSCs	Lentivirus OSKM + shp53RNA (lentivirus O + c-JUN for direct reprogramming)	Abnormal	Not applied	Yes	Yes

Stemness characteristics and oncogenic functions of CSCs

Generation of iPSCs from cancer cells requires the identification of genes that regulate stem cell self-renewal and pluripotency such as *OCT4, SOX2*, and *NANOG*. CSCs require oncogenes or tumor suppressor genes to express oncogenic functions. Both expression states of stemness genes and oncogenes/tumor suppressor genes should be reorganized at the chromatin state by their regulators of epigenetic modification. Thus, three classes of gene sets might provide clues for understanding the reprogramming of cancer cells.

OCT4 is known to be overexpressed in hematological cancers, seminomas, and cancers of the bladder, brain, lung, ovary, pancreas, prostate, kidney, and testicle [28]. OCT4 works synergistically with SOX2 via direct binding to transactivate the target genes [29]. Both *SOX2* and *OCT4* are activators of genes involved in pluripotency, including themselves and *NANOG* [30], and repressors of genes involved in differentiation [31, 32]. Both SOX2 and OCT4 regulate their own transcription by binding the composite elements of SOX–OCT in their enhancers [33].

Overexpression of SOX2 is detected in recurrent prostate cancer, head and neck squamous cell carcinoma, glioblastoma, small-cell lung cancer, and cancers of the breast, liver, pancreas, and stomach [33]. Overexpression of SOX2 increases cell proliferation via cyclin D3, and represses cell cycle regulators such as $p21^{Cip1}$ and $p27^{Kip1}$ [34]. SOX2 promotes the invasion, migration, and metastasis of melanoma, colorectal cancer, glioma, and cancers of the stomach, ovary, and liver through the activation of matric metalloproteinases family, and phosphatidylinositol 3-kinase (PI3K)–RAC-α serine/threonine kinases (AKT)–mammalian target of the rapamycin signaling pathway [35–37].

NANOG is overexpressed in oral squamous cell carcinoma and other types of cancers [38]. NONOG is capable of maintaining pluripotency of ESCs independently of the leukemia inhibitory factor-signal transducers and activator of transcription pathway, which is different from the case of OCT4 [38, 39]. NANOG also controls the cell cycle and proliferation by directly binding to the cyclin D1 promoter for transactivation [40]. NANOG induced the expression of cancer-related genes like CD133 and aldehyde dehydrogenase 1A1 [41]. These stemness transcription factors of SOX2, OCT4, and NANOG co-occupy the promoter regions of about 350 genes in the genome, and OCT4 occupies more than 90% of the promoter regions bound by the OCT4 and SOX2 in human ESCs. These findings suggest that the OCT4–SOX2–NANOG axis is the key cascade for stemness [31].

Reprograming of cancer cells using iPS technology

It has been proposed that oncogenes and tumor suppressor genes should be activated or repressed to generate CSCs. However, the actual oncogenes that can generate CSCs have not been characterized.

Carette et al. [42] reprogrammed a cell line derived from chronic myeloid leukemia (CML) by infecting them with a retrovirus that induced the expression of OCT4, SOX2, KLF4, and MYC (OSKM) followed by the subcutaneous injection of the CML-iPSCs into nonobese/diabetic severe combined immunodeficient (NOD-SCID) mice [Table 1]. They found that the teratomas produced contained differentiated cells in three germ layers, which indicated pluripotency. Whereas the parental CML cell lines were dependent on the BCR–ABL pathway, by contrast, the CML iPSCs were independent of this BCR–ABL signaling and showed resistance to imatinib. However, Cratte et al. did not identify the signaling pathway involved in the suppression of this BCR–ABL cascade. Miyoshi et al. [43] reported on the reprogramming of gastrointestinal cancer cell lines into iPSCs through the OSKM method [Table 1]. Tumors were generated by parenteral injection of gastrointestinal cancer cells into NOD-SCID mice, but not by injection of differentiated cells arising from the iPSCs. These iPSCs expressed increased levels of tumor suppressor genes such as $p16^{Ink4a}$ and p53 upon differentiation.

Striker et al. [44] reported the reprogramming of glioblastoma (GBM) cells to neural stem cells (NSCs) by PiggyBac transposon vectors that expressed OCT4 and KLF4. In these GBM iPSCs, the widespread resetting of epigenetic methylation occurred in cancer-specific methylation variable positions, the GBM tumor suppressor gene CDKN1C ($p57^{Kip2}$), and testin LIM domain protein (TES). The neural progenitor cells (NPCs) differentiated from GBM iPSCs resembled aggressive GBM cells when transplanted into the adult mouse brain [44]. By contrast, non-neural mesodermal progenitors from GBM iPSCs with sustained expression of TES and CDKN1C formed benign tumors, and failed to infiltrate the surrounding regions. These findings suggest that DNA methylation is critical to the expression of these particular genes. Kim et al. [45] generated the iPSC-like cells from pancreatic ductal adenocarcinoma (PDACs) by introducing the genes encoded *OSKM*. One cancer iPS-like clone harbored classical PDAC mutations, including kRAS and $p16^{Ink4a}$ heterozygous deletions and decreased SMAD copy number, and retained the chromosomal alterations seen in the parental cells, and differentiated into all three germ layers during in vitro differentiation in the descendants, although the neural lineages were underrepresented. An in vivo teratoma showed that the iPSC-like cells generated multiple germ layers tissues but preferred to generate endodermal ductal structures.

DNA methylation is another critical epigenetic change. However, the reprogramming of cancer cells into iPSCs shows that only about 50% of cancer-associated epigenetic defects, as defined by a comparison between normal and tumor cells, are stably reset, which suggests that locus-specific changes in the epigenome are required. Reconfiguration of the network of cell-fate transcription factors and downstream developmental epigenetic mechanisms, may effectively silence the cancer-promoting pathways essential for uncontrolled proliferation and infiltration. However, the reciprocal interaction of epigenetic changes and driver mutations of cancer need to be explored in greater detail.

Funato et al. [46] used the pluripotent stem cells to study the role of driver mutations in modeling pediatric brain tumors. Differentiation of human ESCs into NPCs and induced cellular transformation through the overexpression of a constitutively active PDGFRA, TP53 knockdown, or expressing the K27M mutant of histone H3.3 found in pediatric gliomas. Moreover, induced NPC transformation was induced by the combination of different mutations typically observed in human gliomas that collectively affect the signaling of the PI3K, MAPK, and p53 pathways [47].

BMI1 of PRC1 has been shown to be involved in the maintenance and/or self-renewal of many types of stem cells, including embryonic, neural, hematopoietic, and prostate stem cells [48]. BMI1 promotes the proliferation of leukemic stem cells in a mouse model [49], and activates the self-renewal ability of NSCs [50]. BMI1 is known to be directly responsible for the regulation of multiple targets such p16^{Ink4a} and p14^{Arf} [51] and to bind directly to the promoter of *PTEN* gene, which results in the activation of the PI3K–AKT signaling and subsequent stabilization of SNAIL to induce the EMT [52]. BMI1 also occupies the cadherin promoter, which causes E-cadherin repression [52] and cooperates with TWIST1 to promote cancer dedifferentiation and metastasis [53]. In endometrial cancer cells, the loss of BMI1 results in the reduced expression of SOX2 and KLF4 [54]. Overexpression of BMI1 correlates with overexpression of NANOG, high tumor grade status, and increased self-renewal in breast adenocarcinomas [55].

Recently, Kaufhold et al. [56] reported the association of Yin Yang 1 (YY1) and CSC transcription factors and that YY1 might be a transcriptional repressor that acts on CSC-associated transcription factors such as *BMI1*, *SOX2*, and *OCT4*. They also proposed the existence a regulatory loop involving crosstalk between the nuclear factor kB–PI3K–AKT pathway and the downstream controls of target gene products such as YY1, OCT4, SOX2 and BMI1. Taken together, these findings suggest that most of the genes critical for cancer reprogramming belong to the families of (i) stemness genes, (ii) oncogenes/tumor suppressor genes, and (iii) epigenetic-related genes of DNA or histone modification, and (iv) the INK4 locus mediated by PRC family.

Thus, we hypothesized a "two-hit" theory for the generation of CSCs. The first hit introduces stemness and the second hit induces oncogenic features or repression of tumor suppressor function. Both are required for induction and maintenance of CSCs by epigenetic alterations induced by both genes. In this model, the reprogramming can be used as a platform for identification of the functional driver or passenger mutations, and modifications under the activation of stemness genes and the activation of oncogenes (or the repression of tumor suppressor genes) (Fig. 1).

Selective plasticity of CSCs

Cell plasticity is a key issue for the reprogramming of CSCs. Mu et al. [57] and Ku et al. [58] independently reported the role of cell plasticity in cell identity, which allows cancers to thrive. It has been known that hormone deprivation therapy that suppresses androgen receptor (AR) signaling is one of the treatments for metastatic prostate cancer. However, prostate cancers can become resistant to these drugs by losing hormone dependence on androgen. Because androgen stimulates

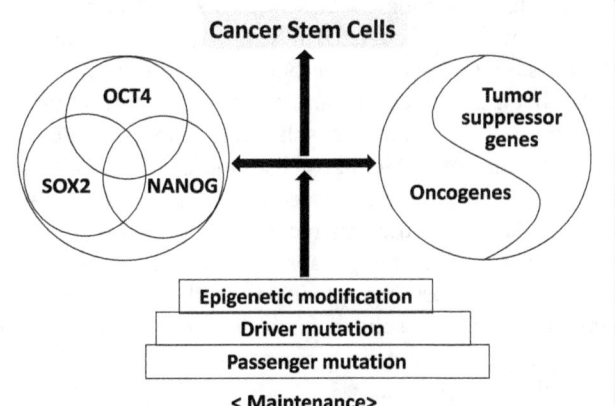

Fig. 1 Schematic representation of hypothetical two-hit theory for crosstalk to generate cancer stem cells by reprogramming. Hypothetical two-hit theory for induction of cancer stem cells was represented. Stemness factors (OCT4, SOX2, and NANOG) and oncogene/tumor suppressor genes (oncogenes such as Myc, KLF4, c-JUN, kRAS, etc.; antioncogenes such as p53, Rb, PTEN, BMI1, EZH2, INK4 family, etc.) and epigenetic modification of DNA methylation and histone modification are required for generation of cancer stem cells by reprogramming. We have reported the feedback control of c-JUN and OCT4 is critical for generation of cancer stem like cells [59]. The oncogene c-JUN transactivated genes encoding OCT4, SOX2, and NANOG [60], and the genes of OCT4, SOX2, and NANOG formed the molecular circuitry for stemness and pluripotency [64], and then OCT4 upregulated the expression of c-JUN gene to form the feedback circuit [59]. Taken together, we hypothesize that these feedback circuit might be regulated by the family of the stemness genes and the family of cancer-related oncogenes or tumor suppressor genes

the growth of prostate cancer cells, decreased production of androgen and/or inhibition of the hormone's action on prostate cancer cells can make a tumor shrink or grow more slowly. Mu et al. [57] reported that the induction of SOX2 expression subsequent to loss of RB1 and TP53 contributes to neuroendocrine differentiation and androgen independence of prostate cancer cells. Ku et al. [58] examined the effects of RB1 and TP53 deletion in a mouse model of metastatic prostate cancer (PTEN loss) and found that EZH2 inhibition restored enzalutamide responsiveness in RB1- and TP53-depleted and AR expressing LNCaP cells. The cell lineage plasticity was determined by the E2F-regulating genes such as SOX2 and EZH2. These data suggest that both tumor suppressor genes, such as RB1, TP53, and PTEN, and the cell cycle regulator E2F-controlled genes, such as SOX2 and EZH2, might be critical for determination of cell lineage plasticity.

Clone selection of CSCs from iPSC-like cells

In an attempt to isolate the CSCs, we have used a new strategy to isolate the clone responsible for generating CSCs among the heterogeneous clones of iPSC-like cells derived from human hepatocyte cell lines [59]. Using the original four Yamanaka's factors plus small hairpin TP53 plasmid, we have generated iPSC-like clones. To identify the possible CSC clones, we have reduced the number of cells that remain competent after tumor formation, as determined by the transplantation of colonies of xenograft-derived iPSC-like cells. One colony comprising about 200 cells finally generated tumors in more than 40% of transplants. We then characterized this colony to determine its tumor-forming capacity. This clone exhibited greater tumor-forming activity and other cancer-related activities such as sphere formation, colony formation, invasion activity, and drug resistance compared with the original liver cancer cells.

To gain further insight into the acquired CSC characteristics of this CSC colony, RNA sequencing was performed and showed that OCT4 and c-JUN expression was greater in this clone than in the original cancer cells. This experiment suggests that both OCT4 and c-JUN are key factors required for the feedback control of each other. Moreover, the two genes—one a stemness gene and the other an oncogene—were also competent in inducing CSCs derived from iPSCs from mouse hepatocytes infected with lentivirus that encoded OCT4 and c-JUN. This combination is interesting because c-JUN is an oncogene and OCT4 is a stemness gene. By themselves, OCT4 and c-JUN showed less transformation activity, but the feedback between OCT4 and c-JUN increased the likelihood of cancer induction. Therefore, we hypothesize that both genes are required to generate liver cancer and that the feedback

regulation of OCT4 and c-JUN might be critical for triggering CSCs.

Future perspectives

This strategy of cancer reprograming is one possible approach for generating CSCs. Chang et al. [60] reported that c-JUN is activated in pluripotent stemness gene promoters such as OCT4, SOX2, and NANOG and promotes the EMT in head and neck cancer cells. We have introduced OCT4 and c-JUN into mouse iPSCs from normal hepatocytes to generate tumor formation [59]. These approaches to induce the feedback regulation of the stemness gene family and oncogene family might provide a novel approach to generate CSC-like clones. Elevated expression of OCT4 and c-JUN was observed in specimens taken from patients with liver cancers. These findings suggest that both genes are possible candidates as future therapeutic targets.

Conclusions

In this review, we have described the methods for generating CSC-like cells from iPSCs from liver cancer cells. The critical point is to isolate the clone with strongest tumor-inducing activity. We have identified the genes of stemness and oncogenes as possible CSC target genes. This approach can now be extended to isolate CSCs and to generate disease- or cancer-specific models with distinct features. However, the efficiency of cell reprogramming from iPSCs to CSCs is lower and each CSCs has been shown to be heterogeneous. Moreover, oncogene induced plasticity including the CSC markers, and the microenvironments controlling this process have still not been elucidated, especially in the cases of the solid tumors [23, 61–63]. Further work is needed to identify and characterize CSC-like cells in other cancers and diseases, which will help to detect the driver and passenger mutations for generating cancers and genetic diseases. The study of the reprogramming of cancer cells should be encouraged to further progress the understanding of cancer and disease biology.

Abbreviations
CSC: Cancer stem cell; EC: Embryonic carcinoma; EMT: Epithelial mesenchymal transition; ESC: Embryonic stem cell; GMB: Glioblastoma; iPSC: Induced pluripotent stem cell; MET: Mesenchymal epithelial transition; MMP: Matrix metalloproteinase; NOD SCID: Nonobese diabetic/severe combined immunodeficient; OSKM: OCT4, SOX2, KLF4 and MYC; PRC: Polycomb repressive complex; YY1: Yin Yang 1

Acknowledgements
We thank CC Ku for drawing the figure and table.

Funding
This work was supported in part by MOST 104-2320-B-037-033-My2, and MOST 104-2314-B-033-002 from the Ministry of Science and Technology; NHRI-Ex102-10109B1, and NHRI-Ex104-10416S1, from the National Health Research Institutes in Taiwan; and KMU-TP103G00, G01, G03, G04, G05,

KMU-TP103A104, KMU-TP104A04, KMU-TP104E24, KMU-TP104PR22, and KMU-DT104001 from Kaohsiung Medical University in Taiwan.

Authors' contributions
KW and CSL contributed to the preparation of this review. All authors KW, CSL, MHT, YHY, CCK, WHL, and KKK read and approved the final manuscript. KKY prepared and revised the final manuscript.

Competing interests
The authors declare that they have no competing interests.

Author details
[1]Graduate Institute of Medicine, Kaohsiung Medical University, Kaohsiung 807, Taiwan. [2]Department of Biological Sciences, National Sun Yat-sen University, Kaohsiung 805, Taiwan. [3]Center of Stem Cell Research, Kaohsiung Medical University, Kaohsiung 807, Taiwan. [4]Department of Surgery, Department of Medicine, Kaohsiung Medical University, Kaohsiung 807, Taiwan. [5]Center of Infectious Diseases and Cancer Research, Kaohsiung Medical University, Kaohsiung 807, Taiwan. [6]Research Center for Environmental Medicine, Department of Medicine, Kaohsiung Medical University, Kaohsiung 807, Taiwan. [7]Faculty of Molecular Preventive Medicine, Graduate School of Medicine, the University of Tokyo, Tokyo 113-0033, Japan. [8]Faculty of Science and Engineering, Tokushima Bunri University, Sanuki 763-2193, Japan.

References
1. Lapidot T, Sirard C, Vormoor J, Murdoch B, Hoang T, Caceres-Cortes J, Minden M, et al. A cell initiating human acute myeloid leukaemia after transplantation into SCID mice. Nature. 1994;367:645–8.
2. Medema JP. Cancer stem cells: the challenges ahead. Nat Cell Biol. 2013;15:338–44.
3. Visvader JE, Lindeman GJ. Cancer stem cells: current status and evolving complexities. Cell Stem Cell. 2012;10:717–28.
4. Yamashita T, Wang XW. Cancer stem cells in the development of liver cancer. J Clin Invest. 2013;123:1911–8.
5. Mani SA, Guo W, Liao MJ, Eaton EN, Ayyanan A, Zhou AY, Brooks M, et al. The epithelial-mesenchymal transition generates cells with properties of stem cells. Cell. 2008;133:704–15.
6. Visvader JE, Lindeman GJ. Cancer stem cells in solid tumours: accumulating evidence and unresolved questions. Nat Rev Cancer. 2008;8:755–68.
7. Hashimoto N, Tsunedomi R, Yoshimura K, Watanabe Y, Hazama S, Oka M. Cancer stem-like sphere cells induced from de-differentiated hepatocellular carcinoma-derived cell lines possess the resistance to anti-cancer drugs. BMC Cancer. 2014;14:722.
8. Marquardt JU, Raggi C, Andersen JB, Seo D, Avital I, Geller D, Lee YH, et al. Human hepatic cancer stem cells are characterized by common stemness traits and diverse oncogenic pathways. Hepatology. 2011;54:1031–42.
9. Chiba T, Kita K, Zheng YW, Yokosuka O, Saisho H, Iwama A, Nakauchi H, et al. Side population purified from hepatocellular carcinoma cells harbors cancer stem cell-like properties. Hepatology. 2006;44:240–51.
10. Ma S, Chan KW, Lee TK, Tang KH, Wo JY, Zheng BJ, Guan XY. Aldehyde dehydrogenase discriminates the CD133 liver cancer stem cell populations. Mol Cancer Res. 2008;6:1146–53.
11. Cardinale V, Renzi A, Carpino G, Torrice A, Bragazzi MC, Giuliante F, DeRose AM, et al. Profiles of cancer stem cell subpopulations in cholangiocarcinomas. Am J Pathol. 2015;185:1724–39.
12. Chen J, McKay RM, Parada LF. Malignant glioma: lessons from genomics, mouse models, and stem cells. Cell. 2012;149:36–47.
13. Vogelstein B, Papadopoulos N, Velculescu VE, Zhou S, Diaz Jr LA, Kinzler KW. Cancer genome landscapes. Science. 2013;339:1546–58.
14. Pon JR, Marra MA. Driver and passenger mutations in cancer. Annu Rev Pathol. 2015;10:25–50.
15. De S, Ganesan S. Looking beyond drivers and passengers in cancer genome sequencing data. Ann Oncol. 2016. doi: 10.1093/annonc/mdw677.
16. Gurdon JB, Wilmut I. Nuclear transfer to eggs and oocytes. Cold Spring Harb Pespect Biol. 2011;3:1–14.
17. Takahashi K, Yamanaka S. Induction of pluripotent stem cells from mouse cancer embryonic and adult fibroblast cultures by defined factors. Cell. 2006;126:663–76.
18. Takahashi K, Tanabe K, Ohnuki M, Narita M, Ichisaka T, Tomoda K, Yamanaka S. Induction of pluripotent stem cells from adult human fibroblasts by defined factors. Cell. 2007;131:861–72.
19. Yu J, Vodyanik MA, Smuga-Otto K, Antosiewicz-Bourget J, Frane JL, Tian S, Nie J, et al. Induced pluripotent stem cell lines derived from human somatic cells. Science. 2007;318:1917–20.
20. Papp B, Plath K. Reprogramming to pluripotency: stepwise resetting of the epigenetic landscape. Cell Res. 2011;21:486–501.
21. Kasai T, Chen L, Mizutani A, Kudoh T, Murakami H, Fu L, Seno M. Cancer stem cells converted from pluripotent stem cells and the cancerous niche. J Stem Cells Regen Med. 2014;10:2–7.
22. Volinia S, Nuovo G, Drusco A, Costinean S, Abujarour R, Desponts C, Garofalo M, et al. Pluripotent stem cell miRNAs and metastasis in invasive breast cancer. J Natl Cancer Inst. 2014;106. doi: 10.1093/jnci/dju324.
23. Curry EL, Moad M, Robson CN, Heer R. Using induced pluripotent stem cells as a tool for modelling carcinogenesis. World J Stem Cells. 2015;7:461–9.
24. Hochedlinger K, Blelloch R, Brennan C, Yamada Y, Kim M, Chin L, Jaenisch R. Reprogramming of a melanoma genome by nuclear transplantation. Genes Dev. 2004;18:1875–85.
25. Camare DA, Mambelli LI, Porcacchia AS, Herkis I. Advances and challenges on cancer cells reprogramming using induced pluripotent stem cells technologies. J Cancer. 2016;7:2296–303.
26. Izgi K, Canatan H, Iskender B. Current status in cancer cell reprogramming and its clinical implications. J Cancer Res Clin Oncol. 2017;143:371–83.
27. Blelloch RH, Hochedlinger K, Yamada Y, Brennan C, Kim M, Mintz B, Chin L, et al. Nuclear cloning of embryonal carcinoma cells. Proc Natl Acad Sci U S A. 2004;101:13985–90.
28. Schoenhals M, Kassambara A, De Vos J, Hose D, Moreaux J, Klein B. Embryonic stem cell markers expression in cancers. Biochem Biophys Res Commun. 2009;383:157–62.
29. Ambrosetti DC, Schöler HR, Dailey L, Basilico C. Modulation of the activity of multiple transcriptional activation domains by the DNA binding domains mediates the synergistic action of Sox2 and Oct-3 on the fibroblast growth factor-4 enhancer. J Biol Chem. 2000;275:23387–97.
30. Kuroda T, Tada M, Kubota H, Kimura H, Hatano SY, Suemori H, Nakatsuji N, et al. Octamer and Sox elements are required for transcriptional cis regulation of Nanog gene expression. Mol Cell Biol. 2005;25:2475–85.
31. Boyer LA, Lee TI, Cole MF, Johnstone SE, Levine SS, Zucker JP, Guenther MG, et al. Core transcriptional regulatory circuitry in human embryonic stem cells. Cell. 2005;122:947–56.
32. Chen X, Xu H, Yuan P, Fang F, Huss M, Vega VB, Wong E, et al. Integration of external signaling pathways with the core transcriptional network in embryonic stem cells. Cell. 2008;133:1106–17.
33. Weina K, Utikal J. SOX and cancer; current research and its implication in the clinic. Clin Transl Med. 2014;3:19.
34. Herreros-Villanueva M, Zhang JS, Koenig A, Abel EV, Smyrk TC, Bamlet WR, de Narvajas AA, et al. SOX2 promotes dedifferentiation and imparts stem cell-like features to pancreatic cancer cells. Oncogenesis. 2013;2:e61.
35. Alonso MM, Diez-Valle R, Manterola L, Rubio A, Liu D, Cortes-Santiago N, Urquiza L, et al. Genetic and epigenetic modifications of Sox2 contribute to the invasive phenotype of malignant gliomas. PLoS One. 2011;6:e26740.
36. Han X, Fang X, Lou X, Hua D, Ding W, Foltz G, Hood L, et al. Silencing SOX2 induced mesenchymal-epithelial transition and its expression predicts liver and lymph node metastasis of CRC patients. PLoS One. 2012;7:e41335.
37. Yang N, Hui L, Wang Y, Yang H, Jiang X. SOX2 promotes the migration and invasion of laryngeal cancer cells by induction of MMP-2 via the PI3K/Akt/mTOR pathway. Oncol Rep. 2014;31:2651–9.
38. Mitsui K, Tokuzawa Y, Itoh H, Segawa K, Murakami M, Takahashi K, Maruyama M, Maeda M, et al. The homeoprotein Nanog is required for maintenance of pluripotency in mouse epiblast and ES cells. Cell. 2003;113:631–42.

39. Chambers I, Colby D, Robertson M, Nichols J, Lee S, Tweedie S, Smith A. Functional expression cloning of Nanog, a pluripotency sustaining factor in embryonic stem cells. Cell. 2003;113:643–55.

40. Han J, Zhang F, Yu M, Zhao P, Ji W, Zhang H, Wu B, et al. RNA interference-mediated silencing of NANOG reduces cell proliferation and induces G0/G1 cell cycle arrest in breast cancer cells. Cancer Lett. 2012;321:80–8.

41. Jeter CR, Liu B, Liu X, Chen X, Liu C, Calhoun-Davis T, Repass J, et al. NANOG promotes cancer stem cell characteristics and prostate cancer resistance to androgen deprivation. Oncogene. 2011;30:3833–43835.

42. Carette JE, Pruszak J, Varadarajan M, Blomen VA, Gokhale S, Camargo FD, Wernig M, et al. Generation of iPSCs from cultured human malignant cells. Blood. 2010;115:4039–42.

43. Miyoshi N, Ishii H, Nagai K, Hoshino H, Mimori K, Tanaka F, Nagano H, et al. Defined factors induce reprogramming of gastrointestinal cancer cells. Proc Natl Acad Sci U S A. 2010;107:40–5.

44. Stricker SH, Feber A, Engström PG, Carén H, Kurian KM, Takashima Y, Watts C, et al. Widespread resetting of DNA methylation in glioblastoma-initiating cells suppresses malignant cellular behavior in a lineage-dependent manner. Genes Dev. 2013;27:654–69.

45. Kim J, Hoffman JP, Alpaugh RK, Rhim AD, Reichert M, Stanger BZ, Furth EE, et al. An iPSC line from human pancreatic ductal adenocarcinoma undergoes early to invasive stages of pancreatic cancer progression. Cell Rep. 2013;3:2088–99.

46. Funato K, Major T, Lewis PW, Allis CD, Tabar V. Use of human embryonic stem cells to model pediatric gliomas with H3.3K27M histone mutation. Science. 2014;346:1529–33.

47. Brennan CW, Verhaak RG, McKenna A, Campos B, Noushmehr H, Salama SR, Zheng S, TCGA Research Network, et al. The somatic genomic landscape of glioblastoma. Cell. 2013;55:462–77.

48. Fasano CA, Dimos JT, Ivanova NB, Lowry N, Lemischka IR, Temple S. shRNA knockdown of Bmi-1 reveals a critical role for p21-Rb pathway in NSC self-renewal during development. Cell Stem Cell. 2007;1:87–99.

49. Lessard J, Sauvageau G. Bmi-1 determines the proliferative capacity of normal and leukaemic stem cells. Nature. 2003;423:255–60.

50. Molofsky AV, He S, Bydon M, Morrison SJ, Pardal R. Bmi-1 promotes neural stem cell self-renewal and neural development but not mouse growth and survival by repressing the p16Ink4a and p19Arf senescence pathways. Genes Dev. 2005;19:1432–7.

51. Park IK, Morrison SJ, Clarke MF. Bmi1, stem cells, and senescence regulation. J Clin Invest. 2004;113:175–9.

52. Song LB, Li J, Liao WT, Feng Y, Yu CP, Hu LJ, Kong QL, et al. The polycomb group protein Bmi-1 represses the tumor suppressor PTEN and induces epithelial-mesenchymal transition in human nasopharyngeal epithelial cells. J Clin Invest. 2009;119:3626–36.

53. Yang MH, Hsu DS, Wang HW, Wang HJ, Lan HY, Yang WH, Huang CH, et al. Bmi1 is essential in Twist1-induced epithelial-mesenchymal transition. Nat Cell Biol. 2010;12:982–92.

54. Dong P, Kaneuchi M, Watari H, Hamada J, Sudo S, Ju J, Sakuragi N. MicroRNA-194 inhibits epithelial to mesenchymal transition of endometrial cancer cells by targeting oncogene BM-1. Mol Cancer. 2011;10:99.

55. Paranjape AN, Balaji SA, Mandal T, Krushik EV, Nagaraj P, Mukherjee G, Rangarajan A. Bmi1 regulates self-renewal and epithelial to mesenchymal transition in breast cancer cells through Nanog. BMC Cancer. 2014;14:785.

56. Kaufhold S, Garbán H, Bonavida B. Yin Yang 1 is associated with cancer stem cell transcription factors (SOX2, OCT4, BMI1) and clinical implication. J Exp Clin Cancer Res. 2016;35:84.

57. Mu P, Zhang Z, Benelli M, Karthaus WR, Hoover E, Chen CC, Wongvipat J, et al. SOX2 promotes lineage plasticity and antiandrogen resistance in TP53- and RB1-deficient prostate cancer. Science. 2017;355:84–8.

58. Ku SY, Rosario S, Wang Y, Mu P, Seshadri M, Goodrich ZW, Goodrich MM, et al. Rb1 and Trp53 cooperate to suppress prostate cancer lineage plasticity, metastasis, and antiandrogen resistance. Science. 2017;355:78–83.

59. Kuo KK, Lee KT, Chen KK, Yang YH, Lin YC, Tsai MH, Wuputra K, et al. Positive feedback loop of OCT4 and c-JUN expedites cancer stemness in liver cancer. Stem Cells. 2016;34:2613–24.

60. Chang CC, Hsu WH, Wang CC, Chou CH, Kuo MY, Lin BR, Chen ST, et al. Connective tissue growth factor activates pluripotency genes and mesenchymal-epithelial transition in head and neck cancer cells. Cancer Res. 2013;73:4147–57.

61. Friedman-Morviski D, Verma IM. Dedifferentiation and reprogramming: origin of cancer stem cells. EMBO Rep. 2014;15:244–53.

62. Rapp UR, Ceteci F, Schreck R. Oncogene-induced plasticity and cancer stem cells. Cell Cycle. 2008;7:45–51.

63. Magee JS, Piskounova E, Morrison SJ. Cancer stem cells: impact, heterogeneity, and uncertainty. Cancer Cell. 2012;21:283–96.

64. Jaenisch R, Young R. Stem cells, the molecular circuitry of pluripotency and nuclear reprogramming. Cell. 2008;132:567–82.

65. Utikali J, Maherali N, Kulalert W, Hochedinger K. Sox2 is dispensable for the reprogramming of melanocytes and melanoma cell into induced pluripotent stem cells. J Cell Sci. 2009;122:3502–10.

28

Biological functions of 12(S)-hydroxyheptadecatrienoic acid as a ligand of leukotriene B$_4$ receptor 2

Toshiaki Okuno[*] and Takehiko Yokomizo

Abstract

Although 12(S)-hydroxyheptadecatrienoic acid (12-HHT) is an abundant fatty acid, it is long considered a byproduct of thromboxane A$_2$ production. We identified a leukotriene B$_4$ receptor 2 (BLT2)-specific agonistic activity in lipid extracts from rat small intestine, and mass spectrometric analysis of partially purified lipids containing BLT2 agonistic activity revealed that 12-HHT is an endogenous ligand of BLT2. In a dextran sulfate sodium (DSS)-induced inflammatory colitis model, BLT2-deficient mice exhibited enhanced intestinal inflammation, possibly due to impaired epithelial barrier function. In a skin wound healing model, BLT2-deficient mice exhibited delayed wound healing via dampened keratinocyte migration. BLT2 also accelerates corneal wound healing, and eye drops containing a non-steroidal anti-inflammatory drug (NSAID) inhibit the production of 12-HHT, resulting in delayed corneal wound healing. Furthermore, BLT2 is expressed in pulmonary epithelial type II cells and vascular endothelial cells in the mouse lung, and BLT2-deficient mice are more susceptible to lung damage by pneumolysin. In this review, we summarize the identification and characterization of 12-HHT as a ligand for BLT2 and discuss recent research on the physiological and pathophysiological roles of the 12-HHT-BLT2 axis. Some side effects of NSAIDs such as delayed wound healing may be caused by reduced 12-HHT production rather than diminished production of prostaglandins.

Keywords: 12-HHT, Barrier function, BLT2, Cyclooxygenase, GPCR, Leukotriene B$_4$, NSAID, Prostaglandin

Background

The prostaglandin (PG) H$_2$ metabolite 12(S)-hydroxyheptadecatrienoic acid (12-HHT, Fig. 1) is biosynthesized by cyclooxygenase (COX) from arachidonic acid [1]. Some G protein-coupled receptors (GPCRs) related to PGs and leukotrienes (LTs), and metabolites of arachidonic acid (AA), were identified in the 1990s [2, 3]. By generating and analyzing gene-deficient mice in which receptors and biosynthetic enzymes for PGs and LTs were disrupted, the biological significance of PGs and LTs has been elucidated [4]. 12-HHT was identified in the 1960s, but it was considered merely as a byproduct of thromboxane (Tx) A$_2$ production [5]. In 2008, we revealed that 12-HHT is an endogenous ligand of BLT2, originally identified as a low-affinity GPCR for leukotriene B$_4$ (LTB$_4$) [6]. Our recent studies demonstrated that the 12-HHT-BLT2 axis contributes to the epithelial barrier

functions of small intestine [7], skin [8], lung [9], and cornea [10]. In this review, we summarize the identification of 12-HHT as a ligand for BLT2, together with recent knowledge of the biological functions of the 12-HHT-BLT2 axis.

Identification of 12-HHT as a natural ligand of BLT2

The second LTB$_4$ receptor, BLT2, was first identified as a low-affinity receptor for LTB$_4$ [11]. Due to the high concentration of LTB$_4$ required for BLT2 activation, we hypothesized that BLT2 might have a high-affinity lipid ligand besides LTB$_4$. To identify the bona fide ligand of BLT2, we extracted lipids from several rat organs and examined their agonistic activities using Chinese hamster ovary (CHO) cells expressing human BLT2. The acetone-soluble fraction of lipids extracted from rat small intestine exhibited a strong agonistic activity toward BLT2. Lipids were separated by high-performance liquid chromatography (HPLC) and the agonistic activities of fractions toward BLT2-expressing CHO cells were analyzed with a

---
* Correspondence: tokuno@juntendo.ac.jp
Department of Biochemistry, Juntendo University School of Medicine, Tokyo, Japan

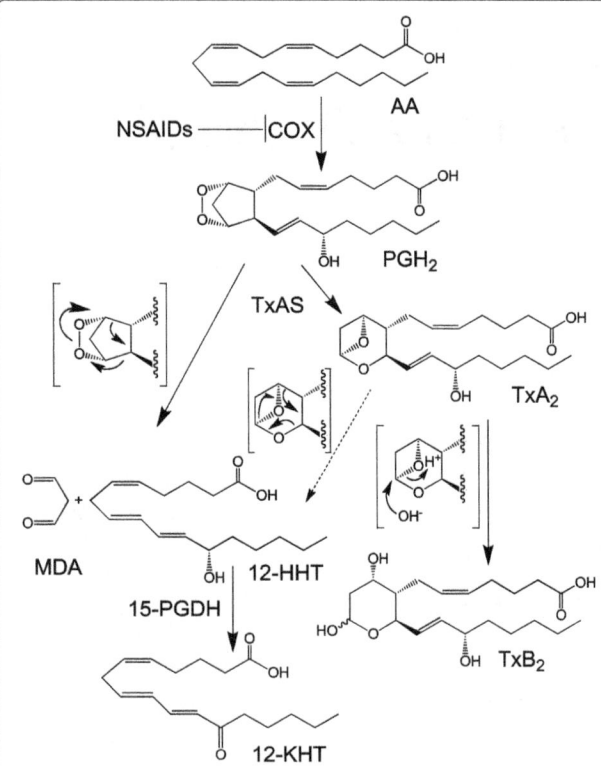

Fig. 1 Biosynthesis and metabolic pathways of 12(S)-hydroxyheptadecatrienoic acid (12-HHT). Thromboxane (Tx) A_2 synthase (TxAS) catalyzes the fragmentation of PGH_2 into 12-HHT and malondialdehyde (MDA). TxA_2 is unstable in aqueous solution and rapidly hydrolyzed to TxB_2, but a proportion of TxA_2 is hydrolyzed to 12-HHT and MDA. 12-HHT is metabolized to 12-keto-heptadecatrienoic acid (12-KHT) by 15-hydroxyprostaglandin dehydrogenase (15-PGDH)

cytosensor microphysiometer that detects acidification of the extracellular fluid caused by proton efflux from activated cells. The fraction containing a strong agonistic activity was analyzed by mass spectrometry (MS) to elucidate the molecular mass and structure of the BLT2 agonistic lipid therein. The combination of exact mass measurement and MS/MS analysis revealed the BLT2 agonist as 12(S)-hydroxyheptadecatrienoic acid (12-HHT), a C17 fatty acid. Commercially available 12-HHT from both Cayman and Biomol (Enzo) activated CHO-BLT2 at a lower concentration than LTB_4 in calcium, cAMP, and chemotaxis assays. The HPLC retention time of authentic 12-HHT and m/z values of MS/MS fragments were identical to those of the agonist extracted from rat small intestine. Furthermore, lipids extracted from small intestine of COX-1-deficient mice displayed much lower agonistic activity than wild-type (WT) mice, suggesting that 12-HHT, a metabolite of COX-1, is an endogenous ligand of BLT2 [6]. Recently, we cloned two zebrafish orthologues of human BLT2, zBLT2a, and zBLT2b, and these receptors were also activated by a

lower concentration of 12-HHT than LTB_4, in a similar fashion to human and mouse BLT2 [12].

Biosynthesis and metabolism of 12-HHT

12-HHT is biosynthesized from the AA metabolite PGH_2 by COX. Thromboxane A synthase (TxAS) catalyzes not only the rearrangement of PGH_2 to TxA_2, it also catalyzes in parallel, and to an almost equimolar amount, its fragmentation into 12-HHT and malondialdehyde (MDA) [13, 14]. During platelet aggregation, large amounts of TxA_2 and 12-HHT are produced by the actions of cytosolic phospholipase $A_2\alpha(cPLA_2\alpha)$, COX-1, and TxAS. 12(S)-Hydroxyeicosatetraenoic acid (12-HETE) is also produced from activated platelets by the action of 12(S)-lipoxygenase (12-LO) [15]. Nonsteroidal anti-inflammatory drug (NSAID) treatment induces the shunting of AA from PG metabolism to 12-HETE production [16]. A high concentration of 12-HETE also activates BLT2 (16), but the biological significance of the 12-HETE-BLT2 axis remains elusive. In addition to catalysis by TxAS, 12-HHT is synthesized from PGH_2 via a non-enzymatic pathway [17]. PGH_2 is extremely unstable and rapidly hydrolyzed to 12-HHT and MDA, or PGE_2, PGD_2, and $PGF_2\alpha$ in aqueous solution. PGH_2 is also rapidly converted to 12-HHT and MDA in the presence of heme or glutathione [13]. TxA_2 is also an unstable metabolite of PGH_2, and most TxA_2 is hydrolyzed to TxB_2, but a proportion of TxA_2 may be hydrolyzed to 12-HHT and MDA (Fig. 1). Additionally, the cytochrome P450 enzyme CYP2S1 that is expressed in macrophages reportedly generates 12-HHT [18, 19], but the contribution of CYP2S1 to 12-HHT production is uncertain. Hecker et al. reported that 12-HHT is preferentially metabolized to a 12-keto derivative by 15-hydroxyprostaglandin dehydrogenase (15-PGDH) [20]. We examined the agonistic activity of 12-keto-heptadecatrienoic acid (12-KHT), which was chemically synthesized by our collaborator [21], toward BLT2, and this was lower than that of 12-HHT (Okuno, unpublished). Eicosanoid profiling using LC-MS/MS with synthetic 12-KHT as a standard for multiple reaction monitoring (MRM) revealed the presence of 12-KHT in various cells and tissues in which 12-HHT is abundant, suggesting that 12-KHT is a metabolite of 12-HHT.

Physiological and pathophysiological roles of the 12-HHT-BLT2 axis

BLT2 is expressed in epithelial cells of intestine and skin keratinocytes in mice [22], suggesting that the 12-HHT-BLT2 axis may contribute to epithelial functions (Table 1). To investigate the roles of BLT2 in intestinal epithelial cells, we analyzed a dextran sulfate sodium (DSS)-induced colitis mouse model. BLT2-deficient mice exhibited enhanced intestinal inflammation, possibly caused by impaired barrier

Table 1 Physiological and pathophysiological roles of the 12-HHT-BLT2 axis

Tissues/cells	In vivo roles of 12-HHT/BLT2	Possible mechanisms
Skin	Acceleration of wound healing	Keratinocyte migration
Cornea	Acceleration of wound healing	Corneal epithelial cell migration
Lung	Protective roles in acute lung injury	Inhibition of CysLT1 signaling
Lung	Suppression of asthma	Reduction of IL-13
Cancer	Chemotherapy resistance	Survival of cancer cells

function [7]. Madin-Darby canine kidney II (MDCK II) cells overexpressing BLT2 exhibited enhanced barrier function when measuring transepithelial electrical resistance (TER) and FITC-dextran leakage. Interestingly, BLT2 was localized to the lateral membrane, and it increased claudin-4 (CLDN4) expression via the Gαi protein-p38 MAPK pathway [23].

To investigate the roles of BLT2 in skin, we evaluated a skin wound healing model. BLT2-deficient mice exhibited delayed wound healing compared with WT mice. Aspirin-treated mice also displayed delayed wound healing, and the delay was abolished in BLT2-deficient mice. TxAS-deficient mice also exhibited partially delayed wound healing, but TxA$_2$/PGH$_2$ receptor (TP)-deficient mice did not show this phenotype. Importantly, a synthetic BLT2 agonist accelerated wound healing in C57BL/6J and diabetic *db/db* mice [8]. We also examined the detailed mechanism of BLT2-dependent acceleration of wound healing. BLT2 stimulation leads to the expression of tumor necrosis factor (TNF)α and interleukin (IL)-1β, both of which stimulate the expression and secretion of metalloproteinases (MMPs) that in turn accelerate keratinocyte migration, possibly by degrading extracellular matrix. These results suggest that

the 12-HHT-BLT2 axis accelerates skin wound healing in vivo (Fig. 2). As described above, NSAIDs such as aspirin inhibit the production of 12-HHT. Our study clearly showed that aspirin-dependent delay in skin wound healing is due to the reduced production of 12-HHT, but not PGs. Reduced 12-HHT levels may therefore explain some side effects of NSAIDs.

Recently, we showed that BLT2 is also expressed in corneal epithelial cells in mice and humans, and the 12-HHT-BLT2 axis accelerates corneal epithelial cell migration and healing of corneal wounds. NSAID-containing eye drops inhibit the production of 12-HHT, which also delays corneal wound healing. These results suggest that the 12-HHT-BLT2 axis accelerates corneal wound healing in a similar manner to skin [10].

Moreover, we found that BLT2 is expressed in pulmonary epithelial type II cells and vascular endothelial cells in the mouse lung. To investigate the roles of BLT2 in lungs, mice were intratracheally treated with pneumolysin (PLY) that induces acute lung injury (ALI). Surprisingly, BLT2-deficient mice were more susceptible to lung damage by PLY, and most BLT2-deficient mice died within minutes, in contrast to intact WT mice. Although the detailed roles of BLT2 in protection against ALI are unclear, we found that PLY treatment induced the production of large amounts of cysteinyl leukotrienes (CysLTs), and a CysLT1 receptor antagonist recovered PLY-induced mortality, vascular permeability, and airway resistance, in both WT and BLT2-deficient mice. These results suggest that the 12-HHT-BLT2 axis suppresses CysLT1 signaling in vascular endothelial cells because production of CysLTs was not affected by BLT2 deficiency (Fig. 3) [9]. In addition, BLT2-knockout (KO) mice exhibited severe eosinophilic lung inflammation in an ovalbumin (OVA)-induced allergic airway disease model. This was explained by enhanced IL-13 production from BLT2-deficient CD4$^+$ cells [24].

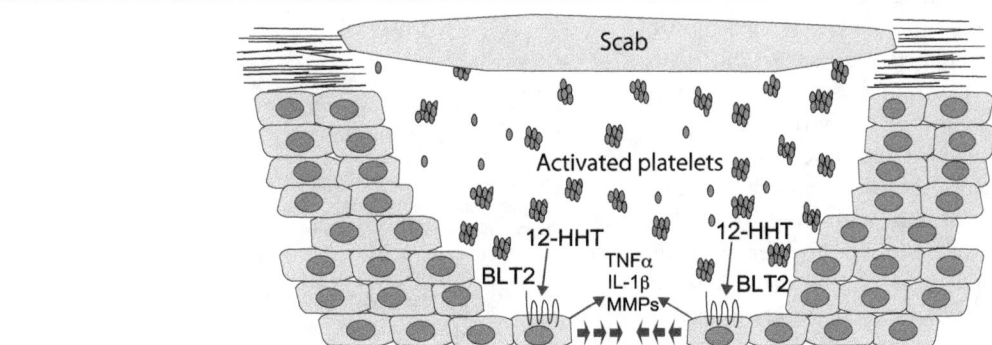

Fig. 2 Roles of the 12-HHT-LTB$_4$ receptor 2 (BLT2) axis in skin wound healing. BLT2 expressed on the surface of keratinocytes is activated by 12-HHT produced by activated platelets. The 12-HHT-BLT2 axis accelerates keratinocyte migration via the production of tumor necrosis factor (TNF)α, interleukin (IL)-1β, and matrix metalloproteinases (MMPs)

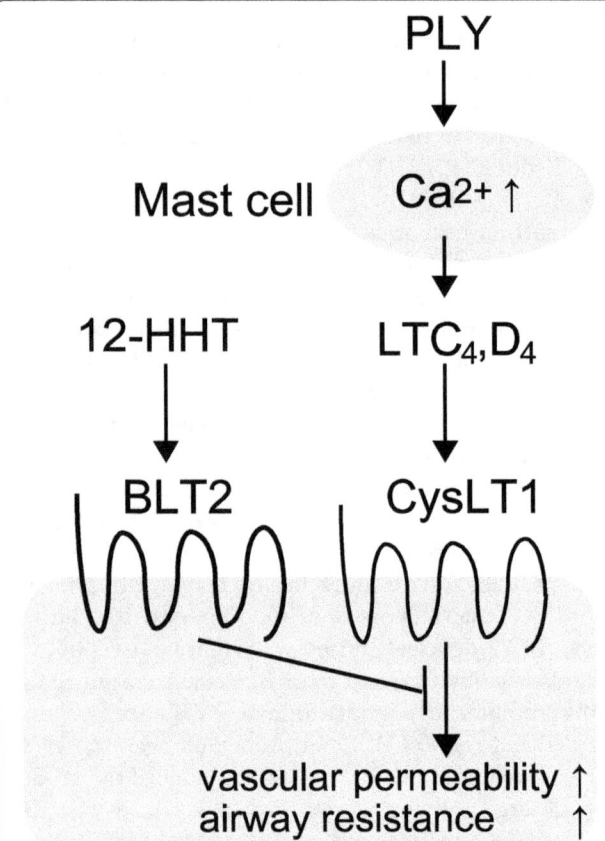

Fig. 3 Roles of the 12-HHT-LTB₄ receptor 2 (BLT2) axis in lung injury. PLY treatment induces the production of large amounts of cysteinyl leukotrienes (CysLTs) from mast cells. The CysLT1 receptor antagonist ameliorates PLY-induced mortality, vascular permeability, and airway resistance. 12-HHT-BLT2 axis suppresses CysLT1 signaling in vascular endothelial cells and smooth muscle cells, but the detailed molecular mechanism is under investigation

Conclusions
For a long time, 12-HHT was considered merely a byproduct of thromboxane biosynthesis, and a biomarker of COX activation. However, we discovered that 12-HHT is an endogenous ligand of BLT2 using unbiased ligand screening and, with others, revealed that the 12-HHT-BLT2 axis mediates various biological functions including the epithelial barrier, wound healing, immunosuppression, and lung protection in vivo. Some side effects of NSAIDs, such as delayed wound healing, may be caused by reduced 12-HHT production rather than diminished PG production.

Abbreviations
12-HHT: 12(S)-Hydroxyheptadecatrienoic acid; ALI: Acute lung injury; BLT2: LTB₄ receptor 2; COX: Cyclooxygenase; CysLT: Cysteinyl leukotriene; LT: Leukotriene; MDA: Malondialdehyde; NSAID: Non-steroidal anti-inflammatory drug; PG: Prostaglandin; PLY: Pneumolysin; Tx: Thromboxane

Acknowledgements
We would like to sincerely thank to all lab members and collaborators.

Funding
This work was supported by MEXT/JSPS KAKENHI (grant numbers 16K08596, 15KK0320, 15H05904, 15H04708, and 18H02627) and the Takeda Science Foundation.

Authors' contributions
TO prepared the manuscript and figures. TY revised the manuscript. TO and TY approved the final manuscript.

Furthermore, 12-HHT-BLT2 signaling is reported to be involved in chemotherapy resistance. F4/80⁺/CD11b^low splenocytes produce 12-HHT following treatment with platinum analogs, which mediates chemotherapy resistance. Interestingly, genetic loss or chemical inhibition of BLT2 prevents 12-HHT-mediated resistance [25]. Combined indomethacin and platinum-based chemotherapy may therefore improve chemo-sensitivity by reducing the production of 12-HHT [26]. We and others reported the roles of BLT2 in cancer cells. Human pancreatic cancer cells express BLT2, and treatment with the BLT2 antagonist or BLT2 knockdown inhibited proliferation and induces apoptosis in pancreatic cancer cells [27–29]. Generation of LTB₄-BLT2-dependent reactive oxygen species (ROS) promotes anti-apoptotic, invasive, and metastatic phenotypes in cancer cells [30–33], suggesting that BLT2 antagonists might be candidates for therapeutic agents against cancer.

References
1. Hamberg M, Samuelsson B. Oxygenation of unsaturated fatty acids by the vesicular gland of sheep. J Biol Chem. 1967;242(22):5344–54.
2. Brink C, Dahlen SE, Drazen J, Evans JF, Hay DW, Nicosia S, et al. International Union of Pharmacology XXXVII. Nomenclature for leukotriene and lipoxin receptors. Pharmacol Rev. 2003;55(1):195–227.
3. Narumiya S, Sugimoto Y, Ushikubi F. Prostanoid receptors: structures, properties, and functions. Physiol Rev. 1999;79(4):1193–226.
4. Back M, Dahlen SE, Drazen JM, Evans JF, Serhan CN, Shimizu T, et al. International Union of Basic and Clinical Pharmacology. LXXXIV: leukotriene receptor nomenclature, distribution, and pathophysiological functions. Pharmacol Rev. 2011;63(3):539–84.
5. John H, Cammann K, Schlegel W. Development and review of radioimmunoassay of 12-S-hydroxyheptadecatrienoic acid. Prostaglandins Other Lipid Mediators. 1998;56(2–3):53–76.
6. Okuno T, Iizuka Y, Okazaki H, Yokomizo T, Taguchi R, Shimizu T. 12(S)-Hydroxyheptadeca-5Z, 8E, 10E-trienoic acid is a natural ligand for leukotriene B4 receptor 2. J Exp Med. 2008;205(4):759–66.
7. Iizuka Y, Okuno T, Saeki K, Uozaki H, Okada S, Misaka T, et al. Protective role of the leukotriene B4 receptor BLT2 in murine inflammatory colitis. FASEB J. 2010;24(12):4678–90.

8. Liu M, Saeki K, Matsunobu T, Okuno T, Koga T, Sugimoto Y, et al. 12-Hydroxyheptadecatrienoic acid promotes epidermal wound healing by accelerating keratinocyte migration via the BLT2 receptor. J Exp Med. 2014;211(6):1063–78.

9. Shigematsu M, Koga T, Ishimori A, Saeki K, Ishii Y, Taketomi Y, et al. Leukotriene B4 receptor type 2 protects against pneumolysin-dependent acute lung injury. Sci Rep. 2016;6:34560.

10. Iwamoto S, Koga T, Ohba M, Okuno T, Koike M, Murakami A, et al. Non-steroidal anti-inflammatory drug delays corneal wound healing by reducing production of 12-hydroxyheptadecatrienoic acid, a ligand for leukotriene B4 receptor 2. Sci Rep. 2017;7(1):13267.

11. Yokomizo T, Kato K, Terawaki K, Izumi T, Shimizu T. A second leukotriene B(4) receptor, BLT2. A new therapeutic target in inflammation and immunological disorders. J Exp Med. 2000;192(3):421–32.

12. Okuno T, Ishitani T, Yokomizo T. Biochemical characterization of three BLT receptors in zebrafish. PLoS One. 2015;10(3):e0117888.

13. Hecker M, Ullrich V. On the mechanism of prostacyclin and thromboxane A2 biosynthesis. J Biol Chem. 1989;264(1):141–50.

14. Hecker M, Haurand M, Ullrich V, Diczfalusy U, Hammarstrom S. Products, kinetics, and substrate specificity of homogeneous thromboxane synthase from human platelets: development of a novel enzyme assay. Arch Biochem Biophys. 1987;254(1):124–35.

15. Vincent JE, Zijlstra FJ, van Vliet H. Determination of the formation of thromboxane B2 (TxB2), 12L-hydroxy-5,8,10 heptadecatrienoic acid (HHT) and 12L-hydroxy-5,8,10,14 eicosatrienoic acid (HETE) from arachidonic acid and of the TxB2 :HHT, TxB2 :HETE and (TxB2 +HHT) :HETE ratio in human platelets. Possible use in diagnostic purposes. Prostaglandins Med. 1980;5(2):79–84.

16. Yokomizo T, Kato K, Hagiya H, Izumi T, Shimizu T. Hydroxyeicosanoids bind to and activate the low affinity leukotriene B4 receptor, BLT2. J Biol Chem. 2001;276(15):12454–9.

17. Matsunobu T, Okuno T, Yokoyama C, Yokomizo T. Thromboxane a synthase-independent production of 12-hydroxyheptadecatrienoic acid, a BLT2 ligand. J Lipid Res. 2013;54(11):2979–87.

18. Fromel T, Kohlstedt K, Popp R, Yin X, Awwad K, Barbosa-Sicard E, et al. Cytochrome P4502S1: a novel monocyte/macrophage fatty acid epoxygenase in human atherosclerotic plaques. Basic Res Cardiol. 2013;108(1):319.

19. Bui P, Imaizumi S, Beedanagari SR, Reddy ST, Hankinson O. Human CYP2S1 metabolizes cyclooxygenase- and lipoxygenase-derived eicosanoids. Drug metab Dispos. 2011;39(2):180–90.

20. Hecker M, Ullrich V. 12(S)-Hydroxy-5,8,10 (Z,E,E)-heptadecatrienoic acid (HHT) is preferentially metabolized to its 12-keto derivative by human erythrocytes in vitro. Eicosanoids. 1988;1(1):19–25.

21. Tojo T, Wang Q, Okuno T, Yokomizo T, Kobayashi Y. Synthesis of (S,5Z,8E,10E)-12-Hydroxyheptadeca-5,8,10-trienoic acid (12S-HHT) and its analogues. Synlett. 2013;24(12):1545–8.

22. Iizuka Y, Yokomizo T, Terawaki K, Komine M, Tamaki K, Shimizu T. Characterization of a mouse second leukotriene B4 receptor, mBLT2: BLT2-dependent ERK activation and cell migration of primary mouse keratinocytes. J Biol Chem. 2005;280(26):24816–23.

23. Ishii Y, Saeki K, Liu M, Sasaki F, Koga T, Kitajima K, et al. Leukotriene B4 receptor type 2 (BLT2) enhances skin barrier function by regulating tight junction proteins. FASEB J. 2016;30(2):933–47.

24. Matsunaga Y, Fukuyama S, Okuno T, Sasaki F, Matsunobu T, Asai Y, et al. Leukotriene B4 receptor BLT2 negatively regulates allergic airway eosinophilia. FASEB J. 2013;27(8):3306–14.

25. Houthuijzen JM, Daenen LG, Roodhart JM, Oosterom I, van Jaarsveld MT, Govaert KM, et al. Lysophospholipids secreted by splenic macrophages induce chemotherapy resistance via interference with the DNA damage response. Nat Commun. 2014;5:5275.

26. van der Velden DL, Cirkel GA, Houthuijzen JM, van Werkhoven E, Roodhart JML, Daenen LGM, et al. Phase I study of combined indomethacin and platinum-based chemotherapy to reduce platinum-induced fatty acids. Cancer Chemother Pharmacol. 2018;81(5):911–21.

27. Hennig R, Osman T, Esposito I, Giese N, Rao SM, Ding XZ, et al. BLT2 is expressed in PanINs, IPMNs, pancreatic cancer and stimulates tumour cell proliferation. Br J Cancer. 2008;99(7):1064–73.

28. Ding XZ, Talamonti MS, Bell RH Jr, Adrian TE. A novel anti-pancreatic cancer agent, LY293111. Anti-Cancer Drugs. 2005;16(5):467–73.

29. Tong WG, Ding XZ, Hennig R, Witt RC, Standop J, Pour PM, et al.

Leukotriene B4 receptor antagonist LY293111 inhibits proliferation and induces apoptosis in human pancreatic cancer cells. Clin Cancer Res. 2002;8(10):3232–42.

30. Lee JW, Kim JH. Activation of the leukotriene B4 receptor 2-reactive oxygen species (BLT2-ROS) cascade following detachment confers anoikis resistance in prostate cancer cells. J Biol Chem. 2013;288(42):30054–63.

31. Cho KJ, Seo JM, Kim JH. Bioactive lipoxygenase metabolites stimulation of NADPH oxidases and reactive oxygen species. Mol Cells. 2011;32(1):1–5.

32. Ryu HC, Kim C, Kim JY, Chung JH, Kim JH. UVB radiation induces apoptosis in keratinocytes by activating a pathway linked to "BLT2-reactive oxygen species". J Invest Dermatol. 2010;130(4):1095–106.

33. Choi JA, Kim EY, Song H, Kim C, Kim JH. Reactive oxygen species are generated through a BLT2-linked cascade in Ras-transformed cells. Free Radic Biol Med. 2008;44(4):624–34.

29

Use of mesenchymal stem cells seeded on the scaffold in articular cartilage repair

Kaoru Yamagata, Shingo Nakayamada and Yoshiya Tanaka[*]

Abstract

Articular cartilage has poor capacity for repair. Once damaged, they degenerate, causing functional impairment of joints. Allogeneic cartilage transplantation has been performed for functional recovery of articular cartilage. However, there is only a limited amount of articular cartilage available for transplantation. Mesenchymal stem cells (MSCs) could be potentially suitable for local implantation. MSCs can differentiate into chondrocytes. Several studies have demonstrated the therapeutic potential of MSCs in the repair of articular cartilage in animal models of articular cartilage damage and in patients with damaged articular cartilage. To boost post-implantation MSC differentiation into chondrocytes, the alternative delivery methods by scaffolds, using hyaluronic acid (HA) or poly-lactic-co-glycolic-acid (PLGA), have developed. In this review, we report recent data on the repair of articular cartilage and discuss future developments.

Keywords: Articular cartilage, Mesenchymal stem cells (MSCs), Scaffold, Poly-lactic-co-glycolic acids (PLGA), Hyaluronic acid (HA)

Background

The articular cartilage plays an important role in the smooth motion of joints. Aging is associated with thinning of the articular cartilage tissue and reduction of its function. Aging is also associated with diminished physical activity, leading to impaired activity of daily living (ADL) and quality of life (QOL). The articular cartilage is a structurally unique tissue, lacking blood vessels and nerves, and is considered to be in a low-nutrient, low-oxygen environment. Furthermore, the inflammatory milieu breaks down the cartilage matrix and induces apoptosis of chondrocytes, leading to irreversible defect in the cartilage, a process that is currently difficult to repair in patients with cartilage degenerative diseases, including rheumatoid arthritis (RA) and osteoarthritis (OA). While certain managements are available to alleviate pain or recover cartilage function, these do not result in recovery once the articular cartilage is damaged. Thus, there is a need to design new techniques for repair of articular cartilage and hence to improve ADL and QOL. In fact, several procedures, such as joint replacement, allogeneic chondrocyte implantation, and implantation of mesenchymal stem

cells (MSCs) seeded on scaffold, have been used in regenerative medicine of the articular cartilage.

Joint replacement bears a heavy burden on patients, and some undesirable effects on the surrounding tissues are sometimes unavoidable. Two types of osteochondral transplantations are considered as alternative techniques. One is autologous osteochondral transplantation, which involves grafting articular cartilage taken from healthy subjects into the affected area [1]. The pathological features of the articular cartilage improve over a short term, whereas the long-term effects are inconsistent [1, 2]. The other technique is allogeneic osteochondral transplantation with the goal of repairing widespread defect in the articular cartilage. In fact, this technique provides improvement of the articular cartilage [3]. However, there remain several issues that need to be discussed, such as the need for adaptation of donor's graft size to the recipient one, assessment of the general health condition, with or without infection [4, 5].

Autologous chondrocyte implantation has been tried also as an alternative strategy. The aim of such treatment is to repair the articular cartilage via implantation of chondrocytes into the affected area after in vitro proliferation of samples prepared from healthy articular cartilage [6]. It has been reported that chondrocytes seeded on a scaffold then implanted into the cartilaginous

---

* Correspondence: tanaka@med.uoeh-u.ac.jp
The First Department of Internal Medicine, School of Medicine, University of Occupational and Environmental Health, Japan, 1-1 Iseigaoka, Yahata-nishi-ku, Kitakyushu 807-8555, Japan

defect can result in the repair of articular cartilage of the knee and ankle tissues within 7–13 and 2–5 years, respectively [7–9]. However, this method has its limitation especially with the use of less than the recommended number of chondrocytes during the implantation process; such cells lose their ability to produce cartilage extracellular matrix (ECM) like hyaline cartilage due to the dedifferentiation of these cells [10–12].

Another promising strategy that has been tested recently is the use of a scaffold alone or bone marrow-derived MSCs seeded on scaffold. MSCs reside in many types of tissues, including bone marrow, adipose, or synovium, and are easy to isolate from these organs. In vitro studies showed that bone marrow-derived MSCs can differentiate into various mesenchymal lineages, including chondrocytes [13]. In vivo studies showed that MSCs contribute to the coverage of articular cartilage, indicating that MSCs are proper tool for implantation to repair the articular cartilage [14–16]. Recently, different types of MSCs other than bone marrow-derived MSCs, including ones derived from synovial tissue, peripheral blood, periosteum, or adipose tissue, have been focused in terms of articular cartilage repair [17–20]. The accumulating evidences demonstrate potential utility of MSCs in the repair of articular cartilage. In particular, it is easy to take large amounts of adipose-derived MSCs (ASC) from fat tissue. However, ability to differentiation of ASC into chondrocytes is poor [21, 22].

In this review, we introduce recent evidences and current status based on mechanism of chondrocyte differentiation and regeneration of the articular cartilage, and then discuss future prospects.

Damage of articular cartilage reflects physical disorder in RA

RA is a systemic autoimmune disease characterized by chronic inflammatory synovitis and progressive joint destruction, which is associated with serious morbidity and mortality [23–25]. Without appropriate treatment, the patients suffer heavy physical disorder associated with limited joint function [24, 25]. Especially, destruction of the articular cartilage, but not bone tissue, correlates with the physical disorder of RA [26, 27]. Clinical or structural remission has recently become an achievable goal through the use of methotrexate (MTX) as the first line disease modifying antirheumatic drug, in addition to tumor necrosis factor (TNF) inhibitors, interleukin-6 (IL-6) inhibitors and cytotoxic T-lymphocyte-associated antigen 4 immunoglobulin fusion protein (CTLA-4Ig), or small-molecular compounds that target Janus kinase (JAK) [28–30]. In this regard, rapid and effective induction of remission is a prerequisite for halting the process of joint destruction. However, it is still difficult to repair damaged or degenerated articular cartilage. Therefore, there is a need for novel treatment strategies, such as regenerative medicine.

Mesenchymal stem cells can differentiate into chondrocytes

The articular cartilage covering the bone heads is composed of chondrocytes and cartilage ECM, which is comprised of aggrecan, proteoglycan, type II, IX, and XI collagen. These tissues, however, show poor self-repair capability. Damage or loss of these tissues often results in functional disorder such as OA. At present, autologous cartilage tissue implantation is applied for functional recovery of articular cartilage tissue [31], but unfortunately, this treatment has the following demerits. First, only a limited amount of osteochondral tissue can be prepared from the patients. Second, the implantation further hurts the residual healthy articular cartilage. Based on the above fact, there is certainly a need to develop novel therapies that can prevent and promote repair of damaged articular cartilage.

Different scaffolds have been designed as the delivery system for the repair of articular cartilage. MSCs reside in various types of tissues, including bone marrow, adipose, synovium, cartilage tissue, and placenta. These cells can differentiate into different types of cells that constitute the joints, including osteoblasts, osteocytes, tenocytes, adipocytes, and chondrocytes [13]. It is anticipated that the use of MSCs residing on scaffolds may help in the regeneration/repair of degenerated or damaged articular cartilage. However, endogenous MSCs have poor ability to repair articular cartilage. Although MSCs are injected intravenously (IV), intra-articularly (IA), or intra-peritoneally (IP), the cells diffuse into the peripheral blood and reside in non-affected area [32–35]. Consequently, such implantation has little effect on the phenotype of the destroyed cartilage tissue. In order to overcome this problem, the transplantation of MSC formed in three dimensional structures, such as cell aggregates and sheets, have been tried [36].

On the other hand, other biological functions of MSCs, such as anti-inflammation, anti-fibrosis, migration, and proliferation, have been reported [32, 33, 37, 38], indicating critical role of MSCs instead of chondrocyte differentiation in cell therapies. In this review, we focus on chondrogenesis related to the repair of articular cartilage.

Chondrogenic differentiation between the 2D and 3D cultures

MSCs in the living body reside in 3dimensional (3D) circumstance. To make implanted MSCs reside in 3D, pre-implantation (IMP) MSCs should be set at 3D, in this case MSCs are seeded on various types of scaffolds. 3D scaffold should be special material, that mimic circumstance in the living body and is proper for cell adhesion, differentiation, proliferation, and formation of cartilage ECM [39].

After harton's jelly (WT)-MSCs were cultured with chondrocyte differentiation medium over 21 days, transcriptional activity of *type II collagen* gene was increased in the culture of 2D (PLGA free monolayer) or 3D with PLGA scaffold [39]. Expression of both *type I collagen* (an osteoblast marker) and *type III collagen* (a fibrocartilage marker) were decreased in 3D whereas their expression were increased in 2D. This indicates that MSCs in 3D, but not 2D, may play role in the formation of hyaline cartilage, but not fibrocartilage or bone tissue.

We have reported that MSCs were cultured with cell growth medium in 2D with cell monolayer (PLGA free) or 3D with PLGA plug scaffold [40]. 3D culture at day 7, but not 2D, up-regulated SOX9 (master regulators of bone and cartilage differentiation). MSCs in 3D culture at day 14, but not 2D, showed positive staining for proteoglycan by safranin O staining. Taken together, 3D-based PLGA promotes efficiently the chondrocyte differentiation of MSCs in vitro without any cytokine stimulation.

Other group showed that compared with 2D culture with MSCs monolayer, collagen-based sponge could enhance differentiation of MSCs into chondrocyte in vitro. This indicates that type II collagen as a cartilage ECM contributes to differentiation of MSCs into chondrocytes.

Thus, these results show significance and generality of 3D MSCs culture with scaffold in chondrogenesis.

PLGA scaffold is required for the repair of articular cartilages

The purpose of implantation is for MSCs to efficiently differentiate into chondrocytes, then express large amounts of cartilage ECM, form hyaline cartilage, and then assimilate into the surrounding tissues. First, a scaffold is required for MSCs to reside on the damaged articular cartilage. Poly-lactic-co-glycolic acids (PLGA) is representative commonly used scaffold composed of both poly-glycolic acid (PGA) and poly-lactic acid (PLA). PLGA has several advantages, such as controlled biodegradability, i.e. it disintegrate in the living body, low immunogenicity, efficient carrier of drugs to the target tissue, forms a scaffold for regeneration of cartilage defect through the support of cell residence and cell differentiation.

Implantation of PLGA alone into the affected joints of a rabbit model of osteochondral defect results in satisfactory repair of the bone and cartilage tissues and results in adequate cover of the defect with cartilage tissue [41]. This finding indicates that endogenous MSCs can adhere to PLGA, and then help in the repair of articular damage. Another in vitro study showed that MSCs seeded on PLGA can differentiate into chondrocytes without any cytokine stimulation [40]. These data emphasize the utility of PLGA as a MSC scaffold to achieve efficient repair of the articular cartilage. On the other hand, bone marrow-derived MSCs obtained from *IL-1Ra* gene knockout mice, which mimic various pathological conditions including RA, have low capacity for

self-renewal or differentiation into osteoblasts compared to the wild-type mice [42]. It is possible that MSCs from RA patients also have poor capacity for differentiation. Thus, it is preferable perhaps to co-implant normal and exogenous MSCs, but not endogenous MSCs, with a scaffold into the affected area in order to achieve a better repair of the articular cartilage in RA. Another study reported the finding of positive staining for proteoglycan in the affected region and the formation of hyaline cartilage-like tissue after implantation of MSC sheet-coated PLGA+MSCs into the cartilage defect into the smooth white tissue of rabbits [43].

While the scaffold enhances residence of MSCs into the local tissue, this can be augmented by the addition of cytokines. For instance, PLGA with transforming growth factor-β3 (TGF-β3) enhanced MSC differentiation into chondrocytes, while implantation of PLGA with stromal-derived factor-1α (SDF-1α) into resulted in repair of the articular cartilage [44, 45]. Thus, implantation of PLGA combined with various cytokines enhances more efficient differentiation of MSCs into articular cartilage.

MSC implantation is relatively safe. One study reported lack of any oncogenesis or infection at 5–137 months after MSC implantation [46]. On the other hand, implantation of polyglycolic acid-hyaluronan with MSCs also induced repair of the damaged articular cartilage [43]. To date, however, the use of PLGA for the repair of articular cartilage remains experimental. Thus, more efficient tools are needed in the future.

Collagen scaffold provides the repair of articular cartilages

Collagen molecules are major components of cartilage ECM, and degraded by collagenases in the living body. Collagen-based material provides proper circumstance for chondrocyte differentiation. Thus, the scaffold is commonly applied for repair strategy of articular cartilage.

Li et al. have reported utility of special tool in the repair of articular cartilage [47]. After rabbit MSCs and collagen are capsuled with microsphere, the tool are applied to implantation into affected area of the osteochondral defect of rabbit. This procedure provided positive staining for type II collagen and glycosaminoglycan (CAG), suggesting formation of hyaline-like tissue. Further, implantation of collagen scaffold alone introduces the repair the osteochondral defect [48]. This finding indicates that the scaffold promotes spontaneous differentiation of endogenous MSCs into chondrocytes.

On the other hand, clinical applications have been tried energetically in addition to studies using animal model. Implantation of collagen gel and MSCs into the athlete, who suffers from knee's pain, results in the formation of hyaline-like tissue, and functional recovery of the articular cartilage [49]. Collectively, these evidences emphasize that collagen materials are a proper and promising scaffold for the repair of the articular cartilage.

Gelatin scaffold is required for the repair of articular cartilages

Hydrogel is 3D polymeric material that can retain large amount of water. The scaffold provides good biocompatibility and can have an affinity with growth factor or cells, such as MSCs. To date hydrogel scaffolds, including agarose or gelatin, have been applied to implantation into the articular cartilage defect with the goal of cartilage repair.

Agarose is polysaccharide composed from the residue of L- and D-galactose. Previously agarose-based 3D-cultures have been performed as a scaffold of MSCs to promote in vitro MSCs chondrogenesis [50]. Implantation of agarose and MSCs into the articular cartilage defect of rabbit resulted in positive staining for type II collagen and proteoglycan, providing the repair of articular cartilage [51]. On the other hand, another group reported the agarose implantation may inhibit spontaneous repair of articular cartilage and further accumulate in the living body due to weak biodegradability. Therefore, this strategy might not been proper for in vivo trial related on the repair of cartilage tissue.

Gelatin is synthesized from denatured collagen, exhibits cell-adhesion and has been be applied in a variety of scaffolds. Thus, gelatin is biodegradable and a promising scaffold for regenerative medicine of articular cartilage.

Ponticiello et al. have reported that human MSCs were seeded on gelatin sponge, and cultured for 21 day,

showing type II collagen staining [52]. After that, the MSCs were implanted into the osteochondral defect of rabbits. Gelatin and MSCs were observed to be very biocompatible, with no evidence of immune response or lymphocytic infiltration at the site. Gelatin is a promising candidate as a carrier matrix for MSC-based cartilage regeneration.

On the other hand, gelatin has disadvantage, such as weakness to mechanical stress. Chemical modification of gelatin via cross-linking with visible light improved the weakness to the stress [53]. In fact, implantation of MSCs seeded on cross-linking gelatin into the osteochondral defect of rabbits provides the repair for the affected area [54]. Taken together, gelatin is an appropriate material to repair articular cartilage applied with MSCs.

Other scaffolds that contribute to the repair of articular cartilage

MSC scaffolds other than PLGA, collagen, or gelatin, such as tricalcium (TCP), PLA, hyaluronic acid (HA), PGA, and fibrin glue, have also been used for implantation into the articular cartilage defect in experimental animal models (Table 1). PLGA is composed of PLA and PGA whilst PGA-hyaluronan is predominantly comprised of PGA and hyaluronan. The both material show biodegradability and help in enhanced residence of MSCs at affected areas. PLGA-based TGF-β3-releasing microspheres is used in terms of the following. PLGA is gradually disintegrate in the living body, subsequently result in release of TGF-β3 and efficient cytokine effect over the long-term. As a result, implanted MSCs are subjected to chondrocyte differentiation.

Table 1 Application of MSC seeded onto various types of scaffolds into animal models of articular cartilage defect

Design for Implantation	Animal model	Follow-up period (months)	Finding	Ref.
BM-MSC seeded on TCP scaffold	Sheep	6	Proteoglycan and type II collagen	[66]
BM-MSC seeded on PLA scaffold	Dog	1.5	Coverage of chondral defect	[67]
BM-MSC seeded on HA scaffold	Mini-pig	3	Coverage of chondral defect	[14]
BMDC seeded on HA scaffold	Goat	6	Coverage of chondral defect, proteoglycan and type II collagen	[55]
BM-MSC seeded on type I collagen scaffold	Sheep	6	Hyaline-like cartilage	[15]
BMDC seeded on PGA or PLGA scaffold	Sheep	3	Hyaline-like cartilage	[16]
BM-MSC seeded on type I collagen scaffold	Sheep	12	Type II collagen	[68]
BM-MSC seeded on HA scaffold	Horse	12	No difference in chondral surface	[56]
BM-MSC seeded on type II collagen scaffold	Pig	2	Hyaline-like cartilage	[69]
BM-MSC suspended in fibrin glue	Goat	6	Improved cartilage tissue	[70]
BM-MSC seeded on PGA-hyaluronan	Rabbit	1.5	Hyaline-like cartilage	[71]
BM-MSC sheet-encapsulated MSC on PLGA scaffold	Rabbit	3	Hyaline-like cartilage	[43]
MSC seeded on PLGA-based TGF-β3-releasing microspheres	Mice	1.5	Hyaline-like cartilage	[72]

BM-MSC bone marrow-derived mesenchymal stem cells, *TCP* tricalcium phosphate, *PLA* polylactic acid, *HA* hyaluronic acid, *PGA* polyglycolic acid, *PLGA* poly-lactic and co-glycolic acids, *TGF-β3* transforming growth factor-β3

HA has been used frequently for implantation of MSCs. Implantation of MSCs-HA into the knee joints of pigs with partial defect in the articular cartilage was followed by efficient covering of the cartilage tissue at 12 weeks followed by the formation of hyaline cartilage-like tissue [14]. However this effect was limited after application of HA alone. Saw et al. [55] reported that the amounts of type II collagen and proteoglycan increased in cartilage defects around the femur tissue after implantation of HA and bone marrow-derived cells (BMDC) in goats. A similar procedure was conducted in pigs. However there was no difference in the repair process of articular cartilage based on MRI imaging between HA and HA + MSC groups at 1 year after implantations [56]. These findings suggest that the efficacy of implantation depends on body size. Further studies to examine changes in cell numbers time of implantation and the implantation tool are required.

Several studies have described the implantation of scaffold and MSCs into affected area in patients with damaged articular cartilage (Table 2). The MRI and arthroscopic findings in patients who had undergone implantation of HA and BMDC with MSCs into the injured joint area showed the formation of new hyaline cartilage-like tissue, which assimilated later into the surrounding tissues within 24 months [57, 58]. Biopsy specimen from these areas showed dense staining for proteoglycan and type II collagen or faint staining for type I collagen, confirming the repair of articular cartilage observed on the MRI images and that the repaired tissue is hyaline cartilage tissue. However, in some cases the results have been the opposite of what was expected.

Table 2 Application of MSC seeded onto different types of scaffolds into patients with damaged articular cartilage

Technique	n; Sex; Age (years) (mean ± SD)	Follow-up period (months)	Finding	Ref.
BM-MSC in type I collagen gel	1; M (31)	12	Hyaline-like cartilage	[49]
BM-MSC within type I collagen gel on a collagen scaffold seeded on PLA scaffold	3; 2 M, 1F (32–45)	18	Coverage of chondral defect	[73]
BMDC suspended in collagen or seeded on HA scaffold	48; 27 M, 21F (28 ± 9)	24–35	Coverage of chondral defect and hypertrophic cartilage	[57]
BMDC seeded on HA scaffold supplemented with platelet-rich fibrin	20; 12 M, 8F (28 ± 9)	29 ± 4	Proteoglycan and type II collagen	[58]
BMDC seeded on HA scaffold supplemented with platelet-rich fibrin	81; 47 M, 34F (30 ± 8)	59 ± 26	Hyaline-like cartilage	[74]
BM-MSC within platelet-rich fibrin glue	5; 4 M, 1F (25)	12	Coverage of chondral defect	[75]
BM-MSC covered by periosteum	72; 38 M, 34F (44 ± 11)	24	Aggrecan and type II collagen	[76]
BMDC with batroxobin covered by type I/III collagen matrix	15; 10 M, 5F (48)	24–38	Coverage of chondral defect	[77]
BM-MSC seeded on type I collagen scaffold supplemented with fibrin glue	2; 2 M (24–25)	30–31	Partial coverage of chondral defect	[78]
Peripheral blood-derived MSC with HA	5; 1 M, 4F (39 ± 11)	10–26	Partial coverage of chondral defect	[79]
BMDC within fibrin glue and coverage with collagen and collagen membrane	1; M; 37 yrs	24	Partial coverage of chondral defect	[80]
BMDC in fibrin glue and coverage with a PGA + HA membrane	9; 5 M, 4F (48 ± 9)	20–24	Hyaline-like cartilage	[81]
BMDC in collagen/platelet paste or seeded on HA or seeded on HA scaffold supplemented with platelet gel	49; 27 M, 22F (28 ± 9)	48	Coverage of chondral defect in 45%	[59]
Peripheral blood-derived MSC and HA	49; 17 M, 32F (37 ± 7)	24	Partial coverage of chondral defect	[18]

BM-MSC bone marrow-derived mesenchymal stem cells, *PLA* polylactic acid, *HA* hyaluronic acid, *PGA* polyglycolic acid

For example, implantation of HA-BMDC-MSCs into the talus was later found to result in the formation of irregular cartilage-like tissue by MRI with little or no assimilation with the residual articular cartilage [59]. Further instrument for implantation is required for the repair of articular cartilage in the affected region.

Optimization of MSC implantation tool required for the repair of articular cartilage

Our in vitro study showed that MSCs seeded on PLGA plug can differentiate into chondrocytes in the growth medium alone, even when MSCs were not cultured in chondrocyte differentiation medium [40]. In order to avoid improper cell differentiation, e.g., osteoblast cells that can trigger ectopic calcification, a special vehicle is needed in advance to direct MSCs into chondrocyte differentiation.

Various mechanisms have been proposed for the differentiation of MSC into chondrocytes. In vitro studies showed that TNF-α, IL-1β, and IL-17 suppress MSC differentiation into chondrocytes [60–64]. Specifically, TNF-α and IL-1β inhibit the smad signaling pathway, and concomitantly down-regulate *Sox9* gene, which encodes master transcriptional factor required for chondrocyte differentiation [61, 62]. On the other hand, IL-17 inhibits the activity of protein kinase A (PKA), leading to low phosphorylation level of SOX9, which consequently inactivate SOX9 [64]. Taken together, pro-inflammatory cytokines do not only inflict damage of joints, but also suppress MSC differentiation into chondrocytes. Notably, stimulation of MSCs, which produce high levels of IL-6, with IL-6R results in the activation of IL-6/IL-6R signaling, which in turn induces the expression of various cartilage-related genes in MSCs, resulting in MSC differentiation into chondrocytes [65].

Based on the above information, it is interesting to study whether implantation of PLGA and IL-6R-treated MSCs contributes to the repair of articular cartilage.

Conclusions

There is a disadvantage in using osteochondral repair as the goal of treatment of articular cartilage tissue damage, since such strategy can negatively affect the residual healthy cartilage tissue. New methods of MSC-based therapy have been tried for the repair of articular cartilage damage. In vitro studies demonstrated that MSCs can differentiate into chondrocytes. Further, 3D culture applied with scaffold enhanced differentiation of MSCs into chondrocytes. In animal models of cartilage damage, the use of local implantation system comprising scaffolds with MSCs, such as

PLGA and HA, can result in repair of the articular cartilage with the formation of new hyaline cartilage-like tissue. Furthermore, implantation of MSCs seeded on scaffold into the damaged articular cartilage of patients resulted in histopathological improvement with regeneration of the cartilage tissue. Further studies are necessary to find optimal implantation vehicles that can result in regeneration of articular cartilage.

Abbreviations
ADL: Activity of daily life; AIA: Antigen-induced arthritis; BMDC: Bone marrow-derived cell; HA: Hyaluronic acid; IL-6R: Interleukin-6 receptor; MSCs: Mesenchymal stem cells; PGA: Polyglycolic acid; PLA: Polylactic acid; PLGA: Poly-lactic and co-glycolic acids; QOL: Quality of life; RA: Rheumatoid arthritis; TCP: Tricalcium phosphate

Acknowledgments
We express our sincere gratitude to all the researchers, collaborators, and technical assistants for contributing to the work cited in this manuscript.

Funding
This work was supported in part by a Grant-In-Aid for Scientific Research from the Ministry of Health, Labor and Welfare of Japan, the Ministry of Education, Culture, Sports, Science and Technology of Japan, Japan Agency for Medical Research and Development, and the University of Occupational and Environmental Health, Japan, through UOEH Grant for Advanced Research.

Authors' contributions
All authors contributed equally to the drafting of the manuscript. All authors read, revised, and approved the final manuscript.

Competing interests
Y. Tanaka, has received consulting fees, speaking fees, and/or honoraria from Daiichi-Sankyo, Astellas, Pfizer, Mitsubishi-Tanabe, Bristol-Myers, Chugai, YL Biologics, Eli Lilly, Sanofi, Janssen, UCB and has received research grants from Mitsubishi-Tanabe, Takeda, Bristol-Myers, Chugai, Astellas, Abbvie, MSD, Daiichi-Sankyo, Pfizer, Kyowa-Kirin, Eisai, Ono. S. Nakayamada, has received speaking fees from Bristol-Myers, UCB, Astellas, Abbvie, Eisai, Pfizer, Takeda and has received research grants from Mitsubishi-Tanabe, Novartis and MSD. K. Yamagata declares no conflict of interest.

References
1. Solheim E, Hegna J, Oyen J, Harlem T, Strand T. Results at 10 to 14 years after osteochondral autografting (mosaicplasty) in articular cartilage defects in the knee. Knee. 2013;20:287–90.
2. Valderrabano V, Leumann A, Rasch H, Egelhof T, Hintermann B, Pagenstert G. Knee-to-ankle mosaicplasty for the treatment of osteochondral lesions of the ankle joint. Am J Sports Med. 2009;37:105S–11S.
3. Levy YD, Gortz S, Pulido PA, McCauley JC, Bugbee WD. Do fresh osteochondral allografts successfully treat femoral condyle lesions? Clin Orthop Relat Res. 2013;471:231–7.
4. Williams SK, Amiel D, Ball ST, Allen RT, Wong VW, Chen AC, et al. Prolonged storage effects on the articular cartilage of fresh human osteochondral allografts. J Bone Joint Surg Am. 2003;85-A:2111–20.

5. Malinin TI, Mnaymneh W, Lo HK, Hinkle DK. Cryopreservation of articular cartilage. Ultrastructural observations and long-term results of experimental distal femoral transplantation. Clin Orthop Relat Res. 1994;303:18–32.

6. Peterson L, Vasiliadis HS, Brittberg M, Lindahl A. Autologous chondrocyte implantation: a long-term follow-up. Am J Sports Med. 2010;38:1117–24.

7. Kon E, Filardo G, Berruto M, Benazzo F, Zanon G, Della Villa S, et al. Articular cartilage treatment in high-level male soccer players: a prospective comparative study of arthroscopic second-generation autologous chondrocyte implantation versus microfracture. Am J Sports Med. 2011;39:2549–57.

8. Nam EK, Ferkel RD, Applegate GR. Autologous chondrocyte implantation of the ankle: a 2- to 5-year follow-up. Am J Sports Med. 2009;37:274–84.

9. Anders S, Goetz J, Schubert T, Grifka J, Schaumburger J. Treatment of deep articular talus lesions by matrix associated autologous chondrocyte implantation - results at five years. Int Orthop. 2012;36:2279–85.

10. Harrison PE, Ashton IK, Johnson WE, Turner SL, Richardson JB, Ashton BA. The in vitro growth of human chondrocytes. Cell Tissue Bank. 2000;1:255–60.

11. Mayne R, Vail MS, Mayne PM, Miller EJ. Changes in type of collagen synthesized as clones of chick chondrocytes grow and eventually lose division capacity. Proc Natl Acad Sci U S A. 1976;73:1674–8.

12. Stokes DG, Liu G, Dharmavaram R, Hawkins D, Piera-Velazquez S, Jimenez SA. Regulation of type-II collagen gene expression during human chondrocyte de-differentiation and recovery of chondrocyte-specific phenotype in culture involves Sry-type high-mobility-group box (SOX) transcription factors. Biochem J. 2001;360:461–70.

13. Pittenger MF, Mackay AM, Beck SC, Jaiswal RK, Douglas R, Mosca JD, et al. Multilineage potential of adult human mesenchymal stem cells. Science. 1999;284:143–7.

14. Lee KB, Hui JH, Song IC, Ardany L, Lee EH. Injectable mesenchymal stem cell therapy for large cartilage defects - a porcine model. Stem Cells. 2007; 25:2964–71.

15. Zscharnack M, Hepp P, Richter R, Aigner T, Schulz R, Somerson J, et al. Repair of chronic osteochondral defects using predifferentiated mesenchymal stem cells in an ovine model. Am J Sports Med. 2010;38:1857–69.

16. Wegener B, Schrimpf FM, Bergschmidt P, Pietschmann MF, Utzschneider S, Milz S, et al. Cartilage regeneration by bone marrow cells-seeded scaffolds. J Biomed Mater Res A. 2010;95:735–40.

17. Koga H, Muneta T, Ju YJ, Nagase T, Nimura A, Mochizuki T, et al. Synovial stem cells are regionally specified according to local microenvironments after implantation for cartilage regeneration. Stem Cells. 2007;25:689–96.

18. Saw KY, Anz A, Siew-Yoke Jee C, Merican S, Ching-Soong Ng R, Roohi SA, et al. Articular cartilage regeneration with autologous peripheral blood stem cells versus hyaluronic acid: a randomized controlled trial. Arthroscopy. 2013;29:684–94.

19. Wakitani S, Goto T, Pineda SJ, Young RG, Mansour JM, Caplan AI, et al. Mesenchymal cell-based repair of large, full-thickness defects of articular cartilage. J Bone Joint Surg Am. 1994;76:579–92.

20. Portron S, Merceron C, Gauthier O, Lesoeur J, Sourice S, Masson M, et al. Effects of in vitro low oxygen tension preconditioning of adipose stromal cells on their in vivo chondrogenic potential: application in cartilage tissue repair. PLoS One. 2013;8:e62368.

21. Kisiday JD, Kopesky PW, Evans CH, Grodzinsky AJ, McIlwraith CW, Frisbie DD. Evaluation of adult equine bone marrow- and adipose-derived progenitor cell chondrogenesis in hydrogel cultures. J Orthopaed Res. 2008;26:322–31.

22. Afizah H, Yang Z, Hui JH, Ouyang HW, Lee EH. A comparison between the chondrogenic potential of human bone marrow stem cells (BMSCs) and adipose-derived stem cells (ADSCs) taken from the same donors. Tissue Eng. 2007;13:659–66.

23. Lee DM, Weinblatt ME. Rheumatoid arthritis. Lancet. 2001;358:903–11.

24. Odegard S, Finset A, Kvien TK, Mowinckel P, Uhlig T. Work disability in rheumatoid arthritis is predicted by physical and psychological health status: a 7-year study from the Oslo RA register. Scand J Rheumatol. 2005;34:441–7.

25. Yelin E. Work disability in rheumatic diseases. Curr Opin Rheumatol. 2007;19:91–6.

26. Kvien TK, Uhlig T. Quality of life in rheumatoid arthritis. Scand J Rheumatol. 2005;34:333–41.

27. Baron R, Kneissel M. WNT signaling in bone homeostasis and disease: from human mutations to treatments. Nat Med. 2013;19:179–92.

28. Kubo S, Yamaoka K, Kondo M, Yamagata K, Zhao J, Iwata S, et al. The JAK inhibitor, tofacitinib, reduces the T cell stimulatory capacity of human monocyte-derived dendritic cells. Ann Rheum Dis. 2014;73:2192–8.

29. Singh JA, Saag KG, Bridges SL Jr, Akl EA, Bannuru RR, Sullivan MC, et al. 2015 American College of Rheumatology guideline for the treatment of rheumatoid arthritis. Arthritis Rheumatol. 2016;68:1–26.

30. Smolen JS, Landewé R, Breedveld FC, Buch M, Burmester G, Dougados M, et al. EULAR recommendations for the management of rheumatoid arthritis with synthetic and biological disease-modifying antirheumatic drugs: 2013 update. Ann Rheum Dis. 2014;73:492–509.

31. Roberts S, Menage J, Sandell LJ, Evans EH, Richardson JB. Immunohistochemical study of collagen types I and II and procollagen IIA in human cartilage repair tissue following autologous chondrocyte implantation. Knee. 2009;16:398–404.

32. Zhang X, Yamaoka K, Sonomoto K, Kaneko H, Satake M, Yamamoto Y, et al. Local delivery of mesenchymal stem cells with poly-lactic-co-glycolic acid nano-fiber scaffold suppress arthritis in rats. PLoS One. 2014;9:e114621.

33. Liang J, Li X, Zhang H, Wang D, Feng X, Wang H, et al. Allogeneic mesenchymal stem cells transplantation in patients with refractory RA. Clin Rheumatol. 2012;31:157–61.

34. Ra JC, Kang SK, Shin IS, Park HG, Joo SA, Kim JG, et al. Stem cell treatment for patients with autoimmune disease by systemic infusion of culture-expanded autologous adipose tissue derived mesenchymal stem cells. J Transl Med. 2011;9:181.

35. Gonzalez MA, Gonzalez-Rey E, Rico L, Buscher D, Delgado M. Treatment of experimental arthritis by inducing immune tolerance with human adipose-derived mesenchymal stem cells. Arthritis Rheum. 2009;60:1006–19.

36. Tasso R, Augello A, Carida' M, Postiglione F, Tibiletti MG, Bernasconi B, et al. Development of sarcomas in mice implanted with mesenchymal stem cells seeded onto bioscaffolds. Carcinogenesis. 2009;30:150–7.

37. Maria AT, Toupet K, Maumus M, Fonteneau G, Le Quellec A, Jorgensen C, et al. Human adipose mesenchymal stem cells as potent anti-fibrosis therapy for systemic sclerosis. J Autoimmun. 2016;70:31–9.

38. Liu L, Chen JX, Zhang XW, Sun Q, Yang L, Liu A, Hu S, et al. Chemokine receptor 7 overexpression promotes mesenchymal stem cell migration and proliferation via secreting chemokine ligand 12. Sci Rep. 2018;8:204.

39. Paduszyński P, Aleksander-Konert E, Zajdel A, Wilczok A, Jelonek K, Witek A, Dzierżewicz Z, et al. Changes in expression of cartilaginous genes during chondrogenesis of Wharton's jelly mesenchymal stem cells on three-dimensional biodegradable poly(L-lactide-co-glycolide) scaffolds. Cell Mol Biol Lett. 2016;21:14.

40. Sonomoto K, Yamaoka K, Kaneko H, Yamagata K, Sakata K, Zhang X, et al. Spontaneous differentiation of human mesenchymal stem cells on poly-lactic-co-glycolic acid nano-fiber scaffold. PLoS One. 2016;11:e0153231.

41. Toyokawa N, Fujioka H, Kokubu T, Nagura I, Inui A, Sakata R, et al. Electrospun synthetic polymer scaffold for cartilage repair without cultured cells in an animal model. Arthroscopy. 2010;26:375–83.

42. Mohanty ST, Kottam L, Gambardella A, Nicklin MJ, Coulton L, Hughes D, et al. Alterations in the self-renewal and differentiation ability of bone marrow mesenchymal stem cells in a mouse model of rheumatoid arthritis. Arthritis Res Ther. 2010;12:R149.

43. Qi Y, Du Y, Li W, Dai X, Zhao T, Yan W. Cartilage repair using mesenchymal stem cell (MSC) sheet and MSCs-loaded bilayer PLGA scaffold in a rabbit model. Knee Surg Sports Traumatol Arthrosc. 2014;22:1424–33.

44. Morille M, Van-Thanh T, Garric X, Cayon J, Coudane J, Noël D, et al. New PLGA-P188-PLGA matrix enhances TGF-beta3 release from pharmacologically active microcarriers and promotes chondrogenesis of mesenchymal stem cells. J Control Release. 2013;170:99–110.

45. Yu Y, Brouillette MJ, Seol D, Zheng H, Buckwalter JA, Martin JA. Use of recombinant human stromal cell-derived factor 1 alpha-loaded fibrin/hyaluronic acid hydrogel networks to achieve functional repair of full-thickness bovine articular cartilage via homing of chondrogenic progenitor cells. Arthritis Rheumatol. 2015;67:1274–85.

46. Wakitani S, Okabe T, Horibe S, Mitsuoka T, Saito M, Koyama T, et al. Safety of autologous bone marrow-derived mesenchymal stem cell transplantation for cartilage repair in 41 patients with 45 joints followed for up to 11 years and 5 months. J Tissue Eng Regen Med. 2011;5:146–50.

47. Li YY, Cheng HW, Cheung KM, Chan D, Chan BP. Mesenchymal stem cell-collagen microspheres for articular cartilage repair: cell density and differentiation status. Acta Biomater. 2014;10:1919–29.

48. Lubiatowski P, Kruczynski J, Gradys A, Trzeciak T, Jaroszewski J. Articular cartilage repair by means of biodegradable scaffolds. Transplant Proc. 2006; 38:320–2.

49. Kuroda R, Ishida K, Matsumoto T, Akisue T, Fujioka H, Mizuno K, et al. Treatment of a full-thickness articular cartilage defect in the femoral condyle of an athlete with autologous bone-marrow stromal cells. Osteoarthr Cartil. 2007;15:226e231.

50. Awad HA, Wickham MQ, Leddy HA, Gimble JM, Guilak F. Chondrogenic differentiation of adipose-derived adult stem cells in agarose, alginate, and gelatin scaffolds. Biomaterials. 2004;25:3211–22.

51. Diduch DR, Jordan LC, Mierisch CM, Balian G. Marrow stromal cells embedded in alginate for repair of osteochondral defects. Arthroscopy. 2000;16:571–7.

52. Ponticiello MS, Schinagl RM, Kadiyala S, Barry FP. Gelatin-based resorbable sponge as a carrier matrix for human mesenchymal stem cells in cartilage regeneration therapy. J Biomed Mater Res. 2000;52:246–55.

53. Hoch E, Schuh C, Hirth T, Tovar GE, Borchers K. Stiff gelatin hydrogels can be photo-chemically synthesized from low viscous gelatin solutions using molecularly functionalized gelatin with a high degree of methacrylation. J Mater Sci Mater Med. 2012;23:2607–17.

54. Mazaki T, Shiozaki Y, Yamane K, Yoshida A, Nakamura M, Yoshida Y, et al. A novel, visible light-induced, rapidly cross-linkable gelatin scaffold for osteochondral tissue engineering. Sci Rep. 2014;4:4457.

55. Saw KY, Hussin P, Loke SC, Azam M, Chen HC, Tay YG, et al. Articular cartilage regeneration with autologous marrow aspirate and hyaluronic acid: an experimental study in a goat model. Arthroscopy. 2009;25:1391–400.

56. McIlwraith CW, Frisbie DD, Rodkey WG, Kisiday JD, Werpy NM, Kawcak CE, et al. Evaluation of intra-articular mesenchymal stem cells to augment healing of microfractured chondral defects. Arthroscopy. 2011;27:1552–61.

57. Giannini S, Buda R, Vannini F, Cavallo M, Grigolo B. One-step bone marrow-derived cell transplantation in talar osteochondral lesions. Clin Orthop Relat Res. 2009;467:3307–20.

58. Buda R, Vannini F, Cavallo M, Grigolo B, Cenacchi A, Giannini S. Osteochondral lesions of the knee: a new one-step repair technique with bone-marrow-derived cells. J Bone Joint Surg Am. 2010;92:2–11.

59. Giannini S, Buda R, Battaglia M, Cavallo M, Ruffilli A, Ramponi L, et al. One-step repair in talar osteochondral lesions: 4-year clinical results and t2-mapping capability in outcome prediction. Am J Sports Med. 2013;41:511–8.

60. Sitcheran R, Cogswell PC, Baldwin AS Jr. NF-kappaB mediates inhibition of mesenchymal cell differentiation through a posttranscriptional gene silencing mechanism. Genes Dev. 2003;17:2368–73.

61. Baugé C, Legendre F, Leclercq S, Elissalde JM, Pujol JP, Galéra P, et al. Interleukin-1 beta impairment of transforming growth factor beta1 signaling by downregulation of transforming growth factor b receptor type II and up-regulation of Smad7 in human articular chondrocytes. Arthritis Rheum. 2007;56:3020–32.

62. Roman-Blas JA, Stokes DG, Jimenez SA. Modulation of TGF-beta signaling by proinflammatory cytokines in articular chondrocytes. Osteoarthr Cartil. 2007;15:1367–77.

63. Baugé C, Attia J, Leclercq S, Pujol JP, Galéra P, Boumédiene K. Interleukin-1beta upregulation of Smad7 via NF-kappaB activation in human chondrocytes. Arthritis Rheum. 2008;58:221–6.

64. Kondo M, Yamaoka K, Sonomoto K, Fukuyo S, Oshita K, Okada Y, et al. IL-17 inhibits chondrogenic differentiation of human mesenchymal stem cells. PLoS One. 2013;8:e79463.

65. Kondo M, Yamaoka K, Sakata K, Sonomoto K, Lin L, Nakano K, et al. Contribution of the Interleukin-6/STAT-3 signaling pathway to Chondrogenic differentiation of human Mesenchymal stem cells. Arthritis Rheumatol. 2015;67:1250–60.

66. Guo X, Wang C, Zhang Y, Xia R, Hu M, Duan C, et al. Repair of large articular cartilage defects with implants of autologous mesenchymal stem cells seeded into beta-tricalcium phosphate in a sheep model. Tissue Eng. 2004;10:1818–29.

67. Wayne JS, McDowell CL, Shields KJ, Tuan RS. In vivo response of polylactic acid-alginate scaffolds and bone marrow-derived cells for cartilage tissue engineering. Tissue Eng. 2005;11:953–63.

68. Marquass B, Schulz R, Hepp P, Zscharnack M, Aigner T, Schmidt S, et al. Matrix-associated implantation of predifferentiated mesenchymal stem cells versus articular chondrocytes: in vivo results of cartilage repair after 1 year. Am J Sports Med. 2011;39:1401–12.

69. Zhang Y, Wang F, Chen J, Ning Z, Yang L. Bone marrow-derived mesenchymal stem cells versus bone marrow nucleated cells in the treatment of chondral defects. Int Orthop. 2012;36:1079–86.

70. Bekkers JE, Tsuchida AI, van Rijen MH, Vonk LA, Dhert WJ, Creemers LB, et al. Single-stage cell-based cartilage regeneration using a combination of chondrons and mesenchymal stromal cells: comparison with microfracture. Am J Sports Med. 2013;41:2158–66.

71. Patrascu JM, Krüger JP, Böss HG, Ketzmar AK, Freymann U, Sittinger M, et al. Polyglycolic acid-hyaluronan scaffolds loaded with bone marrow-derived mesenchymal stem cells show chondrogenic differentiation in vitro and cartilage repair in the rabbit model. J Biomed Mater Res B Appl Biomater. 2013;101:1310–20.

72. Morille M, Toupet K, Montero-Menei CN, Jorgensen C, Noël D. PLGA-based microcarriers induce mesenchymal stem cell chondrogenesis and stimulate cartilage repair in osteoarthritis. Biomaterials. 2016;88:60–9.

73. Wakitani S, Nawata M, Tensho K, Okabe T, Machida H, Ohgushi H. Repair of articular cartilage defects in the patello-femoral joint with autologous bone marrow mesenchymal cell transplantation: three case reports involving nine defects in five knees. J Tissue Eng Regen Med. 2007;1:74–9.

74. Giannini S, Buda R, Cavallo M, Ruffilli A, Cenacchi A, Cavallo C, et al. Cartilage repair evolution in post-traumatic osteochondral lesions of the talus: from open field autologous chondrocyte to bone-marrow-derived cells transplantation. Injury. 2010;41:1196–203.

75. Haleem AM, Singergy AA, Sabry D, Atta HM, Rashed LA, Chu CR, et al. The clinical use of human culture-expanded autologous bone marrow mesenchymal stem cells transplanted on platelet-rich fibrin glue in the treatment of articular cartilage defects: a pilot study and preliminary results. Cartilage. 2010;1:253–61.

76. Nejadnik H, Hui JH, Feng Choong EP, Tai BC, Lee EH. Autologous bone marrow-derived mesenchymal stem cells versus autologous chondrocyte implantation: an observational cohort study. Am J Sports Med. 2010;38(6):1110.

77. Gobbi A, Karnatzikos G, Scotti C, Mahajan M, Mazzucco L, Grigolo B. One-step cartilage repair with bone marrow aspirate concentrated cells and collagen matrix in full-thickness knee cartilage lesions: results at 2-year follow-up. Cartilage. 2011;2:286–99.

78. Kasemkijwattana C, Hongeng S, Kesprayura S, Rungsinaporn V, Chaipinyo K, Chansiri K. Autologous bone marrow mesenchymal stem cells implantation for cartilage defects: two cases report. J Med Assoc Thail. 2011;94:395–400.

79. Saw KY, Anz A, Merican S, Tay YG, Ragavanaidu K, Jee CS, et al. Articular cartilage regeneration with autologous peripheral blood progenitor cells and hyaluronic acid after arthroscopic subchondral drilling: a report of 5 cases with histology. Arthroscopy. 2011;27:493–506.

80. Gigante A, Cecconi S, Calcagno S, Busilacchi A, Enea D. Arthroscopic knee cartilage repair with covered microfracture and bone marrow concentrate. Arthrosc Tech. 2012;1:e175–e80.

81. Enea D, Cecconi S, Calcagno S, Busilacchi A, Manzotti S, Kaps C, et al. Single-stage cartilage repair in the knee with microfracture covered with a resorbable polymer-based matrix and autologous bone marrow concentrate. Knee. 2013;20:562–9.

Permissions

All chapters in this book were first published in I&R, by BioMed Central; hereby published with permission under the Creative Commons Attribution License or equivalent. Every chapter published in this book has been scrutinized by our experts. Their significance has been extensively debated. The topics covered herein carry significant findings which will fuel the growth of the discipline. They may even be implemented as practical applications or may be referred to as a beginning point for another development.

The contributors of this book come from diverse backgrounds, making this book a truly international effort. This book will bring forth new frontiers with its revolutionizing research information and detailed analysis of the nascent developments around the world.

We would like to thank all the contributing authors for lending their expertise to make the book truly unique. They have played a crucial role in the development of this book. Without their invaluable contributions this book wouldn't have been possible. They have made vital efforts to compile up to date information on the varied aspects of this subject to make this book a valuable addition to the collection of many professionals and students.

This book was conceptualized with the vision of imparting up-to-date information and advanced data in this field. To ensure the same, a matchless editorial board was set up. Every individual on the board went through rigorous rounds of assessment to prove their worth. After which they invested a large part of their time researching and compiling the most relevant data for our readers.

The editorial board has been involved in producing this book since its inception. They have spent rigorous hours researching and exploring the diverse topics which have resulted in the successful publishing of this book. They have passed on their knowledge of decades through this book. To expedite this challenging task, the publisher supported the team at every step. A small team of assistant editors was also appointed to further simplify the editing procedure and attain best results for the readers.

Apart from the editorial board, the designing team has also invested a significant amount of their time in understanding the subject and creating the most relevant covers. They scrutinized every image to scout for the most suitable representation of the subject and create an appropriate cover for the book.

The publishing team has been an ardent support to the editorial, designing and production team. Their endless efforts to recruit the best for this project, has resulted in the accomplishment of this book. They are a veteran in the field of academics and their pool of knowledge is as vast as their experience in printing. Their expertise and guidance has proved useful at every step. Their uncompromising quality standards have made this book an exceptional effort. Their encouragement from time to time has been an inspiration for everyone.

The publisher and the editorial board hope that this book will prove to be a valuable piece of knowledge for researchers, students, practitioners and scholars across the globe.

List of Contributors

Satoshi Kubo and Yoshiya Tanaka
The First Department of Internal Medicine, School of Medicine, University of Occupational and Environmental Health, 1-1 Iseigaoka, Yahata-nishi-ku, Kitakyushu, Fukuoka 807-8555, Japan

Hussein Abdellatif, Dalia M. Saleh, Huda Eltahry and Kamal G. Botros
Anatomy and Embryology Department, Faculty of Medicine, University of Mansoura, Mansoura, Egypt

Gamal Shiha
Internal Medicine Department, Faculty of Medicine, University of Mansoura, Mansoura, Egypt
Egyptian Liver Research Institute and Hospital (ELRIAH), Mansoura, Egypt

Takahiko Horiuchi and Hiroshi Tsukamoto
Kyushu University Beppu Hospital, Beppu, Japan
Kyushu University Graduate School of Medical Sciences, Fukuoka, Japan

Minoru Tanaka
Department of Regenerative Medicine, Research Institute, National Center for Global Health and Medicine, Tokyo, Japan

Atsushi Miyajima
Institute of Molecular and Cellular Biosciences, The University of Tokyo, Tokyo, Japan

Takao Ito and Tatsushi Igaki
Laboratory of Genetics, Graduate School of Biostudies, Kyoto University, Yoshida-Konoecho-cho, Sakyo-ku, Kyoto 606-8501, Japan

Tomoko Fujita and Shuh Narumiya
Center for Innovation in Immunoregulatory Technology and Therapeutics, Faculty of Medicine, Kyoto University, Yoshida Konoecho, Sakyo-ku, Kyoto 606-8501, Japan

Yuki Fujita and Toshihide Yamashita
Department of Molecular Neuroscience, Graduate School of Medicine, Osaka University, 2-2 Yamadaoka, Suita, Osaka, Japan

Seiji Okada
Department of Advanced Initiatives, Graduate School of Medical Sciences, Kyushu University, 3-1-1 Maidashi, Higashi-ku, Fukuoka 812-8582, Japan
Orthopaedics, Graduate School of Medical Sciences, Kyushu University, Fukuoka, Japan

Taira Maekawa and Yasuo Miura
Department of Transfusion Medicine and Cell Therapy, Kyoto University Hospital, 54 Kawaharacho, Shogoin, Sakyo-ku, Kyoto 606-8507, Japan

Noriko Sugino
Department of Transfusion Medicine and Cell Therapy, Kyoto University Hospital, 54 Kawaharacho, Shogoin, Sakyo-ku, Kyoto 606-8507, Japan
Department of Hematology/Oncology, Graduate School of Medicine, Kyoto University, Kyoto 606-8507, Japan

Akifumi Takaori-Kondo
Department of Hematology/Oncology, Graduate School of Medicine, Kyoto University, Kyoto 606-8507, Japan

Tatsuo Ichinohe
Department of Hematology and Oncology, Research Institute for Radiation Biology and Medicine, Hiroshima University, Hiroshima 734-8553, Japan

Shingo Nakayamada and Yoshiya Tanaka
The First Department of Internal Medicine, School of Medicine, University of Occupational and Environmental Health, 1-1 Iseigaoka, Yahata-nishi, Kitakyushu 807-8555, Japan

Yutaka Kuroda and Shuichi Matsuda
Department of Orthopaedic Surgery, Graduate School of Medicine, Kyoto University, Shogoin, Kawahara-cho 54, Sakyo-ku, Kyoto 606-8507, Japan

Haruhiko Akiyama
Department of Orthopaedic Surgery, Gifu University, Gifu, Japan

Satoru Morikawa and Taneaki Nakagawa
Department of Dentistry and Oral Surgery, Keio University School of Medicine, 35 Shinanomachi, Shinjuku-ku, Tokyo 160-8582, Japan

Takazumi Yasui
Department of Dentistry and Oral Surgery, Keio University School of Medicine, 35 Shinanomachi, Shinjuku-ku, Tokyo 160-8582, Japan
Department of Physiology, Keio University School of Medicine, 35 Shinanomachi, Shinjuku-ku, Tokyo 160-8582, Japan
Department of Dentistry and Oral Surgery, Kawasaki Municipal Kawasaki Hospital, 12-1 Shinkawadori, Kawasaki-ku, Kawasaki, Kanagawa 210-0013, Japan

Hideyuki Okano
Department of Physiology, Keio University School of Medicine, 35 Shinanomachi, Shinjuku-ku, Tokyo 160-8582, Japan

Yo Mabuchi
Department of Physiology, Keio University School of Medicine, 35 Shinanomachi, Shinjuku-ku, Tokyo 160-8582, Japan
Department of Biochemistry and Biophysics, Graduate School of Health Care Sciences, Tokyo Medical and Dental University, 1-5-45 Yushima Bunkyo-ku, Tokyo 113-8510, Japan

Yumi Matsuzaki
Department of Physiology, Keio University School of Medicine, 35 Shinanomachi, Shinjuku-ku, Tokyo 160-8582, Japan
Department of Cancer Biology, Faculty of Medicine, Shimane University, 89-1 Enya-cho, Izumo, Shimane 693-8501, Japan

Katsuhiro Onizawa
Department of Dentistry and Oral Surgery, Kawasaki Municipal Kawasaki Hospital, 12-1 Shinkawadori, Kawasaki-ku, Kawasaki, Kanagawa 210-0013, Japan

Chihiro Akazawa
Department of Biochemistry and Biophysics, Graduate School of Health Care Sciences, Tokyo Medical and Dental University, 1-5-45 Yushima Bunkyo-ku, Tokyo 113-8510, Japan

Takahisa Noma, Koji Ohmori and Masakazu Kohno
Department of Cardiorenal and Cerebrovascular Medicine, Faculty of Medicine, Kagawa University, Kagawa 761-0793, Japan

Ryo Kawakami
Department of Cardiorenal and Cerebrovascular Medicine, Faculty of Medicine, Kagawa University, Kagawa 761-0793, Japan
Department of Clinical Gene Therapy, Graduate School of Medicine, Osaka University, Kagawa 565-0871, Japan

Ryuichi Morishita
Department of Clinical Gene Therapy, Graduate School of Medicine, Osaka University, Kagawa 565-0871, Japan

Hironori Nakagami
Department of Health Development and Medicine, Graduate School of Medicine, Osaka University, 2-2 Yamada-oka, Suita 565-0871, Osaka, Japan

Hideki Arimochi, Yuki Sasaki, Akiko Kitamura and Koji Yasutomo
Department of Immunology and Parasitology, Graduate School of Medicine, Tokushima University, 3-18-15 Kuramoto, Tokushima 770-8503, Japan

Haiko Karsjens and Eckhard Lammert
Institute of Metabolic Physiology, Heinrich-Heine University, Düsseldorf, Germany
Institute for Beta Cell Biology, Leibniz Center for Diabetes Research, German Diabetes Center (DDZ), Düsseldorf, Germany

Jan Eglinger
Institute of Metabolic Physiology, Heinrich-Heine University, Düsseldorf, Germany
Institute for Beta Cell Biology, Leibniz Center for Diabetes Research, German Diabetes Center (DDZ), Düsseldorf, Germany
Current address: Friedrich Miescher Institute for Biomedical Research, Basel, Switzerland

Hiroyasu Sato and Yoshitaka Taketomi
Lipid Metabolism Project, The Tokyo Metropolitan Institute of Medical Science, 2-1-6 Kamikitazawa, Setagaya-ku, Tokyo 156-8506, Japan

Makoto Murakami
Lipid Metabolism Project, The Tokyo Metropolitan Institute of Medical Science, 2-1-6 Kamikitazawa, Setagaya-ku, Tokyo 156-8506, Japan
AMED-CREST, Japan Agency for Medical Research and Development, Tokyo 100-0004, Japan

Naoe Kaneko, Tomoyuki Iwasaki, Yuki Ito, Shinnosuke Morikawa, Naoko Nakano, Mie Kurata and Junya Masumoto
Department of Pathology, Ehime University Graduate School of Medicine and Proteo-Science Center, Shitsukawa 454, Toon 791-0295, Ehime, Japan

Hiroyuki Takeda
Divison of Proteo-Drug-Discovery Sciences, Ehime University Proteo-Science Center, Bunkyocho 3, Matsuyama 790-8577, Ehime, Japan

Tatsuya Sawasaki
Division of Cell-free Sciences, Ehime University Proteo-Science Center, Bunkyocho 3, Matsuyama 790-8577, Ehime, Japan

Akihiro Yamashita, Yoshihiro Tamamura, Miho Morioka, Nobuyuki Shima and Noriyuki Tsumaki
Cell Induction and Regulation Field, Department of Clinical Application, Center for iPS Cell Research and Application, Kyoto University, Kyoto, Japan

Peter Karagiannis
International Public Communications Office, Center for iPS Cell Research and Application, Kyoto University, Kyoto, Japan

Yoshihide Asano
Department of Dermatology, Graduate School of Medicine, University of Tokyo, 7-3-1 Hongo, Bunkyo-ku, Tokyo 113-8655, Japan

Gurjeet Kaur, Vishakha Grover, Nandini Bhaskar, Rose Kanwaljeet Kaur and Ashish Jain
Department of Periodontology, Dr Harvansh Singh Judge Institute of Dental Sciences and Hospital, Panjab University, Sector-25, Chandigarh, India

Toshinori Okinaga, Wataru Ariyoshi and Tatsuji Nishihara
Division of Infections and Molecular Biology, Department of Health Promotion, Kyushu Dental University, Kitakyushu, Fukuoka 803-8580, Japan

Junya Kaneko
Division of Infections and Molecular Biology, Department of Health Promotion, Kyushu Dental University, Kitakyushu, Fukuoka 803-8580, Japan
Division of Oral and Maxillofacial Surgery, Department of Science of Physical Functions, Kyushu Dental University, Kitakyushu, Fukuoka 803-8580, Japan

Hisako Hikiji
School of Oral Health Sciences, Kyushu Dental University, Kitakyushu, Fukuoka 803-8580, Japan

Daigo Yoshiga, Manabu Habu and Kazuhiro Tominaga
Division of Oral and Maxillofacial Surgery, Department of Science of Physical Functions, Kyushu Dental University, Kitakyushu, Fukuoka 803-8580, Japan

Atsushi Otsuka and Chisa Nakashima
Department of Dermatology, Kyoto University Graduate School of Medicine, 54 Shogoin-Kawara, Sakyo, Kyoto 606-8507, Japan

Pawinee Rerknimitr
Department of Dermatology, Kyoto University Graduate School of Medicine, 54 Shogoin-Kawara, Sakyo, Kyoto 606-8507, Japan
Division of Dermatology, Department of Medicine, Faculty of Medicine, Skin and Allergy Research Unit, Chulalongkorn University, Bangkok, Thailand

Kenji Kabashima
Department of Dermatology, Kyoto University Graduate School of Medicine, 54 Shogoin-Kawara, Sakyo, Kyoto 606-8507, Japan

Singapore Immunology Network (SIgN) and Institute of Medical Biology, Agency for Science, Technology and Research (A*STAR), Biopolis, Singapore

Kiyomi Tsuji-Tamura
Department of Cell Differentiation, Institute of Molecular Embryology and Genetics, Kumamoto University, Kumamoto 860-0811, Japan
Present Address: Oral Biochemistry and Molecular Biology, Department of Oral Health Science, Faculty of Dental Medicine and Graduate School of Dental Medicine, Hokkaido University, Sapporo 060-8586, Japan

Minetaro Ogawa
Department of Cell Differentiation, Institute of Molecular Embryology and Genetics, Kumamoto University, Kumamoto 860-0811, Japan

Koichiro Watanabe, Yasuaki Ikuno, Yumi Kakeya, Hirotaka Kito, Aoi Matsubara, Mizuki Kaneda, Yu Katsuyama and Hayato Naka-Kaneda
Department of Anatomy, Shiga University of Medical Science, Seta Tsukinowa-cho, Otsu, Shiga 520-2192, Japan

Hidetoshi Masumoto
Clinical Translational Research Program, RIKEN Center for Biosystems Dynamics Research, 2-2-3 Minatojima-minamimachi, Chuo-ku, Kobe, Hyogo 650-0047, Japan
Clinical Translational Research Program, RIKEN Center for Developmental Biology, Kobe, Japan
Department of Cell Growth and Differentiation, Center for iPS Cell Research and Application (CiRA), Kyoto University, 53 Shogoin Kawahara-cho, Sakyo-ku, Kyoto 606-8507, Japan
Department of Cardiovascular Surgery, Kyoto University Graduate School of Medicine, Kyoto, Japan

Jun K. Yamashita
Department of Cell Growth and Differentiation, Center for iPS Cell Research and Application (CiRA), Kyoto University, 53 Shogoin Kawahara-cho, Sakyo-ku, Kyoto 606-8507, Japan

Jaicy Jacob, Namdev More, Kiran Kalia and Govinda Kapusetti
Department of Medical Devices, National Institute of Pharmaceutical Education and Research, Ahmedabad 380054, India

Kenly Wuputra, Ming-Ho Tsai, Chia-Chen Ku and Wen-Hsin Lin
Graduate Institute of Medicine, Kaohsiung Medical University, Kaohsiung 807, Taiwan

Chang-Shen Lin
Graduate Institute of Medicine, Kaohsiung Medical University, Kaohsiung 807, Taiwan
Department of Biological Sciences, National Sun Yat-sen University, Kaohsiung 805, Taiwan

Ya-Han Yang and Kung-Kai Kuo
Center of Stem Cell Research, Kaohsiung Medical University, Kaohsiung 807, Taiwan
Department of Surgery, Department of Medicine, Kaohsiung Medical University, Kaohsiung 807, Taiwan

Kazunari K. Yokoyama
Graduate Institute of Medicine, Kaohsiung Medical University, Kaohsiung 807, Taiwan
Center of Stem Cell Research, Kaohsiung Medical University, Kaohsiung 807, Taiwan
Center of Infectious Diseases and Cancer Research, Kaohsiung Medical University, Kaohsiung 807, Taiwan

Research Center for Environmental Medicine, Department of Medicine, Kaohsiung Medical University, Kaohsiung 807, Taiwan
Faculty of Molecular Preventive Medicine, Graduate School of Medicine, the University of Tokyo, Tokyo 113-0033, Japan
Faculty of Science and Engineering, Tokushima Bunri University, Sanuki 763-2193, Japan

Toshiaki Okuno and Takehiko Yokomizo
Department of Biochemistry, Juntendo University School of Medicine, Tokyo, Japan

Kaoru Yamagata, Shingo Nakayamada and Yoshiya Tanaka
The First Department of Internal Medicine, School of Medicine, University of Occupational and Environmental Health, Japan, 1-1 Iseigaoka, Yahata-nishi-ku, Kitakyushu 807-8555, Japan

Index

www.ingramcontent.com/pod-product-compliance
Lightning Source LLC
Chambersburg PA
CBHW080413190526
45161CB00003B/223